Chronic Myelogenous Leukemia

HEMATOLOGY

Series Editors

Kenneth M. Brinkhous, M.D.
Department of Pathology
University of North Carolina
School of Medicine
Chapel Hill, North Carolina

Sanford A. Stass, M.D.
Hematopathology Program
The University of Texas System Cancer Center
M. D. Anderson Hospital and Tumor Institute
Houston, Texas

Volume 1 Prostaglandins and Leukotrienes: Blood and Vascular Cell Function, *Jonathan M. Gerrard*

Volume 2 Hematopoietic Stem Cells, *edited by David W. Golde and Fumimaro Takaku*

Volume 3 Bone Marrow Transplantation: Biological Mechanisms and Clinical Practice, *edited by Dirk W. van Bekkum and Bob Löwenberg*

Volume 4 Myelofibrosis: Pathophysiology and Clinical Management, *edited by S. M. Lewis*

Volume 5 Plasma Fibronectin: Structure and Function, *edited by Jan McDonagh*

Volume 6 The Acute Leukemias: Biologic, Diagnostic, and Therapeutic Determinants, *edited by Sanford A. Stass*

Volume 7 Hemostasis and Animal Venoms, *edited by Hubert Pirkle and Francis S. Markland, Jr.*

Volume 8 Hematopoiesis: Long-Term Effects of Chemotherapy and Radiation, *edited by Nydia G. Testa and Robert Peter Gale*

Volume 9 Coagulation and Bleeding Disorders, *edited by Theodore S. Zimmerman and Zaverio M. Ruggeri*

Chronic Myelogenous Leukemia

Molecular Approaches to Research and Therapy

edited by

ALBERT B. DEISSEROTH
RALPH B. ARLINGHAUS
The University of Texas M. D. Anderson Cancer Center
Houston, Texas

Marcel Dekker, Inc. New York • Basel • Hong Kong

Library of Congress Cataloging-in-Publication Data

Chronic myelogenous leukemia: molecular approaches to research and therapy/
edited by Albert B. Deisseroth, Ralph Arlinghaus.
p. cm. -- (Hematology; v. 13)
Includes bibliographical references.
Includes index.
ISBN 0-8247-8352-2 (alk. paper)
1. Acute myelocytic leukemia--Molecular aspects. I. Deisseroth, Albert B. II. Arlinghaus, Ralph. III. Series: Hematology (New York, N.Y.); v. 13.
[DNLM: 1. Leukemia, Myeloid, Chronic--genetics. 2. Leukemia, Myeloid, Chronic--therapy. W1 HE873 v. 13 / WH 250 C5565]
RC643.C492 1991
616.99'419--dc20
DNLM/DLC
for Library of Congress 90-13850
CIP

This book is printed on acid-free paper.

MARCEL DEKKER, INC.
270 Madison Avenue, New York, New York 10016

Current printing (last digit):
10 9 8 7 6 5 4 3 2 1

PRINTED IN THE UNITED STATES OF AMERICA

Series Introduction

For most of this century, hematology has followed a pattern of major scientific discoveries, improved understanding of disease, and rapid application of new knowledge in the clinic. The rate of advance continues at an accelerating pace, so that all but the most zealous have difficulty in keeping up with the literature in even a limited area of specialized interest. As the explosive development of knowledge continues apace, it is a continuing challenge to keep abreast of significant new developments as they impact on clinical and laboratory hematology. The Hematology series is designed to help in this respect, by providing up-to-date and expert presentations on important subject areas in our field. It is hoped that these works, both individually and collectively, will become important volumes for updating information and for reference for the clinician, investigator, teacher, and student, and in this manner contribute to the advancement of hematology.

This volume of the series is devoted to the basic cellular and molecular derangements in chronic myelogenous leukemia and to the impact of this newer knowledge on diagnosis and assessing efficacy of treatment. It has been over 30 years since Nowell and Hungerford described the Philadelphia chromosome as the marker for chronic myelogenous leukemia. Retrospectively, this discovery looms up as a major breakthrough that has pointed the way for an astounding series of advances, documented in this book, that makes chronic myelogenous leukemia as well understood as any malignancy. The chapters in this volume present a fascinating and readable story of the unfolding of molecular and biological events that underlie the proliferative leukemic process and that determine the course of disease. A large body of new information has developed, thanks to the application of the modern technologies of molecular genetics, immunology, and cell biology. At the conceptual level, there is detailed understanding of many aspects of pathogenesis of chronic myelogenous leukemia, such as the possible role of an abnormal gene product, and its activated protein tyrosine kinase activity, in upsetting normal intracellular regulatory mechanisms of cell proliferation and maturation. At the applied level, the polymerase chain reaction has been successfully used to detect minimal residual disease after treatment, indicating the presence of abnormal cells at low concentration heretofore not detectable.

This book presents a comprehensive picture of current knowledge of chronic mylogenous leukemia and provides an introduction for understanding the new developments that most certainly lie ahead in this active field. The authors and editors are authorities in their various subject areas, and with their contributions to this volume they further advance the subject.

Kenneth M. Brinkhous
Series Coeditor

Preface

It has been 100 years since Virchow first reported the morphological diagnosis of chronic myelogenous leukemia (CML). During this time, momentous changes have occurred in the tools that are available to study this disease and to conduct its diagnosis and treatment. We are currently passing through a revolution in biology and medicine that has not only produced techniques necessary to diagnose the precise defects in genetically unstable evolving leukemic populations of neoplastic hematopoietic cells, but that has also allowed us to develop the tools to intervene decisively in the therapy of these disorders.

Therefore, it is incumbent upon us to link these great events that are occurring at the interface of biology and medicine. Nowhere in biology or medicine has more progress been made in the last 10 years in the understanding of a disease at a molecular level than in chronic myelogenous leukemia. The molecular signature of this disease, the BCR-ABL chimeric gene, has been identified and characterized in great detail. We are now studying the biological targets of this abnormal, tyrosine-specific protein kinase, and the factors concerned with its unregulated activity.

We are fortunate to have collected leaders from a number of fields to bring together all the information on the molecular biology and clinical behavior of CML in order to clarify the directions for future research. We hope that you, the reader, will find this to be an exciting adventure in molecular medicine.

Albert B. Deisseroth
Ralph B. Arlinghaus

Contributors

D. Frank Andrews III Division of Oncology, Department of Medicine, University of Washington and Fred Hutchinson Cancer Research Center, Seattle, Washington

Ralph B. Arlinghaus Ph.D. Department of Molecular Pathology, The University of Texas M. D. Anderson Cancer Center, Houston, Texas

Randy L. Bennett McArdle Laboratory for Cancer Research, University of Wisconsin–Madison, Madison, Wisconsin

Alain Berrebi, Ph.D. Hematology Unit, Kaplan Hospital, Rehovot, Israel

Anna Butturini, M.D. Department of Pediatrics, University of Parma, Parma, Italy

Eli Canaani, Ph.D. Department of Chemical Immunology, The Weizmann Institute of Science, Rehovot, Israel

Bayard Clarkson, M.D. Hematology/Lymphoma Service, Department of Medicine, Memorial Sloan-Kettering Cancer Center, New York, New York

Steven J. Collins, M.D. Molecular Medicine Program, Fred Hutchinson Cancer Research Center, Seattle, Washington

Carlo Croce The Wistar Institute, Philadelphia Pennsylvania

Albert B. Deisseroth, M.D., Ph.D. Department of Hematology, The University of Texas M. D. Anderson Cancer Center, Houston, Texas

David S. Durica, Ph.D. Department of Zoology, University of Oklahoma, Norman, Oklahoma

Stephen G. Emerson, M.D., Ph.D. Department of Internal Medicine and Pediatrics, The University of Michigan Medical Center, Ann Arbor, Michigan

Elena Fainstein, M.D. Department of Chemical Immunology, The Weizmann Institute of Science, Rehovot, Israel

Alexander Fefer, M.D. Division of Oncology, Department of Medicine, University of Washington and Fred Hutchinson Cancer Research Center, Seattle, Washington

Min-Zhuang Fu, M.D., Ph.D. Department of Hematology, The University of Texas M. D. Anderson Cancer Center, Houston, Texas

Robert Peter Gale, M.D., Ph.D. Division of Hematology and Oncology, Center for Health Sciences, School of Medicine, University of California, Los Angeles, California

Frank B. Gertler McArdle Laboratory for Cancer Research, University of Wisconsin–Madison, Madison, Wisconsin

John M. Goldman, M.D. Department of Hematology, Royal Postgraduate Medical School, London, England

John Groffen, Ph.D. Section of Molecular Diagnosis, Department of Pathology, Children's Hospital of Los Angeles, University of Southern California, Los Angeles, California

Susan C. Guba, M.D. Department of Internal Medicine, The University of Michigan Medical Center, Ann Arbor, Michigan

Jordan U. Gutterman, M.D. The University of Texas M. D. Anderson Cancer Center, Houston, Texas

Nora Heisterkamp, Ph.D.* Section of Molecular Genetics, Department of Pediatrics, Children's Hospital of Los Angeles, Univeristy of Southern California, Los Angeles, California

Mark J. Henkemeyer McArdle Laboratory for Cancer Research, University of Wisconsin–Madison, Madison, Wisconsin

C. V. Herst, Ph.D. Oncore Analytics, Houston, Texas

**Current affiliation*: Section of Molecular Diagnosis, Department of Pathology, Children's Hospital of Los Angeles, Los Angeles, California

F. Michael Hoffmann, Ph.D. McArdle Laboratory for Cancer Research, University of Wisconsin–Madison, Madison, Wisconsin.

O. M. Zack Howard, Ph.D.† Department of Hematology, The University of Texas M. D. Anderson Cancer Center, Houston, Texas

Man-ling Hu, Ph.D. Department of Hematology, The University of Texas M. D. Anderson Cancer Center, Houston, Texas

Elizabeth A. Johnson, Ph.D. Department of Hematology, The University of Texas M. D. Anderson Cancer Center, Houston, Texas

Hagop M. Kantarjian, M.D. The University of Texas M. D. Anderson Cancer Center, Houston, Texas

Michael J. Keating, M.D. Department of Hematology, The University of Texas M. D. Anderson Cancer Center, Houston, Texas

Razelle Kurzrock, M.D. Department of Clinical Immunology and Biological Therapy, The University of Texas M. D. Anderson Cancer Center, Houston, Texas

Ming-Sheng Lee, M.D. Division of Laboratory Medicine, The University of Texas M. D. Anderson Cancer Center, Houston, Texas

David Leibowitz, M.D. Department of Medicine and Medical Genetics, School of Medicine, Indiana University, Indianapolis, Indiana

Wanjun Li, Ph.D. Department of Molecular Pathology, The University of Texas M. D. Anderson Cancer Center, Houston, Texas

Timothy M. Lopez, M.D. Department of Hematology, The University of Texas M. D. Anderson Cancer Center, Houston, Texas

Tracy Gross Lugo, Ph.D. Department of Microbiology, Howard Hughes Medical Institute, University of California, Los Angeles, California

Christophe Marcelle Department of Chemical Immunology, The Weizmann Institute of Science, Rehovot, Israel

†*Current affiliation*: Biological Carcinogenesis and Development Program, Frederick Cancer Research Facility, National Cancer Institute, Frederick, Maryland.

James A. McCubrey, Ph.D. Department of Microbiology and Immunology, School of Medicine, East Carolina University, Greenville, North Carolina

Christine Morris, Ph.D.* Section of Molecular Genetics, Department of Pediatrics, Children's Hospital of Los Angeles, University of Southern California, Los Angeles, California

John J. Nemunaitis Division of Oncology, Department of Medicine, University of Washington and Fred Hutchinson Cancer Research Center, Seattle, Washington

Nikolaos J. Paslidis, M.D. Department of Hematology, The University of Texas M. D. Anderson Cancer Center, Houston, Texas

Miron Prokocimer, M.D. Hematology Division, Beilinson Medical Center, Sackler School of Medicine, Tel-Aviv University, Petah Tikva, Israel

E. Premkumar Reddy, Ph.D. The Wistar Institute, Philadelphia, Pennsylvania

Margaret F. Romine, Ph.D. Department of Hematology, The University of Texas M. D. Anderson Cancer Center, Houston, Texas

David Seong, M.D. Department of Hematology, The University of Texas M. D. Anderson Cancer Center, Houston, Texas

Scott K. Shore, Ph.D. The Wistar Institute, Philadelphia, Pennsylvania

Simon H. Sims, Ph.D. Department of Hematology, The University of Texas M. D. Anderson Cancer Center, Houston, Texas

Jack W. Singer, M.D. Division of Oncology, Department of Medicine, University of Washington and Fred Hutchinson Cancer Research Center, Seattle, Washington

Sanford A. Stass, M.D. Division of Laboratory Medicine, The University of Texas M. D. Anderson Cancer Center, Houston, Texas

Linda S. Steelman Department of Microbiology and Immunology, School of Medicine, East Carolina University, Greenville, North Carolina

---

**Current affiliation*: Section of Molecular Diagnosis, Department of Pathology.

Annabel Strife Laboratory of Hematopoietic Cell Kinetics, Memorial Sloan-Kettering Cancer Center, New York, New York

Moshe Talpaz, M.D. Department of Clinical Immunology and Biological Therapy, The University of Texas M. D. Anderson Cancer Center, Houston, Texas

E. Donnall Thomas, M.D. Division of Oncology, Department of Medicine, University of Washington and Fred Hutchinson Cancer Research Center, Seattle, Washington

Andrzej Wedrychowski, Ph.D. Department of Hematology, The University of Texas M. D. Anderson Cancer Center, Houston, Texas

Carol A. Westbrook, M.D., Ph.D. Department of Medicine, University of Chicago, Chicago, Illinois

Owen N. Witte, M.D. Department of Microbiology, Howard Hughes Medical Institute, University of California, Los Angeles, California

Kun Wu, M.D. University of Nebraska Medical Center, Omaha, Nebraska

Tianying Yuan, M.D. Department of Hematology, The University of Texas M. D. Anderson Cancer Center, Houston, Texas

Contents

PART I
Introduction to the Biological and Clinical Understanding of Chronic Myelogenous Leukemia

1
Discordant Maturation in Chronic Myelogenous Leukemia

Bayard Clarkson and Annabel Strife *Memorial Sloan-Kettering Cancer Center, New York, New York*

INTRODUCTION

There has recently been extraordinary progress in our understanding of chronic myelogenous leukemia (CML). During the last several years, the new findings arising from dissection of the genetic abnormalities at the molecular level have received the most attention, but there have also been important new observations arising from clinical investigations and from studies of the biologic behavior of the leukemic cells. As a result of this new knowledge, CML is probably now as well understood as any human neoplasm.

In this chapter we first review the most important observations at different levels of investigation relevant to understanding the pathogenesis of CML and then propose a general unifying hypothesis to integrate and explain these observations. Although the present state of knowledge is sufficient to permit one to develop a plausible comprehensive hypothesis, which we have called discordant maturation, there is as yet very little information about what the specific abnormalities might be. The task ahead, to correctly fill in all the pieces of the puzzle, is clearly going to be formidable. We hope that setting forth a general hypothesis at this juncture will help stimulate interest and focus attention on the most important areas that still require experimental solutions.

Chronic myelogenous leukemia was first recognized as a clinical entity around the middle of the last century. The first published description of CML appeared in 1845 in a paper entitled "Case of hypertrophy of the spleen and liver in which death took place from suppuration of the blood" (1). The next year Virchow published his classic paper entitled "Weisses Blut und Milztumoren" (2), in which he recognized that the "white blood" and splenic enlargement did not represent a suppurative process but rather were manifestations of a distinct disease entity, thereafter called leukemia. He later distinguished between the splenic form of leukemia (CML) and one in which lymphadenopathy was more prominent (chronic lymphocytic leukemia, CLL). The early reports of "splenic" leukemia undoubtedly described patients with classic CML, but some of them also probably included patients with other myeloproliferative disorders. In the ensuing years, CML was gradually distinguished from myelofibrosis and other myeloproliferative diseases on the basis of differing clinical and pathologic features, but the first real clue to its pathogenesis was the landmark discovery in 1960 by Nowell and Hungerford of an abnormally small chromosome, the Philadelphia (Ph) chromosome (3).

GENETIC ABNORMALITIES

It soon became apparent that about 90% of patients who presented with clinical features of CML had the Ph chromosome in most of their marrow metaphases, but about 10% with similar clinical manifestations did not; the subsequent literature has customarily referred to Ph-positive and Ph-negative CML. A decade after the Ph chromosome was first described and shortly after the introduction of chromosome banding techniques, the Ph chromosome was identified as a number 22 chromosome (4). A few years later, in 1973, Rowley showed that the Ph anomaly was not due to a simple deletion but rather resulted from translocation of the distal segment of the long arm of chromosome 22 to the distal portion of the long arm of chromosome 9 [t(9;22) (q34;q11)] (5). Although it was generally presumed that the translocation was reciprocal, this was not confirmed at the molecular level until another decade had passed, when it was demonstrated that the c-*abl* oncogene was transposed from its normal position (q34) on chromosome 9 to a specific breakpoint cluster region (*bcr*) on chromosome 22 (q11) (6,7). The transposed c-*abl* and rearranged *bcr* gene on 22q11 form a new fusion *bcr-abl* gene that transcribes a novel chimeric 8.5 kb mRNA (8), which in turn encodes a hybrid 210 kD phosphoprotein $p210^{bcr\text{-}abl}$ (9). The chimeric transcript and its protein product are larger than the corresponding normal c-*abl* mRNA (6 and 7 kb) and its protein $p145^{c\text{-}abl}$, and the $p210^{bcr\text{-}abl}$ has altered tyrosine kinase activity similar to that of the Abelson murine leukemia virus product, $p160^{v\text{-}abl}$ (10). Because the $p160^{v\text{-}abl}$ tyrosine-specific kinase activity is known to be necessary for cellular transformation (11), it has been suggested that the p210$^{bcr\text{-}abl}$ tyrosine kinase activity may also have an essential role in the pathogenesis of CML (12).

The molecular events just described are so consistent that it seems highly likely that they have a critical and probably a primary causal role in the pathogenesis of CML. However, before one can reasonably reach this conclusion, several issues must first be addressed:

1. Are the variant Ph chromosome translocations that have been described compatible with such a theory?
2. What about Ph-negative CML?
3. Is there a pre-existent genetic abnormality prior to the t(9;22) translocation?
4. What molecular events determine blastic transformation?
5. Where does Ph-positive acute leukemia fit?

Variant Translocations

Since the standard t(9;22) translocation was described, several hundred variant chromosomal translocations have been reported. There are differences in the incidence of variants in different geographic regions and among different ethnic groups, but the overall ratio of variant to standard translocations appears to be about 1:25 (13–15). If the deleted segment of 22q is translocated to any chromosome other than 9, the variant is classified as simple, whereas if three or more chromosomes are interchanged (usually including 22 and 9) it is called a complex variant. Because almost every chromosome in addition to 9 and 22 has been involved in variant translocations, it appears the involvement of these other chromosomes is random and not crucial to the pathogenesis of CML. Sometimes the Ph chromosome is not recognizable microscopically (i.e., "masked") but can nevertheless be shown by molecular techniques to be involved. With the use of high-resolution banding and in situ hybridization techniques, it has been shown that almost all the variants, both simple and complex and including the masked Ph abnormalities, also involve juxtaposition of c-*abl* (transposed from chromosome 9) and the rearranged *bcr* gene on 22 to form a functional fused *bcr-abl* gene (6,16–19). There appears to be no difference in the clinical course or survival duration of patients with variant compared to standard translocations (14, 15). Thus the preponderance of evidence suggests that formation of the novel *bcr-abl* fusion gene and its translation product, p210$^{bcr\text{-}abl}$, are probably consistent and necessary events in the pathogenesis of CML.

Ph-Negative CML

Most recent publications on CML state rather loosely that about 5-10% of patients with CML are Ph negative; higher percentages were usually estimated in the older literature. As noted earlier, some of the presumed Ph-negative patients have a masked Ph chromosome, and their clinical features and the crucial molecular changes, including *bcr* rearrangement and transcription of *bcr-abl* mRNA, are indistinguishable from those of Ph-positive CML (20–22). Rare patients have also been reported who are Ph negative initially but in whom the Ph translocation later appears (23). In contrast, the Ph-positive clone was shown to disappear in a CML patient 4 years after diagnosis, to be replaced by subpopulations of cells with other clonal abnormalities and cells with normal karyotypes (24). Still other Ph-negative cases, including juvenile CML (25), chronic myelomonocytic leukemia, and various other myeloproliferative disorders, have simply been misdiagnosed as CML; the clinical and laboratory findings in such patients differ from those of Ph-positive CML, and they usually have a shorter survival (26–28). When such cases are excluded, there remain only rare cases of true Ph-negative CML whose clinical and laboratory characteristics are indistinguishable from those of classic Ph-positive patients (28–30). Although the exact incidence is uncertain, such cases do exist and we have also observed several patients with clinical and laboratory features typical of Ph-positive CML during the last several years at our center but whose marrow cells lacked the Ph chromosome and had no *bcr* rearrangement. In keeping with the general experience, these patients responded poorly to chemotherapy and their survival was shorter than the 3–4 year average for patients with Ph-positive CML.

Is the Occurrence of the t(9;22) Translocation in a Pluripotent Stem Cell the Primary Causal Event?

It has been convincingly demonstrated that Ph-positive CML is a clonal disorder caused by a somatic mutation in a single pluripotent stem cell in patients heterozygous for glucose-6-phosphate dehydrogenase (G6PD) (31), and the clonal origin of the disease has subsequently been amply confirmed using other techniques (32). The transformed Ph-positive stem cell is capable of generating cells of multiple lineages, including granulocytes, monocyte-macrophages, erythrocytes, megakaryocytes, and sometimes B cells (31,33,34). T cells are almost always Ph negative during the chronic phase (34,35), although there are a few reports of involvement of T cell progenitors during the chronic phase and of T cells during the acute phase (36,37). Marrow fibroblasts (38) and residual normal hematopoietic stem cells also lack the Ph chromosome (39–42).

A critical question is whether the t(9;22) translocation is the primary event in the causation of CML or whether there may have been a pre-existent abnormality in the clonally transformed (Ph-positive) stem cell, as well as perhaps in other Ph-negative stem cells. Fialkow and his colleagues proposed a multistep pathogenetic model for CML (43,44), suggesting that at least some of the Ph-negative progenitor cells are clonal and represent an earlier stage in the evolution of the leukemic clone that precedes the acquisition of the t(9;22) abnormality. However, although this concept has been widely accepted, the supporting evidence for it is far from conclusive. Considerable contrary evidence has been reported, demonstrating that the Ph-negative progenitors are nonclonal and arguing that they are probably normal, although it is recognized that it is very difficult if not impossible to prove that a cell is totally "normal" (39,40,45-50). The question of whether the t(9;22) translocation is the primary causal abnormality is of crucial importance, but the issue will remain unsettled until more convincing evidence is put forth to support the multistep model, such as the demonstration of a predisposing molecular lesion in the Ph-negative stem cells. In the meantime, despite widespread acceptance of the multistep concept of pathogenesis, we are not aware of any compelling evidence that this concept is correct, and we consider it more reasonable to assume that the 9;22 translocation is indeed the primary causal event. The translocation may be merely an accidental event occurring during division, or in some cases radiation or other injuries may predispose to its occurrence.

What Molecular Events Determine Blastic Transformation?

The precise breakpoint within *bcr* is unique for most CML patients but usually occurs between exons 2 and 3 or between exons 3 and 4 (7,51). Numerous investigators have searched for a correlation between the exact molecular site of the *bcr* breakpoint and the clinical course of CML (51-56). The results of some of these investigations are conflicting, but recent data suggest that although there is no correlation between the site of the breakpoint and the phase of CML and that no change in the location of the breakpoint occurs with progression of the disease, patients with a 3′ breakpoint may have a significantly shorter chronic phase than those with a 5′ breakpoint (53,55,56). Serial studies in additional patients will be necessary to confirm these findings.

Approximately 10% of patients with Ph-positive CML in the chronic phase have additional karyotypic abnormalities at the time of diagnosis (57-59). The presence of such additional abnormalities is an independent prognostic criterion with an adverse, but unusually delayed, influence on survival (59). When large numbers of marrow metaphases are examined with modern banding methods, or if patients are studied later in the chronic phase, the frequency of additional abnormalities rises; by the time the disease has evolved to the blastic phase about 80% of patients have additional chromosomal abnormalities (60-63).

As the disease progresses from the chronic phase to an accelerated or blastic phase, the progenitor cells develop a partial or complete block in their ability to undergo maturation. The direction of differentiation and the level and completeness of maturation arrest during blastic transformation are variable: myeloblastic, promyelocytic, monoblastic, erythroblastic, megakaryoblastic, early B cell, and rarely T cell types of transformations have all been described, as have mixed, sequential, and biphenotypic myeloid-lymphoid types (60,64-68). The blastic phenotype may depend on the level of progenitor cell in which the secondary transforming event occurs, or possibly, as is discussed later, it may be governed in part by the secondary event itself, such as the activation of a particular oncogene.

The most frequent secondary karyotypic abnormalities are hyperdiploidy, hypodiploidy, reduplication of the Ph chromosome (+Ph), trisomy 8 (+8), +19, +21, isochromosome 17 [i(17q)], and loss or gain of the Y chromosome (–Y or +Y) (19,59-61). Most earlier studies failed to show a correlation between the specific karyotypic abnormality and the blastic phenotype, but recently several specific correlations similar to those found in acute leukemia have been recognized. For example, t(15;17) occurs both in the promyelocytic (M3) type of acute nonlymphoblastic leukemia (ANLL) and in the promyelocytic type of blastic CML (69,70), and abnormalities of 3q are found both in ANLL with abnormal thrombopoiesis and in megakaryoblastic transformation of CML (19,71). In the majority of lymphoid transformations, the blasts have the same phenotype [common acute lymphocytic leukemia antigen ($CALLA^+$)], Ia^+, and TdT^+ as in the common pre-B cell type of acute lymphoblastic leukemia (ALL). An additional Ph and loss of the Y are common findings in both myeloid and lymphoid transformation, but +8, +19, and i(17q) changes are confined to the former and are absent or very rare in lymphoid transformations (72-75).

It is evident that multiple additional cytogenetic abnormalities may be associated with conversion from the chronic to blastic phases of CML. Some of the evolutionary changes are more closely associated with certain types of transformation than others, but no consistent molecular genetic abnormalities have yet been identified that are comparable to the highly consistent abnormal *bcr-abl* gene found in chronic-phase CML.

While some investigators have failed to find *ras* mutations in CML (76), other investigators using sensitive assay systems have described a multiplicity of *ras* mutations, both early and late in the course of the disease (77,78). The data suggest that there is considerable instability of the *ras* genes and that the cells containing mutations do not necessarily have a proliferative advantage (78). Amplification of c-*myc* and elevated expression of c-*myc* mRNA (79) have also been reported in CML, but these findings appear to be infrequent. Abnormalities in the structure or regulation of expression of the p53 gene have been reported in some patients with CML (80-82). Although structural alterations of the p53 gene are rare in chronic-phase CML, they are relatively common in the accelerated or blastic phases (81,82). The p53 gene is now thought to have a dominant negative role in suppressing transformation and tumor progression in many systems (83-85). Mutations in the p53 gene occur frequently in a number of human tumors in addition to CML, and these mutations are thought to interfere with the suppressive role of the normal p53 product, resulting in tumor progression (84,85). The p53 gene is located on chromosome 17p, and isochromosome 17q alterations are common in blastic transformation as already noted; correlative cytogenetic and molecular studies should eventually answer how frequently p53 mutations might occur in the absence of morphologically evident chromosomal changes.

Ph-Positive Acute Leukemia

It has been recognized for many years that some patients presenting with acute leukemia may have a cytogenetic abnormality that is morphologically indistinguishable from the Ph chromosome (86-89). The Ph is infrequent in ANLL, but it occurs in about 20% of adults and perhaps 5% of children with ALL (37, 67,89-97). It is generally agreed that such patients have a very poor prognosis (93-99).

During the last decade or so, there has been an ongoing controversy about whether Ph-positive ALL is a separate disease entity or whether it merely represents a de novo presentation of lymphoblastic transformation of Ph-positive CML (i.e., either following a short, clinically undiagnosed chronic phase or after rapid progression to blastic phase without an intervening clinically recognizable chronic phase). The arguments, based on clinical or laboratory features favoring one or the other view (22,51,67,72,74,89-98), were inconclusive and are not recapitulated here.

Recent molecular studies suggest that the proponents of both views may be partly right (or partly wrong), although the issue is still not completely settled (22,51,100-110). More patients must be studied to determine the true incidence of the specific molecular abnormalities, but it appears that only a small minority of children and perhaps half of adults with Ph-positive ALL are indistinguishable from Ph-positive CML patients in blastic phase. In these patients the breakpoints occur either between the second and third or between the third and fourth exons of the *bcr* region, resulting in the two common variants of the fused *bcr-abl* gene seen typically in Ph-positive CML, both of which are associated with the expression of a $p210^{bcr\text{-}abl}$ hybrid protein. In the remaining Ph-positive ALL patients the breakpoint occurs 5′ of the *bcr* region within the large first intron of the *bcr* gene; in this case the first exon of *bcr* (instead of exons 2 or 3 as in CML) is linked to *abl*, resulting in a smaller 185-190 kD protein (12,51,100-110). The downstream *abl* sequences are the same in both types of Ph^+ ALL, and thus the *abl* portions of the p185/190 and p210 proteins are homologous; however, although both proteins share sequences encoded by the first *bcr* exon, the p185/190 protein lacks other *bcr* information present in the p210 protein. A child has recently been reported with Ph^+ leukemia with features of both ALL and CML who coexpressed both p185 and p210 mRNA transcripts (111). It has been suggested that alternative or aberrant splicing in *bcr-abl* mRNA, resulting in a switch in production of $p210^{bcr\text{-}abl}$ into $p185/190^{bcr\text{-}abl}$, may be responsible for acute transformation (112), but it is not yet clear how often this may occur (113).

It has recently been shown that by modifying and extending the polymerase chain reaction (PCR) (114) to include RNA as the starting template, the unique leukemia-specific mRNA sequences can be greatly amplified (115). With this highly sensitive procedure it is possible to distinguish between the different types of Ph-positive ALL without the necessity of molecular cloning and using relatively few cells (112,113,116). When this method is more widely applied we can anticipate rapid improvements in the accuracy and specificity of diagnostic tests as well as in follow-up examinations to detect minimal numbers of leukemic cells after treatment.

Whereas the majority of blastic transformations of CML are myeloid, Ph-positive cases presenting as acute leukemias have more commonly been diagnosed as ALL (12,51,94–110). However, Ph^+ ANLL also occurs in about 1-2% of cases of ANLL (51,86,97,117-119). Ph^+ ALL has been reported to be a clonal disease involving progenitor cells whose only detected phenotypic expressions were those of the lymphoid lineage (120), but in recent studies in which the leukemic cells from Ph^+ acute leukemias have been carefully examined by various methods, including morphologic studies, immunologic markers, progenitor cell assays, ultrastructural cytochemistry, and cytogenetic and molecular techniques, many cases have been shown to have concurrent expression of both lymphoid and myeloid phenotypes (121–126). In one recent study, the cases diagnosed as Ph^+ ANLL were reported to have greater multilineage potentiality and/or lineage promiscuity than those diagnosed as Ph^+ ALL (127), suggesting Ph^+ ANLL may result from clonal expansion of a more undifferentiated stem cell than in ALL. However, since the criteria for making the primary diagnosis of ANLL or ALL differ in different reports, such interpretations should be regarded with caution until more cases have been examined using uniform diagnostic criteria.

It is hardly surprising that the leukemic cells from patients with blastic transformation of CML may have mixed-lineage phenotypes, because in such cases the acute-phase clone almost certainly evolved from further transformation of a multipotential chronic-phase stem cell (31). However, myeloid and mixed-lineage phenotypes have also been observed in Ph^+ acute leukemia with p185/190 c-*abl* expression, indicating that the latter molecular abnormality is also not necessarily restricted to the lymphoid lineage (124,126,128).

Not many patients have yet had specific molecular diagnoses prior to treatment or been followed long enough to know how the different molecular types of Ph-positive acute leukemia may differ in their response to treatment. However, based on the overall experience in treatment of Ph^+ ALL and assuming the two types occur with about equal frequency at least in adults, it appears that both types respond poorly to treatment and have shorter survival than do most other types of ALL (67,93,97-98,129,130). Again, there are as yet few studies correlating molecular types with therapeutic response in Ph^+ ALL, Ph^+ ANLL, or blastic transformation of Ph^+ CML, but complete remissions may occur in all these Ph^+ leukemias following effective chemotherapy with temporary disappearance of Ph^+ cells from the marrow, although the remissions are usually of short duration (66,67,72,74,92-99,131-133). Complete remissions with temporary disappearance of Ph^+ metaphases from the marrow as well as in colonies grown in vitro (134), appear to be much more common in Ph^+ ALL than in blastic CML, but additional studies are needed to correlate the molecular diagnoses with the clinical responses to different treatment protocols.

One important biologic difference may distinguish leukemias with p185/190*bcr-abl* and p210*bcr-abl* expression. p210*bcr-abl* expression can clearly be associated with either a chronic or an acute form of leukemia; moreover, with effective chemotherapy, patients who have progressed from the chronic to the blastic phase or patients presenting de novo with Ph^+ acute leukemia may sometimes revert temporarily to a (Ph^+) chronic phase (in addition to sometimes undergoing complete remissions) (67,93,133). On the other hand, until very recently it was generally assumed that the translocation resulting in p185/190*bcr-abl* expression was found only in patients with acute leukemia. Although there are as yet no documented reports of patients presenting with acute leukemia with p185/190*bcr-abl* expression who have reverted to the chronic phase following treatment, there is a recent report of two patients in chronic phase with deletion of central *bcr* sequences, one of whom had 7kb chimeric ALL type mRNA (135). Thus no definite conclusions can be drawn until more information is available on the frequency of this occurrence.

The available evidence thus suggests that the genetic abnormality that results in p185/190*bcr-abl* expression, although not entirely lineage specific, is much more apt to be associated with acute leukemia, but p210*bcr-abl* expression may be found in either acute or chronic leukemia. It is uncertain whether this difference in the biologic behavior of the transformed cells is solely due to the molecular differences already noted or whether additional abnormalities, as yet unrecognized, must occur before the p210 type of Ph^+ leukemia can present as an acute leukemia, as presumably occurs during the transition of CML from the chronic to the blastic phase. However, as will be discussed later in connection with infection of cells with recombinant retroviruses containing *bcr-abl* constructs, recent studies suggest that the information contained in the *bcr* gene, which is present in the p210 protein but is missing from the p185/190 protein, may be responsible for both differences in tyrosine kinase activity and in transforming potency.

It has been emphasized in several recent reports (19,22) that one cannot explain all the variations in disease behavior on the basis of the slight molecular genetic differences that have been described, and doubtless additional abnormalities will be found that influence the behavior of the leukemic cells. Nevertheless, the *bcr-abl* abnormalities are so highly consistent that it appears very likely they may have a primary causative role. Moreover, the possiblility cannot yet be excluded that minor differences in the amount of genetic information transcribed may even determine whether the leukemic cells lose their ability to mature.

BIOLOGIC ABNORMALITIES

The natural history, clinical features, and conventional laboratory findings of CML are well known, and because there are many comprehensive reviews of these topics (58,130,136–139), in this chapter we limit our discussion to those observations about the biologic behavior of the disease that are relevant to understanding its pathogenesis. If one accepts the proposition that the genetic lesions described earlier are primarily causal, it is equally important to understand the biologic consequences of the specific molecular abnormalities that result in a single transformed cell and its progeny eventually becoming dominant and replacing the entire normal hematopoietic population.

As mentioned earlier, there is convincing evidence that the Ph^+ leukemic population results from a monoclonal expansion of a single pluripotential stem cell (31-36,45-47,140). The granulocytes, monocytes, erythrocytes, and megakaryocytes and some B cells all arise from the leukemic clone (31,33,34). During the chronic phase of the disease the leukemic cells retain their capacity for relatively normal differentiation and maturation, and only rather subtle abnormalities occur, as is described later. Based on serial examinations of survivors of the atomic bomb explosions in Japan (141), it was estimated that an average of 8 years elapsed between the initial stem cell mutation and progression of the disease to a symptomatic phase with a white blood cell (WBC) count of 100×10^9 per L. Such estimates are clearly very crude, but they are nevertheless consistent with previous observations, all of which suggest there is usually a period of at least several years between the original transformation and development of symptomatic disease (137). The duration of the preclinical phase is undoubtedly highly variable, as is the course of the disease after diagnosis (130). Four infants, 1-2 years old, with chronic-phase Ph^+ CML have recently been diagnosed at our institution, and there are reports of even younger infants with this diagnosis, the youngest being only 3 months old (142,143). It is thus clear that the preclinical evolution of CML can sometimes take place in less than 1 or 2 years, but it should be kept in mind that the leukemic mass in tiny infants is much smaller than in adults in whom at least several years are probably generally required for the original Ph^+ cell to expand to a clinically significant number.

The leukemic clone has a clear proliferative advantage over the normal myeloid progenitors, because by the time the disease is diagnosed almost all the proliferating cells in the marrow are derived from the Ph-positive clone (39,40,42, 144,145). Only rarely do the leukemic and normal populations remain more or less evenly balanced for long periods (39,40,144,146). During the chronic phase of the disease, the leukemic population's proliferative advantage appears to be only marginal because of the long period required for it to replace the normal hematopoietic population. In the chronic phase, the proliferative parameters of the leukemia cells differ only minimally from those of normal hematopoietic cells, and CML has been likened to a minimal deviation tumor (147).

Cytokinetic Abnormalities

There is no evidence that the Ph^+ leukemic progenitor cells are totally unregulated in their growth or that they proliferate more rapidly than do normal progenitors. To the contrary, it has been consistently found from measurements of kinetic parameters that the leukemic cells proliferate at about the same rate or more slowly than comparable normal progenitors. Although there is considerable variability among patients, almost all kinetic studies performed during the chronic phase of CML have shown that, on the average, the DNA synthesis time of both blood and marrow myelocytes in CML is about the same as that of normal marrow granulocyte precursors (148,149), but the leukemic precursors have lower mitotic indices, a lower fraction of cells in DNA synthesis, longer generation times, slower emergence times of the maturing cells, and longer transit times in the maturation compartments than do comparable normal precursors (147–159). For example, in untreated chronic-phase CML, the average pulse [^{3}H]-thymidine ([^{3}H] TdR) labeling index (LI) of the Ph^+ myeloblasts in the marrow (which measures the fraction of blasts actively engaged in DNA synthesis using the exogenous thymidine "salvage" pathway) is about 20% (151,155,156,158); this is only about half the mean LI value of 40–50% found for marrow myeloblasts in DNA synthesis in normal subjects (160,161). Similarly, although the number of myeloid committed precursors or colony-forming cells (CFUc) in CML are always greatly increased in the blood and usually also increased in the marrow compared to CFUc in normal individuals (157,158), the mean fraction of CML CFUc in DNA synthesis, as determined by the [^{3}H] thymidine suicide method, is only about 20%, or again approximately half the value (~40%) found for CFUc in normal marrow (157).

Stryckmans and his colleagues (161–163) found a relationship between the WBC count and the [^{3}H] thymidine LI in chronic-phase CML; when the WBC was >40,000 cells per mm^3 the mean myeloblast LI was about 20%, whereas after treatment when the WBC was <20,000 per mm^3, the average myeloblast LI was 46% or in the same range as that of myeloblasts in normal subjects. When treatment was discontinued and the disease relapsed, the LI of the CML myeloblasts again decreased (161). All the marrow metaphases remained Ph-positive during this study, so the normal LI values in CML patients with low WBC counts were not due to repopulation of the marrow with normal cells. A similar relationship to extent of disease was found for CML CFUc, with the fraction of CFUc in DNA synthesis returning from decreased to normal values during remission (157,161,163). Stryckmans also observed that unlike the myeloblasts, the LI of CML myelocytes was not influenced by the WBC count, and he suggested that both CML and normal myelocytes may no longer be under regulatory control (161,163).

It thus appears that the slower proliferative parameters of the CML intermediate-level precursors (i.e., CFUc and blasts but not myelocytes) may be related at least in part to the high cell density in the marrow in vivo (147,159,163). All cells, both normal and neoplastic, are inhibited in their growth at high cell densities, although the density at which growth arrest occurs varies greatly among different populations and the mode of growth inhibition may also differ depending on the conditions (164,165). The general tendency of Ph^+ populations is to undergo progressive expansion, but CML patients often show stabilization of their WBC counts and the size of their spleens for many months without treatment, although the levels at which these parameters stabilize may vary considerably among patients. CML cells are thus still subject to feedback regulation, although curtailment of cell production occurs at higher than normal cell densities (155,159). The Ph^+ cell "cytostat" appears to be set at a higher level than normal. Although the mode of density-dependent inhibition and the specific defect in Ph^+ progenitors are unknown, it is likely that the abnormality is somehow related to the cells' discordant maturation as will be discussed later.

In untreated chronic-phase CML, not only is the increased cell density in the marrow a constant feature, but the total mass of myeloid tissue is invariably expanded, sometimes enormously, with active cell production usually occurring in the spleen and sometimes also in the liver and other organs (155,158,166). Although generally many immature cells are present in the blood and their fraction in S phase is similar or only slightly lower than that in the marrow, because their mitotic index is almost invariably lower in the blood, the immature cells apparently must return to the marrow or spleen to divide (155,161–163). The rate of cell production is similar in the marrow and spleen, and in patients with extensive splenic involvement the majority of circulating immature granulocytes may originate in the spleen (155,166).

Leukocyte kinetic studies (167–170) have shown that the size of the total blood granulocyte pool (TBGP) may be 10-100 times greater than normal; both the circulating granulocyte pool (CGP) and marginated granulocyte pool (MGP) are grossly expanded. If only the mature granulocytes (bands and polymorphonuclear cells) are considered, the increase is between 3- and 30-fold (171).

Using a variety of isotopic labeling procedures, it has been consistently found that the mature granulocytes in chronic-phase CML have a markedly slower rate of disappearance from the blood than do normal mature granulocytes (155,158, 168–176). Interpretation of the slow granulocyte disappearance rate in CML is confounded by the presence of many circulating immature granulocytes and by the abnormal granulocyte traffic and distribution patterns in CML (155,158,

163,166,173,175-177). However, by irradiating the immature cells to minimize their contribution, the blood transit time of the CML polymorphonuclear cells was still 2-4 times longer than normal (171). The granulocyte turnover rate (GTR, i.e., GTR = TBGP divided by average granulocyte transit time in the blood) was also usually found to be substantially increased in CML (1-14 times normal) (168,171). Cross-transfusion experiments also showed that normal mature granulocytes transfused into CML patients disappear normally and that CML mature granulocytes transfused into cancer patients disappear more slowly than normal (168,170,171).

Although the complexity of the system makes data interpretation and calculation of precise values difficult, the overall evidence from these studies strongly suggests that CML mature granulocytes have an intrinsic abnormality that results in their having a significantly increased life span (163,168,171). However, it is generally agreed that their prolonged life span is not of sufficient magnitude to solely account for the huge increase in the WBC count and greatly expanded TBGP in CML, and that therefore production of granulocytes must also be substantially increased (147,155,158,159,171). The vast increase in the number of proliferating precursors in the marrow, blood, spleen, and other organs can undoubtedly account for the increased production, even though the proliferative rate of these precursors during advanced disease is less than that of normal precursors, as noted earlier.

In the course of leukokinetic studies, it was observed that, as in the case of the myeloblast and CFUc S-phase fractions already noted, the other abnormal cytokinetic parameters (i.e., TBGP, GTR, and transit time) also tend to return toward normal values during remission (168,170,175), despite persistence of the Ph chromosome in all bone marrow mitoses (178). It has been suggested (163, 179) that because all these abnormalities are reversible following restoration of more normal levels of granulopoiesis following treatment, they may be more closely linked to the increased total body granulocyte cell mass (which could result in the premature release of immature myeloid cells into the blood from the marrow and spleen), rather than being directly linked to the pathogenesis of the disease. However, as is discussed later, the reversibility may not necessarily mean an "either/or" relationship, and a more complex explanation may pertain.

Regulation of Myelopoiesis in CML

Blood granulocyte levels have sometimes been observed to undergo cyclic fluctuations in normal individuals (180,181), although most normal people do not have obvious oscillations, probably because of the damping action of granulocyte reserves in the marrow (182). Pronounced cyclic oscillations have been observed following injury to the marrow by cytotoxic drugs (183) and in cyclic neutropenia (184). In idiopathic neutropenia, marked cyclic fluctuations of the absolute neutrophil counts have been observed during prolonged treatment with a constant low dose of granulocyte-stimulating factor (G-CSF) (185).

Cyclic oscillations of the blood granulocytes have also been observed in CML, occurring both spontaneously (186–189) and during treatment with hydroxyurea administered at a constant dose (190); the amplitude and length of the individual cycles in CML were considerably greater than in normal subjects or patients with cyclic neutropenia. In normal subjects and cyclic neutropenic patients, the amplitude of the cycles is relatively small and the length of the cycles is generally about 20 days (180–184); it has been noted that 20 days is about twice the time estimated for a stem cell to produce polymorphonuclear leukocytes (154). During treatment of a patient with idiopathic neutropenia with a constant low dose of G-CSF, the cycle length was about 40 days and the amplitude gradually lessened with continuing treatment (185). In CML, the amplitudes of individual cycles have sometimes been very large (i.e., $>$100,000 per mm^3) and the lengths of the cycles have varied between 30 and 110 days (186–189). Thus, although there is considerable variability among patients, both the amplitudes and lengths of the cycles in CML are usually much greater than in normal subjects or patients with neutropenia.

There are several possible explanations, but increased cycle amplitude and duration are just what would be expected if an increased number of divisions occurred during passage through the maturation compartments as we have postulated occurs in CML (50). The occurrence of cyclic oscillations in CML provides strong evidence that the leukemic population is responsive to normal regulatory controls. In one CML patient who was studied serially, an inverse relationship was found between the WBC counts and the level of colony-stimulating factor (189).

Competition Between CML and Normal Hematopoietic Populations and Influence of Treatment

Findings at Diagnosis

Based on studies in patients who are heterozygous for glucose-6-phosphate dehydrogenase (31,44) and those with chromosomal mosaicism (45,47,140), the evidence is quite convincing that the Ph^+ stemline originates from the transformation of a single multipotential stem cell. As mentioned earlier, it may take about 8 years from the time of the original transforming event until the Ph^+ population has expanded to the point at which the disease becomes symptomatic (141); it has been estimated that the leukemic population may number 5 trillion or more cells at the time of diagnosis (147,155,159,168). Although the proliferative advantage of the Ph^+ population may be only marginal in view of the long preclinical course of the disease, by the time of diagnosis the leukemic population has almost invariably achieved almost complete dominance over the normal hematopoietic population. Even in asymptomatic patients almost all the dividing cells in the marrow are Ph^+ in the great majority of patients (39,40-42, 144,145); only in an occasional patient does the normal population coexist with the Ph population for long periods without the influence of therapy (39,40,144-147).

In addition to direct cytogenetic examination of marrow and peripheral blood, numerous cytogenetic studies have been performed on colonies growing in semisolid media derived from marrow and peripheral blood cells of CML patients. In short-term cultures, the great majority of progenitors committed to forming myeloid and erythroid colonies belong to the Ph^+ clone, and colonies derived from normal Ph-negative progenitors are rare (40,191-196). However, in long-term cultures, Ph-negative progenitors can usually be detected (41,195, 196), presumably because the conditions allow sufficient time for the quiescent normal progenitors, which have been suppressed by the dominant leukemic population in vivo, to begin proliferating. The long-term culture conditions in fact often favor the normal cells, allowing them to proliferate longer than the Ph^+ progenitors, which die early.

Effects of Treatment

With conventional treatment with relatively low doses of busulfan, hydroxyurea, or other cytotoxic drugs, it is usually possible to control the leukocyte count and reduce the size of the spleen during the chronic phase of the disease, but the marrow metaphases usually remain largely Ph^+ and repopulation with Ph-negative cells has only been observed occasionally (197-202). Conventional treatment at best has only a marginal effect in improving survival, and our experiences with conservative treatment at Memorial Hospital is similar to that at other institutions. In a retrospective review conducted around 1970, we found that the median survival of patients with CML seen between 1948 and 1967 was only 31 months (203), the same as Minot et al. had found in 1924 (204).

In an effort to improve survival and to see if it would be possible to obtain complete hematologic and cytogenetic remissions with regularity, in 1970 we started treating patients with CML more aggressively with the then newly designed L-5 protocol (205,206). This protocol consisted of splenic irradiation followed by splenectomy, repeated courses of arabinosylcytosine and 6-thioguanine, L-asparaginase and vincristine, and hydroxyurea; further chemotherapy depended on the results of cytogenetic analysis after completing the intensive phase of treatment. About one-fourth of the chronic-phase patients had complete remissions with disappearance of Ph^+ metaphases from the marrow, and another 17% had partial remissions with significant reduction in Ph^+ marrow metaphases (39,207). Most of the cytogenetic responses lasted only a few months, but in two patients the response lasted over 3 years (39). We subsequently tried two other more intensive treatment protocols for chronic-phase

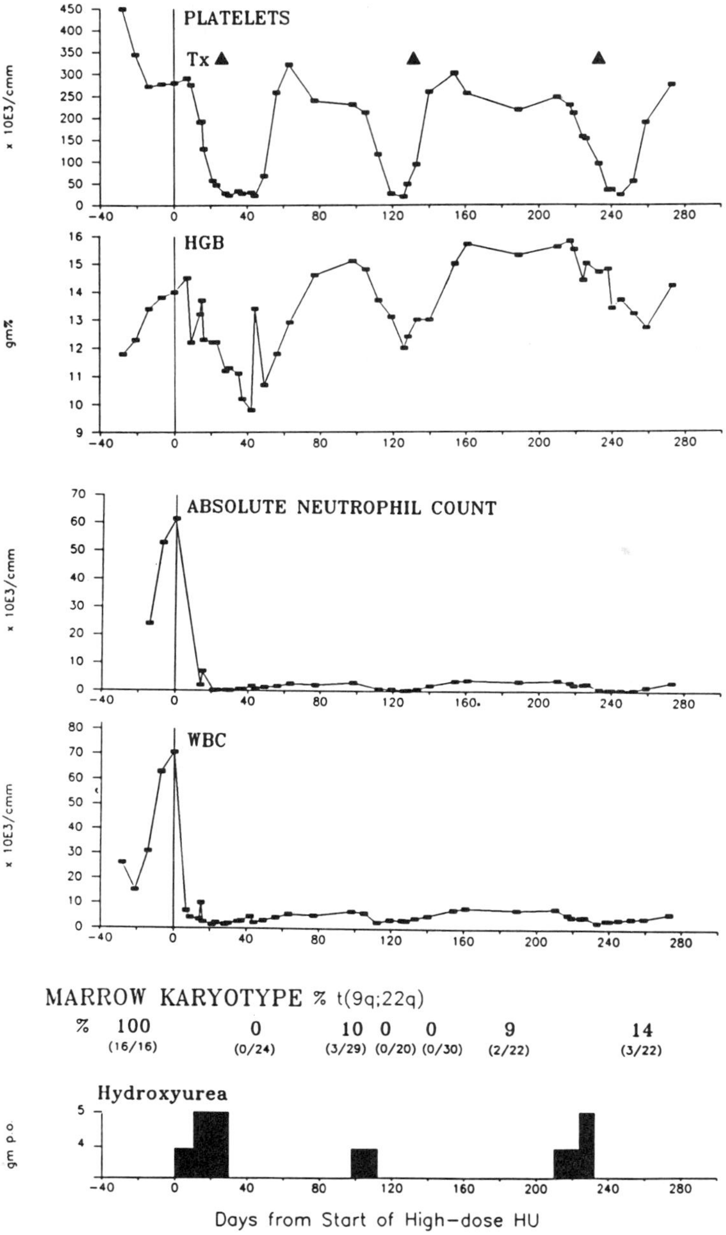

Figure 1 Effects of moderately high doses of hydroxyurea on blood cell counts and marrow cytogenetics in a patient with typical Ph^+ chronic-phase CML.

CML, but the final results were no better than with the L-5 protocol (40,207-209). Patients who had a significant reduction in Ph^+ cells lived longer than non-responding patients, but there was at best only a slight improvement in overall survival, and with one possible exception, no patients were cured (39,207). Similar results have been observed at other centers with different intensive chemotherapy protocols (145,210-213).

If it is true that the Ph^+ population somehow inhibits proliferation of normal hematopoietic progenitors, as is presumably the case since almost all the dividing cells in the marrow are Ph^+ at diagnosis, then it is expected that, at least with the initial course of treatment, effective doses of cell cycle-specific agents, such as hydroxyurea or arabinosylcytosine, should selectively kill the leukemic progenitors and have relatively little effect on the quiescent normal stem cells. Indeed, it has recently been shown that transient remissions with temporary reduction or disappearance of Ph^+ metaphases in the marrow can sometimes be achieved by treatment with chronic administration of low-dose arabinosylcytosine (214,215) or short-term intensive treatment with relatively high doses of hydroxyurea (216). An example of such a response to high-dose hydroxyurea is shown in Figure 1. The problem of course is how to maintain the remission once it is achieved, because once the normal progenitors resume division, they too are killed by the drug.

Clinical trials of various interferon preparations, or of interferon plus chemotherapy, have also produced complete or partial remissions in CML, some of which have been quite durable (42,217-222). However, it is not yet clear whether any of the interferons have substantially altered the course of the disease, and a longer period of observation is necessary.

Results of Bone Marrow Transplantation

The only form of treatment for CML that may have been curative with any regularity so far is supralethal doses of total-body irradiation and/or chemotherapy followed by rescue with allogeneic (223-227) or syngeneic (228,229) bone marrow transplantation (BMT). In the different reported series, 45-70% of patients transplanted in the chronic phase have had long-term disease-free survival, with the results becoming progressively worse if the transplants are performed in the accelerated or blastic phases. Autologous stem cell transplantation using cryopreserved peripheral blood or bone marrow stem cells obtained during the chronic phase has also been attempted to restore accelerated or blastic disease to the chronic phase, but the results have generally been of only marginal benefit (230-232).

One of the serious complications following allogeneic bone marrow transplantation is graft-versus-host disease (GVHD), and various methods have been used to remove T cells from the donor marrow in vitro prior to transplantation since

T cells appear to be largely responsible for GVHD. T cell depletion has proven to be highly effective in preventing or reducing the severity of GVHD, but unfortunately it has also been found to be associated with both an increased risk of graft failure and a high leukemic relapse rate (226,233-235). Acute GVHD does not appear to influence the relapse rate, but chronic GVHD does. Allografted patients who develop chronic GVHD have a lower relapse rate (~10%) than do patients receiving syngeneic transplants or allografted patients without GVHD (~20-30%). Presumably the difference represents some type of antileukemic effect associated with GVHD. Moreover, because the relapse rate with T cell-depleted allografts is even higher (~40-50%), T cells may also contribute to an antileukemic effect. As is mentioned later, however, the mechanism by which T cells, natural killer (NK) cells, or other cytotoxic cells may exert such an antileukemic effect is not well understood.

Patients in whom the bone marrow was studied serially after transplantation in chronic-phase CML have shown a variety of cytogenetic patterns (233-237). The patients may remain in complete remission with either all donor cells (complete chimeras) or as mixed chimeras with varying proportions of both donor and normal (Ph-negative) host cells, or their leukemia may relapse. Leukemic relapse may occur early or late (i.e., before or after 6-12 months). Relapse is commonly manifested by re-establishment of chronic-phase disease, but acute-phase relapse may also occur occasionally, usually accompanied by other chromosomal abnormalities. There are two reports (238,239) of the appearance of leukemia in donor lymphoid blast cells following bone marrow transplantation performed during a second chronic phase (one of which was Ph^+), but this is apparently a very rare occurrence since leukemia in donor cells has not been reported in any of the recent large series of CML patients who have been transplanted during their first chronic phase.

In some cases, Ph^+ cells have been observed to persist or to come and go spontaneously in the absence of hematologic relapse or to appear and then disappear entirely again after 6-12 months without treatment (224-227, 233-237). The true incidence of such transient or persistent cytogenetic relapses unaccompanied by clinical relapse is difficult to determine from the available reports; the reported incidence varies considerably in different series, undoubtedly depending on such factors as the timing and frequency of karyotypic studies, the number of metaphases examined, the length of follow-up, and whether the marrow graft was depleted of T cells. Overall the combined incidence of transient relapse plus persistent cytogenetic relapse without hematologic relapse appears to occur in approximately 10-20% of patients (233-237), but most of the reports have fairly short follow-up and the incidence may fall if late hematologic relapse occurs. In most patients with cytogenetic relapse without clinical relapse, less than 10% of the cells are Ph^+; if greater than 30% Ph^+ cells are detected, clinical relapse is the usual outcome. A similar phenomenon has not been noted with any such regularity after marrow transplantation in acute leukemia in which reappearance of any leukemic metaphases appears almost invariably to herald a hematologic relapse (240).

Competition of Normal and Leukemic Stem Cells After Transplantation

The events resulting in repopulation of the marrow following BMT offer an unparalleled opportunity to observe the competition of normal donor stem cells and normal and leukemic host stem cells. The vast majority of the host's hematopoietic cells, both normal and leukemic, are destroyed by the total-body irradiation and high doses of cytotoxic drugs, and the cells in the marrow graft already committed to maturation soon die after a limited number of divisions. The marrow thus remains almost empty of hematopoietic cells for several weeks or longer except for the transplanted donor stem cells and, in cases of mixed chimerism, the relatively few normal and/or leukemic host stem cells that survive the preparative treatment. Because it is not possible to predict which individuals may be destined to develop CML, except in such unusual circumstances as accidental exposure to irradiation, the events following BMT afford the next best opportunity to study differences in the behavior of competing normal and leukemic stem cells; this is especially true in syngeneic grafts in which immunologic defenses do not complicate the repopulation kinetics.

Perhaps the most interesting (and largely unanticipated) observation so far has been the occurrence of transient or fluctuating leukemic relapse without the hematologic relapse mentioned earlier. To date this phenomenon has mostly been detected by cytogenetic methods whose level of sensitivity is only about 1-10%, depending on how many metaphases are examined (233-237). Moreover, because the marrow may remain hypocellular for long periods after BMT, it is usually difficult to find many cells in metaphase for analysis. Newer molecular diagnostic methods are beginning to be applied and should provide valuable additional information about the competition between the normal and leukemic populations. DNA restriction length polymorphisms (RFLPs) is a highly sensitive method to distinguish between individuals (241-243) and will probably supplement or replace existing markers, such as the Y chromosome in the case of sex-mismatched individuals or autosomal heteromorphisms, for the detection of chimerism (235,244). The polymerase chain reaction (114,115) is capable of detecting 1 Ph^+ cell per 10^3 (245) or per 10^5 (246) nonleukemic cells, and when this method is applied after transplantation it is likely that the true incidence of subclinical leukemic relapse is even higher than has heretofore been detected.

One may suppose that since CML originates in a single stem cell, any surviving stem cell should be capable of reproducing the disease, although this may require a number of years. However, there are several possible explanations whereby leukemic cells could persist without causing resurgence of clinically evident relapse.

The evidence for immunologic defense mechanisms has already been mentioned, whereby T cells or other natural cytotoxic cells contained in the marrow graft kill or inhibit the growth of the surviving Ph^+ cells. Numerous immunologic investigations have been carried out during different stages of CML, including evaluation of general immune responsiveness (247), immune reactivity to autochthonous or allogeneic CML antigens or to other leukemic antigens (248-251), loss of expression of myeloid differentiation antigens (252), presence of circulating immune complexes (253-255), and impaired suppressor or cytotoxic cell activity (256-258), and several clinical immunotherapy trials have been conducted (259-261). However, it is difficult to decipher from these investigations exactly what immune defenses are operative in killing or inhibiting the growth of the leukemic cells.

Studies are continuing at several institutions, including our own, to evaluate the impairment of function of natural killer and other cytotoxic cells in suppressing the growth of Ph^+ cells in CML and in examining possible ways to potentiate their antileukemic activity (262-266). However, it is not yet clear if any of the immunotherapeutic maneuvers that have been proposed will be successful. Because the evidence mentioned earlier from the bone marrow transplantation experience suggests that immune defenses may play a role in preventing relapse, such investigations are clearly worth pursuing. However, it will probably first be necessary to reach a better understanding of how NK and other cytotoxic cells function (267-270), how they can recognize CML cells as abnormal, and how they might be defective in CML before an effective form of immunotherapy can be developed.

Another possible explanation for the subclinical persistence of Ph^+ cells after transplantation is that the high doses of irradiation and cytotoxic drugs used in the conditioning regimen may have caused sufficient sublethal damage to the leukemic stem cells to render them incapable of unlimited proliferation. There is indeed suggestive evidence that this may occur. Chromosomal abnormalities consistent with radiation-induced damage have been observed in host cells (both Ph^+ and Ph negative) after transplantation (235), and it is quite possible that these changes are associated with impaired reproductive potential. Moreover, it has been observed that many of the patients in whom Ph^+ cells reappear after transplantation remain stable and require little or no treatment to prevent progression of their disease. This indolent behavior of the leukemic cells after BMT is in distinct contrast to their more aggressive behavior prior to transplantation and suggests they may have been injured by the irradiation and/or intensive chemotherapy.

Finally, two possible alternative explanations are compatible with our hypothesis of discordant maturation:

1. All the most primitive Ph stem cells capable of reproducing the disease could have been destroyed by the intensive pretransplant treatment, and the persistent Ph^+ cells are those in later maturation compartments, which are capable only of limited proliferation.
2. Only a very few of the earliest Ph stem cells survived, and it may require several years for them to reassume dominance as in the original evolution of the disease.

With more careful study and longer follow-up, it may eventually be possible to determine which of these explanations is correct; none of them are mutually exclusive and it is quite possible that several factors may be operative.

MORPHOLOGIC, BIOCHEMICAL, AND FUNCTIONAL ABNORMALITIES OF LEUKEMIC CELLS IN CML

During the chronic phase of the disease the leukemic cells function fairly normally and are able to support life largely in the absence of normal hematopoietic cells, which they have replaced. All the myeloid lineages are involved in CML, but expansion of the granulocyte lineage is usually most striking; a possible explanation for the less obvious involvement of the erythroid lineage is discussed later. Many patients at diagnosis are largely asymptomatic. Symptoms occur when the spleen becomes grossly enlarged, the WBC count becomes sufficiently elevated to cause leukostasis, significant anemia develops, or abnormalities of the platelets result in thrombotic or hemorrhagic complications. In the absence of extreme blood cell counts or other unusual manifestations, such as hyperbasophilia, patients have few symptoms because the leukemic cells are able to carry out all their normal functions fairly effectively, such as transporting oxygen, killing invading microorganisms, and maintaining hemostasis. Nevertheless, numerous subtle morphologic, biochemical, and functional abnormalities of the leukemic cells have been described, which we now summarize.

Morphologic Abnormalities

A number of morphologic abnormalities have been observed by the light microscope in CML granulocytes, erythrocyte precursors, and megakaryocytes (137, 271-273). These include hypersegmentation, hyposegmentation, abnormal lobulation, and ring-shaped nuclei of the polymorphonuclear leukocytes; binucleate myelocytes; multinuclearity, nuclear fragments, and karyorrhexis of the erythroblasts; and large mononuclear forms, multiple small separated nuclei, and micro forms of the megakaryocytes (273). The dysplastic changes occur in the chronic phase of CML more frequently than in normal subjects and become even more prominent as the disease approaches blastic transformation; the appearance of hyposegmented neutrophils and micromegakaryocytes in particular appear to herald blastic transformation (273,274). Another abnormality occurring in CML that is never observed in normal granulocytes is the presence of both eosinophilic and basophilic granules in the same cell (275,276). Such hybridoid cells with dual granulation were found with varying frequency in all cases of CML examined and occurred in both mature segmented cells and immature nonsegmented cells. It was concluded that lineage infidelity may occur in mature as well as immature cells because the progenitors of the chimeric granulocytes follow false genetic programs (276).

Electron microscopic studies have also revealed that maturation is faulty in developing CML cells. Especially significant is the observation that there is asynchrony between maturation of the cytoplasm and the nucleus, with the former proceeding more rapidly (277–279). Asano and Kawahara observed that CML promyelocytes contain a greater than normal number of granules but their nuclei remain immature (277). Anderson observed the same asynchrony in the rate of maturation of the nucleus and cytoplasmic organelles in CML myelocytes (278). Vainchenker et al. found that cytoplasmic maturation of CML megakaryocytes in plasma clot cultures proceeds as in normal megakaryocytes with platelet shedding but nuclear maturation lags, resulting in hypoploid megakaryocytes (279).

Ultrastructural investigation of the stromal component of the marrow microenvironment in chronic-phase CML has shown that the venous sinuses are well preserved but the sinus endothelium has significantly more pores than normal, with some pores of larger than normal diameter (280,281). A decrease in the percentage of the endothelial cell layer covered by the adventitial cell layer (adventitial cell cover rate) was also noted (280,281). These changes undoubtedly contribute to the increased passage of immature CML cells through the marrow-blood barrier (282), which normally prevents immature cells from passing into the circulation.

Biochemical and Functional Abnormalities

Circulating polymorphonuclear neutrophils in CML have been shown to have a large number of biochemical and functional abnormalities. In reviewing these abnormalities, it is well to keep in mind the evidence already cited that (1) maturation of CML cells is asynchronous, with cytoplasmic maturation proceeding more rapidly than nuclear maturation; and (2) CML cells are prematurely released from the marrow before maturation is complete. In general, the abnormalities described are quantitative rather than qualitative and represent mean values of the total mature granulocyte population. As such, they do not reveal what proportion of the circulating segmented CML granulocytes have reached full maturity and exhibit biochemical and functional characteristics typical of normal circulating granulocytes. The biochemical abnormalities include low neutrophil alkaline phosphatase (NAP) activities (283–285); subnormal contents of lactoferrin (286) and lysozyme (287); hypersialylation of the membrane proteins due to increased activity of a specific sialyltransferase (288); reduced total gangliosides and neutral glycosphingolipid content of the cell membrane compared to normal neutrophils (289); and quantitative changes in many of the cellular proteins, including granule proteins (290–292) and some of the plasma membrane protein constituents (292–293).

Functional defects of CML circulating polymorphonuclear neutrophils that have been described include subnormal adhesiveness to glass (294,295) and nylon (296) surfaces; delayed emigration to extravascular sites (297–299); impaired phagocytic and bacteriocidal activities (290,300–307); and reduced motility and defective chemotaxis compared to normal neutrophils (308).

Leukocytes from untreated patients with CML or those in relapse are agglutinated with concanavalin A (ConA), but leukocytes from normal subjects, patients with granulocytosis, and CML patients in remission are not (309). The enhanced agglutinability of CML leukocytes appears to be due to defective endocytosis of the fluorescein isothiocyanate ConA ligand so that it remains on the cell surface (310), and the impaired internalization may in turn be due to differences in transmembrane ConA binding proteins and in their interaction with the cytoskeleton (311). Granulocytes from untreated CML patients have higher electrophoretic mobilities (EPM) than normal circulating granulocytes but similar to those of immature cells from normal bone marrow (312). Both the CML and normal granulocytes are heterogeneous with respect to their surface charge density as reflected by their EPM. Normal mature bone marrow granulocytes have higher EPM than do normal peripheral blood granulocytes; the surface charge normally decreases as the myeloid cells mature in the marrow and is further reduced before their release into the blood, and this process is incomplete in CML owing to the premature release of immature cells into the circulation.

The abnormalities of CML granulocytes return toward normal when the disease is brought into hematologic remission by treatment (313). Moreover, many of the abnormalities can be modulated in vitro. For example, maturation of CML granulocytes induced by retinoic acid can curtail hypersialylation (314). The aberrant sialylation of membrane glycoproteins in CML granulocytes appears to be responsible for their decreased adhesion to nylon wool and decreased binding to the chemotactic peptide, *N*-formyl-methionyl-leucyl-phenylalanine (fMLP) (288,315). Normal granulocytes show a rapid transient rise in intracellular free cytosolic calcium ($[Ca^{2+}]$) after stimulation with fMLP, whereas untreated chronic-phase CML granulocytes have a decrease in $[Ca^{2+}]$ (316). This abnormality is reversible since neuraminidase-treated CML granulocytes or CML granulocytes from patients treated with chemotherapy show an increase in $[Ca^{2+}]$ after fMLP stimulation similar to that seen in normal granulocytes (316).

Another example of a reversible defect is the decreased neutrophil alkaline phosphatase activity (NAP). NAP activity is uniformly low in patients with CML at diagnosis but increases during infections or when the leukocyte count is reduced with chemotherapy (283,313). CML granulocytes have been shown to recover NAP activity in vitro by treatment with exogenous granulocyte growth factors (e.g., rhG-CSF) (317) or in the presence of monocytes that produce soluble growth factors (285).

Pedersen (313) and other investigators (294,312,318-320) have emphasized that many if not all of the biochemical and functional abnormalities of CML leukocytes, including impaired adhesiveness, extravascular emigration, phagocytic and bacteriocidal activities, NAP activities, hypersialylation, reduced lactoferrin and lysozyme contents, are mutually linked characteristics related to the degree of neutrophil maturation. For example, band forms have lower NAP activities and are less capable of adhering, emigrating, and phagocytizing than segmented forms; marrow segmented cells phagocytize less actively than circulating segmented cells; and the density of sialoproteins decreases and adhesiveness increases as the neutrophil matures (312-316). Therefore, even among morphologically indistinguishable normal polymorphonuclear cells there is heterogeneity in the degree of maturation (i.e., marrow versus circulating polymorphonuclear cells). The asynchronous nuclear-cytoplasmic maturation of CML cells coupled with the premature release of CML cells from the marrow could result in a proportion of circulating morphologically mature CML cells resembling normal marrow mature neutrophils.

ABNORMALITIES OF GROWTH OF CML PROGENITOR CELLS IN VITRO

Numerous experiments have been conducted by ourselves and other investigators to investigate the growth characteristics of CML progenitors in vitro and compare them with the behavior of normal progenitor cells. Because it was our own studies (40,50,321,322) that led us to develop the concept of discordant maturation, we show examples of representative experiments to illustrate why we believe this concept offers the most reasonable explanation for the experimental results. We then summarize the results of our studies and those of other investigators and attempt to show that they are all compatible with the concept of discordant maturation.

Marrow Cellularity and Differential Counts

As previously noted, the total blood granulocyte pool in CML is usually increased 10- to 100-fold (168), and the bone marrow is invariably described as hypercellular at diagnosis. Although there are no accurate comparative measurements of the total bone marrow myeloid mass in CML and normal subjects, based on both core bone marrow biopsies and aspirates, we have found that the

Table 1 Bone Marrow Differential Counts: CML and Normal[a]

	Bl	Pro	Myel	Meta	B&P	Ery	Ly	Other
Normal[b]	1.2	3.0	8.7	11.0	33.5	19.1	9.8	13.7
CML[c]	1.9	3.2	21.8	18.0	45.3	3.4	1.9	4.5
CML/ normal	–	–	2.5	1.6	1.4	0.18	0.19	–

[a]Bl, myeloblasts; Pro, promyelocytes; Myel, myelocytes; Meta, metamyelocytes; B&P, bands and polymorphonuclear leukocytes; Ery, erythrocyte precursors, all stages; Ly, lymphocytes; Other: monocytes, plasma cells, megakaryocytes, reticulum cells, and unidentified cells.
[b]Mean values based on sternal aspirations, 750 adults, male and female. [*Handbook of Biological Data* (edited by W. S. Spector), W. B. Saunders, Philadelphia, 1956, p. 172.]
[c]Mean values based on 24 newly diagnosed chronic-phase patients with CML with no more than 4% blasts in the marrow.

total cell count per unit volume of marrow is increased in CML an average of about threefold (40). Differential cell counts of the bone marrow of normal subjects and CML patients as reported in standard medical and hematology textbooks show considerable variability both among individual subjects and in the mean values. In Table 1 we have taken as normal values the mean differential cell count from one of the largest reported series (323), which was based on sternal marrow aspirates in 750 adults. For CML we used the mean values of differential counts of marrow aspirates in 24 newly diagnosed untreated patients with chronic-phase Ph^+ CML seen recently at Memorial Hospital; the median values were very similar to the means. Patients who had received any treatment were excluded. It is evident from Table 1 that the percentages of myeloblasts and promyelocytes in CML are similar to normal, but there are increased proportions of more mature granulocytes (myelocytes, metamyelocytes, bands, and polymorphonuclear cells) compared to normal. The percentages of lymphocytes and erythrocyte precursors in CML marrow were only about one-fifth of those in normal marrow.

Core Bone Marrow Biopsies

Short-term cultures of core bone marrow biopsies afford a good method to compare the growth characteristics of normal and leukemic populations under conditions similar to those existing in vivo (40). The core biopsies were flushed of loosely adherent cells and then cultured in methylcellulose over an agar underlayer containing peripheral blood leukocytes as a source of growth factors. In the experiments summarized in Table 2, at each time point the core was transferred to a new culture and the cells that had emanated from the core into

Table 2 Cells Emanating from CML and Normal Core Bone Marrow Biopsies Cultured in Methylcellulose[a]

	Total cell number emanating from cores, % CML number at 3 days		Maturation index					
			BP/Bl[b]			BP/Bl + Pro[b]		
Days	CML	Normal	CML	Normal	(CML/normal)[c]	CML	Normal	(CML/normal)[c]
0–3	100	36	16.2	13.8	(1.2)	5.1	3.9	(1.3)
3–10	10	6	19.3	3.0	(6.4)	5.3	1.6	(3.3)
10–17	3	3	21.3	4.9	(4.3)	8.0	2.1	(3.8)
17–24	2	2	29.0	20.3	(1.4)	17.4	5.6	(3.1)

[a]The values shown are the means of seven CML and four normal core bone marrow biopsies.
[b]BP, Neutrophilic, eosinophilic, and basophilic bands and polymorphonuclear cells; Bl, blasts; Pro, promyelocytes.
[c]Ratio of CML maturation index to normal maturation index.
Source: Reprinted from Strife, A., and Clarkson, B. (1988). *Semin. Hematol. 25*:1–19.

Table 3 Absolute Number of CML CFU-GM per 10^6 Nucleated Marrow Cells Shown as a Percentage of the Number Obtained from Normal Marrow[a]

Group	% Normal GM colonies			
	3 days	7 days	14 days	21 days
A: total CFU-GM				
Total	360	270	112	108
>50 cells	–	24	23	21
B: HLA-DR + CFU-GM[b]				
Total	95	82	81	54
>50 cells	–	17	15	15

[a]Five normal and five CML marrows.
[b]Mean differentials of DR + populations: normal and CML, blasts 54 and 56%; promyelocytes, 28 and 23%; myelocytes, 11 and 7%, respectively.

the methylcellulose during that time period were harvested and analyzed for their total cell number, morphologic composition, and pulse [^{3}H] thymidine labeling indices.

Table 2 shows the mean total cell number emanating from the cores as a percentage of the number emanating from the CML cores and the maturation indices during each time interval of culture (50,321). Although the mean production of total cells emanating from the CML cores was almost three times the number from normal cores during the first 3 days, the CML cores produced the same number of cells as did the normal cores after 10 days in culture. The mean absolute number of myeloblasts produced by the CML cores was less than from normal cores for all time periods except between 0 and 3 days (not shown). The absolute number of promyelocytes was slightly greater than normal for the first 10 days of culture but less than normal after that (50,321). The progressive decrease in the immature myeloid cells emanating from the CML cores was balanced by an increased production of more mature myeloid cells (myelocytes, metamyelocytes, bands, and polymorphonuclear granulocytes) during all time periods of culture, resulting in increased maturation indices of the CML populations.

There was no significant difference in the [^{3}H] TdR pulse LIs of neutrophilic precursors (myeloblasts → myelocytes) emanating from the CML and normal cores across the time periods of culture, but there was a significant interaction effect due to a decrease over time in the [^{3}H] TdR LIs for cells emanating from the CML cores, whereas no such decrease occurred in the LIs of normal cells (40).

Production of CFU-GM By CML and Normal Marrow

In another set of experiments we determined the total number of granulocyte-macrophage colonies (CFU-GM) produced by both total light density and HLA-DR^+ CML and normal marrow cells; the light density (<1.075 g/mL) marrow fraction contains >95% of the CFU-GM, and the more primitive progenitors are concentrated in the HLA-DR+ fraction in normal marrow (322). The source of granulocyte-monocyte colony-stimulating factor (CSF) in these experiments was a selected lot of Mo T cell line conditioned medium (MoCM), which in our hands provides optimal stimulation of colony growth (50,324). The absolute number of GM colonies produced per 10^6 nucleated CML and normal bone marrow cells were calculated, and the results are summarized in Table 3 (322). Table 3 shows the mean absolute number of CML CFU-GM colonies per 10^6 light-density nucleated bone marrow cells as a percentage of the number obtained from normal marrow. Although CML marrows generated about three times more total GM colonies than normal marrows through 7 days, they produced the same number at 14 and 21 days. The major difference was in the proliferative potential of the CFU-GM derived from CML marrows. CML CFU-GM generated only 21-24% of the number of large colonies (>50 cells) generated by normal CFU-GM. The persistence of small GM colonies for up to 21 days in culture is probably due to the increased life span of the morphologically more mature Ph^+ cells. The increase in production of CML granulocytes thus appears to be mainly due to granulocyte progenitors with limited proliferative potential.

HLA-DR-positive CFU-GM populations were obtained by sorting partially enriched marrow progenitor cells derived from the same marrow populations shown in Table 3 in a fluorescence-activated cell sorter (FACS-IV) (322). The DR^+ populations were examined using a fluorescent microscope, and the mean percentage positive was >90%. The differentials of the DR^+ populations derived from normal and CML marrows were very similar (mean number blasts plus promyelocytes = 82 and 79%, respectively). The results are shown in Table 3 as the mean absolute number of CML DR^+ CFU-GM per 10^6 nucleated bone marrow cells as a percentage of the number of normal DR^+ CFU-GM. In contrast to the total CFU-GM population from CML marrow, there was no increase in the number of DR^+ CFU-GM relative to normal. Consistent with the total CFU-GM populations, CML DR^+ CFU-GM had far less proliferative potential, producing only about 16% of the number of large GM colonies generated by normal DR^+ CFU-GM from 7 to 21 days. The lack of increase in number or proliferative capacity of CML DR^+ CFU-GM compared to normal DR^+ CFU-GM again suggests that the progenitor population mainly responsible for the expansion of the granulocyte mass in CML is a more mature GM progenitor population. The cells still having proliferative potential that were excluded from the DR^+ populations were the more mature DR^- blasts and promyelocytes and

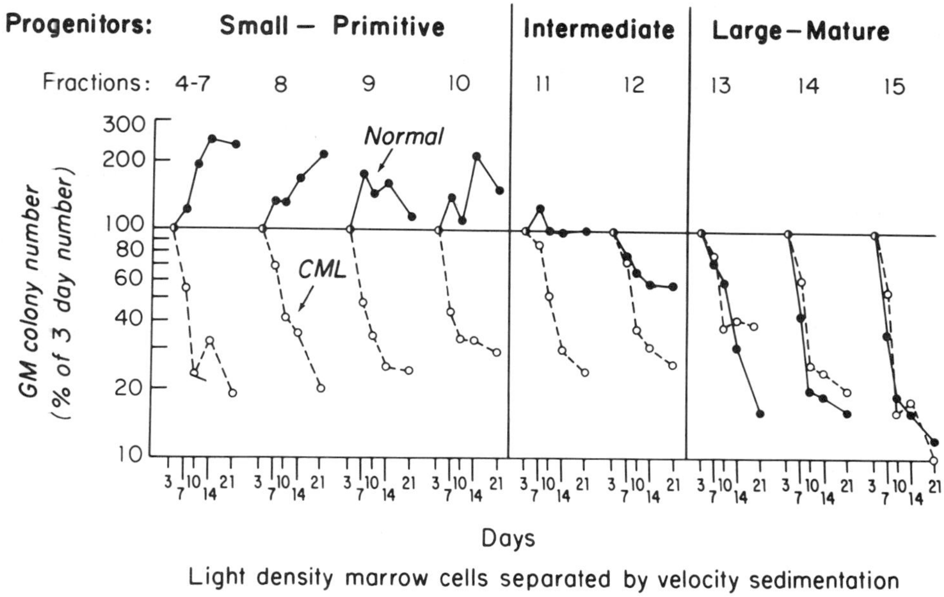

Figure 2 Percentage change in the number of CFU-GM with time in normal (●) and CML (○) marrow fractions. The number of colonies (or aggregates) present at 3 days was taken as 100%. (Modified from Strife et al., *Blood 62*:389–397, 1983.)

essentially all the myelocytes, and the data suggest that it is these latter mature progenitors that are the major source of increased granulocyte production in CML (50,322).

Comparison of Subpopulations of Normal and CML CFU-GM Separated By Velocity Sedimentation

In other experiments, light-density bone marrow cells from normal and CML donors were separated on the basis of cell size by velocity sedimentation in an isokinetic gradient of Ficoll. As previously reported (321), progenitor cells differing in size also differ in their degree of maturation, with the most primitive progenitors residing primarily in the small cell fractions and the mature progenitors residing primarily in the larger cell fractions. Each fraction was cloned, and the numbers of developing CFU-GM colonies from each fraction were determined beginning at 3 days and at subsequent times through 21 days (321).

The results are summarized in Figure 2. The number of GM aggregates present at 3 days is shown as 100%, and the percentage of increase or decrease from this value was determined on subsequent days. The patterns of development

Table 4 Percentage of the Total Number of GM Colonies Derived from Primitive (F4–10), Intermediate (F11–12), and Mature (F13–15) GM Progenitor Cells (CFU-GM) at Each Time Point[a]

	% Total number of GM colonies		
Progenitors	3 Days	7 Days	13 Days
Normal			
Primitive	8	18	42
Intermediate	17	36	29
Mature	75	46	29
CML			
Primitive	3	3	3
Intermediate	15	18	20
Mature	82	79	77

[a]The results are derived from five CML patients and five normal donors. Light-density marrow cells were separated by velocity sedimentation in an isokinetic gradient of Ficoll.

of GM colonies derived from normal and CML mature (large) progenitors were similar. The peak number of GM colonies was reached at 3 days, and the number decreased steadily on subsequent days owing to the limited proliferative potential of most of these mature progenitors. However, there was a pronounced deviation in behavior of CML primitive (small) progenitors. Whereas GM colonies derived from normal primitive progenitors continued to increase in number and size from that present at 3 days, the number of GM colonies derived from CML primitive progenitors steadily decreased in number, exhibiting the same limited proliferative capacity as the mature progenitors (321). There was no difference in the differential counts of the primitive normal and CML fractions that would explain this deviation. We also examined the morphologic composition of over 2400 colonies derived from both the CML and normal fractions to determine if the deviation in behavior could be explained by differences in the distribution or composition, but there were no differences in the distribution or composition of colonies derived from the normal and CML fractions (321).

Based on the pattern of development of colonies as shown in Figure 2, we pooled fractions 4–10, 11-12, and 13–15 and calculated the percentage of the total number of GM colonies derived from primitive, intermediate, and mature GM progenitor cells at each time point (321). The results are shown in Table 4. At all culture times, 77% or more of the total GM colonies from CML marrow were derived from the mature progenitor population and only 3% came from the primitive progenitor fraction. In contrast, although 75% of the normal GM colonies present at 3 days were derived from mature progenitors, the contribu-

Table 5 Ratio of the Median Absolute Number of GM Colonies Derived from Each CML CFU-GM Subpopulation to the Median Absolute Number Derived from Each Normal CFU-GM Subpopulation

	CML/normal				
	3 Days	7 Days	10 Days	14 Days	21 Days
Small (fractions 4–10)	0.9	0.1	0.2	0.2	0.1
Intermediate (fractions 11–12)	2.7	0.6	0.5	0.8	0.3
Large (fractions 13–15)	4.1	2.7	2.7	2.3	1.1
Total	3.4	1.4	1.3	1.0	0.5

Source: Reprinted from Strife, A., and Clarkson, B. (1988). *Semin. Hematol.* *25*:1–19.

tion of the normal mature progenitors decreased with time concomitantly with an increasing contribution by normal primitive progenitors to 42% at 14 days.

In Table 5 the absolute number of GM colonies derived from each CML progenitor subpopulation is compared to the absolute number derived from the comparable normal subpopulation (50,321). It is evident from this comparison that the CML large (mature) progenitor subpopulation is mainly responsible for producing the increased total number of GM colonies obtained from CML marrow during the first 10 days of culture. In contrast, the small (primitive) CML progenitor population produced only a small fraction (0.1-0.2) of the colonies generated from the comparable normal progenitor population at all culture times after 3 days.

In accord with these results, in an earlier study we observed that in some CML patients whose marrow cells on direct cytogenetic analysis were 100% Ph positive in short-term cultures, normal Ph-negative GM progenitors could be detected in the small (primitive) progenitor cell fraction from both marrow and blood prior to treatment (40). Presumably the cell dilutions employed in preparing the progenitors for culture and the limited proliferative potential of the Ph^+ progenitors in the small cell fraction permitted the detection of small numbers of these previously quiescent normal Ph-negative progenitors. However, the continuing active proliferation of the Ph^+ large (mature) progenitors obscured detection of any Ph-negative cells that may have been present in the mature progenitor fraction.

Comparison of Enriched Normal and CML Progenitor Cell Populations

Using density separations and a panel of monoclonal antibodies followed by immunoadherence or immune rosetting, we depleted normal and CML bone marrows of accessory and maturing cells by these negative selection procedures to

Table 6 Comparison of the Growth Patterns of Primitive Normal and Primitive CML GM Progenitors with Mature Normal GM Progenitors

	% Number of 3 day colonies		
		14 Day	
GM Progenitors	3 Day, total %	Total %	>100 Cells %
Primitive normal	100	88	70
Blasts, 77%			
Promyelocytes, 10%			
Primitive CML	100	36	15
Blasts, 78%			
Promyelocytes, 17%			
Mature normal	100	55	43
Blasts, 75%			
Promyelocytes, 20%			

obtain highly enriched populations of progenitor cells (322,324). The enriched progenitor cell populations were then further separated into subpopulations in Pretlow's isokinetic gradient of Ficoll utilizing a centrifugal field to separate the progenitors on the basis of cell size and maturity, as noted earlier.

Granulopoiesis

The results of a typical experiment comparing the growth patterns of primitive normal and primitive CML CFU-GM progenitors with the growth pattern of mature normal progenitors are shown in Table 6 (322). The differentials of the three populations are similar (75-78% blasts and 10-20% promyelocytes) and are therefore appropriate for comparison. The results are shown as a percentage of the number of GM colonies present at 3 days (100%) that were still present at 14 days of culture; also shown is the percentage of the 3 day number of colonies that achieved a size greater than 100 cells at 14 days. Of the 3 day GM colonies derived from primitive normal progenitors, 88% were still present at 14 days, and 70% of the 3 day colonies achieved a size greater than 100 cells. In contrast, only 36% of the 3 day GM colonies derived from primitive CML progenitors were still present at 14 days and only 15% of the 3 day colonies grew to greater than 100 cells. Even the mature normal progenitors had a greater proliferative potential than the CML primitive progenitors, with 43% of the 3 day colonies growing to >100 cells. These observations again strongly suggest that the most mature proliferating cells (i.e., late blasts, late promyelocytes, and myelocytes) are largely responsible for the expansion of the Ph-positive population.

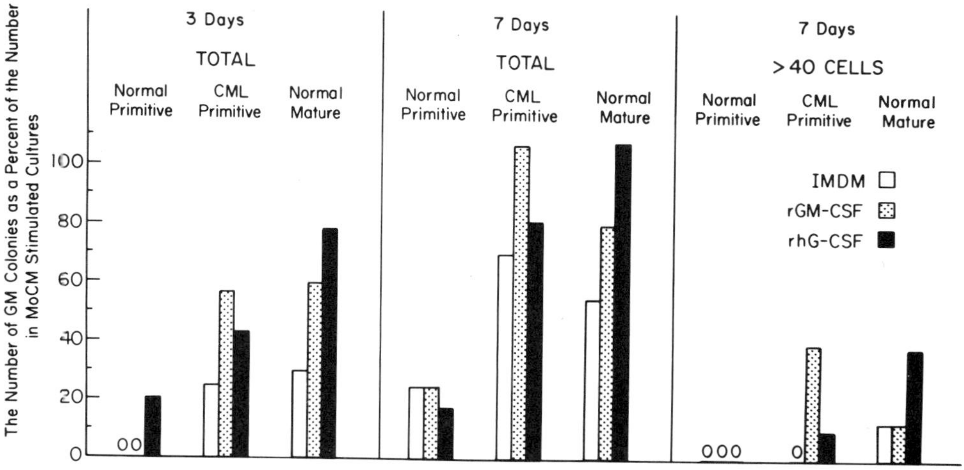

Figure 3 The same progenitor populations shown in Table 6 and described in the text were studied for their response to growth factors. The number of CFU-GM in Iscove's modified Dulbecco's medium (IMDM; which contains no CSF) and rGM-CSF- and rhG-CSF-stimulated cultures are shown as a percentage of the number of GM colonies present in MoCM-stimulated cultures (100%). (Strife et al., *Cancer Res. 48*:1035–1041, 1988.)

The hematopoietic growth factors GM-CSF and G-CSF have been shown to primarily affect the growth of relatively mature progenitor cells (324). Additional experiments were conducted to determine the responsiveness of enriched primitive and mature normal and CML progenitors to these growth factors (322). Figure 3 shows the growth of the same progenitor cell populations shown in Table 6 in IMDM cultures (Iscove's modified Dulbecco's medium containing no CSF) and in cultures stimulated by rGM-CSF and rhG-CSF. The results are shown as a percentage of the number of GM colonies in MoCM-stimulated cultures, taken as 100%.

The normal primitive (small) progenitor population contained a small subpopulation of CFU-GM (25%) evident at 7 days, which was able to divide to a limited degree in the absence of CSF (IMDM control); rGM-CSF and rhG-CSF did not increase either the size or number of these GM colonies. In contrast, the majority of CML primitive (small) GM progenitors (from comparable populations) were able to divide to a limited degree in the absence of CSF (70% at 7 days), and these CML primitive progenitors responded to rGM-CSF and rhG-CSF. The normal mature (large) GM progenitors behaved very similarly to the primitive CML progenitors. Of the normal mature progenitors, 55% (at 7 days) began to divide in the absence of CSF, and these normal mature (large) GM

Table 7 Effect of Delayed Addition of Erythropoietin (EPO) on Subpopulations of Normal and CML Erythroid Progenitors (BFU-E) Cloned in the Absence of BPA (Erythroid Stimulating Factors)

	% Number in MoCM-stimulated cultures	
EPO	Normal (mean)	CML (mean)
Initial		
Primitive	48	93
Intermediate	75	86
Mature	119	119
48 h		
Primitive	4	58
Intermediate	7	63
Mature	4	44

progenitors also responded to rGM-CSF and rhG-CSF. That the CML primitive GM progenitors responded better to rGM-CSF and the normal mature GM progenitors responded better to rhG-CSF is most likely only a reflection of the composition of the individual progenitor populations (eosinophilic versus neutrophilic) since rhG-CSF does not stimulate eosinophilic colonies (324). The observation that the CML primitive progenitors behave similarly to normal mature progenitors suggests that the growth characteristics of the CML primitive CFU-GM are not unique but rather resemble the growth characteristics of normal mature CFU-GM (322).

Erythropoiesis

We have consistently observed that the majority of CML erythroid colonies (BFU-E) and CML mixed granulocyte-monocyte-erythroid colonies (CFU-GEM) are significantly smaller than normal and therefore exhibit the same limited proliferative capacity as do CML GM progenitors (50,322). In Table 7 the effect of the delayed addition of erythropoietin (EPO) is shown on enriched subpopulations of normal and CML BFU-E cloned in the absence of BPA (burst-promoting activity or erythroid-stimulating factors) (322). The number of BFU-E in cultures without BPA is shown as a percentage of the number in cultures that were stimulated by MoCM (which contains BPA). When erythropoietin was added to the cultures initially, only 48% of the normal primitive BFU-E could respond to EPO without a source of BPA but the requirement for BPA diminished with increasing maturity of the normal BFU-E. In contrast, 93% of the primitive CML BFU-E were capable of responding to EPO initially in the absence of BPA, thus indicating a more advanced stage of maturation.

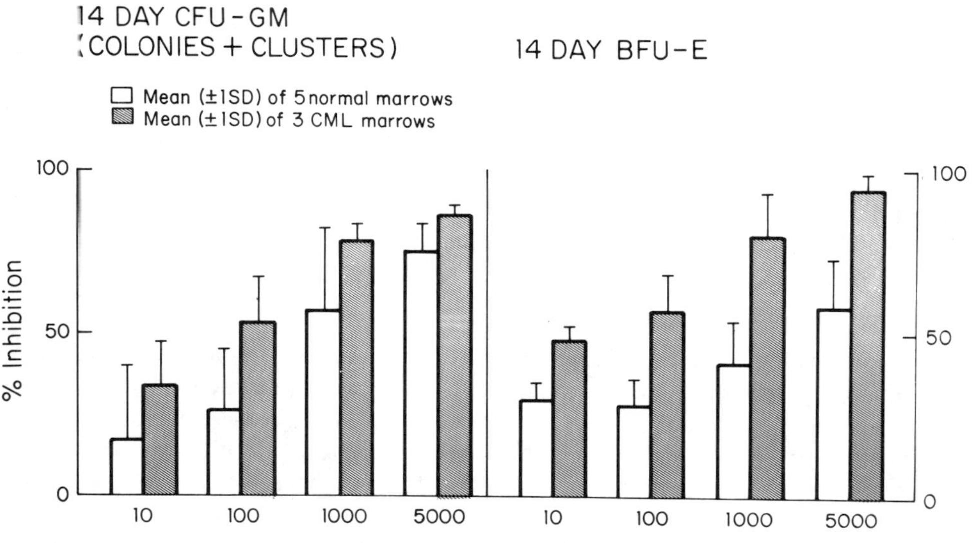

(a)

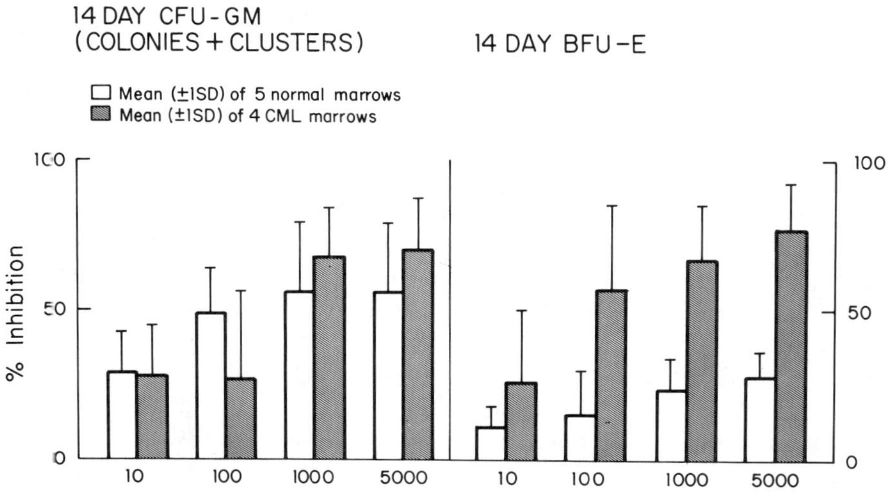

(b)

Figure 4 Effect of the continuous presence of rIFN-α (a) and rIFN-γ (b) on the growth of CFU-GM and BFU-E derived from highly enriched normal and CML hematopoietic progenitor cell populations obtained by negative selection using immunoadherence or immune rosetting. The cell populations were cloned at 800–5000 cells per mL, and quadruplicate cultures were scored at 14 days. (Unpublished observations: Wisniewski, D., Strife, A., and Clarkson, B.)

An even more marked difference was seen between normal and CML BFU-E grown in the absence of BPA, when EPO addition was delayed for 48 h. Only a minor population of the normal BFU-E (4–7%) was able to survive in the absence of BPA when deprived of EPO for 48 h, whereas a much larger proportion of CML BFU-E (44–63%) were able to survive in the absence of BPA. The most likely explanation for the difference is that most of the CML erythroid progenitors had already formed EPO-receptor complexes that were sufficient to sustain them for a limited period of EPO deprivation, whereas the majority of normal progenitors had not yet done so (50,322).

Inhibitory Effects of Interferon and Tumor Necrosis Factor

As noted earlier, it has been shown that both the natural and recombinant interferons can produce hematologic remissions in CML, and in conjunction with the clinical trials, comparative studies have been conducted by several groups on the inhibitory effects of the various interferons on normal and CML marrow cells in vitro. To avoid confusion with indirect effects that may be mediated through other cells, we compared the direct effects of recombinant α- and γ-interferon on highly enriched progenitor cells from normal and CML marrows.

The results are shown in Figure 4. Both normal and CML progenitors are directly inhibited by α-interferon, and the inhibition is dose dependent (Figure 4a). CFU-GM and BFU-E from CML patients appeared slightly more sensitive than normal precursors in these experiments, but additional studies are required to determine if this difference is significant. Both normal and CML progenitors are also inhibited by γ-interferon in a dose-dependent fashion, and the CML BFU-E were more sensitive (Figure 4b). Although not reflected in the data shown in Figure 4, it should be emphasized that increasing concentrations of both interferons resulted not only in a reduction in the number of colonies but also a decrease in the size of the colonies remaining at a given dose concentration; this was especially true of the erythroid colonies. Since under our culture conditions we have consistently observed that the great majority of untreated CML erythroid colonies are strikingly smaller than those from normal bone marrow, more of the CML colonies fall below the counting threshold on treatment with interferon.

These observations may explain why CML progenitors appear to be more sensitive to inhibition by interferon and may at least in part account for interferon's therapeutic effect in vivo. Another interesting explanation for interferon's therapeutic activity has recently been suggested (325). In contrast to normal progenitors, CML progenitors are deficient in expression of the cell surface cytoadhesion molecule LFA-3, which could contribute to giving the CML cells a proliferative advantage in vivo by rendering them less capable of adhering to regulatory cells or matrix molecules. α-Interferon was found to induce expression of cell surface LFA-3 on CML progenitors, thus correcting the deficiency in LFA-3

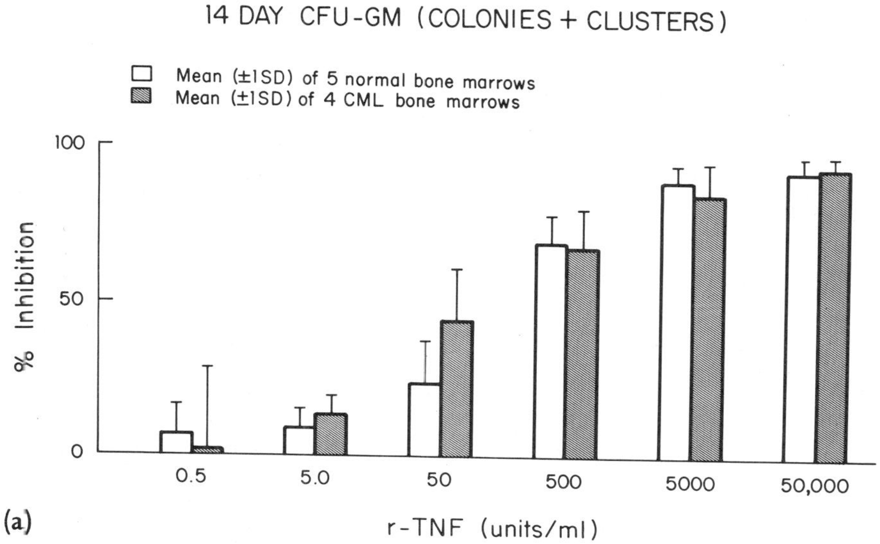

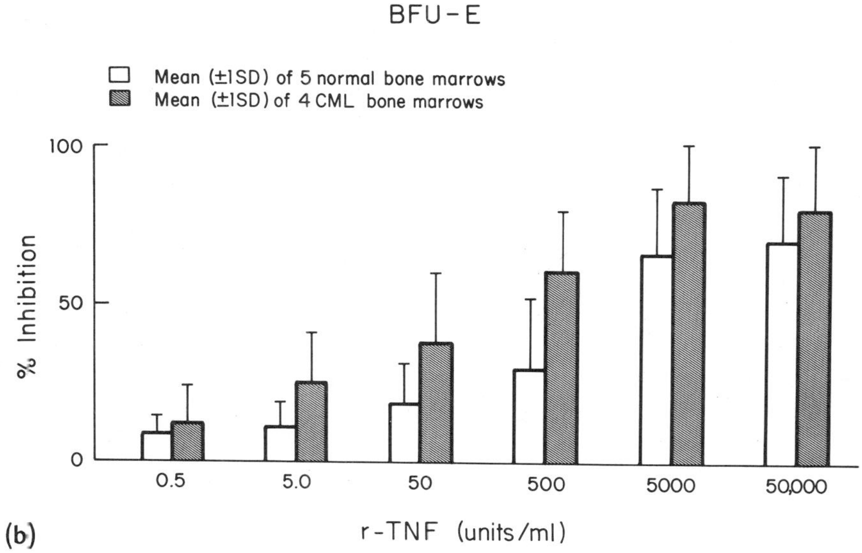

Figure 5 Effect of continuous presence of rTNF-α on growth of CFU-GM (a) and BFU-E (b) derived from highly enriched normal and CML hematopoietic progenitor cell populations obtained by negative selection using immunoadherence or immune rosetting. The cell populations were cloned at 800–5000 cells per mL, and quadruplicate cultures were scored at 14 days. (Modified from Wisniewski et al. *Cancer Res. 47*:4788–4794, 1987.)

or other related cytoadhesion proteins and thereby reducing their proliferative advantage (325).

We also compared the effects of recombinant tumor necrosis factor (TNF) on enriched CML and normal progenitors (326). CFU-GM are directly inhibited by TNF; for both normal and CML, significant inhibition began at 50 units/mL and no significant differences in sensitivity were observed (Figure 5a). BFU-E from CML appeared slightly more sensitive to TNF than normal BFU-E (Figure 5b), but the differences may not be statistically significant; moreover, because of the differences in colony size, the increased sensitivity may be more apparent than real, as already noted.

Summary of Experimental Observations

The most important observations from our studies discussed here and from other studies we have previously reported (40,50,321,322,326) can be summarized as follows:

1. The majority of CML progenitor cells have less proliferative potential than comparable normal progenitors.
2. Compared to normal, CML core bone marrow biopsies produced greater numbers of mature cells but fewer immature cells.
3. CML marrows contain increased numbers of mature HLA-DR-negative GM progenitors with limited proliferative potential, but there is no increase in primitive CML progenitors.
4. The behavior of CML primitive progenitors resembles that of normal mature progenitors in their limited proliferative capacity and responsiveness to growth factors that act on mature progenitors.
5. The mature CML progenitors are mainly responsible for the increased total number of GM colonies generated by CML marrows during the first week to 10 days of culture.
6. CML and normal progenitors respond to the same growth and inhibitory factors, indicating that CML progenitors are subject to the same regulatory controls as normal progenitors.

Results of Other Investigations

In reviewing the literature, we found considerable additional evidence from studies reported by other investigators that were consistent with our own findings that the major abnormality in CML is not unregulated proliferation of primitive progenitors but rather greatly increased production of mature progenitors with limited proliferative potential, although different interpretations of the results were sometimes suggested.

Consistent with our velocity sedimentation findings, Miller et al. (327) observed that although the peak of normal GM colonies shifted from the large progenitor cell fractions at 7 days to the small progenitor cell fractions at 14 days, no such shift was observed in the case of CML progenitors. Olofsson and Nilsson found that CML primitive CFU-GM had a markedly reduced self-renewal capacity relative to normal primitive CFU-GM (328). Several groups have shown that although retinoic acid (RA) enhances the clonal growth of normal CFU-GM (329–331), there is either no enhancing effect or an inhibitory effect is observed on the growth of CML CFU-GM colonies and clusters (329,332,333). This suggests that RA, which is known to induce differentiation in some hematopoietic cells (334), may have a more potent influence in causing the more mature CML CFU-GM to terminally differentiate than is the case with less mature normal progenitors. Lepine and Messner (335) found that, compared to normal pluripotent progenitors (CFU-GEM), a higher percentage of CML CFU-GEM were actively cycling, thus resembling the more mature type of murine CFU-GEM with less self-renewal capacity. Kerk et al. have shown that there are two classes of CFU-GEM in the mouse that differ in their proliferative state and self-renewal capacity (336). The more primitive CFU-GEM are initially in a quiescent state and have a greater self-renewal capacity, whereas the more mature CFU-GEM are capable of immediately proliferating and have a lower self-renewal capacity. As previously reported (324), we have also observed that human normal marrow CFU-GEM progenitor cells are heterogeneous with regard to their level of maturation and responsiveness to rGM-CSF. rGM-CSF acted primarily on the most mature CFU-GEM derived from the large progenitor population and had negligible activity on CFU-GEM derived from the small (primitive) progenitor population (324). Therefore, the observation that a higher fraction of CML CFU-GEM were cycling suggests a higher proportion of the CFU-GEM in CML is of the more mature variety.

The limited proliferative capacity of Ph^+ progenitors has also been demonstrated in long-term marrow cultures. Coulombel et al. showed that Ph^+ progenitors have less proliferative potential and decline more rapidly in long-term cultures than normal progenitors (195). A higher percentage of the Ph^+ progenitors were found to be cycling (337) similarly to mature normal progenitors with low proliferative potential in long-term culture (338). Finally, in keeping with the increased proportion of more mature granulocyte progenitors in CML, other investigators have also observed an increased ratio of mature to primitive erythroid progenitors in CML marrow compared to normal marrow (339,340).

Numerous studies have been conducted seeking differences in the regulation of growth of normal and CML progenitors in addition to those already mentioned. Except for the subtle differences previously described in the progenitors' responsiveness to selected growth and inhibitory factors (i.e., G-CSF, GM-CSF,

BPA, EPO, interferon, TNF, and RA), which may merely reflect differences in the state of maturation of the normal and leukemic progenitors, all the studies we have been able to find have shown that CML and normal progenitors respond to the same regulators. The reports of cyclic oscillations of CML granulocytes in vivo, which provide strong evidence for their feedback regulation, have already been described, and the results of comparative in vitro studies also suggest that CML and normal progenitors are sensitive to the same stimulatory and inhibitory factors (341-346). There are reports of decreased sensitivity of CML progenitors to certain negative feedback regulators, such as lactoferrin and prostaglandin E_1 (286,347,348), but the evidence is inconclusive and interpretations other than differing sensitivities of the progenitors have been suggested as responsible for the experimental differences observed (344-346,349).

Platelet-derived growth factor (PDGF) (350-352) and transforming growth factor β (TGF-β) (353-355) are regulatory proteins present in normal platelets that are mitogenic for cells of mesenchymal origin and are thought to have an important role in wound healing. It has been proposed that, if abnormally expressed, PDGF (356,357) and TGF-β (358,359) may contribute to causing malignant transformation.

PDGF has been shown to promote the growth of normal erythropoietic and pluripotent progenitor cells in vitro (360,361), perhaps acting indirectly via marrow mesenchymal cells (362,363), and it can also stimulate purified CML peripheral blood progenitors, although the latter require higher concentrations than normal marrow progenitors for maximal stimulation (364). In view of the close sequence homology between the β chain of PDGF and the transforming protein of simian sarcoma virus (356,357) and the fact that the cellular homolog (c-*sis*) of the transforming viral gene (v-*cis*) is translocated from chromosome 22 to chromosome 9 in CML, it has been proposed that excessive expression of the translocated c-*sis* oncogene could directly or indirectly contribute to overproduction of CML progenitors (365). Canaani et al. (366) were unable to demonstrate c-*sis* expression in either normal or CML hematopoietic cells, but Romero and his coworkers (367) recently reported that both c-*cis* and c-*abl* are expressed in the accelerated and blastic phases of CML.

It has also been suggested that TGF-β may play a role in the pathogenesis of CML. TGF-β-like activity can be detected in normal sera, and this activity is reported to be enhanced in the sera of CML patients (368); moreover, several human myeloid leukemic cell lines, including three blastic CML lines, have been shown to express TGF-β transcripts constitutively (369). There are also reports that there may be an unidentified factor in normal human sera that enhances the growth of CML but not normal CFU-GM (370) and that sera from CML patients, but not normal sera, contain an activity that greatly increases the number of normal CFU-GM in the presence of human placental conditioned media (371). These preliminary results clearly require confirmation and extension before their significance can be evaluated.

Despite recent advances in the purification of various growth factors and in determining their modes of action, it is apparent from the foregoing discussion that there is only rudimentary understanding of how hematopoietic progenitors are regulated in their growth, differentiation, and maturation. The investigations that have been carried out so far are at an early stage, and a great deal of work lies ahead before it is possible to develop a comprehensive understanding of hematopoietic regulation, which is clearly extremely complicated. It is nevertheless evident from the studies that have been conducted that CML and normal progenitors respond similarly to all the purified stimulatory and inhibitory factors that have been examined and that any differences in responsiveness are merely quantitative. Thus from the standpoint of the present discussion, the important conclusion is that CML progenitors are subject to the same kinds of regulation as are normal progenitors and that any differences are very subtle. In the future, when the intricacies of hematopoietic regulation are more fully understood at the molecular level, it may be possible to define precisely the specific subtle differences that may exist.

DISCORDANT MATURATION HYPOTHESIS

Summary of Evidence for Discordant Maturation and Its Consequences

As discussed earlier, ultrastructural analyses of CML cells have revealed an asynchronism in the maturation of the nucleus and cytoplasmic organelles (277–279), with cytoplasmic maturation consistently more rapid than nuclear maturation. Our hypothesis of discordant maturation (50) proposes that this asynchrony has three important consequences:

1. CML progenitors have a reduced proliferative potential because fewer are recycling as primitive progenitors relative to those entering the later maturation compartment.
2. The lag in nuclear maturation enables the mature CML progenitors to undergo more than the normal number of divisions in the mature compartment not under growth regulatory control, resulting in the expansion of the leukemic population.
3. The mature cells have an increased life span due to the lag in nuclear maturation. Although CML myeloid cells are capable of complete maturation, many circulating morphologically mature cells functionally and biochemically have not yet reached full maturity.

It has long been puzzling why the expansion of Ph^+ leukemic cells is typically associated with the granulocytic lineage and, in approximately half the patients, an increase in platelet production, whereas the Ph^+ erythroid population is not expanded. In fact, most patients at the time of diagnosis are slightly to moderately anemic (137). A possible explanation may lie in considering some distinctive features of erythropoiesis that differ from those of granulopoiesis. One critical difference is that the end product of erythropoiesis is an anucleate red cell. As the erythroid progenitors go through the process of division and maturation, there is progressive degeneration of the nucleus that ends in denucleation of the end cell, thus preventing any possibility of continuing cell division. There is evidence that the mean corpuscular hemoglobin concentration (MCHC) is one of the factors responsible for inactivating the erythroid nucleus, thus causing cessation of cellular division (372–374). If cytoplasmic maturation of the Ph^+ erythroid progenitors is more rapid than nuclear maturation, the critical MCHC (possibly 20 g/dL) would be reached at an earlier than normal stage of nuclear maturation and nuclear division would cease prematurely, resulting in a reduced number of cell divisions. At this critical hemoglobin concentration, hemoglobin enters the nucleus through pores in the nuclear membrane (375,376) and is thought to react with receptive nucleoproteins, inducing chromosomal inactivation and nuclear condensation (372,375,376). A similar nuclear-cytoplasmic asynchrony occurs in the megaloblastic anemias (373,374). In the case of the microcytic anemias, the opposite asynchrony occurs. In the latter, hemoglobin synthesis is slow and therefore it takes longer than normal to reach the critical MCHC. As a result, more cell divisions occur before nuclear inactivation. Since the red cell volume is decreasing with each successive division, this results in small (microcytic) cells (373,374).

A comparison of the effects of discordant maturation on granulopoiesis and erythropoiesis in CML can be summarized as follows:

1. Both CML granulopoietic and erythropoietic progenitors have a reduced proliferative potential due to less recycling as primitive progenitors relative to those entering the later maturation compartment. As was shown from our experimental observations, CML BFU-E were similar to CML CFU-GM in that they both were much smaller and at a more advanced stage of maturation than comparable populations of normal BFU-E and CFU-GM.
2. Whereas the lag in nuclear maturation allows mature granulopoietic progenitors to expand in the mature compartment not under growth regulatory control, the lag in erythroid nuclear maturation (relative to cytoplasmic maturation) results in the critical MCHC being reached at an earlier than normal stage of nuclear maturation. The latter results in nuclear division ceasing prematurely before the normal number of cell divisions occurs, thus resulting in a reduction in red cell production.
3. The mature granulocytic cells (polymorphonuclear cells) have an increased life span due to the lag in nuclear maturation, but this does not occur in the anucleate mature red cell. Thus the increased life span of the granulo-

cytes contributes to the increase in granulocyte mass, but no such increase occurs in the erythroid lineage.

The experimental observations just cited are all consistent with the conclusion that abnormal maturation rather than unregulated growth is the main biologic defect in CML. We have been unable to find convincing evidence to the contrary in the literature; although there are numerous references to the presumed occurrence of unregulated growth of CML stem cells or later progenitor cells, these appear merely to be presumptions without sound experimental basis. Since no good methods are available to quantitatively assess the proliferative kinetics of human stem cells, the possibility cannot definitely be excluded that Ph^+ stem cells proliferate faster or that a greater proportion of them recycle than do normal stem cells. However, such a possibility is at best remote because it is totally inconsistent with all the available experimental data with regard to the behavior of early and late progenitors in which it is possible to make measurements (i.e., CFU-GEM → myelocytes). All the in vivo kinetic studies and cell culture studies have consistently shown that CML progenitors proliferate more slowly and have less self-renewal capacity than normal progenitors. When the CML population density is reduced in vivo by chemotherapy or in vitro by experimental manipulation, the rate of proliferation of CML precursors may be similar to that of normal precursors, but even under conditions of lowered cell density it is never faster. The kinetic studies have also demonstrated that the most primitive CML precursors that can be measured are still subject to normal regulatory controls and that the major expansion of the leukemic population takes place as a result of additional divisions in the later maturation compartments, which are no longer subject to regulatory control.

Hypothetical Models of Normal and Leukemic Hematopoiesis

Various hematopoietic cell multiplication models have been proposed, including tangential and logarithmic and various combinations thereof (159,377,378). The asynchronous logarithmic or clonal succession model, as originally proposed by Kay (377), is probably the most popular since it is supported by considerable experimental evidence based on repopulating assays in animals (379-381) and because it appears to afford the animal the most protection in the event of injury to the hematopoietic system. According to the clonal succession theory, normal hematopoiesis is maintained by sequential activation of different stem cell clones rather than through a continuing static contribution of the entire stem cell pool. Such a system implies there is always a large resting stem cell reserve that is somewhat protected from injury by virtue of its quiescent state but can be mobilized if the actively cycling cells are damaged or to meet other demands. Other experimental data favor an alternative system in which the entire stem cell pool contributes to maintaining hematopoiesis (382-384). Whereas some models (159, 385) suggest there may be degrees of stemness, with some stem cells having less proliferative potential or being more restricted in their choice of lineage than others, other evidence favors a stochastic model in which a stem cell, although pluripotent, can commit to produce cells exclusively of one lineage as well as of multiple lineages (380,386,387).

Hypothetical models of cell multiplication in CML have been constructed by our group as well as by other investigators (147,159,388,389), but all these models are seriously flawed because of incorrect assumptions, erroneous concepts, and the failure to accurately represent the dynamic interplay between proliferation and maturation (50). We are currently designing a new model that, we hope, will correct these deficiencies and integrate the process of maturation with proliferation.

Regardless of which normal hematopoietic cell multiplication model is correct, there is good evidence that relatively few normal stem cells are required for repopulation of animals. Minimal estimates for mice have ranged from one stem cell per 10^4-10^5 marrow cells (383,390), and it has been shown experimentally that only about 6-30 CFU-S are needed for hematopoietic reconstitution of lethally irradiated mice using untreated marrow cells (147,391-393). Since the true stem cells constitute only a subset of CFU-S (394), it appears that very few stem cells are required for repopulation of mice. In experiments using retrovirus-mediated gene transfer techniques to mark stem cells and track them after transplantation in irradiated or stem cell-deficient recipients (380,395,396), it has also been shown that very few stem cell clones, perhaps only one or two, are capable of producing the majority of mature hematopoietic cells in mice.

Thus the situation in CML or other types of leukemia in which the entire leukemic population is descended from a single cell may not be as different from normal hematopoiesis as has heretofore been commonly thought. The transforming event may induce a relatively minor alteration in a stem cell, causing it to undergo a subtle behavioral change, which gives it a slight advantage over the normal stem cells and over a long period of time enables the Ph^+ clone to replace the normal population.

Hypothesis of Discordant Maturation as the Primary Biologic Defect in CML

The evidence derived from our studies as well as those of other investigators cited here has led us to propose that the primary biologic defect in CML that results in an increased mass of myeloid cells is not unregulated proliferation but rather discordant maturation (50,322). According to the discordant maturation hypothesis, the altered tyrosine kinase activity of the p210*bcr-abl* protein changes the normal pattern of protein phosphorylation in the signal transduction pathways, resulting in subtle distortion in the transmission of critical regulatory messages. All the *abl* proteins have tyrosine kinase activity, but they differ in the way they utilize themselves as substrates and in their specific activities, suggesting they may function differently (9,12,105,106,109). Moreover, the altered *abl* proteins of both Ph^+ CML and Ph^+ ALL share many features with the altered v-*abl* protein of the Abelson murine leukemia virus whose tyrosine kinase activity is essential for transformation (9), and many of the protein tyrosine kinases serve as receptors and signal transducers for hormones and growth factors. It is therefore quite reasonable to assume that the altered tyrosine kinase activities of the p210 and p185/190 proteins are capable of transforming human stem cells or at least in causing subtle alterations in the regulation of their proliferation and maturation. It has been hypothesized by several investigators that events controlling the induction of differentiation and maturation occur during specific phases of the cell cycle (397-399). We assume that some of the proteins that are abnormally phosphorylated are key regulating proteins that control the genes that normally direct the orderly sequence of proliferation and maturation of the myeloid progenitors. Because these regulatory proteins undergo subtle conformational changes as a result of their abnormal phosphorylation they become faulty regulators, and some of the critical genes are either not turned on and off in the correct temporal sequence or their transcription is otherwise altered in some fashion, as yet unknown.

The results of this subtle disregulation of genetic programming are that there is asynchronous development of the nucleus and cytoplasm and the various dysplastic, biochemical, and cytokinetic changes that have been described take place. Because these abnormalities are relatively minor, the cells are able to carry out most of their essential functions. In general, the biochemical and functional abnormalities described are quantitative and represent mean values of the total mature granulocyte population. As such, they do not reveal what proportion of segmented CML granulocytes have reached full maturity and exhibit normal biochemical and functional characteristics. Because of the lag in nuclear maturation and associated dysplastic changes, the partially mature CML precursors, which are no longer under regulatory control, go through one or more additional divisions during passage through the maturation compartments than do the comparable normal precursors and also have an increased life span, thus further contributing to the increase in myeloid mass.

Once the leukemic population has overexpanded to the extent that the normal cell density in the marrow is exceeded, the normal stem cells are suppressed. The mechanism of suppression of normal hematopoiesis is poorly understood, but it is undoubtedly complex, just as is the positive control of hematopoiesis. Whatever the mechanism, because the Ph^+ progenitors differ only slightly from normal progenitors, it is reasonable to assume that the latter must recognize the leukemic cells as normal and cease cell production as they ordinarily do when the normal maximum permitted cell density is reached.

The molecular events responsible for transforming the original stem cell in CML, which permits it to undergo an enormous uniclonal expansion and eventually to become dominant over the normal population, do not bring about these changes by permitting unregulated proliferation of the affected cells as seen in classic experimental examples of complete malignant transformation (400,401). The initial t(9;22) translocation in CML instead causes only subtle alterations in the cells' biologic behavior, giving them only a slight proliferative advantage over the normal cells, somewhat analogous to those seen in other premalignant lesions, such as junctional nevi of the skin or adenomatous polyps of the colon. Because the cells comprising the latter lesions naturally have only very limited migratory capacity, they remain fixed in situ, whereas the transformed stem cell in CML, being naturally highly migratory, quickly disseminates its progeny throughout the entire hematopoietic system. Many benign tumors undergo malignant progression during which additional genetic abnormalities occur, causing progressive loss of the cells' ability to mature and resulting in blastic-phase CML or in malignant melanoma or colonic cancer (402,403). The secondary genetic abnormalities associated with malignant progression are generally less consistent than the primary event (402). Whereas no single additional abnormality has been identified as CML progresses from the chronic to the blastic phase, as already noted about 80% of patients acquire additional chromosomal abnormalities.

Evidence from Experimental Systems Supporting the Hypothesis

The Abelson virus was originally isolated from a murine B cell lymphoma and was subsequently found to be highly efficient in rapidly transforming early B cells and NIH 3T3 cells, apparently directly inducing their full transformation dramatically in a single step (404). However, other studies have shown that the Abelson virus may cause more subtle phenotypic changes in various cell types. Although essential for oncogenic progression, the Abelson virus may not be sufficient for inducing all the features associated with full transformation. For example, pre-B cells infected with Abelson virus have been isolated that have only limited oncogenic potential but express viral kinase at the same levels as fully transformed cells (405). It has also been shown that Abelson can infect and stimulate erythroid precursors to form colonies and differentiate in the absence of erythropoietin (406) and that Abelson-infected mast cells lose their dependence on interleukin-3 (IL-3) (407,408). Witte has recently reviewed these findings and suggested that the viral kinase may function in a pleiotropic fashion with effects on multiple signaling pathways (409). It is therefore quite reasonable to postulate that the first stage of transformation of human stem cells in CML may be due to altered kinase activity of $p210^{bcr\text{-}abl}$ that would cause only subtle changes in the cell's behavior.

It was noted earlier that many of the biochemical and kinetic changes of chronic-phase CML cells can be reversed by treatment with various substances, including cytotoxic drugs, growth factors, neuraminidase, and *cis*-retinoic acid (161-163,313-317). In many tumor cell lines, including some transformed by the *ras* or *sis* oncogenes, it has been shown that by activating one or more of the signal transduction systems the cells can be forced to undergo "reverse transformation," with restoration of normal morphologic features and growth characteristics (410). The transformed phenotype can be attenuated by activation of protein kinase A or protein kinase C, and this modulation is accompanied by phosphorylation of unique proteins and changes in the phosphoinositide cycle (410).

Experimental Approaches to Defining the Specific Abnormalities Responsible for Discordant Maturation

If altered p210$^{bcr\text{-}abl}$ protein tyrosine kinase activity is indeed the primary abnormality responsible for the Ph^{+} population's disocrdant maturation and its achieving dominance over the normal population, the next task is to determine the specific abnormalities in the transduction pathways and in gene expression. This is a daunting undertaking because of the multiplicity of protein kinases, phosphoproteins, and genes involved in regulating the growth, differentiation, and maturation of myeloid (as well as other) cells. Most of the protein kinases and regulatory proteins have not yet even been identified, let alone characterized with regard to their specific functions and regulatory roles. Moreover, undoubtedly many of the genes involved in regulating myeloid progenitors have also not yet been identified, and the specific regulatory functions of even those that have been recognized remain largely obscure, as do the mechanisms controlling their transcription.

Signal transduction (411-414) and regulation of gene transcription (415-417) are highly complicated processes, and very little is as yet known about the specific genes involved in normal myeloid growth and differentiation, let alone what regulatory distortions may occur as a result of abnormal protein phosphorylation in CML. At least 40 genes are known to be involved in regulating cell cycle progression in the budding and fission yeasts (418), and it has been estimated that at least several hundred genes may have a role in the control of growth and differentiation of mammalian cells (419). Hunter has suggested that there may be over a thousand protein kinases that function in a fashion analogous to transistors in electrical circuits to regulate the biologic circuitry of the cell and that any one sophisticated circuit may include a hundred or more protein kinase "chips" (420). Protein phosphatases may have equally important roles in the regulation of protein function (412).

Abnormalities in Signal Transduction

Although the task of unraveling the specific regulatory defects in CML is undoubtedly a formidable undertaking, the altered tyrosine kinase activity of the unique p210$^{bcr\text{-}abl}$ protein is an important clue. Protein tyrosine kinases are much less numerous than protein serine or threonine kinases, and many of the former function as receptors and signal transducers for growth factors of hematopoietic as well as other types of cells (420). Phosphorylation and dephosphorylation of specific proteins involving tyrosine residues is undoubtedly important in controlling the differentiation or activation of many types of cells, including these of the granulocyte lineage (421-423). For example, platelets express high levels of c-*src* protein kinase activity (424) and activation of c-*src* kinase occur when HL-60 cells are induced to differentiate to granulocytes or macrophages (425). Normal human polymorphonuclear leukocytes contain higher levels of cytosolic tyrosine kinase and membrane-associated phosphotyrosine phosphatase activities than are found in HL-60 cells, suggesting that both activities increase during differentiation of myeloid cells (426). Treatment of mature polymorphonuclear leukocytes with fMLP or phorbol esters causes a significant decrease in tyrosine phosphatase activity and increased phosphorylation of some protein bands, indicating that activation of tyrosine kinase and inhibition of phosphatase may also have important roles in the response of mature granulocytes to such stimulation (426).

The search for specific abnormalities in phosphotyrosine-containing proteins in CML has only begun recently. Using phosphotyrosine antibodies, immunoprecipitation and gel electrophoretic techniques, altered tyrosine phosphorylation of a number of proteins in addition to p210 has been shown to occur in CML-derived cell lines, fresh CML cells, and in *bcr-abl* virus-infected cells (427-432). However, the results reported by different groups are inconsistent with regard to some of the phosphotyrosine-containing proteins, possibly because of technical differences (431), and it is not yet clear whether some of the proteins may also be present in normal immature progenitors. Much work is required before it is possible to identify, purify, and define the specific roles of the critical proteins that may be responsible for misregulation of Ph^+ cells.

Gene Transfection Experiments

Another experimental approach that has been used to try to identify specific changes resulting from p210 or p185 kinase activity has been to infect cells with retroviral constructs encoding for p210$^{bcr\text{-}abl}$ or p185$^{bcr\text{-}abl}$. Whereas the v-*abl* product p160 readily transforms NIH 3T3 fibroblasts, the p210$^{bcr\text{-}abl}$ protein does not; cell lines expressing high levels of p210 were morphologically normal (433). When helper virus *gag* determinants were fused to the *bcr-abl* protein, the *gag-bcr-abl* protein was then able to transform NIH 3T3 cells, probably because the *gag* sequences contain an NH_2-terminal myristyl fatty acid moiety that determines membrane localization. It appears that if a myristylation site or hydrophobic domain is lacking, the protein is not anchored to the cell membrane but remains in the cytoplasm, where it is unable to induce transformation (433). In other experiments (434) it was found that, by combining a retroviral gene transfer system with a long-term murine bone marrow culture system selective for the growth and differentiation of early B cells, cells expressing high levels of p210 tyrosine kinase became dominant in the culture and led to clonal outgrowths of immature lymphoid cells. Although the expression of p210 stimulated growth, it was not generally sufficient for full oncogenic behavior. The degree of oncogenicity was variable; although all the cloned cell lines had high p210 expression, only some of them progressed to a fully malignant phenotype as manifested by increased cloning efficiency and the ability to induce tumors in syngeneic mice (434).

In a recent review (80), Clark et al. state that their observations are quite consistent with our discordant maturation hypothesis in that the immature lymphocytes expressing p210 have much slower transformation kinetics and are markedly less tumorigenic than cells transformed with the v-*abl* oncogene. In other experiments it was shown that when an additional oncogene such as v-*myc* or *p53*, was coexpressed with p210 or v-*abl*, the transformed cells were more tumorigenic than when only one gene was expressed, and it was suggested these observations may be relevant to the blastic transformation of CML (80). Lugo et al. (432) have recently reported that infection of fibroblasts with p185-virus results in much greater tyrosine kinase activity and transforming potency than does infection with p210-virus.

Coexpression of two oncogenes has been shown to be complementary in producing more complete transformation in rodent cells (435,436) and in avian cells, both in vitro and in vivo (437,438). In one exceptional case, chick myelomonocytic cells doubly transformed by v-*myc* plus either v-*myb* or v-*Myb,ets* were indistinguishable from cells transformed by either v-*myb* or v-*myb,ets* alone even when they expressed high levels of v-*myc* protein (439). It was concluded that the probable explanation was that although v-*myc* induced only proliferation without affecting differentiation, because v-*myb* induces both proliferation and a block or reversal of differentiation, v-*myb* has a dominant effect over v-*myc*.

More typically in the case of transforming viruses, such as AEV or MH2, which contain two oncogenes, it is the combination of a cytoplasmic and a nuclear oncogene that leads to enhanced oncogenicity (438). Different oncogene combinations can cooperate in different ways to alter the growth and differentiation of chick hematopoietic cells. Some oncogenes (e.g., v-*erb*B, v-*myc*, and v-*myb*) can disrupt growth control by induction of self-renewal capacity in differentiated cells, some (v-*mil* and v-*crb*B) act by making cells independent of growth factors by autocrine or nonautocrine mechanisms, and still others (v-*erb*A and v-*myb*) can act by blocking or reverting differentiation (438).

Much less is known about the transformation of human hematopoietic progenitors than of avian progenitor cells. The avian leukemia viruses are very efficient in transforming avian progenitors in vitro; moreover, transforming experiments can readily be performed in vivo in newborn chicks to determine whether comparable types of transformation occur, which is usually the case (438). As Graf has emphasized (438), the fact that some of the avian transforming viruses acquired two different oncogenes is probably based on the selective pressure imposed by the original investigators to isolate pathogens with very high oncogenic potential.

Not only are experiments comparable to those in chicks obviously impossible in humans, but it appears to be much more difficult to introduce genetic material into early human progenitor cells by retroviral gene transfer or electroporation techniques. Although the evidence is much less compelling than in the well-controlled avian systems, coexpression of two oncogenes may also be implicated in causing blastic transformation in CML. As previously noted, it has been suggested that coexpression of p210 and c-*myc* or *ras* or alteration in *p53* gene structure and expression may have a concomitant molecular role in the evolution of blastic transformation in CML (76-85). However, there is at present very little information about the molecular events responsible for blastic progression in CML and we must await additional experimental evidence.

Daley and Baltimore (440) recently reported that the gene for p210$^{bcr\text{-}abl}$ can function as a dominant oncogene in that it can transform the murine bone marrow-derived lymphoblastoid IL-3-dependent Ba/F3 cell line so it grows in the absence of IL-3 and induces tumors in nude mice. p210 did not trigger endogenous expression of IL-3 or other growth factors in an autocrine fashion but rather provided the stimulus for Ba/F3 proliferation normally provided through the IL-3 signal transduction pathway (440). The mechanisms by which the cells acquire IL-3 independence is not known, but possibly p210$^{bcr\text{-}abl}$ directly phosphorylates the IL-3 receptor (409) or an intermediate protein involved in signal transduction (441,442), thus autostimulating the pathway normally used by the hormone-receptor complex (443). The modes of action of IL-3 by which it affects cellular metabolism to control the growth and differentiation of hematopoietic progenitor cells are very complex and several ways have been described by which IL-3 dependence can be abrogated (444-446). A number of cytokines with both positive and negative effects on the growth of hematopoietic progenitors have recently been shown to induce rapid tyrosine or serine phosphorylation, strongly suggesting that such phosphorylations have key roles in the transduction of cytokine signals (443,447,448).

Very recently, Daley et al. (449) have reported that murine bone marrow infected with a retrovirus encoding p210$^{bcr\text{-}abl}$ and transplanted into irradiated syngeneic recipients results in several hematologic tumors, among which is a myeloproliferative disease resembling the chronic phase of CML. Heisterkamp et al. (450) have also very recently reported generating 10 mice transgenic for a *bcr/abl* p190 DNA construct, 8 of which died of acute leukemia (2 myeloid and 6 lymphoid) 10 to 58 days after birth.

Genes Involved in Programming Normal and Leukemic Myeiopoiesis

It is apparent from the foregoing review that there is as yet almost no information about what specific abnormalities may occur in the signal transduction pathways as a result of the t(9;22) translocation, and knowledge is equally incomplete about what genes are misregulated in the chronic or acute phases of CML.

A large number of proto-oncogenes have been reported to be expressed in normal human myeloid cells and in the myeloid leukemias, including c-*abl*, c-*ras*^{H}, c-*myc*, c-*myb*, c-*fes*, c-*fos*, c-*ras*^{K}, c-*erb*, c-*fms*, c-*cis*, c-*src*, and c-*fgr* (451–462), but very little is as yet known about their specific functions and regulatory roles. In some of the early studies no correlation was found between the expression of particular oncogenes and hematopoietic lineage (451,452), but subsequent studies have shown that expression of some genes (e.g., c-*myb*, c-*erb*, c-*fos*, c-*fes*, c-*src*, and c-*fgr*) are more characteristic of myelopoiesis or myeloid leukemias than of normal or neoplastic lymphopoiesis (454–459,461,462). The expression of some genes varies with the state and direction of differentiation. For example, in some myeloid cell lines, expression of c-*myc* and c-*myb* is greater in immature than mature cells and falls with induction of differentiation; c-*fos* is induced during monocyte-macrophage differentiation of some (but not all) monocytic lines but not during the induction of granulocytic differentiation (459). In other experiments, when normal murine monocytic cells or human myeloid leukemic cells at different stages of differentiation were examined for the expression of *src*-related proto-oncogenes, it was found that c-*fgr* is expressed at its highest levels in the differentiated normal monocytic or leukemic myelomonocytic cells but the highly related c-*src* gene was expressed in myeloid leukemia cells at all stages of differentiation (462). When normal monocytic cells were stimulated with the monocyte colony-stimulating factor CSF-1, c-*fgr* transcripts (but not c-*src* or c-*yes* transcripts) were selectively induced, suggesting that the c-*fgr* tyrosine kinase has a unique function in controlling the proliferation of differentiated monocytes distinct from that of other tyrosine kinases (462).

There is very little information concerning specific abnormalities of gene expression in CML cells beyond what has already been noted. Some proto-oncogenes (i.e., c-*myc*, c-*ras*, c-*fos*, and *p53*) are expressed in a cell cycle-dependent manner in that their expression is markedly increased when quiescent (G_0) cells are stimulated by mitogens to enter the G_1 phase of the cell cycle in preparation for division. In one recent study comparing acute leukemic and CML cells (460), the expression of c-*myc* and three other G_1-specific genes were compared to that of the H3 S-phase-specific gene that encodes histone H3; it was reasoned that if the ratio of expression of G_1- to S-phase genes increased rather than remaining constant, this would support the concept that the G_1 genes were deregulated.

However it was found that although the G_1 genes were overexpressed in CML cells, in keeping with their predominantly cycling status, H3 expression was increased in parallel. Thus, in contrast to the findings in the leukemic cells from 9 of 10 AML patients in which c-*myc* expression was disproportionately elevated with respect to H3, no evidence of deregulation of the cell cycle genes could be detected in CML cells (460). These findings are of course quite consistent with our conclusion that deregulation of proliferation is not the underlying defect in the chronic phase of CML.

Relevance of the Hypothesis to Other Neoplasms

Many spontaneous human neoplasms in addition to CML have highly specific genetic abnormalities (60,243,402,403,463-471). Nonrandom chromosomal translocations are most common, but additions, deletions, gene rearrangements and amplifications, and mutations of proto-oncogenes have also been reported. Some of the abnormalities in particular types of tumors [e.g., t(14;18), t(8;14), and t(15;17)] are so consistent that, as in the case of the t(9;22) translocation, it is probable that they are the primary causative lesions and, moreover, that they determine the biologic behavior of the tumor (402,469-471). Additional chromosomal changes frequently occur when the different tumors undergo malignant progression, but again, as in the case of CML, the secondary changes tend to be less specific and consistent than the primary abnormalities (402,471). It is probable that discordant maturation rather than unregulated growth is also the primary biologic abnormality in a number of other human neoplasms. This is especially likely in slowly growing tumors in which the majority of cells are partially mature, and which require only a relatively small input from an early stem cell compartment (50). Examples of such tumors include follicular lymphoma, multiple myeloma, myelodysplastic syndromes, and some types of acute nonlymphoblastic leukemia.

Although our discordant maturation hypothesis for CML was arrived at independently and originated from our own clinical and laboratory investigations, in reviewing the literature we have found that conceptually similar theories under different names have been proposed for other tumors by several previous investigators (472-475). Potter has recently re-emphasized that his theory of "blocked ontogeny" may require only a partial block in differentiation (476). His theory stemmed from an entirely different source than CML, namely extensive data on enzyme levels in Morris hepatomas, but the partially blocked ontogeny theory as it has evolved (476) is remarkably similar to the discordant maturation hypothesis we have proposed for CML. We believe the latter term best describes the biologic abnormality in CML for the reasons given in this chapter, but the semantics are perhaps less important than recognizing the concept that the primary abnormality in CML and probably many other neoplasms is due to faulty gene expression, which in turn may be due to minor errors in signal transduction and gene regulation. CML is an excellent target tumor for further investigation because it has a highly consistent primary genetic abnormality, the *bcr-abl* gene, and because the product of this gene is a qualitatively different protein with uniquely altered enzymatic activity. Since it is highly probable that the altered tyrosine kinase activity has a critical role in causing error in signal transduction and gene regulation, the p210 protein provides an important first clue as to how the genes directing myelopoiesis are misregulated.

SUMMARY

In this chapter, we have presented a unifying hypothesis of the pathogenesis of CML that states that the primary biologic abnormality in the chronic phase of the disease is uncoordinated maturation of the nucleus in relation to the maturation of the cytoplasm rather than uncontrolled proliferation. It is proposed that the altered tyrosine kinase activity of the chimeric $p210^{bcr\text{-}abl}$ protein causes abnormal phosphorylation of some of the critical regulatory proteins in the signal transduction pathways. As a result of their altered phosphorylation (or dephosphorylation), the regulatory proteins become faulty regulators of the genes that normally direct the orderly proliferation, differentiation, and maturation of myeloid progenitors. This subtle disregulation of the genetic programming of myelopoiesis results in uncoupled or discordant development of the nucleus and cytoplasm and in various related dysplastic, biochemical, and functional changes. Because the abnormalities are relatively minor, the Ph^+ progenitors are still responsive to normal regulatory factors and the mature Ph^+ cells are still able to perform their essential functions. The morphologically mature circulating Ph^+ granulocytes are a heterogeneous population with different degrees of maturation. While they are capable of fully maturing, because of their asynchronous nuclear-cytoplasmic development and premature release from the marrow, a portion of the circulating morphologically mature Ph^+ granulocytes have biochemical and functional characteristics resembling those of normal marrow mature granulocytes. With appropriate stimulation the partially mature cells can be induced to undergo more complete maturation.

Because of the lag in nuclear maturation, the partially mature Ph^+ granulocyte precursors, which are no longer under regulatory control, go through one or more additional divisions during passage through the intermediate or later maturation compartments than do comparable normal precursors, and they also have increased longevity, thus further contributing to expansion of the granulocyte mass. In a similar fashion the delayed nuclear maturation and discordant cytoplasmic maturation of megakaryocytes frequently result in increased platelet production. However, discordant maturation during erythropoiesis has a different consequence, probably because the end stage of maturation in the red cell lineage is an anucleate cell. The concentration of cellular hemoglobin is thought to be one of the factors responsible for inactivating the erythroid nucleus. The more rapid cytoplasmic maturation in Ph^+ erythroid progenitors, relative to nuclear maturation, results in the critical concentration of hemoglobin being reached at an earlier than normal stage of nuclear maturation, and as a result chromosomal inactivation and nuclear condensation occur prematurely. The effect of this is fewer than the normal number of cell divisions and consequently reduced red cell production. Moreover, in contrast to the increased life span of the mature Ph^+ granulocyte, there is no such increase in the longevity of the anucleate Ph^+ red cell. Thus discordant maturation results in anemia rather than leukocytosis or thrombocytosis.

We have reviewed the pertinent literature describing the many cytokinetic, morphologic, biochemical, and functional abnormalities that occur in CML, and we have found that all the observations are compatible with the concept that discordant maturation is the primary abnormality in CML rather than unregulated growth. Recent gene transfer experiments are also consistent with this hypothesis. Whereas the v-*abl* product p160 can rapidly cause full malignant transformation of several cell types, including fibroblasts and lymphoblasts, the $p210^{bcr\text{-}abl}$ protein does not transform fibroblasts and causes only partial transformation of lymphoblasts; immature lymphocytes expressing high levels of p210 generally have only limited oncogenic potential.

Many examples in experimental animal systems show that coexpression of two oncogenes leads to enhanced oncogenicity, and it has been suggested that activation of one or more additional oncogenes may be responsible for blastic transformation in CML. Several candidate oncogenes have been implicated, but more evidence is required before any definite conclusions can be made about what molecular events are responsible for blastic progression. It appears that secondary abnormalities associated with blastic transformation are much less consistent than the primary t(9;22) translocation.

If the t(9;22) translocation and the resultant altered $p210^{bcr\text{-}abl}$ tyrosine kinase activity are indeed the primary abnormalities responsible for the CML cells' discordant maturation and their achieving dominance over the normal population, the next task is to determine what specific abnormalities occur in the transduction pathways and in the regulation of gene expression. Very little is known about the genes responsible for programming normal myelopoiesis, and there is a similar dearth of knowledge about which protein kinases and proteins may be involved in regulating these genes, let alone what specific abnormalities may occur in CML. The task ahead is thus formidable and requires a major effort by many investigators. However, it is clearly worth the undertaking: it may have far-reaching significance because discordant maturation may also be the primary biologic abnormality in other spontaneous human tumors.

ACKNOWLEDGMENTS

We would like to thank Su De Meritt and Claire Jacobus for their expert help in the preparation of this manuscript.

NOTE: This chapter was completed in February 1989 and the literature cited does not extend beyond that date except for a few very recent references to new findings of considerable importance and relevance.

REFERENCES

1. Bennett, J. H. (1845). Case of hypertrophy of the spleen and liver in which death took place from suppuration of the blood. *Edinburgh Med. Surg. J. 64*:413.
2. Virchow, R. (1846). Weisses Blut und Milztumoren. *Med. Z. 15*:157.
3. Nowell, P. C., and Hungerford, D. A. (1960). Chromosome studies on normal and leukemic human leukocytes. *JNCI 25*:85–109.
4. Caspersson, T., Gahrton, G., Lindsten, J., and Zech, L. (1970). Identification of the Philadelphia chromosome on a number 22 by quinacrine mustard fluorescence analysis. *Exp. Cell Res. 63*:238–240.
5. Rowley, J. D. (1973). A new consistent chromosomal abnormality in chronic myelogenous leukaemia identified by quinacrine, fluorescence and Giemsa staning (letter). *Nature 243*:290–293.
6. Bartram, C. R., de Klein, A., Hagemeijer, A., van Agthoven, T., Geurts von Kessel, A., Bootsma, D., Grosveld, G., Ferguson-Smith, M. A., Davies, T., Stone, M., Heisterkamp, N., Stephenson, J. R., and Groffen, J. (1983). Translocation of c-*abl* oncogene correlates with the presence of a Philadelphia chromosome in chronic myelocytic leukaemia. *Nature 306*:277–280.
7. Groffen, J., Stephenson, J. R., Heisterkamp, N., de Klein, A., Bartram, C. R., and Grosveld, G. (1984). Philadelphia chromosomal breakpoints are clustered within a limited region, *bcr*, on chromosome 22. *Cell 36*:93–99.
8. Shtivelman, E., Lifshitz, B., Gale, R. P., and Canaani, E. (1985). Fused transcript of *abl* and *bcr* genes in chronic myeloid leukaemia. *Nature 315*: 550–554.
9. Konopka, J. B., Watanabe, S. M., and Witte, O. N. (1984). An alteration of the human c-*abl* protein in K562 leukemia cells unmasks associated tyrosine kinase activity. *Cell 37*:1035–1042.
10. Konopka, J. B., and Witte, O. N. (1985). Detection of c-*abl* tyrosine kinase activity in vitro permits direct comparison of normal and altered *abl* gene products. *Mol. Cell. Biol. 5*:3116–3123.
11. Rosenberg, N. E., Clark, D. R., and Witte, O. N. (1980). Abelson murine leukemia virus mutants deficient in kinase activity and lymphoid cell transformation. *J. Virol. 36*:766–774.

12. Clark, S. S., McLaughlin, J., Crist, W. M., Champlin, R., and Witte, O. (1987). Reports: Unique forms of the *abl* tyrosine kinase distinguish Ph^1-positive CML from Ph^1-positive ALL. *Science 235*:85–88.
13. Heim, S., Billström, R., Kristoffersson, U., Mandahl, N., Strömbeck, B., and Mitelman, F. (1985). Variant Ph translocations in chronic myeloid leukemia. *Cancer Genet. Cytogenet. 18*:215–227.
14. Sandberg, A. A., Gemmill, R. M., and Hecht, B. K. (1986). The Philadelphia chromosome: A model of cancer and molecular cytogenetics. *Cancer Genet. Cytogenet. 21*:129–146.
15. De Braekeleer, M. (1986). Breakpoint distribution in variant Philadelphia translocations in chronic myeloid leukemia. *Cancer Genet. Cytogenet. 23*: 167–170.
16. Hagemeijer, A., de Klein, A., Gödde-Salz, E., Turc-Carel, C., Smit-Elisabeth, M. E., van Agthoven, A. J., and Grosveld, G. C. (1985). Translocation of c-*abl* to "masked" Ph in chronic myeloid leukemia. *Cancer Genet. Cytogenet. 18*:95–104.
17. De Braekeleer, M. (1987). Variant Philadelphia translocations in chronic myeloid leukemia. *Cytogenet. Cell Genet. 44*:215–222.
18. Ohyashiki, K., Ohyashiki, J. H., Kinniburgh, A. J., Rowe, J., Miller, K. B., Raza, A., Preisler, H. D., and Sandberg, A. A. (1987). Transposition of breakpoint cluster region (3^1 *bcr*) in CML cells with variant Philadelphia translocations. *Cancer Genet. Cytogenet. 26*:105–115.
19. Bernstein, R. (1988). Cytogenetics of chronic myelogenous leukemia. *Semin. Hematol. 25*:20–34.
20. Bartram, C. R., and Carbonell, F. (1986). *bcr* Rearrangement in Ph-negative CML (letter). *Cancer Genet. Cytogenet. 21*:183–184.
21. Morris, C. M., Reeve, A. E., Fitzgerald, P. H., Hollings, P. E., Beard, M. E. J., and Heaton, D. C. (1986). Genomic diversity correlates with clinical variation in Ph^1 negative chronic myeloid leukemia. *Nature 320*:281–283.
22. Dreazen, O., Klisak, I., Rassool, F., Goldman, J. M., Sparkes, R. S., and Gale, R. P. (1987). Do oncogenes determine clinical features in chronic myeloid leukaemia? *Lancet 1*:1402–1405.
23. Lisker, R., Casas, L., Mutchinick, O., Lopez-Ariza, B., and Labardini, J. (1982). Patient with chronic myelogenous leukemia and late appearing Philadelphia chromosome. *Cancer Genet. Cytogenet. 6*:275–277.
24. Hagemeijer, A., Smit, E. M. E., Löwenberg, B., and Abels, J. (1979). Chronic myeloid leukemia with permanent disappearance of the Ph chromosome and development of new clonal subpopulations. *Blood 53*:1–14.
25. Altman, A. J., Palmer, C. G., and Bazhner, R. L. (1974). Juvenile "chronic granulocytic" leukemia: A panmyelopathy with prominent monocytic involvement and circulating monocyte colony-forming cells. *Blood 43*:341–350.
26. Pugh, W. C., Pearson, M., Vardiman, J. W., and Rowley, J. D. (1985). Philadelphia chromosome-negative chronic myelogenous leukemia: A morphological reassessment. *Br. J. Haematol. 60*:457–467.

27. Travis, L. P., Pierre, R. V., and De Wald, G. W. (1986). Ph[1] negative chronic granulocytic leukemia: A nonentity. *Am. J. Clin. Pathol. 85*:186–193.
28. Kantarjian, H. M., Keating, M. J., Walters, R. S., McCredie, K. B., Smith, T. L., Talpaz, M., Beran, M., Cork, A., Trujillo, J. M., and Freireich, E. J. (1986). Clinical and prognostic features of Philadelphia chromosome-negative chronic myelogenous leukemia. *Cancer 58*:2023–2030.
29. Ezdinli, E. Z., Sokol, J. E., Crosswhile, L., and Sandberg, A. A. (1970). Philadelphia chromosome positive and negative chronic myeloid leukemia. *Ann. Intern. Med. 72*:175–182.
30. Cervantes, F., and Rozman, C. (1982). A multivariate analysis of prognostic factors in chronic myeloid leukemia. *Blood 60*:1298–1309.
31. Fialkow, P. J., Jacobson, R. J., Papayannopoulou, T., Penfold, G. K., Jacobson, R. T., and Hansen, J. A. (1977). Chronic myelocytic leukemia: Clonal origin in a stem cell common to the granulocyte, erythrocyte, platelet and monocyte/macrophage. *Am. J. Med. 63*:125–130.
32. Yoffe, G., Chinault, A. C., Talpaz, M., Blick, M. B., Kantarjian, H. M., Taylor, K., and Spitzer, G. (1987). Clonal nature of Philadelphia chromosome positive and negative chronic myelogenous leukemia by DNA hybridization analysis. *Exp. Hematol. 15*:725–728.
33. Martin, P. J., Najfeld, V., and Hansen, J. A. (1980). Involvement of the B-lymphoid system in chronic myelogenous leukaemia. *Nature 287*:49–50.
34. Nitta, M., Kato, Y., Strife, A., Wachter, M., Fried, J., Perez, A., Jhanwar, S., Duigou-Osterndorf, R., Chaganti, R. S. K., and Clarkson, B. (1985). Incidence of involvement of the B and T lymphocyte lineages in chronic myelogenous leukemia. *Blood 66*:1053–1061.
35. Bartram, C. R., Raghavachar, A., Anger, B., Stain, C., and Bettelheim, P. (1987). T lymphocytes lack rearrangement of the *bcr* gene in Philadelphia chromosome positive chronic myelocytic leukemia. *Blood 69*:1682–1685.
36. Fauser, A. A., Kanz, L., Bross, K. J., and Löhr, G. W. (1985). T cells and probably B cells arise from the malignant clone in chronic myelogenous leukemia. *J. Clin. Invest. 75*:1080–1082.
37. Dreazen, O., Canaani, E., and Gale, R. P. (1988). Molecular biology of chronic myelogenous leukemia. *Semin. Hematol. 25*:35–49.
38. Maniatis, A. K., Amsel, S., Mitus, W. J., and Coleman, N. (1969). Chromosome pattern of bone marrow fibroblasts in patients with chronic granulocytic leukaemia. *Nature 222*:1278–1279.
39. Cunningham, I., Gee, T., Dowling, M., Chaganti, R., Bailey, R., Hopfan, S., Bowden, L., Turnbull, A., Knapper, W., and Clarkson, B. (1979). Results of treatment of Ph[1] chronic myelogenous leukemia with an intensive treatment regimen (L-5). *Blood 53*:375–395.
40. Goto, T., Nishikori, M., Arlin, Z., Gee, T., Kempin, S., Burchenal, J., Strife, A., Wisniewski, D., Lambek, C., Little, C., Jhanwar, S., Chaganti, R., and Clarkson, B. (1982). Growth characteristics of leukemic and normal hematopoietic cells in Ph[1]+ chronic myelogenous leukemia and effects of intensive treatment. *Blood 59*:793–808.

41. Dubé, I. D., Kalousek, D. K., and Coulombel, L. (1984). Cytogenetic studies in early myeloid progenitor compartments in Ph[1]-positive chronic myeloid leukemia. II. Long term culture reveals the persistence of Ph[1]-negative progenitors in treated as well as newly diagnosed patients. *Blood 63*:1172–1177.
42. Talpaz, M., Kantarjian, H. M., McCredie, K. B., Trujillo, J. M., Keating, M. J., and Gutterman, J. U. (1986). Chronic myelogenous leukemia: Hematologic remission and cytogenetic improvements induced by recombinant alpha A interferon. *N. Engl. J. Med. 314*:1065–1069.
43. Fialkow, P. J., Martin, P. J., and Najfeld, V. (1981). Evidence of a multistep pathogenesis of chronic myelogenous leukemia. *Blood 58*:158–163.
44. Martin, P. J., Najfeld, V., and Fialkow, P. J. (1982). Review article: B-lymphoid cell involvement in chronic myelogenous leukemia: Implications for the pathogenesis of the disease. *Cancer Genet. Cytogenet. 6*:359–368.
45. Fitzgerald, P. H., Pickering, A. F., and Eiby, J. R. (1971). Clonal origin of the Philadelphia chromosome and chronic myeloid leukemia. Evidence from a sex chromosome mosaic. *Br. J. Haematol. 21*:473–480.
46. Singer, J. W., Arlin, Z. A., Najfeld, V., Adamson, J. W., Kempin, S. J., Clarkson, B. D., and Fialkow, P. J. (1980). Restoration of nonclonal hematopoiesis in chronic myelogenous leukemia (CML) following a chemotherapy-induced loss of the Ph[1] chromosome. *Blood 56*:356–360.
47. Chaganti, R. S. K., Bailey, R. B., Jhanwar, S. C., Arlin, Z. A., and Clarkson, B. D. (1982). Chronic myelogenous leukemia in the monosomic cell line of a fertile Turner syndrome mosaic (45,X/46,XX). *Cancer Genet. Cytogenet. 5*:215–221.
48. Dubé, I. D., Arlin, Z. A., Kalousek, D. K., Eaves, C. J., and Eaves, A. C. (1984). Concise report: Nonclonal hemopoietic progenitor cells detected in long-term marrow cultures from a Turner syndrome mosaic with chronic myeloid leukemia. *Blood 64*:1284–1287.
49. Hogge, D. E., Coulombel, L., Kalousek, D. K., Eaves, C. J., and Eaves, A. C. (1987). Nonclonal hemopoietic progenitors in a G6PD heterozygote with chronic myelogenous leukemia revealed after long-term marrow culture. *Am. J. Hematol. 24*:389–394.
50. Strife, A., and Clarkson, B. (1988). Biology of chronic myelogenous leukemia: Is discordant maturation the primary defect? *Semin, Hematol. 25*:1–19.
51. Kurzrock, R., Gutterman, J. U., and Talpaz, M. (1988). The molecular genetics of Philadelphia chromosome-positive leukemias. In *Mechanisms of Disease* (F. H. Epstein, ed.). *N. Engl. J. Med. 319*:990–998.
52. Schaefer-Rego, K., Dudek, H., Popenoe, D. (1987). CML patients in blast crisis have breakpoints localized to a specific region of the BCR. *Blood 70*:448–455.
53. Shtalrid, M., Talpaz, M., Kurzrock, R., Kantarjian, H., Trujillo, J., Gutterman, J., Yoffe, G., and Blick, M. (1988). Analysis of breakpoints within the *bcr* gene and their correlation with the clinical course of Philadelphia-positive chronic myelogenous leukemia. *Blood 72*:485–490.

54. Dreazen, O., Berman, M., and Gale, R. P. (1988). Molecular abnormalities of *bcr* and c-*abl* in chronic myelogenous leukemia associated with a long chronic phase. *Blood 71*:797–799.
55. Mills, K. I., MacKenzie, E. D., and Birnie, G. D. (1988). The site of the breakpoint within the *bcr* is a prognostic factor in Philadelphia-positive CML patients. *Blood 72*:1237–1241.
56. Dubé, I., Dixon, J., Beckett, T., Grossman, A., Weinstein, M., Benn, P., McKeithan, T., Norman, C., and Pinkerton, P. (1989). Location of breakpoints within the major breakpoint cluster region (*bcr*) in 33 patients with *bcr* rearrangement-positive chronic myeloid leukemia (CML) with complex or absent Philadelphia chromosomes. *Genes, Chromosomes & Cancer 1*:106–111.
57. Sonta, S., and Sandberg, A. A. (1977). Chromosomes and causation of human cancer and leukemia. XXVIII. Value of detailed chromosome studies on large numbers of cells in CML. *Am. J. Hematol. 3*:121–126.
58. Kantarjian, H. M., Smith, T. L., McCredie, K. B., Keating, M. J., Walters, R. S., Talpaz, M., Hester, J. P., Bligham, G., Gehan, E., and Freireich, E. J. (1985). Chronic myelogenous leukemia: A multivariate analysis of the associations of patient characteristics and therapy with survival. *Blood 66*: 1326–1335.
59. Sokal, J. E., Gomez, G. A., Baccarani, M., Tura, S., Clarkson, B. D., Cervantes, F., Rozman, C., Carbonell, F., Anger, B., Heimpel, H., Nissen, N. I., and Robertson, J. E. (1988). Prognostic significance of additional cytogenetic abnormalities at diagnosis of Philadelphia chromosome-positive granulocytic leukemia. *Blood 72*:294–298.
60. Sandberg, A. A. (1980). *The Chromosomes in Human Cancer and Leukemia*. Elsevier North Holland, New York, p. 185.
61. Whang-Peng, J., and Knutsen, T. (1982). Chromosomal abnormalities. In *Chronic Granulocytic Leukaemia* (M. T. Shaw, ed.), Praeger, Eastbourne, U.K., p. 49.
62. Swolin, B., Weinfeld, A., Westin, J., Waldenström, J., and Magnusson, B. (1985). Karyotypic evolution in Ph-positive chronic myeloid leukemia in relation to management and disease progression. *Cancer Genet. Cytogenet. 18*:65–79.
63. Singh, S., Wass, J., Vincent, P. C., Young, G. A. R., and Gunz, F. W. (1986). Significance of secondary cytogenetic changes in patients with Ph-positive chronic granulocytic leukemia in the acute phase. *Cancer Genet. Cytogenet. 21*:209–220.
64. Griffin, J. D., Todd, R. F., Ritz, J., Nadler, L. M., Canellos, G. P., Rosenthal, D., Gallivan, M., Beveridge, R. P., Weinstein, H., Karp, D., and Schlossman, S. F. (1983). Differentiation patterns in the blastic phase of chronic myeloid leukemia. *Blood 61*:85–91.
65. Griffin, J. D., Tantravahi, R., Canellos, G. P., Wisch, J. S., Reinherz, E. L., Sherwood, G., Beveridge, B. P., Daley, J. F., Lane, H., and Schlossman, S. (1983). T-cell surface antigens in a patient with blast crisis of chronic myeloid leukemia. *Blood 61*:640–644.

66. Janossy, G., Woodruff, R. K., Pipard, M. J., Prentice, G., Hoffbrand, A. V., Paxton, A., Lister, T. A., Bunch, C., and Greaves, M. F. (1979). Relation of "lymphoid" phenotype and response to chemotherapy incorporating vincristine-prednisolone in the acute phase of Ph^1 positive leukemia. *Cancer 43*:426–434.
67. Jain, K., Arlin, Z., Mertelsmann, R., Gee, T., Kempin, S., Koziner, B., Middleton, A., Jhanwar, S., Chaganti, R., and Clarkson, B. (1983). Philadelphia chromosome and terminal transferase-positive acute leukemia: Similarity of terminal phase of chronic myelogenous leukemia and de novo presentation. *J. Clin. Oncol. 1*:669–676.
68. Herrmann, F., Ludwig, W. D., and Kolecki, P. (1984). Blast crisis in CML showing early T-lymphoblastic transformation. *Br. J. Haematol. 56*:175–176.
69. Berger, R., Bernheim, A., Daniel, M. T., and Flandrin, G. (1983). t(15;17) in a promyelocytic form of chronic myeloid leukemia blastic crisis. *Cancer Genet. Cytogenet. 8*:149–152.
70. Hogge, D. W., Misawa, S., Schiffer, C. A., and Testa, J. R. (1984). Promyelocytic blast crisis in chronic granulocytic leukemia with 15;17 translocation. *Leuk. Res. 8*:1019–1023.
71. Bernstein, R., Bagg, H., Pinto, M., Lewis, D., and Mendelow, B. (1986). Chromosome 3q21 abnormalities associated with hyperactive thrombopoiesis in acute blastic transformation of chronic myeloid leukemia. *Blood 68*: 652–647.
72. O'Malley, F. M., and Garson, O. M. (1985). Chronic granulocytic leukemia: Correlation of blastic transformation type with karyotypic evolution. *Am. J. Hematol. 20*:313–323.
73. Yao, E. (1985). Chromosomal abnormalities in lymphoid crisis of chronic myelogenous leukemia. *Cancer Genet. Cytogenet. 16*:235–243.
74. Parreira, L., Kearney, L., Rassool, F., Babapulle, V. B., Matutes, E., Parreira, A., Tavares de Castro, J., Goldman, J. M., and Catovsky, D. (1986). Correlation between chromosomal abnormalities and blast phenotype in the blast crisis of Ph-positive CGL. *Cancer Genet. Cytogenet. 22*:29–34.
75. Alimena, G., De Cuia, M. R., Diverio, D., Gastaldi, R., and Nanni, M. (1987). The karyotype of blastic crisis. *Cancer Genet. Cytogenet. 26*:39–50.
76. Clark, S. S., Crist, W. M., and Witte, O. N. (1989). Molecular pathogenesis of Ph-positive leukemia. *Annu. Rev. Med. 40*:113–122.
77. Liu, E., Hjelle, B., and Bishop, J. M. (1988). Transforming genes in chronic myelogenous leukemia. *Proc. Natl. Acad. Sci. USA 85*:1952–1956.
78. Rovera, G., Reichard, B. A., Hudson, S., Bittenbender, S., Yamada, M., Tournay, O., and Preisler, H. D. (1989). Point mutations in both transforming and non-transforming codons of the *N-ras* proto-oncogene of Ph+ leukemias. *Oncogene 4*:867–872.
79. McCarthy, D. M., Goldman, J. M., Rasool, F. V., Graham, S. V., and Birnie, G. D. (1984). Genomic alterations involving the c-*myc* proto oncogene during the evolution of a case of chronic granulocytic leukemia. *Lancet 2*:1312.
80. Lübbert, M., Miller, C. W., Crawford, L., and Koeffler, H. P. (1988). p53 in chronic myelogenous leukemia. Study of mechanisms of differential expression. *J. Exp. Med. 167*:873–886.

81. Ahuja, H., Bar-El., M., Advani, S. H., Benchimol, S., and Cline, M. J. (1989). Alterations in the p53 gene and the clonal evolution of the blast crisis of chronic myelocytic leukemia. *Proc. Natl. Acad. Sci. USA 86*:6783–6787.
82. Mashal, R., Shtalrid, M., Talpaz, M., Kantarjian, H., Smith, L., Beran, M., Cork, A., Trujillo, J. Gutterman, J., and Deisseroth, A. (1990). Rearrangement and expression of p53 in the chronic phase and blast crisis of chronic myelogenous leukemia. *Blood 75*:180–189.
83. Finlay, C. A., Hinds, P. W., and Levine, A. J. (1989). The p53 proto-oncogene can act as a suppressor of transformation. *Cell 57*:1083–1093.
84. Nigro, J. M., Baker, S. J., Preisinger, A. C., Jessup, J. M., Hostetter, R., Cleary, K., Bigner, S. H., Davidson, N., Baylin, S., Devilee, P., Glover, T., Collins, F. S., Weston, A., Modali, R., Harris, C. C., and Vogelstein, B. (1989). Mutations in the p53 gene occur in diverse human tumor types. *Nature 342*:705–708.
85. Lane, D. P., and Benchimol, S. (1990). p53: oncogene or anti-oncogene? (Review). *Genes & Development 4*:1–8.
86. Whang-Peng, J., Henderson, R. S., Knutsen, T., Freireich, E. J., and Gart, J. J. (1970). Cytogenetic studies in acute myelocytic leukemia with special emphasis on the occurrence of the Ph^1 chromosome. *Blood 36*:448–457.
87. Clarkson, B., Fried, J., Strife, A., Safai, Y., Ota, K., and Ohkita, T. (1970). Studies of cellular proliferation in human leukemia. III. Behavior of leukemic cells in three adults with acute leukemia given continuous infusions of ^{3}H·Thymidine for 8 or 10 days. *Cancer 25*:1237–1260.
88. Secker-Walker, L. M., Summersgill, B. M., Swansbury, G. J., Lawler, S. D., Chessells, J. M., and Hardisty, R. M. (1976). Philadelphia positive blast crisis masquerading as acute lymphoblastic leukaemia in children. *Lancet 2*:1405.
89. Bloomfield, C. D., Lindquist, L. L., Brunning, R. D., Yunis, J. J., and Coccia, P. F. (1978). The Philadelphia chromosome in acute leukemia. *Virchows Arch [Cell Pathol.] 29*:81–91.
90. Janossey, G., Roberts, M., and Greaves, M. F. (1976). Target cell in chronic myeloid leukemia and its relationship to acute lymphoid leukemia. *Lancet 2*:1059–1061.
91. Peterson, L. C., Bloomfield, C. D., and Brunning, R. D. (1976). Blast crisis as an initial or terminal manifestation of chronic leukemia. *Am. J. Med. 60*: 209–220.
92. Bloomfield, C. D., Peterson, L. C., Yunis, J. J., and Brunning, R. D. (1977). The Philadelphia chromosome (Ph^1) in adults presenting with acute leukemia: A comparison of Ph^{1+} and Ph^{1-} patients. *Br. J. Haematol. 36*: 347–358.
93. Catovsky, E. (1979). Ph^1 positive acute leukaemia and chronic granulocyte leukemia. One or two diseases. *Br. J. Haematol. 42*:493–498.
94. Rowley, J. D. (1980). Ph^1 positive leukemia including chronic myelogenous leukemia. *Clin. Haematol. 9*:55–86.
95. Bloomfield, C. D., Rowley, J. D., Goldman, A. I., Lawler, S. D., Secker Walker, L. M., and Mitelman, F. (1983). Chromosomal abnormalities and their clinical significance in acute lymphoblastic leukemia. Third International Workshop on Chromosomes in Leukemia. *Cancer Res. 43*:868–873.

96. Parakash, O., and Yunis, J. J. (1984). High resolution chromosomes of t(9;22) positive leukemias. *Cancer Genet. Cytogenet. 11*:361–367.
97. Look, A. T. (1985). The emerging genetics of acute lymphoblastic leukemia: Clinical and biologic implications. *Semin. Oncol. 12*:92–104.
98. Clarkson, B., Ellis, S., Little, C., Gee, T., Arlin, Z., Mertelsmann, R., Andreeff, M., Kempin, S., Koziner, B., Chaganti, R., Jhanwar, S., McKenzie, S., Cirrincione, C., and Gaynor, J. (1985). Acute lymphoblastic leukemia in adults. *Semin. Oncol. 12*:160–179.
99. Gaynor, J., Chapman, C., Little, C., McKenzie, S., Miller, W., Andreeff, M., Arlin, Z., Berman, E., Kempin, S., Gee, T., and Clarkson, B. (1988). A cause-specific hazard rate analysis of prognostic factors among 199 adults with acute lymphoblastic leukemia: The Memorial Hospital experience since 1969. *J. Clin. Oncol. 6*:1014–1030.
100. Rorenhuis, S., Smets, L. A., Slater, R. M., Behrendt, H., and Veerman, A. J. P. (1985). Distinguishing the Philadelphia chromosome of acute lymphoblastic leukaemia from its counterpart in chronic myelogenous leukaemia. *N. Engl. J. Med. 313*:51.
101. Erikson, J., Griffin, C. A., Ar-Rushdi, A., Valtieri, M., Hoxie, J., Finan, J., Emanuel, B. S., Rovera, G., Nowell, P. C., and Croce, C. M. (1986). Heterogeneity of chromosome 22 breakpoint in Philadelphia positive (Ph^{1+}), acute lymphocytic leukemia. *Proc. Natl. Acad. Sci. USA 83*:1807.
102. Gale, R. P., and Goldman, J. M. (1988). Workshop Letter: Rapid progress in chronic myelogenous leukemia. *Leukemia 2*:321–324.
103. De Klein, A., Hagemeijer, A., and Bartram, C. R. (1986). *bcr* rearrangement and translocation of the c-*abl* oncogene in Philadelphia positive acute lymphoblastic leukemia. *Blood 68*:1369–1375.
104. Chan, L. C., Karhi, K. K., Heisterkamp, N., Eridani, S., Powles, R., Lawler, S. D., Groffen, J., Foulkes, J. G., Greaves, M. F., and Wiedemann, L. M. (1987). A novel *abl* protein expressed in Philadelphia chromosome positive acute lymphoblastic leukaemia. *Nature 325*:635–637.
105. Hermens, A., Heisterkamp, N., von Lindern, M., von Baal, S., Meijer, D., van der Plas, D., Wiedemann, L. M., Groffen, J., Bootsma, D., and Grosveld, G. (1987). Unique fusion of *bcr* alpha c-*abl* genes in Philadelphia chromosome positive acute lymphoblastic leukemia. *Cell 51*:33–40.
106. Fainstein, E., Marcelle, C., Rosner, A., Canaani, E., Gale, R. P., Dreazen, O., Smith, S. D., and Croce, C. M. (1987). A new fused transcript in Philadelphia positive acute lymphocytic leukaemia. *Nature 330*:386–388.
107. Kurzrock, R., Shtalrid, M., Romero, P., Kloetzer, W. S., Talpaz, M., Trujillo, J. M., Blick, M., Beran, M., and Gutterman, J. U. (1987). A novel c-*abl* protein in Ph^1 positive acute lymphoblastic leukemia. *Nature 235*:631-635.
108. Walker, L. C., Ganesan, T. S., Dhut, S., Gibbons, B., Lister, T. A., Rothbard, J., and Young, B. D. (1987). Novel chimeric protein expressed in Philadelphia positive acute lymphoblastic leukaemia. *Nature 329*:851–853.
109. Rubin, C. M., Carrino, J. J., Dickler, M. N., Leibowitz, D., Smith, S. D., and Westbrook, C. A. (1988). Heterogeneity of genomic fusion of BCR and ABL in Philadelphia chromosome-positive acute lymphoblastic leukemia. *Proc. Natl. Acad. Sci. USA 85*:2795–2799.

110. Secker-Walker, L. M., Cooke, H. M. G., Browett, P. J., Shippey, C. A., Norton, J. D., Coustan-Smith, E., and Hoffbrand, A. V. (1988). Variable Philadelphia breakpoints and potential lineage restriction of *bcr* rearrangement in acute lymphoblastic leukemia. *Blood 72*:784–791.
111. Shannon, K., Chang, S., Morley, B., Smith, S. D., Kawasaki, E., Russo, C., and Kan, Y. W. (1988). Simultaneous expression of CML and all types of mRNA transcripts in Philadelphia (Ph′) chromosome-positive leukemia. *Blood* (Suppl. 1) *72*:225a (abstract 812).
112. Carrino, J. J., Westbrook, C. A., Hooberman, A. L., and Leibowitz, D. (1988). Long-range splicing within the BCR-ABL gene may play a role in acute transformation in BCR-rearranged Ph^1 ALL. *Blood* (Suppl. 1)*72*: 176a (Abstract 613).
113. Hermans, A., Selleri, L., Gow, J., and Grosveld, G. C. (1988). Concise Report: Absence of alternating splicing in *bcr-abl* mRNA in chronic myeloid leukemia cell lines. *Blood 72*:2066–2069.
114. Saiki, R. K., Scharf, S., Faloona, F., Mullis, K. B., Horn, G. T., Erlich, H. A., and Arnheim, N. (1985). Enzymatic amplification of β-globin genomic sequences and restriction site analysis for diagnosis of sickle cell anemia. *Science 230*:1350–1354.
115. Kawasaki, E. S., Clark, S. S., Coyne, M. Y., Smith, S. D., Champlin, R., Witte, O. N., and McCormick, F. P. (1988). Diagnosis of chronic myeloid and acute lymphocytic leukemias by detection of leukemia-specific mRNA sequences amplified in vitro. *Proc. Natl. Acad. Sci. USA 85*:5698–5702.
116. Hermans, A., Gow, J., Selleri, L., von Lindern, M., Hagemeijer, A., Wiedemann, L. M., and Grosveld, G. (1988). *bcr-abl* oncogene activation in Philadelphia chromosome-positive acute lymphoblastic leukemia. *Leukemia 2*: 628–633.
117. Sasaki, M., Kondo, K., and Tomiyasu, T. (1983). Cytogenetic characterization of ten cases of Ph^1-positive acute myelogenous leukemia. *Cancer Genet. Cytogenet. 9*:119–128.
118. Mitelman, F. (1985). *Catalog of Chromosome Aberrations in Cancer*, 2nd ed. Alan R. Liss, New York.
119. Berger, R., Flandrin, G., Bernheim, A., Le Coniat, M., Vecchione, D., Pacot, A., Derré, J., Valensi, S., Sigaux, F., and Ochoa-Noguera, M. E. (1987). Cytogenetic studies on 519 consecituve de novo nonlymphocytic leukemias. *Cancer Genet. Cytogenet. 29*:9–21.
120. Dow, L. W., Martin, P., Moohr, J., Greenberg, M., Macdougall, L. G., Najfeld, V., and Fialkow, P. J. (1985). Evidence for clonal development of childhood acute lymphocytic leukemia. *Blood 66*:902–907.
121. Janosey, G., Woodruff, R. K., Paxton, A., Greaves, M. F., Capellaro, D., Kirk, B., Innes, E. M., Eden, O. B., Lewis, C., Catovsky, D., and Hoffbrand, A. V. (1978). Membrane marker and cells separation studies in Ph^1-positive leukemia. *Blood 51*:861–877.
122. Parkin, J. L., McKenna, R. W., and Brunning, R. D. (1982). Philadelphia chromosome-positive blastic leukemia: Ultrastructural and ultracytochemical evidence of basophil and mast cell differentiation. *Br. J. Haematol. 52*: 663–677.

123. Nowell, P. C., Wilmoth, D., Hoxie, J., and Lyss, A. P. (1984). Ph^1-positive acute leukemia with a 17q;21q translocation. *Cancer Genet. Cytogenet.* *12*:51–55.
124. Tachibana, M., Raimondi, S. C., Lauer, S. J., Sartain, P., and Dow, L. W. (1987). Evidence for a multipotential stem cell disease in some childhood Philadelphia chromosome-positive acute lymphoblastic leukemia. *Blood* *70*:1458–1461.
125. Turhan, A. G., Eaves, C. J., Kalousek, D. K., Eaves, A. C., and Humphries, R. K. (1988). Concise Report: Molecular analysis of clonality and *bcr* rearrangements in Philadelphia chromosome-positive acute lymphoblastic leukemia. *Blood 71*:1495–1498.
126. Kurzrock, R., Shtalrid, M., Talpaz, M., Kloetzer, W. S., and Gutterman, J. U. (1987). Expression of c-*abl* in Philadelphia-positive acute myelogenous leukemia. *Blood 70*:1584–1588.
127. Chen, S. J., Flandrin, G., Daniel, M.-T., Valensi, F., Baranger, L., Grausz, D., Bernheim, A., Chen, Z., Sigaux, F., and Berger, R. (1988). Philadelphia-positive acute leukemia: Lineage promiscuity and inconsistently rearranged breakpoint cluster region. *Leukemia 2*:261–273.
128. Hirsch-Ginsberg, C., Childs, C., Chang, K-S., Beran, M., Cork, A., Reuben, J., Freireich, E. J., Chang, L. C. M., Bollum, F. J., Trujillo, J., and Stass, S. A. (1988). Phenotypic and molecular heterogeneity in Philadelphia chromosome-positive acute leukemia. *Blood 71*:186–195.
129. Marks, S. M., Baltimore, D., and McCaffrey, R. (1978). Terminal transferase as a predictor of initial responsiveness to vincristine and prednisone in blastic chronic myelogenous leukemia. *N. Engl. J. Med. 298*:812–814.
130. Sokal, J. E., Baccarani, M., Russo, D., and Tura, S. (1988). Staging and prognosis in chronic myelogenous leukemia. *Semin. Hematol. 25*:49–61.
131. Mastrangelo, R., Zuelzer, W. W., and Thompson, R. I. (1967). The significance of the Ph′ chromosome in acute myeloblastic leukemia: Serial cytogenetic studies in a critical case. *Pediatrics 40*:834–841.
132. Arlin, Z., Chaganti, R. S. K., Gee, T., and Clarkson, B. (1977). Complete remission of the blastic phase of chronic myelogenous leukemia (blCML). *Proc. Am. Assoc. Cancer Res 18*:196 (abstract 782).
133. Berman, E., Raymond, G., Gee, T. S., Kempin, S., Andreeff, M., Gulati, S., Kolitz, J., Gabrilove, J., Young, C. Y., and Clarkson, B. D. (1988). Results of a randomized trial comparing idarubicin (IDR)/cytosine arabinoside (ARA-C) with daunorubicin (DNR)/ARA-C in adult patients (PTS) with untreated acute nonlymphocytic leukemia (ANLL). *Blood* (Suppl. 1) *72*: 189a (abstract 667).
134. Kitano, K., Sato, Y., Suda, T., and Miura, Y. (1988). Difference of cell lineage expression of haematopoietic progenitor cells in Philadelphia-positive acute lymphoblastic leukaemia and chronic myelogenous leukemia. Br. J. Haematol. 70:21–26.
135. Selleri, L., von Lindern, M., Hermans, A., Meijer, D., Torelli, G., and Grosveld, G. (1990). Chronic myeloid leukemia may be associated with several *bcr-abl* transcripts including the acute lymphoid leukemia-type 7kb transcript. *Blood 75*:1146–1153.

136. Koeffler, H. P., and Golde, D. W. (1981). Chronic myelogenous leukemia: New concepts. *N. Engl. J. Med. 304*:1201–1269.
137. Wintrobe, M. M., Lee, G. R., Boggs, D. R., Bithell, T. C., Foerster, J., Athens, J. W., and Lukens, J. N. (eds.) (1981). Chronic myeloid leukemia. In *Clinical Hematology*, 8th ed. Lea & Febiger, Chap. 64, Philadelphia, pp. 1565–1595.
138. Champlin, R., Gale, R. P., Foon, K. A., and Gold, D. W. (1986). Chronic leukemias: Oncogenes, chromosomes and advances in therapy. *Ann. Intern. Med. 104*:671–688.
139. Clarkson, B. (1988). The chronic leukemias. In *Cecil Textbook of Medicine*, 18th ed. (J. B. Wyngaarden and L. H. Smith, Jr., eds.). W. B. Saunders, eds.). Philadelphia, pp. 988–1001.
140. Moore, M. A. S., Ekert, H., Fitzgerald, M. D., and Carmichael, A. 91974). Evidence for the clonal origin of chronic myeloid leukemia from a sex chromosome mosaic: Clinical, cytogenetic and marrow culture studies. *Blood 43*:15–22.
141. Kamada, N., and Uchino, H. (1978). Chronologic sequence in appearance of clinical and laboratory findings characteristic of chronic myelocytic leukemia. *Blood 51*:843–850.
142. Esposito, L., Di Tullio, M. T., Rea, F., and Citarella, O. (1972). La leucemia mieloide cronica nella infanzia. Rilievi clinico ematologici e citogenetici. *Pediatria 80*:229–246.
143. Saffhill, R., Dexter, T. M., Muldal, S., Testa, N. G., Morris Jones, P., and Joseph, A. (1976). Short Communication: Terminal deoxynucleotidyl transferase in a case of Ph^1 positive infant chronic myelogenous leukaemia. *Br. J. Cancer 33*:664–667.
144. Sokal, J. E. (1980). Significance of Ph^1-negative marrow cells in Ph^1-positive chronic granulocytic leukemia. *Blood 56*:1072–1076.
145. Kantarjian, H. M., Vellekoop, L., and McCredie, K. B. (1985). Intensive combination chemotherapy (ROAP 10) and splenectomy in the management of chronic myelogenous leukemia. *J. Clin. Oncol. 3*:192–200.
146. Canellos, G. P., and Whang-Peng, J. (1972). Philadelphia-chromosome-positive preleukemic state. *Lancet 2*:1227–1228.
147. Clarkson, B. R., Strife, A., Fried, J., and Gulati, S. (1986). Cytokinetics and cancer treatment. In *Proceedings of the General Motors Cancer Research Foundation* (Monograph) (E. J. Freireich and E. Frei, eds.). J. B. Lippincott, Philadelphia, pp. 131–182.
148. Stryckmans, P., Cronkite, E. P., Fache, F., Fliedner, T. M., and Ramos, J. (1966). Deoxyribonucleic acid synthesis time or erythropoietic and granulopoietic cells in human beings. *Nature 211*:717–720.
149. Vincent, P. C., Cronkite, E. P., Greenberg, M. L., Kirsten, C., Schiffer, L. M., and Stryckmans, P. A. (1969). Leukocyte kinetics in chronic myeloid leukemia. I. DNA synthesis time in blood and marrow myelocytes. *Blood 33*:843–850.
150. Killmann, S. A., Cronkite, E. P., Robertson, J. S., Fliedner, T. M., and Bond, V. P. (1963). Estimation of phases of the life cycle of leukemic cells

from labeling in human beings in vivo with tritiated thymidine. *Lab. Invest. 12*:671–684.

151. Schmid, J. R., Kiely, J. M., Tauxe, W. N., and Owen, C. A. Jr. (1966). Cell proliferation in leukemia during relapse and remission. I. DNA and RNA synthesis of leukemic cells in the bone marrow in vitro. *Acta Haematol. (Basel) 36*:313–322.
152. Rondanelli, G. E., Magliulo, E., Giraldi, A., and Cario, E. P. (1967). The chronology of the mitotic cycle of human granulocytopoietic cells. *Blood 30*:557–568.
153. Killman, S. A. (1968). Acute leukemia. The kinetics of leukemic blast cells in man. An analytical review. *Semin. Hematol. 1*:38–102.
154. Cronkite, E. P., and Vincent, P. C. (1970). Granulocytopoiesis. In *Hemopoietic Cellular Proliferation* (F. Stohlman, ed.), Grune & Stratton, New York, pp. 211–228.
155. Ogawa, M., Fried, J., Sakai, Y., Strife, A., and Clarkson, B. D. (1970). Studies of cellular proliferation in human leukemia. VI. The proliferative activity, generation time, and emergence time of neutrophilic granulocytes in chronic granulocytic leukemia. *Cancer 25*:1031–1049.
156. Baccarini, M., and Killmann, S. A. (1972). Cytokinetic studies in chronic myeloid leukaemia: Evidence for early presence of abnormal myeloblasts. *Scand. J. Haematol. 9*:283–292.
157. Moore, M. A. S., Williams, N., and Metcalf, D. (1973). In vitro colony formation by normal and leukemic human hematopoietic cells: Characterization of the colony forming cells. *JNCI 50*:603–623.
158. Vincent, P. C. (1974). Cell kinetics of the leukemias. In *Leukemia*, 3rd ed. (F. Gunz and A. G. Bailie, eds.). Grune & Stratton, New York, pp. 189–221.
159. Clarkson, B., and Rubinow, S. I. (1977). Growth kinetics in human leukemia. In *Growth Kinetics and Biochemical Regulations of Normal and Malignant Cells* (B. Drewinko and R. Humphrey, eds.). Williams & Wilkins, Baltimore, pp. 591–628.
160. Greenberg, M. L., Chanana, A. D., Cronkite, E. P., Giacomelli, G., Rai, K. R., Schiffer, L. M., Stryckmans, P. A., and Vincent, P. C. (1972). The generation time of human leukemic myeloblasts. *Lab. Invest. 26*:245–252.
161. Stryckmans, P., Debusscher, L., and Socquet, M. (1976). Regulation of bone marrow myeloblast proliferation in chronic myeloid leukemia. *Cancer Res. 36*:3034–3038.
162. Stryckmans, P., Debusscher, L., Peltzer, T., and Socquet, M. (1975). Variations of the proliferative activity of leukemic myeloblasts related to the stage of the disease. In *Unclassifiable Leukemias* (M. Bessis and G. Brecher, eds.). Springer-Verlag, New York, p. 239.
163. Stryckmans, P. A., Debusscher, L., and Collard, E. (1977). Cell kinetics in chronic granulocytic leukaemia (CGL). *Clin. Haematol. 6*:21–40.
164. Todo, A., Strife, A., Fried, J., and Clarkson, B. D. (1971). Proliferative kinetics of human hematopoietic cells during different growth phases in vitro. *Cancer Res. 31*:1330–1340.

165. Yen, A., Fried, J., and Clarkson, B. (1977). Alternative modes of population growth inhibition in a human lymphoid cell line growing in suspension. *Exp. Cell Res. 107*:325–341.
166. Clarkson, B. D., Ota, K., O'Connor, A., and Karnofsky, D. A. (1963). Production of granulocytes by the spleen in chronic granulocytic leukemia (CGL) (abstract). *J. Clin. Invest. 42*:924.
167. Mauer, A. M., and Jarrold, T. (1963). Granulocyte kinetic studies in patients with proliferative disorders of the bone marrow. *Blood 22*:125–138.
168. Athens, J. W., Raab, S. O., Haab, O. P., Boggs, D. R., Ashenbrucker, H., Cartwright, G. E., and Wintrobe, M. M. (1965). Leukokinetic studies. X. Blood granulocyte kinetics in chronic myelocytic leukemia. *J. Clin. Invest. 44*:765–777.
169. Chervenick, P. A., and Boggs, D. R. (1968). Granulocyte kinetics in chronic myelocytic leukemia. *Ser. Haematol. 1*:24–37.
170. Galbraith, P. R. (1966). Studies on the longevity, sequestration and release of the leukocytes in chronic myelogenous leukemia. *J. Assoc. Med. Can. 95*:511–521.
171. Galbraith, P. R., and Abu-Zahra, H. T. (1972). Granulopoiesis in chronic granulocytic leukaemia. *Br. J. Haematol. 22*:135–143.
172. Perry, S., Moxley, J. H., III, Weiss, G. H., and Zelen, M. (1966). Studies of leukocyte kinetics by liquid scintillation counting in normal individuals and in patients with chronic myelocytic leukemia. *J. Clin. Invest. 45*:1388–1399.
173. Duvall, C. P., and Perry, S. (1968). The use of 51-chromium in the study of leukocyte kinetics in chronic myelocytic leukemia. *J. Lab. Clin. Med. 71*:614–628.
174. Cronkite, E. P. (1968). Normal human granulocytopoiesis. In *The Proliferation and Spread of Neoplastic Cells*. Williams & Wilkins, Baltimore, pp. 281–294.
175. Uchida, T. (1971). Leukokinetic studies in peripheral blood. II. Granulocyte kinetics in chronic myelocytic leukemia. *Acta Haematol. Jpn. 34*:186–204.
176. Scott, J. L., McMillan, R., Davidson, J. G., and Marino, J. V. (1971). Leukocyte labeling with ^{51}chromium. II. Leukocyte kinetics in chronic myeloid leukemia. *Blood 38*:162–173.
177. Moxley, J. H., Perry, S., Weiss, G. H., and Zelen, M. (1965). Return of leucocytes to the bone marrow in chronic myelocytic leukaemia. *Nature 208*:1281–1282.
178. Whang, J., Frei, E., III, Tjio, J. H., Carbone, P. P., and Brecher, G. (1963). The distribution of the Philadelphia chromosome in patients with chronic myelogenous leukemia. *Blood 22*:664–673.
179. Stryckmans, P. A. (1974). Current concepts in chronic myelogenous leukemia. *Semin. Hematol. 11*:101–127.
180. Morley, A. A. (1966). A neutrophil cycle in healthy individuals. *Lancet 2*:1220–1222.

181. Morley, A. A., King-Smith, E. A., and Stohlman, F., Jr. (1970). The oscillatory nature of hemopoiesis. In *Hemopoietic Cellular Proliferation* (F. Stohlman, Jr., ed.). Grune & Stratton, New York, pp. 3–14.
182. King-Smith, E. A., and Morley, A. (1970). Computer simulation of granulopoiesis-normal and impaired granulopoiesis. *Blood 36*:254–262.
183. Morley, A., and Stohlman, F., Jr. (1970). Cyclophosphamide-induced cyclical neutropenia. An animal model of a human periodic disease. *N. Engl. J. Med. 282*:643–646.
184. Morley, A. A., Carew, J. P., and Baikie, A. G. (1967). Familial cyclical neutropenia. *Br. J. Haematol. 13*:719–738.
185. Jakubowski, A. A., Souza, L., Kelly, F., Fain, K., Budman, D., Clarkson, B., Bonilla, M. A., Moore, M. A. S., and Gabrilove, J. (1989). Effects of human granulocyte colony-stimulating factor in a patient with idiopathic neutropenia. *N. Engl. J. Med. 320*:38–42.
186. Morley, A. A., Baikie, A. G., and Galton, D. A. G. (1967). Cyclic leucocytosis as evidence for retention of normal homoeostatic control in chronic granulocytic leukaemia. *Lancet 2*:1320–1323.
187. Shadduck, R. K., Winkelstein, A., and Nunna, N. G. (1972). Cyclic leukemic cell production in CML. *Cancer 29*:399–401.
188. Vodopick, H., Rupp, E. M., Edwards, C. L., Goswitz, F. A., and Beauchamp, J. J. (1972). Spontaneous cyclic leukocytosis and thrombocytosis in chronic granulocytic leukemia. *N. Engl. J. Med. 286*:284–290.
189. Gatti, R. A., Robinson, W. A., Deinard, A. S., Nesbit, M., McCullough, J. J., Ballow, M., and Good, R. A. (1973). Cyclic leukocytosis in chronic myelogenous leukemia: New perspectives on pathogenesis and therapy. *Blood 41*:771–782.
190. Kennedy, B. J. (1970). Cyclic leukocyte oscillations in chronic myelogenous leukemia during hydroxyurea therapy. *Blood 35*:751–760.
191. Shadduck, R. K., and Nankin, H. R. (1971). Cellular origin of granulocyte colonies in chronic myeloid leukaemia. *Lancet 2*:1097–1098.
192. Chervenick, P. A., Ellis, L. D., Pan, S. F., and Lawson, A. L. (1971). Human leukemic cells: In vitro growth of colonies containing the Philadelphia (Ph′) chromosome. *Science 174*:1134–1136.
193. Moore, M. A. S., and Metcalf, D. (1973). Cytogenetic analysis of human acute and chronic myeloid leukemic cells cloned in agar culture. *Int. J. Cancer 11*:143–152.
194. Singer, J. K., Fialkow, P. J., Steinman, L., Najfeld, V., Stein, S. J., and Robinson, W. A. (1979). Chronic myelocytic leukemia (CML): Failure to detect residual normal committed stem cells in vitro. *Blood 53*:264–268.
195. Coulombel, L., Kalousek, D. K., Eaves, C. J., Gupta, C. M., and Eaves, A. C. (1983). Long-term marrow culture reveals chromosomally normal hematopoietic progenitor cells in patients with Philadelphia chromosome-positive chronic myelogenous leukemia. *N. Engl. J. Med. 308*:1493–1498.
196. Dube, I. D., Gupta, C. M., Kalousek, D. K., and Eaves, A. C. (1984). Cytogenetic studies of early myeloid progenitor compartments in Ph^1-positive chronic myeloid leukemia (CML): Persistence of Ph^1-negative committed

progenitors that are suppressed from differentiating in vivo. *Br. J. Haematol. 56*:633–644.

197. Fitzgerald, P. H., Adams, A., and Gunz, F. W. (1963). Chronic granulocytic leukemia and the Philadelphia chromosome. *Blood 21*:183–196.
198. Maurice, P. A., Alberto, P., Ferrier, S., and Freund, M. (1971). Leucémie myélocytaire chronique: "Guérison" apparente depuis plus de 9 ans, consécutive à une hypoplasie médullaire thérapeutique. *Schweiz. Med. Wochenschr. 101*:1781–1782.
199. Canellos, G. P., Whang-Peng, J., Schnipper, L., and Brown, C. H., III (1972). Prolonged cytogenetic and hematologic remission of blastic transformation in chronic granulocytic leukemia. *Cancer 30*:288–293.
200. Finney, R., McDonald, G. A., Baikie, A. G., and Douglas, A. S. (1972). Chronic granulocytic leukemia with Ph′ negative cells in the bone marrow and a ten year remission after busulfan therapy. *Br. J. Haematol. 23*:283–288.
201. Brandt, L., Mitelman, F., Panani, A., and Lenner, H. C. (1976). Extremely long duration of chronic myeloid leukaemia with Ph′ negative and Ph′ positive bone marrow cells. *Scand. J. Haematol. 16*:321–325.
202. Golde, D. W., Bersch, N. L., and Sparkes, R. S. (1976). Chromosomal mosaicism associated with prolonged remission to chronic myelogenous leukemia. *Cancer 37*:1849–1852.
203. Monfardini, S., Gee, T., Fried, J., and Clarkson, B. (1973). Survival in chronic myelogenous leukemia: Influence of treatment and extent of disease at diagnosis. *Cancer 31*:492–501.
204. Minot, J. B., Buckman, T. E., and Isaacs, R. (1924). Chronic myelogenous leukemia: Age, incidence, duration and benefit derived from irradiations. *JAMA 82*:1489–1494.
205. Dowling, M., Jr., Haghbin, T., Gee, T., Wakonig-Vaartaga, T., and Clarkson, B. (1973). Attempt to induce true remissions in chronic myelocytic leukemia (CML). *Cancer Chemother. Rep.* Part 1, *57*:102 (abstract 50).
206. Dowling, M. D., Hopfan, S., Knapper, W. H., Vaartaja, T., Gee, T., Haghbin, M., and Clarkson, B. D. (1974). Attempt to induce true remission in chronic myelogenous leukemia (CML). *Proc. Am. Soc. Clin. Oncol. 15*:189 (abstract 822).
207. Clarkson, B. (1985). Editorial: Chronic myelogenous leukemia: Is aggressive treatment indicated? *J. Clin. Oncol. 3*:135–139.
208. Arlin, Z., Kempin, S., Gee, T., Goto, T., Chaganti, R., Koenigsberg, E., and Clarkson, B. (1979). Induction of true remission in Philadelphia chromosome positive ($Ph^{1}+$) chronic myelogenous leukemia (CML) with the L15 protocol. *Proc. Am. Soc. Clin. Oncol. 20*:339 (abstract C-198).
209. Arlin, Z. A., Mertelsmann, R., Berman, E., Gee, T., Kurland, E., Chaganti, R. S. K., Jhanwar, S. C., Moore, M. A. S., and Clarkson, B. D. (1985). 13-*cis*-retinoic acid does not increase the true remission rate and the duration of true remission (induced by cytotoxic chemotherapy) in patients with chronic phase chronic myelogenous leukemia. *J. Clin. Oncol. 3*:473–476.
210. Fuscaldo, K. E., Brodsky, I., Kahn, S. B., and Conroy, J. F. (1977). CGL:

Effect of sequential chromosomal analysis, splenectomy, and intensive chemotherapy of survival (abstract). *Proc. Am. Soc. Clin. Oncol. 18*:294.
211. Smalley, R. V., Vogel, J., Huguley, C. M., and Miller, D. (1977). Chronic granulocytic leukemia: Cytogenetic conversion of the bone marrow with cycle-specific chemotherapy. *Blood 50*:107–113.
212. Sharp, J. C., Wayne, A. W., and Crofts, M. (1979). Karyotypic conversion in Ph^1-positive chronic myeloid leukaemia with combination chemotherapy. *Lancet 1*:1370–1372.
213. Hester, J. P., Waddell, C. C., and Coltman, C. A. (1984). Response of chronic myelogenous leukemia patients to COAP-splenectomy. A Southwest Oncology Group Study. *Cancer 54*:1977–1982.
214. Sokal, J. E., Leong, S. S., and Gomez, G. A. (1987). Preferential inhibition by cytarabine of CFU-GM from patients with chronic granulocyte leukemia. *Cancer 59*:197–202.
215. Sokal, J. E., Gockerman, J. P., and Bigner, S. H. (1987). Evidence for a selective antileukemic effect of cytosine arabinoside in chronic granulocytic leukemia. *Blood* (Suppl. 1) *70*:237a (abstract 805).
216. Kolitz, J., Kempin, S., Berman, E., Jhanwar, S., Arlin, Z., Gee, T., and Clarkson, B. (1989, in press). Cytogenetic response in chronic myelogenous leukemia with high-dose hydroxyurea. *Proc. Am. Assoc. Clin. Oncol. 8*: 208.
217. Talpaz, M., Kantarjian, H. M., McCredie, K. B., Keating, M. J., Trujillo, J., and Gutterman, J. (1987). Clinical investigation of human alpha interferon in chronic myelogenous leukemia. *Blood 69*:1280–1288.
218. Niederle, N., Kloke, O., and Osieka, K. R. (1987). Interferon alfa-2b in the treatment of chronic myelogenous leukemia. *Semin. Oncol. 14*:29–35.
219. Bergsagel, D. E., Haas, R. H., and Messner, H. A. (1986). Interferon alfa-2b in the treatment of chronic granulocytic leukemia. *Semin. Oncol. 13*:29–34.
220. McGlave, P., Mamus, S., Vilen, B., and Dewald, G. (1987). Effect of recombinant gamma interferon on chronic myelogenous leukemia bone marrow progenitors. *Exp. Hematol. 5*:331–335.
221. Kurzrock, R., Talpaz, M., Kantarjian, H., Walters, R., Saks, S., Trujillo, J. M., and Gutterman, J. U. (1987). Therapy of chronic myelogenous leukemia with recombinant interferon-gamma. *Blood 70*:943–947.
222. Kantarjian, H. M., Talpaz, M., Keating, M. J., Walters, R. S., McCredie, K. B., Freireich, E. J., and Gutterman, J. U. (1988). Combined nodality therapy with intensive chemotherapy (DOAP) followed by alpha interferon (IFN-A) maintenance in chronic myelogenous leukemia (CML). *Proc. Am. Assoc. Cancer Res. 29*:210 (abstract 836).
223. Speck, B., Bortin, M. M., and Champlin, R. (1984). Occasional survey. Allogeneic bone marrow transplantation for chronic myelogenous leukemia. *Lancet 2*:665–668.
224. Thomas, E. D., Clift, R. A., and Fefer, A. (1986). Marrow transplantation for the treatment of chronic myelogenous leukemia. *Ann. Intern. Med. 104*:155–163.

225. Goldman, J. M., Apperley, J. F., and Jones, L. (1986). Bone marrow transplantation for patients with chronic myelogenous leukemia. *N. Engl. J. Med. 314*:202–207.
226. Champlin, R. E., Goldman, J. M., and Gale, R. P. (1988). Bone marrow transplantation in chronic myelogenous leukemia. *Semin. Hematol. 25*: 74–80.
227. Martin, P. J., Clift, R. A., Fisher, L. D., Buckner, C. D., Hansen, J. A., Appelbaum, F. R., Doney, K. D. S., Sullivan, K. M., Witherspoon, R. P., Stort, R., and Thomas, E. D. (1988). HLA-identical marrow transplantation during accelerated-phase chronic myelogenous leukemia: Analysis of survival and remission duration. *Blood 72*:1978–1984.
228. Fefer, A., Cheever, M. A., and Greenberg, P. D. (1982). Treatment of chronic granulocytic leukemia with chemoradiotherapy and transplantation of marrow from identical twins. *N. Engl. J. Med. 306*:63–68.
229. Jones, L., Thein, S. L., and Jeffreys, A. J. (1987). Identical twin marrow transplantation for five patients with chronic myeloid leukemia: Role of DNA finger printing to confirm monozygosity in three cases. *Eur. J. Haematol. 39*:144–147.
230. Vogler, W. R., Winton, E. F., and James, S. (1983). Autologous marrow transplantation after karyotypic conversion to normal in blastic phase of chronic myelogenous leukemia. *Am. J. Med. 75*:1080–1084.
231. Phillips, G. L., and Herzig, G. P. (1984). Intensive chemotherapy, total body irradiation and autologous marrow transplantation for chronic granulocytic leukemia blast phase. *J. Clin. Oncol. 2*:379–384.
232. Haines, M. E., Goldman, J. M., and Worsley, A. M. (1984). Chemotherapy and autografting for chronic granulocytic leukemia in transformation: Probable prolongation of survival for some patients. *Br. J. Haematol. 58*: 711–721.
233. Bretagne, S., Vidaud, M., Kuentz, M., Cordonnier, C., Henni, T., Vinci, G., Goossens, M., and Vernant, J. P. (1987). Concise Report: Mixed blood chimerism in T cell depleted bone marrow transplant recipients: Evaluation using DNA polymorphisms. *Blood 70*:1692–1695.
234. Arthur, C. K., Apperley, J. F., Guo, A. P., Rassool, F., Gao, L. M., and Goldman, J. M. (1988). Cytogenetic events after bone marrow transplantation for chronic myeloid leukemia in chronic phase. *Blood 71*:1179–1186.
235. Offit, K., Burns, J. P., Cunningham, I., Jhanwar, S. C., Black, P., Kernan, N. A., O'Reilly, R. J., and Chaganti, R. S. K. (1990). Cytogenetic analysis of chimerism and leukemia relapse in chronic myelogenous leukemia patients after T cell-depleted bone marrow transplantation. *Blood 75*: 1346-1355.
236. Cooperative Study Group on Chromosomes in Transplanted Patients (A. Zaccaria, G. Rosti, and N. Testoni, Study Organizers) (1988). Cytogenetic follow-up of 100 patients submitted to bone marrow transplantation for Philadelphia chromosome-positive chronic myeloid leukemia. *Eur. J. Haematol. 40*:50–57.

237. Walker, H., Singer, C. R. J., and Patterson, J. (1986). The significance of host hemopoietic cells detected by cytogenetic analysis of bone marrow from recipients of bone marrow transplants. *Br. J. Haematol. 62*:385–391.
238. Marmont, A., Frassoni, F., Bacigalupo, A., and Podesta, M. (1984). Recurrence of Ph positive leukemia in donor cells after bone marrow transplantation for chronic granulocytic leukemia. *N. Engl. J. Med. 310*:903–906.
239. Smith, J. L., Heerema, N. A., and Provisor, A. J. (1985). Leukaemic transformation of engrafted bone marrow cells. *Br. J. Haematol. 60*:415–422.
240. Zaccaria, A., Rosti, G., and Testoni, N. (1987). Chromosome studies in patients with acute nonlymphocytic or acute lymphocytic leukemia submitted to bone marrow transplantation. Results of an European Cooperative Study. *Cancer Genet. Cytogenet. 26*:51–58.
241. Botstein, D., White, R., Skolnick, M., and Davis, R. L. (1980). Construction of a genetic linkage map in man using restriction fragment polymorphisms. *Am. J. Hum. Genet. 32*:314–331.
242. Donis-Keller, H., Barker, D., Knowlton, R., Schumm, J., and Braman, J. (1986). Application of RFLP probes to genetic mapping and clinical diagnosis in humans. In *DNA Probes. Applications in Genetic and Infectious Disease and Cancer*. Current Communications in Molecular Biology, Vol. 73. Cold Spring Harbor Laboratory, Cold Spring Harbor, New York, p. 81.
243. Chaganti, R. S. K., Allen, G. J., Doucette, L. A., and Long, L. I. (1988). The role of molecular genetics in diagnostic and prognostic evaluation of cancer and leukemia. In *Nucleid Acid Probes in Diagnosis of Human Genetic Diseases*. Alan R. Liss, New York, pp. 55–81.
244. Sparkes, R. S. (1981). Cytogenetic analysis of human bone marrow transplantation. *Cancer Genet. Cytogenet. 4*:345–352.
245. Dobrovic, A., Trainor, K. J., and Morley, A. A. (1988). Concise Report: Detection of the molecular abnormality in chronic myeloid leukemia by use of the polymerase chain reaction. *Blood 72*:2063–2065.
246. Lee, M., Chang, K. S., Freireich, E., Talpzaz, M., Kantargian, H., Trujillo, J., and Stass, S. (1988). Detection of minimal residual chimeric BCR/ABL transcripts by modified polymerase chain reaction (PCR). *Blood* (Suppl. 1) *72*:282a (abstract 982).
247. Joshi, C. S., Gollerkeri, M. P., and Gangal, S. G. (1975). Evaluation of general immune responsiveness in cancer patients. *Indian J. Med. Res. 63*:315–322.
248. Gangal, S. G., Damle, N. K., Khare, A. G., and Advani, S. H. (1979). Cellular sensitization in chronic myeloid leukaemia patients to leukaemic blast antigens. *Br. J. Cancer 40*:391–396.
249. Damle, N. K., Khare, A. G., Advani, S. H., and Gangal, S. G. (1979). Leukemia associated in vitro cell mediated immunity in chronic myeloid leukemia patients in remission. *Indian J. Exp. Biol. 17*:1376–1379.
250. Khare, A. G., Advani, S. H., and Gangal, S. G. (1981). In vitro cellular immune reactivity of soluble antigens obtained from cultured leukemic cells in chronic myeloid leukemia. *Indian J. Exp. Biol. 19*:524–527.

251. Karande, A. A., Advani, S. H., and Gangal, S. G. (1983). In vitro induction of chronic myeloid leukemia associated immune reactivity in normal human lymphocytes by xenogeneic immune RNA. *Neoplasma 30*:403–409.
252. Todd, M. B., Waldron, J. A., Jennings, T. A., Rome, L. S., Markowitz, S. D., Holford, T. R., Gardner, J. P., Wolak, J. P., and Malech, H. L. (1987). Loss of myeloid differentiation antigens precedes blastic transformation in chronic myelogenous leukemia. *Blood 70*:122–131.
253. Mod, A., Carpentier, N., Fust, G., Lambert, P. H., Miescher, H., and Hollan, S. R. (1980). Serial measurement of circulating immune complexes in the sera of patients with leukemia. *J. Clin. Lab. Immunol. 4*:15.
254. Saranath, D., Advani, S., and Gangal, S. (1983). Circulating immune complexes in chronic myeloid leukemia patients at various stages of the disease. *Leuk. Res. 7*:771–777.
255. Chhajlani, V., Zingde, S., Adwani, S., and Gothoskar, B. (1983). Circulating immune complexes in chronic myeloid leukemia: Turbidimetric measurement and two-dimensional electrophoretic analysis. *Leuk. Res. 7*:565–573.
256. Khare, A. G., Advani, S. H., and Gangal, S. G. (1981). In vitro generation of lymphocytotoxicity to autochthonous leukaemic cells in chronic myeloid leukaemia. *Br. J. Cancer 43*:13–18.
257. Somasundaram, R., Advani, S. H., and Gangal, S. G. (1983). Concanavalin A induced suppressor cell activity and autorosette forming cells in chronic myeloid leukemia patients. *Br. J. Cancer 48*:783–790.
258. Dabholkar, M., Advani, S., Tatake, R., and Gangal, S. (1986). Natural and antibody-dependent cellular cytotoxicity in chronic myeloid leukemia patients in remission. *Leuk. Res. 10*:203–209.
259. Ramchandar, K., Baker, M. A., and Taub, R. N. (1975). Antibody responses to leukemia-associated antigens during immunotherapy of chronic myelocytic leukemia. *Blood 46*:845–854.
260. Sokal, J. E., Aungst, C. W., Synderman, M., and Gomez, G. (1977). Immunotherapy of chronic myeloid leukemia: Effect of different vaccination schedule. *Clin. Haematol. 6*:129–139.
261. Advani, S. H., Gulwani, B., Ghogale, S. G., Shetye, M. R., and Gangal, S. G. (1985). Effect of administration of BCG, levamisole and irradiated leukemic cells on immune status and remission status in chronic myelogenous leukemia. *Oncology 42*:275–281.
262. Fujimiya, Y., Bakke, A., Cheng Chang, W., Linker-Israeli, M., Udis, B., Horwitz, D., and Pattengale, P. K. (1986). Natural killer-cell immunodeficiency in patients with chronic myelogenous leukemia. I. Analysis of the defect using the monoclonal antibodies HNK-1 (LEU-7) and B73.1. *Int. J. Cancer 37*:639–649.
263. Lotzova, E., Savary, C. A., and Herberman, R. B. (1987). Induction of NK cell activity against fresh human leukemia in culture with interleukin 2. *J. Immunol. 138*:2718–2727.
264. Fujimiya, Y., Weng-Cheng, C., Bakke, A., Horwitz, D., and Pattengale, P. K. (1987). Natural killer (NK) cell immunodeficiency in patients with

chronic myelogenous leukemia. II. Successful cloning and amplification of natural killer cells. *Cancer Immunol. Immunother. 24*:213–220.

265. Keever, C. A., Hauch, M., Barnett, L., Bordignon, C., Cunningham, I., Castro-Malaspina, H., and O'Reilly, R. J. (1988). The potentiation of NK cell mediated anti-leukemia activity following BMT. *Blood* (Suppo. 1) *72*: 393a (abstract 1483).
266. Verfaillie, C., Miller, W., Kay, N., and McGlave, P. (1988). ALAK cells in chronic myelogenous leukemia: A population of nonmalignant cells with potent antitumor activity. *Blood* (Suppl. 1) *72*:233a (abstract 841).
267. Brunet, J. F., Dosseto, M., Denizot, F., Martei, M-G., Clark, W. R., Haggi, T. M., Ferrier, P., Nabholz, M., Schmitt-Verhulst, A-M., Lucianni, M-F., and Goldstein, P. (1986). The inducible cytotoxic T-lymphocyte-associated gene transcript CTLA-1: Sequence and gene localization to mouse chromosome 14. *Nature 322*:269–271.
268. Boulet, A. M., Erwin, C. R., and Rutter, W. J. (1986). Cell-specific enhancers in the rat exocrine pancreas. *Proc. Natl. Acad. Sci. USA 83*:3599-3603.
269. Benfy, P. N., Yin, F. H., and Leder, P. (1987). Cloning of mast cell protease, RMCPII. *J. Biol. chem. 262*:5377–5384.
270. Bleackley, R. C., Lobe, C. G., Duggan, B., Ehrman, N., Fregeau, C., Meier, M., Letellier, M., Havele, C., Shaw, J., and Paetkau, V. (1988). The isolation and characterization of a family of serine protease genes expressed in activated cytotoxic T-lymphocytes. *Immunol. Rev. 103*:5–19.
271. Darte, J. M., Dacie, J. V., and McSorley, J. G. A. (1952). Pelger-like leucocytes in chronic myeloid leukemia. *Acta Haematol. (Basel) 12*:117.
272. Langenhuijsen, M. M. A. C. (1984). Neutrophils with ring-shaped nuclei in myeloproliferative disease. *Br. J. Haematol. 58*:277.
273. Matsuo, T., Tomonoaga, M., Kuriyama, K., Yao, E., Nonaka, H., Jinnai, I., Jubashi, T., Yoshida, Y., Amenomori, T., and Ichimaru, M. (1986). Prognostic significance of the morphological dysplastic changes in chronic myelogenouss leukemia. *Leuk. Res. 10*:331–337.
274. Lingg, G., Schmalzl, F., Breton-Gorius, J., Tabilio, A., Schaefer, H. E., Geissler, D., Schweiger, M., and Kirchmair, W. (1985). Megakaryoblastic micromegakaryocytic crisis in chronic myeloid leukemia. *Blut 51*:275-285.
275. Doan, C. A., and Reinhart, H. L. (1941). The basophil granulocyte, basophilocytosis and myeloid leukemia basophil and "mixed granule" types: an experimental clinical and pathological study with the report of a new syndrome. *Am. J. Clin. Pathol. 11*:1–33.
276. Mlynek, M.-L., and Leder, L.-D. (1986). Lineage infidelity in chronic myeloid leukemia: Demonstration and significance of hybridoid leukocytes. *Virchows Arch [Cell Pathol.] 51*:107–114.
277. Asano, M., and Kawahara, I. (1968). Ultramicroscopic characteristics of bone marrow cells in human chronic myeloid leukemia. *Med. J. Shinshu Univ. 13*:109–126.

278. Anderson, D. R. (1966). Ultrastructure of normal and leukemic leukocytes in human peripheral blood. *J. Ultrastruct. Res.* (Suppl.) *9*:1–42.
279. Vainchenker, W., Guichard, J., and Deschamps, J. F. (1982). Megakaryocyte cultures in the chronic phase and in the blast crisis of chronic myeloid leukaemia: Studies on the differentiation of the megakaryocyte progenitors and on the maturation of megakaryocytes in vitro. *Br. J. Haematol.* *51*:131–146.
280. Kuto, F., Nagaoka, T., Watanabe, Y., Hayashi, M., Horasawa, Y., Hirasawa, Y., and Tokuhiro, H. (1984). Chronic myelocytic leukemia: Ultrastuctural histopathology of bone marrow from patients in the chronic phase. *Ultrastruct. Pathol.* *6*:307–317.
281. Nagaoka, T., Kuto, F., Watanabe, Y., Fujino, Y., Hirasawa, Y., and Tokuhiro, H. (1986). Bone marrow sinus and cell egress in human leukaemia: A morphometric study of core biopsies using wide-field electron microscopy. *Br. J. Haematol.* *63*:737–747.
282. Tavassoli, M. (1979). The marrow-blood barrier. *Br. J. Haematol.* *41*:297–302.
283. Perillie, P. E., and Finch, S. C. (1961). Alkaline phosphatase activity of exudative leukocytes in acute leukemia. *Blood* *18*:572–580.
284. Pedersen, B., and Hayhoe, F. G. J. (1971). Relation between phagocytic activity and alkaline phosphatase content of neutrophils in chronic myeloid leukaemia. *Br. J. Haematol.* *21*:257–260.
285. Matsuo, T. (1986). In vitro modulation of alkaline phosphatase activity in neutrophils from patients with chronic myelogenous leukemia by monocyte-derived activity. *Blood* *67*:492–497.
286. Broxmeyer, H. D., Mendelsohn, N., and Moore, M. A. S. (1977). Annormal granulocyte feedback regulation of colony forming and colony stimulating activity-producing cells from patients with chronic myelogenous leukemia. *Leuk. Res.* *1*:3–12.
287. Odeberg, H., Olofsson, T., and Olsson, I. (1975). Granulocyte function in chronic granulocytic leukaemia. I. Bacterial and metabolic capabilities during phagocytosis in isolated granulocytes. *Br. J. Haematol.* *29*:427–441.
288. Baker, M. A., Taub, R. N., and Kanani, A. (1985). Increased activity of a specific sialyltransferase in chronic myelogenous leukemia. *Blood* *66*: 1068–1071.
289. Nojiri, H., Takaku, F., and Ohta, M. (1985). Changes in glycosphingolipid composition during differentiation of human leukemic granulocytes in chronic myelogenous leukemia compared with in vitro granulocytic differentiation of human promyelocytic leukemia cell line HL-60. *Cancer Res.* *45*:6100–6106.
290. Oloffson, T., Odeberg, H., and Olsson, I. (1976). Granulocyte function in chronic granulocytic leukemia. II. Bactericidal capacity, phagocytic rate, oxygen consumption, and granule protein composition in isolated granulocytes. *Blood* *48*:581–593.

291. Evans, W. H., Bednarek, J. M., and Alvarez, V. L. (1985). Direct analysis of differentiation proteins in normal and leukemic human granulocytosis by high-performance liquid chromatography. *JNCI 75*:227–235.
292. Bednarek, J. M., Knight, R. D., Taylor, G., and Evans, W. H. (1988). Progressive loss of phenotypic proteins in mature granulocytes before the onset of blast crisis in human chronic myelogenous leukemia. *JNCI 80*:251–257.
293. Zingde, S. M., Mungikar, A. M., Chhajlani, V., Advani, S. H., and Gothoskar, B. P. (1985). Plasma membranes from normal and chronic myeloid leukemic granulocytes: Isolation and two-dimensional polyacrylamide gel electrophoretic analysis. *Cancer Biochem. Biophys. 7*:333–342.
294. Brandt, L. (1965). Adhesiveness to glass and phagocytic activity of neutrophilic leukocytes in myeloproliferative diseases. *Scand. J. Haematol. 2*:126–136.
295. Penny, R., Galton, D. A. G., Scott, J. T., and Eisen, V. (1966). Studies on neutrophile function. I. Physiological and pharmacological aspects. *Br. J. Haematol. 12*:623–632.
296. Taub, R. N., Baker, M. A., and Madyastha, K. R. (1980). Masking of neutrophil surface lectin-binding sites in chronic myelogenous leukemia (CML). *Blood 55*:294–298.
297. Perillie, P. E., and Finch, S. (1960). The local exudative cellular response in leukemia. *J. Clin. Invest. 39*:1353–1357.
298. Senn, H. J., Rhomberg, W. U., and Jungi, W. F. (1971). Störung der leukozytären Abwehrfunktion als paraneoplastiches Syndrom bei Hämoblastosen. *Schweiz Med. Wochenschr. 101*:466–470.
299. Banerjee, T. K., Senn, H., and Holland, J. F. (1972). Comparative studies on localized leukocyte mobilization in patients with chronic myelocytic leukemia. *Cancer 29*:637–644.
300. Penny, R., and Galton, D. A. G. (1966). Studies on neutrophil function. II. Pathological aspects. *Br. J. Haematol. 12*:633–645.
301. Rosner, F., Valmont, J., Kozinn, P. J., and Caroline, L. (1970). Leukocyte function in patients with leukemia. *Cancer 25*:835–842.
302. Goldman, J. M., and Catovsky, D. (1972). Function of the phagocytic leukocytes in leukemia. *Br. J. Haematol.* (Suppl.) *23*:223–230.
303. Whittaker, J. A., Khurshid, M., and Hughes, H. R. (1974). Neutrophil function in chronic granulocytic leukemia before and after busulphan treatment. *Br. J. Haematol. 28*:541–549.
304. Brandt, L. (1976). Studies on the phagocytic activity of neutrophilic leukocytes with special reference to chronic myeloproliferative conditions and megaloblastic anemia. *Scand. J. Haematol.* (Suppl. 2), p. 41.
305. El-Maallem, H., and Fletcher, J. (1979). Defective hydrogen-peroxide production in chronic granulocytic neutrophils. *Br. J. Haematol. 41*:49–55.
306. Corberand, J., Laharraque, P., Deharrard, B., Nyuyen, F., and Pris, J. (1980). Phagocytosis in myeloproliferative disorders. *Am. J. Clin. Pathol. 74*:301–305.

307. Anklesaria, P. N., Advani, S. H., and Bhisey, A. N. (1985). Studies on granulocyte functions in patients with chronic myeloid leukemia. *Tumori 71*: 317–324.
308. Anklesaria, P. N., Advani, S. H., and Bhisey, A. N. (1985). Defective chemotaxis and adherence in granulocytes from chronic myeloid leukemia (CML) patients. *Leuk. Res. 9*:641–648.
309. Bhisey, A. N., Rao, S. G. A., Advani, S. H., and Ray, V. (1980). Agglutination of granulocytes from chronic myeloid leukaemia by concanavalin A. *Acta Haematol. (Basel) 63*:211–216.
310. Zingde, S. M., Anklesaria, P. N., Advani, S. H., Bhisey, A. N., and Gothoskar, B. P. (1987). Differential endocytosis of fluorescein isothiocyanate-concanavalin A by normal and chronic myeloid leukemic granulocytes. *Blut 55*:81–88.
311. Zingde, S. M., Advani, S. H., and Gothoskar, B. P. (1987). Plasma membrane proteins from human normal and chronic myeloid leukemic granulocytes: Identification and partial characterization of the concanavalin A-binding and detergent resistant proteins. *Blut 55*:89–100.
312. Anklesaria, P. N., and Bhisey, A. N. (1985). Studies on electrophoretic mobility of leucocytes from chronic myeloid leukemia patients. *Indian J. Exp. Biol. 23*:609–612.
313. Pedersen, B. (1982). Annotation: Functional and biochemical phenotype in relation to cellular age of differentiated neutrophils in chronic myeloid leukaemia. *Br. J. Haematol. 51*:339–344.
314. Taub, R. N., Hindenburg, A. A., and Baker, M. A. (1985). Brief Communication: Regeneration of membrane sialic acid after neuraminidase treatment of leukemic granulocytes. *Leuk. Res. 19*:507–510.
315. Baker, M. A., Kanani, A., Hindeburg, A., and Taub, R. N. (1986). Changes in the granulocyte membrane following chemotherapy for chronic myelogenous leukemia. *Br. J. Haematol. 62*:431–438.
316. Kanani, A., May, C., Sutherland, D. R., Hindenburg, A., Taub, R. N., Mills, G. B., and Baker, M. A. (1987). Altered rise of FMLP stimulated free cystolic calcium [Ca^{2+}] in CML granulocytes. *Blood* (Suppl. 1) *70*:90a (abstract 214).
317. Yuo, A., Kitagawa, S., Okabe, T., Urabe, A., Komatsu, Y., Itoh, S., and Takaku, F. (1987). Recombinant human granulocyte colony-stimulating factor repairs the abnormalities of neutrophils in patients with myelodysplastic syndromes and chronic myelogenous leukemia. *Blood 70*:404–411.
318. Tornyos, K. (1967). Phagocytic activity of cells of the inflammatory exudate in human leukemia. *Cancer Res. 27*:1756–1760.
319. Jungi, W. F., Meuret, G., and Senn, H. J. (1974). Granulozyten-clearance und granulozytenkinetik bei myeloproliferativen syndromen. *Schweiz. Med. Wochenschr. 104*:133–135.
320. Oseas, R., Yang, H-H., Baehner, R. L., and Boxer, L. A. (1981). Lactoferrin: A promoter of polymorphonuclear leukocyte adhesiveness. *Blood 57*: 939–945.

321. Strife, A., Lambek, C., Wisniewski, D., Arlin, Z., Thaler, H., and Clarkson, B. (1983). Proliferative potential of subpopulations of granulocyte-macrophage progenitor cells in normal subjects and chronic myelogenous leukemia patients. *Blood 62*:389–397.
322. Strife, A., Lambek, C., Wisniewski, D., Wachter, M., Gulati, S. C., and Clarkson, B. D. (1988). Discordant maturation as the primary biological defect in chronic myelogenous leukemia. *Cancer Res. 48*:1035–1041.
323. Spector, W. S. (1956). *Handbook of Biological Data*. W. B. Saunders, Philadelphia.
324. Strife, A., Lambek, C., Wisniewski, D., Gulati, S., Gasson, J. C., Golde, D. W., Welte, K., Gabrilove, J. L., and Clarkson, B. (1987). Activities of four purified growth factors on highly enriched human hematopoietic progenitor cells. *Blood 69*:1508–1523.
325. Upadhyaya, G., Deisseroth, A. B., and Emerson, S. G. (1988). CML progenitor cells are deficient in cell surface LFA-3: Modulation by alpha-interferon in vitro and in vivo. *Blood* (Suppl. 1) *72*:231a (abstract 836).
326. Wisniewski, D., Strife, A., Atzpodien, J., and Clarkson, B. D. (1987). Effects of recombinant human tumor necrosis factor on highly enriched hematopoietic progenitor cell populations from normal human bone marrow and peripheral blood and bone marrow from patients with chronic myeloid leukemia. *Cancer Res. 47*:4788–4794.
327. Miller, A. M., Gross, M. A., and Yunis, A. A. (1978). Alterations in the properties of the myeloid colony forming unit in chronic myelocytic leukemia. *Blood 52*:290a.
328. Oloffson, T., and Nilsson, B. (1986). Defective recloning capacity of granulocyte-macrophage colony-forming cells in chronic myeloid leukaemia. *Scand. J. Haematol. 36*:168–175.
329. Aglietta, M., Piacibello, W., and Stacchini, A. (1985). In-vitro effect of retinoic acid on normal and chronic myeloid leukemia granulopoiesis. *Leuk. Res. 9*:879–883.
330. Douer, D., and Koeffler, H. P. (1982). Retinoic acid enhances colony stimulating factor induced clonal growth of normal human myeloid progenitor cells in vitro. *Exp. Cell Res. 138*:193–198.
331. Koeppler, H., and Robinson, W. A. (1982). The effect of 6 retinoids on granulocyte colony formation in human bone marrow cultures (abstract). *Blut 45*:214.
332. Moore, M. A. S., Mertelsmann, R., and Pelus, L. M. (1981). Phenotypic evaluation of chronic myeloid leukemia. *Blood Cells 7*:217–236.
333. Nadkarni, K. S., Joshi, K. S., Kothari, V. C., Advani, S. H., and Rao, S. G. A. (1984). Effect of retinoic acid on bone-marrow committed stem cells (CFU-c) from chronic myeloid leukemia patients. *Tumori 70*:503–505.
334. Breitman, T. R. (1981). Induction of terminal differentiation of HL-60 and fresh leukemic cells by retinoic acid. In *Growth of Cells in Hormonally Defined Media* (September 1-4, 1981). Cold Spring Harbor Laboratory, Cold Spring Harbor, New York, p. 101.

335. Lepine, J., and Messner, H. A. (1983). Pluripotent hemopoietic progenitors (CFU-GEMM) in chronic myelogenous leukemia. *Int. J. Cell Cloning 1*:230–239.
336. Klerk, D. K., Henry, E. A., and Eaves, A. C. (1985). Two classes of primitive pluripotent hematopoietic progenitor cells: Separation by adherence. *J. Cell. Physiol. 125*:127–134.
337. Eaves, A. C., Cashman, J. D., and Gaboury, L. A. (1986). Unregulated proliferation of primitive chronic myeloid leukemia progenitors in the presence ofnormal marrow adherent cells. *Proc. Natl. Acad. Sci. USA 83*:5306-5310.
338. Cashman, J., Eaves, A. C., and Eaves, C. J. (1985). Concise Report: Regulated proliferation of primitive hematopoietic progenitor cells in long-term human marrow cultures. *Blood 66*:1002–1005.
339. Eaves, A. C., and Eaves, C. J. (1979). Abnormalities in the erythroid progenitor compartments in patients with chronic myelogenous leukemia (CML). *Exp. Hematol. 7*:65–75.
340. Singer, J. W., Adamson, J. W., and Arlin, Z. A. (1981). Chronic myelogenous leukemia: In vitro studies of hematopoietic regulation in a patient undergoing intensive chemotherapy. *J. Clin. Invest. 67*:1593–1598.
341. Golde, D. W., Byers, L. A., and Cline, M. J. (1974). Chronic myelogenous leukemia cell growth and maturation in liquid culture. *Cancer Res. 34*: 419–423.
342. Metcalf, D., Moore, M. A. S., Sheriden, J. W., and Spitzer, G. (1974). Responsiveness of human granulocyte leukemic cells to colony stimulating factor. *Blood 43*:847–859.
343. Metcalf, D. (1984). The clonal culture in vitro of human leukaemic cells. In *The Leukaemic Cell* (D. Catovsky, ed.). Churchill Livingstone, Edinburgh, pp. 220–252.
344. Cannistra, S. A., Herrmann, F., Davis, R., Nichols, K., and Griffin, J. D. (1986). Relationship between HLA-DR expression by normal myeloid progenitor cells and inhibition of colony growth by prostaglandin E. *J. Clin. Invest. 77*:13–20.
345. Richman, C. M., and Johnson, G. D. (1987). Granulocyte/macrophage progenitor cells from peripheral blood and bone marrow differ in their response to prostaglandin E_1. *Blood 70*:1792–1796.
346. Dowding, C. R., Gordon, M. Y., and Goldman, J. M. (1988). Increased DR antigen expression by committed hemopoietic progenitor cells but not primitive progenitor cells in chronic myeloid leukemia. *Exp. Hematol. 16*: 171–175.
347. Broxmeyer, H. D., Smithyman, A., Eger, R. R., Meyers, P. A., and De Souza, M. (1978). Identification of lactoferrin as the granulocyte derived inhibitor of colony stimulating activity production. *J. Exp. Med. 148*:1052.
348. Pelus, L. M., Broxmeyer, H. E., Clarkson, B. D., and Moore, M. A. S. (1980). Abnormal responsiveness of granulocyte macrophage committed colony forming cells from patients with chronic myeloid leukemia to inhibition by prostaglandin E1. *Cancer Res. 40*:2512.

349. Rao, S. G. A., Nadkarni, K. S., Joshi, K., Kothari, V., and Advani, S. H. (1984). Normal responsiveness of granulocyte macrophage committed stem cells from patients with chronic myeloid leukemia to proliferation inhibition by prostaglandin E 1. *Indian J. Exp. Biol. 22*:340–342.
350. Ross, R. J., Glomset, J., Kariya, B., and Harker, L. (1974). A platelet dependent serum factor that stimulates the proliferation of arterial smooth muscle cells in vitro. *Proc. Natl. Acad. Sci. USA 71*:1207–1210.
351. Heldin, C. H., Wasteson, A., and Westermark, B. (1977). Partial purification and characterization of platelet factors stimulating the multiplication of normal glial cells. *Exp. Cell. Res. 109*:429–437.
352. Siefert, R. S., Schwarz, S. M., and Bowen-Pope, D. F. (1984). Developmentally regulated production of platelet-derived growth factor like molecules. *Nature 311*:669–671.
353. Anzano, M. A., Roberts, A. B., Smith, J. M., Sporn, M. B., and De Larco, J. E. (1983). Sarcoma growth factor from conditioned medium of virally transformed cells is composed of both type alpha and type beta transforming growth factors. *Proc. Natl. Acad. Sci. USA 80*:6264–6268.
354. Kaplan, P. L., Anderson, M., and Ozanne, B. (1982). Transforming growth factor(s) production enables cells to grow in the absence of serum: An autocrine system. *Proc. Natl. Acad. Sci. USA 79*:485–489.
355. Child, B. J., Proper, J. A., Tucker, R. F., and Moses, H. L. (1982). Serum contains platelet derived transforming growth factor PTGF. *Proc. Natl. Acad. Sci. USA 79*:5312–5316.
356. Waterfield, M., Scrace, G., Whittle, N., Stroobant, P., Johnsson, A., Wasteson, A., Westermark, B., Heldin, C. H., Huang, J. S., and Deuel, T. F. (1983). Platelet derived growth factor is structurally related to the putative transforming protein $p28^{sis}$ of simian sarcoma virus. *Nature 30*:35.
357. Doolittle, R. F., Hunkapiller, M. W., Hood, L. E., Devare, S. G., Robbins, K. C., Aaronson, S. A., and Antoniades, H. N. (1983). Simian sarcoma virus, v-*sis* is derived from the gene (or genes) encoding a platelet derived growth factor. *Science 221*:275.
358. Kaplan, P. L., and Ozanne, B. (1983). Cellular responsiveness to growth factor co-relates with the cell's ability to express the transformed phenotype. *Cell 33*:937–938.
359. Roberts, A. B., Frolik, C. A., Anzano, M. A., and Sporn, M. B. (1983). Transforming growth factors from neoplastic and non-neoplastic tissues. *Fed. Proc. 42*:2621–2626.
360. Daniak, N., Davies, G., Kalmanti, M., Lawler, J., and Kulkarni, V. (1983). Platelet derived growth factor promotes proliferation of erythropoietic progenitor cells in vitro. *J. Clin. Invest. 71*:1206.
361. Michalevicz, R., Francis, G. E., Price, G. M., and Hoffbrand, A. V. (1985). The role of platelet derived growth factor on human pluripotent progenitor (CFU-GEMM) growth in vitro. *Leuk. Res. 9*:399.
362. Delwiche, F., Raines, E., Powell, J., Ross, R., and Adamson, J. (1985). Platelet derived growth factor enhances in vitro erythropoiesis via stimulation of mesenchymal cells. *J. Clin. Invest. 76*:137.

363. Michalevicz, R., Katz, F. E., Stoobant, P., Tindle, R. W., and Hoffbrand, A. V. (1986). Platelet derived growth factor stimulates growth of highly purified multipotent haemopoietic progenitors. *Br. J. Haematol. 63*:591.
364. Katz, F. E., Michalevicz, R., Lam, G., Hoffbrand, A. V., and Goldman, J. M. (1987). Effect of platelet-derived growth factor on enriched populations of haemopoietic progenitors from patients with chronic myeloid leukaemia. *Leuk. Res. 2*:339–344.
365. Francis, G. E., Michalevicz, R., and Wickramasinghe, R. G. (1983). Chronic myeloid leukemia and the Philadelphia translocation: Do the *sis* oncogene and platelet derived growth factor provide the ink? *Leuk. Res. 7*:817.
366. Canaani, E., Gale, R. P., Steiner-Saltz, D., Berrebi, A., Aghai, E., and Januszewicz, E. (1984). Altered transcription of an oncogene in chronic myeloid leukaemia. *Lancet 1*:593–595.
367. Romero, P., Blick, M., Talpaz, M., Murphy, E., Hester, J., and Gutterman, J. (1986). Concise Report: c-*sis* and c-*abl* expression in chronic myelogenous leukemia and other hematologic malignancies. *Blood 67*:839–841.
368. Kothari, V., Advani, S. H., and Rao, S. G. A. (1986). Growth factors in chronic myelogenous leukemia. *Cancer Lett. 32*:285–292.
369. Lopez, A. R., Lyding, J., and Deisseroth, A. (1988). Transforming growth factor beta expression in human leukemia cell lines. *Blood* (Suppl. 1) *72*: 124a (abstract 405).
370. Frassoni, F., Repetto, M., Piaggio, G., Podesta, M., and Marmont, A. M. (1987). Human serum-dependent survival of GM-CFCs in vitro from patients with chronic granulocytic leukemia. *Leuk. Res. 11*:3–6.
371. Rao, S. G. A., Kothari, V., Nadkarni, K., Ahuja, H., and Advani, S. (1987). Evidence for the presence in sera from chronic myelogenous leukemia patients of an activity that enhances the number of normal bone marrow-derived granulocyte/monocyte committed stem cell colonies. *Nouv. Rev. Fr. Hematol. 29*:231–236.
372. Stohlman, F., Jr. (1970). Kinetics of erythropoiesis. In *Regulation of Hematopoiesis*, Vol. 1, *Red Cell Production* (A. S. Gordon, ed.). Appleton-Century-Crofts, New York, Chap. 14, pp. 317–326.
373. Wintrobe, M. M., Lee, G. R., Boggs, D. R., Bithell, T. C., Foerster, J., Athens, J. W., and Lukens, J. N. (eds.) (1981). Erythropoiesis. In *Clinical Hematology*, 8th ed. Lea & Febiger, Philadelphia, Chap. 64, pp. 108–135.
374. Jandl, J. H. (1987). Physiology of red cells. In *Blood—Textbook of Hematology*, 1st ed. Little, Brown, Boston, Chap. 2, pp. 49–109.
375. Tooze, J., and Davies, H. G. (1963). The occurrence and possible significance of haemoglobin in the chromosomal regions of mature erythrocyte nuclei of the newt *Triturus cristatus cristatus. J. Cell Biol. 16*:501–511.
376. Orlic, D. (1970). Ultrastructural analysis of erythropoiesis. In *Regulation of Hematopoiesis*, Vol. 1, *Red Cell Production* (A. S. Gordon, ed.), Appleton-Century-Crofts, New York, Chap. 12, pp. 271–296.
377. Kay, H. E. M. (1965). How many cell generations? *Lancet 2*:418–419.

378. Lajtha, L. G., and Oliver, R. (1960). Cell production and its regulation. In *Ciba Foundation Symposium on Haemopoiesis*. (G. E. M. Wolstenholme and M. Cameron, eds.). London, pp. 289–324.
379. Hellman, S., Botnick, L. E., and Hannon, E. C. (1978). Proliferative capacity of murine hematopoietic stem cells. *Proc. Natl. Acad. Sci. USA 75*: 490–494.
380. Lemischka, I. R., Raulet, D. H., and Mulligan, R. C. (1986). Developmental potential and dynamic behavior of hematopoietic stem cells. *Cell 45*:917–927.
381. Mintz, B., Anthony, K., and Litwin, S. (1984). Monoclonal derivation of mouse myeloid and lymphoid lineages from totipotent hematopoietic stem cells experimentally engrafted in fetal hosts. *Proc. Natl. Acad. Sci. USA 81*:7835–7839.
382. Buescher, E. S., Alling, D. W., and Fallin, J. I. (1986). Use of an X-linked human neutrophil marker to estimate timing of lyonization and site of the dividing stem cell pool. *J. Clin. Invest. 76*:1581–1584.
383. Harrison, D. E., Lerner, C., and Hoppe, P. C. (1987). Large numbers of primitive stem cells are active simultaneously in aggregated embryo chimeric mice. *Blood 69*:773–777.
384. Micklem, H. S., Ansell, J. D., and Wayman, J. E. (1983). The clonal organization of hematopoiesis in the mouse. *Prog. Immunol. 5*:633–644.
385. Abramson, S., Miller, R. G., and Phillips, R. A. (1977). The identification in adult bone marrow of pluripotent and restricted stem cells of the myeloid and lymphoid systems. *J. Exp. Med. 145*:1567–1579.
386. Leary, A. G., and Ogawa, M. (1987). Concise Report: Blast cell colony assay for umbilical cord blood and adult bone marrow progenitors. *Blood 69*:953–956.
387. Nakahata, T., Gross, A.J., and Ogawa, M. (1982). A stochastic model of self-renewal and commitment to differentiation of the primitive hemopoietic stem cells in culture. *J. Cell. Physiol. 113*:455–458.
388. Grossman, Z. (1986). Open Forum: The stem cell concept revisited: Self-renewal capacity is a dynamic property of hemopoietic cells. *Leuk. Res. 10*:937–950.
389. Grossman, Z. (1986). A new approach to the evolution of the blastic crisis from chronic myelocytic leukemia: Dynamic interplay of cellular alterations and a changing microenvironment. *EMBO J. 5*:671–677.
390. Boggs, D. R., Boggs, S. S., and Saxe, D. F. (1982). Hematopoietic stem cells with high proliferative potential: Assay of their concentration in marrow by the frequency and duration of cure of W/W^v mice. *J. Clin. Invest. 70*:242–253.
391. Stiff, P. J., and Koester, A. R. (1987). In vitro chemoseparation of leukemic cells from murine bone marrow using VP16-213: Importance of stem cell assays. *Exp. Hematol. 15*:263–268.
392. Jones, R. J., Sharkis, S. J., Celano, P., Colvin, O. M., Rowley, S. D., and Sensenbrenner, L. L. (1987). Progenitor cell assays predict hematopoietic reconstitution after syngeneic transplantation in mice. *Blood 70*:1186–1192.

393. Spangrude, G. J., Heimfeld, S., and Weissman, I. L. (1988). Research Articles: Purification and characterization of mouse hematopoietic stem cells. *Science 241*:58–62.

394. Nakano, T., Waki, N., Asai, H., and Kitamura, Y. (1989). Effect of 5-fluorouracil on "primitive" hematopoietic stem cells that reconstitute whole erythropoiesis of genetically anemic W/W^v mice. *Blood 73*:425–430.

395. Dick, J. E., Magli, M. C., and Huszar, D. (1985). Introduction of a selectable gene into primitive stem cells capable of long-term reconstitution of the hemopoietic system of W/W^v mice. *Cell 42*:71–79.

396. Keller, G., Paige, C., and Gilboa, E. (1985). Articles: Expression of a foreign gene in myeloid and lymphoid cells derived from multipotent hematopoietic precursors. *Nature 318*:149–154.

397. Tanaka, M., Levy, J., Terada, M., Breslow, R., Rifkind, R. A., and Marks, P. A. (1975). Induction of erythroid differentiation in murine virus infected erythroleukemia cells by highly polar compounds. *Proc. Natl. Acad. Sci. USA 72*:1003–1006.

398. Yen, A., and Chiao, J. W. (1983). Control of cell differentiation during proliferation. I. Monocytic differentiation of HL-60 promyelocytes. *Exp. Cell Res. 146*:87–93.

399. Boyd, A. W., and Metcalf, D. (1984). Induction of differentiation in HL60 leukaemic cells: A cell cycle dependent all-or-none event. *Leuk. Res. 8*: 27–43.

400. Pastan, I., and Willingham, M. (1978). Cellular transformation and the morphologic phenotype of transformed cells. *Nature 274*:645–650.

401. Tooze, J. (ed.) (1984). *The Molecular Biology of Tumor Viruses*, 2nd ed. Cold Spring Harbor Laboratory, Cold Spring Harbor, New York.

402. Clarkson, B. D. (In press, 1989). Leukemias and lymphomas: Clinical overview: Molecular assays for chromosomal rearrangements. Proceedings of the September 7-11, 1988, Cold Spring Harbor Meeting on Cancer Cells, The Molecular Diagnostics of Human Cancer (M. E. Furth and M. F. Greaves, eds.) Published as Clincal Perspective: Molecular assays for chromosomal rearrangements: Leukemias and lymphomas. *Cancer Cells* 7:1-7.

403. Vogelstein, B., Fearon, E. R., Hamilton, S. R., Kern, S. E., Preisinger, A. C., Leppert, M., Nakamura, Y., White, R., Smits, A. M. M., and Bos, J. L. (1988). Genetic alterations during colorectal-tumor development. *N. Engl. J. Med. 319*:525–532.

404. Rosenberg, N., and Baltimore, D. (1980). Abelson virus. In *Viral Oncology* (G. Klein, ed.). Raven Press, New York, pp. 187–203.

405. Whitlock, C. A., Ziegler, S. F., and Witte, O. N. (1983). Progression of the transformed phenotype in clonal lines of Abelson virus-infected lymphocytes. *Mol. Cell. Biol. 3*:596–604.

406. Waneck, G. L., and Rosenberg, N. (1981). Abelson leukemia viruses induces lymphoid and erythroid colonies in infected fetal cell cultures. *Cell 26*:79–89.

407. Cook, W. D., Metcalf, D., Nicola, N. A., Burgess, A. W., and Walker, F. (1985). Malignant transformation of a growth factor-dependent myeloid cell line by Abelson virus without evidence of an autocrine mechanism. *Cell 41*:685–693.
408. Pierce, J. H., DiFiore, P. P., Aaronson, S. A., Potter, M., Humphrey, J., Scott, A., and Ihle, J. N. (1985). Neoplastic transformation of mast cells by Abelson MuLV: Abrogation of IL-3 dependence by nonautocrine mechanism. *Cell 41*:677–683.
409. Witte, O. N. (1986). Functions of the *abl* oncogene. *Cancer Surv. 5*:183–197.
410. Lockwood, A. H., Murphy, S. K., Borislow, S., Lazarus, A., and Pendergast, M. (1987). Cellular signal transduction and the reversal of malignancy. *J. Cell. Biochem. 33*:237–255.
411. Hunter, T., and Cooper, J. A. (1986). Viral oncogenes and tyrosine phosphorylation. In *The Enzymes*, Vol. XVII, Control by Phosphorylation, Part A (P. D. Boyer and E. G. Krebs, eds.). Academic Press, New York, pp. 192–237.
412. Hunter, T. (1989). Protein-tyrosine phosphatases: The other side of the coin. (Minireview). *Cell 58*:1013-1016.
413. Nishizuka, Y. (1986). Studies and perspectives of protein kinase C. *Science 233*:305–312.
414. Watson, J. D., Wigler, M., and Feramisco, J. (eds.) (1988). Abstracts From The Molecular Biology of Signal Transduction—Cold Spring Harbor Symposium: May 25-June 1, 1988. Cold Spring Harbor Laboratory, Cold Spring Harbor, New York.
415. Varmus, H. (1987). Oncogenes and transcriptional control. *Science 238*: 1337–1339.
416. Weinberg, R. A. (1989). Oncogenes and the Molecular Origins of Cancer. Cold Spring Harbor Laboratory Press, Cold Spring Harbor, New York.
417. Bentley, D. L., and Groudine, M. (1988). Sequence requirements for premature termination of transcription in the human c-*myc* gene. *Cell 53*: 245–256.
418. Draetta, G., and Beach, D. (1988). Activation of *cdc*2 protein kinase during mitosis in human cells. Cell cycle-dependent phosphorylation and subunit rearrangement. *Cell 54*:17–26.
419. Weinstein, I. B. (1987). Growth factors, oncogenes, and multistage carcinogenesis. *J. Cell. Biochem. 33*:213–224.
420. Hunter, T. (1987). Review: A thousand and one protein kinases. *Cell 50*: 823–829.
421. Anderson, N. L., Gemmell, M. A., Coussens, P. M., Murao, S.-I., and Huberman, E. (1985). Specific protein phosphorylation in human promyelocytic HL-60 leukemia cells susceptible or resistant to induction of cell differentiation by phorbol-12-myristate-13-acetate. *Cancer Res. 45*:4955.
422. Hunter, T., and Cooper, J. A. (1985). Protein-tyrosine kinases. *Annu. Rev. Biochem. 54*:897–930.

423. Hayakawa, T., Suzuki, K., Suzuki, S., Andrews, P. C., and Babior, B. M. (1986). A possible role for protein phosphorylation in the activation of the respiratory burst in human neutrophils. *J. Biol. Chem. 261*:9109.
424. Golden, A., Nemeth, S. P., and Brugge, J. S. (1986). Blood platelets express high levels of the pp60$^{c\text{-}src}$-specific tyrosine kinast activity. *Proc. Natl. Acad. Sci. USA 83*:852.
425. Barnekow, A., and Gessler, M. (1986). Activation of the pp60$^{c\text{-}src}$ kinase during differentiation of monomyelocytic cells in vitro. *EMBO J. 5*: 701.
426. Kraft, A. S., and Berkow, R. L. (1987). Tyrosine kinase and phosphotyrosine phosphatase activity in human promyelocytic leukemia cells and human polymorphonuclear leukocytes. *Blood 70*:356–362.
427. Naldini, L., Stacchini, A., Cirillo, D. M., Aglietta, M., Gavosto, F., and Comoglio, P. M. (1986). Phosphotyrosine antibodies identify the p210$^{c\text{-}abl}$ tyrosine kinase and proteins phosphorylated on tyrosine in human chronic myelogenous leukemia cells. *Mol. Cell. Biol. 6*:1803–1811.
428. Evans, J. P. M., Wickremasinghe, R. G., and Hoffbrand, A. V. (1987). Letter: Tyrosine protein kinase substrates in Philadelphia-positive human chronic granulocytic leukemia derived cell lines (K562 and BV173): Detection by using an immunoblotting technique. *Leukemia 1*:524–525.
429. Evans, J. P., Wickremasinghe, R. G., and Hoffbrand, A. V. (1987). Preliminary Communication: Detection of tyrosine protein kinase substrates in fresh leukemia cells and normal blood cells using an immunoblotting technique. *Leukemia 1*:782–785.
430. Ogawa, R., Ohtsuka, M., and Watanabe, Y. (1986). Complement-mediated lysis of K562 human leukemic cells by antibodies to phosphotyrosine and identification of cell surface proteins phosphorylated on tyrosine. *Cancer Res. 46*:2507–2510.
431. Huhn, R. D., Posner, M. R., Rayter, S. I., Foulkes, J. G., and Frackleton, A. R., Jr. (1987). Cell lines and peripheral blood leukocytes derived from individuals with chronic myelogenous leukemia display virtually identical proteins phosphorylated on tyrosine residues. *Proc. Natl. Acad. Sci. USA 84*:4408–4412.
432. Lugo, T. G., Pendergast, A-M., Muller, A. J., and Witte, O. N. (1990). Tyrosine kinase activity and transformation potency of *bcr-abl* oncogene products. *Science 247*:1079–1082.
433. Daley, G. Q., McLaughlin, J., Witte, O. N., and Baltimore, D. (1987). The CML-specific P210 *bcr/abl* protein, unlike v-*abl*, does not transform NIH/3T3 fibroblasts. *Science 237*:532–535.
434. McLaughlin, J., Chianese, E., and Witte, O. N. (1987). In vitro transformation of immature hematopoietic cells by the P210 BCR/ABL oncogene product of the Philadelphia chromosome. *Proc. Natl. Acad. Sci. USA 84*: 6558–6562.
435. Parada, L. F., Land, H., Weinberg, R. A., Wolf, D., and Rotter, V. (1984). Cooperation between genes encoding p53 tumor antigen and *ras* in cellular transformation. *Nature 312*:649.

436. Jenkins, J. R., Rudge, K., and Currie, G. A. (1984). Cellular immortalization by a cDNA clone encoding the transformation-associated phosphoprotein p53. *Nature 312*:651–654.
437. Damm, K., Beug, H., Graf, T., and Vennström, B. (1987). A single point mutation in *erb*A restores the erythroid transforming potential of a mutant avian erythroblastosis virus (AEV) defective in both *erb*A and *erb*B oncogenes. *EMBO J. 6*:375–382.
438. Graf, T. (1988). Review: Leukemias as a multistep process: Studies with avian retroviruses containing two oncogenes. *Leukemia 2*:127–131.
439. Ness, S. A., Beug, H., and Graf, T. (1987). v-*myb* dominance over v-*myc* in doubly transformed chick myelomonocytic cells. *Cell 51*:41–50.
440. Daley, G. Q., and Baltimore, D. (1988). Transformation of an interleukin 3-dependent hematopoietic cell line by the chronic myelogenous leukemia-specific $p210^{bcr/abl}$ protein. *Proc. Natl. Acad. Sci. 85*:9312–9316.
441. Garland, J. M. (1988). Rapid phosphorylation of a specific 33-kDa protein (p33) associated with growth stimulated by murine and rat IL3 in different IL3-dependent cell lines, and its constitutive expression in a malignant independent clone. *Leukemia 2*:94–102.
442. Garland, J. M., Kinnaird, A., and Elliott, K. (1988). Open Forum: Cell stimulation by interleukin 3 is a novel process of signal transduction: The rolling cell cycle and its implications for leukemic transformation. *Leukemia 2*:476–480.
443. Sorensen, P. H. B., Mui, A. L.-F., Murthy, S. C., and Krystal, G. (1989). Interleukin-3, GM-CSF, and TPA induce distinct phosphorylation events in an interleukin 3-dependent multipotential cell line. *Blood 73*:406–418.
444. Leary, A. G., Yang, Y-C., Clark, S. C., Gasson, J. C., Golde, D. W., and Ogawa, M. (1987). Recombinant gibbon interleukin 3 supports formation of human multilineage colonies and blast cell colonies in culture: Comparison with recombinant human granulocyte-macrophage colony-stimulating factor. *Blood 70*:1343–1348.
445. Ihle, J. N., Keller, J., Rein, A., Cleveland, J., and Rapp, U. (1985). Interleukin-3 regulation of the growth of normal and transformed hematopoietic cells. *Cancer Cells 3*:211–219.
446. Dean, M., Cleveland, J. L., Rapp, U. R., and Ihle, J. N. (1987). Role of myc in the abrogation of IL3 dependence of myeloid FDC-P1 cells. *Oncogene Research 1*:279–296.
447. Evans, J. P. M., Mire-Sluis, A. R., Hoffbrand, A. V., and Wickremasinghe, R. G. (1990). Binding of G-CSF, GM-CSF, tumor necrosis factor-alpha, and gamma-interferon to cell surface receptors on human myeloid leukemia cells triggers rapid tyrosine and serine phosphorylation of a 75-Kd protein. *Blood 75*:88–95.
448. Isfort, R. J., and Ihle, J. N. (1990). Multiple hematopoietic growth factors signal through tyrosine phosphorylation. *Growth Factors 2*:213–220.
449. Daley, G. Q., Van Etten, R. A., and Baltimore, D. (1990). Induction of chronic myelogenous leukemia in mice by the $P210^{bcr\text{-}abl}$ gene of the Philadelphia chromosome. *Science 247*:824–830.

450. Heisterkamp, N., Jenster, G., ten Hoeve, J., Zovich, D., Pattengale, P. K., and Groffen, J. (1990). Acute leukaemia in bcr/abl transgenic mice. *Nature 344*:251–253.
451. Roy-Burman, P., Devi, B. G., and Parker, J. W. (1983). Differential expression of c-*erb*B, c-*myc* and c-*myb* oncogene loci in human lymphomas and leukemias. *Int. J. Cancer 32*:185–191.
452. McClain, K. L. (1984). Expression of oncogenes in human leukemias. *Cancer Res. 44*:5382–5389.
453. Slamon, D. J., deKernion, J. B., Verma, I. M., and Cline, M. J. (1984). Expression of cellular oncogenes in human malignancies. *Science 224*: 256–262.
454. Rosson, D., and Tereba, A. (1983). Transcription of hematopoietic-associated oncogenes in childhood leukemia. *Cancer Res. 43*:3912–3918.
455. Blick, M., Westin, E., and Gutterman, J. (1984). Oncogene expression in human leukemia. *Blood 64*:1234–1239.
456. Nienhuis, A. W., Bunn, H. F., and Turner, P. H. (1985). Expression of the human c-*fms* proto-oncogenes in hematopoietic cells and its deletion in the 5q-syndrome. *Cell 42*:421–428.
457. Ferrari, S., Torelli, U., Selleri, L., Donelli, A., Venturelli, D., Moretti, L., and Torelli, G. (1985). Expression of human c-*fes* onc-gene occurs at detectable levels in myeloid but not in lymphoid cell populations. *Br. J. Haematol. 59*:21–25.
458. Mavillo, F., Sposi, N. M., and Petrini, M. (1986). Expression of cellular oncogenes in primary cells from human acute leukemias. *Proc. Natl. Acad. Sci. USA 83*:4394–4398.
459. Koeffler, H. P. (1986). Human acute myeloid leukemia lines: Models of leukemogenesis. *Semin. Hematol. 23*:223–236.
460. Calabretta, B., Venturelli, D., Kaczmarek, L., Narni, F., Talpaz, M., Anderson, B., Beran, M., and Baserga, R. (1986). Altered expression of G_1-specific genes in human malignant myeloid cells. *Proc. Natl. Acad. Sci. USA 83*:1495–1498.
461. Rowley, P. T., and Skuse, G. R. (1987). Concise Review: Oncogene expression in myelopoiesis. *Int. J. Cell Cloning 5*:255–266.
462. Willman, C. L., Stewart, C. C., Griffith, J. K., Stewart, S. J., and Tomasi, T. B. (1987). Differential expression and regulation of the c-*src* and c-*fgr* protooncogenes in myelomonocytic cells. *Proc. Natl. Acad. Sci. USA 84*: 4480–4484.
463. Yunis, J. J. (1986). Chromosome and oncogene rearrangements in leukemia and lymphoma. *Monogr. Pathol. 27*:91–96.
464. Yunis, J. J., Frizzera, G., Oken, M. M., McKenna, J., Theologides, A., and Arnesen, M. (1987). Multiple recurrent genomic defects in follicular lymphoma: A possible model for cancer. *N. Engl. J. Med. 316*:79–84.
465. Nowell, P. C. (1986). Mechanisms of tumor progression. *Cancer Res. 46*: 2203–2207.
466. Chaganti, R. S. K. (1987). Cytogenetics of leukemia and lymphoma. In *Malignant Lymphoma* (C. W. Berard, R. F. Dorfman, and N. Kaufman,

eds.). Williams & Wilkins, Baltimore, pp. 184–203.

467. Richardson, M. E., Quanguang, C., Filippa, D. A., Offit, K., Hamptom, A., Kodura, P. R. K., Jhanwar, S. C., Lieberman, P. H., Clarkson, B. D., and Chaganti, R. S. K. (1987). Intermediate-to-high-grade histology of lymphomas carrying t(14;18) is associated with additional nonrandom chromosome changes. *Blood 70*:444–447.
468. Sandberg, A. A., Turc-Carel, C., and Gemmill, R. M. (1988). Chromosomes in solid tumors and beyond. *Cancer Res. 48*:1049–1059.
469. Levine, E. G., Arthur, D. C., Frizzera, G., Peterson, B. A., Hurd, D. D., and Bloomfield, C. D. (1988). Cytogenetic abnormalities predict clinical outcome in non-Hodgkin lymphoma. *Ann. Intern. Med. 108*:14–20.
470. Chaganti, R. S. K., Doucette, L. A., Offit, K., Filippa, D. A., Allen, G. J., Condon, M. R., Jhanwar, S. C., Clarkson, B. D., and Lieberman, P. H. (1989). Specific translocation in non-Hodgkin's lymphoma: Incidence, molecular detection, and histological and clinical correlations. *Cancer Cells 7*:33-36.
471. Chaganti, R. S. K., and Klein, E. A. (1990). The cytogenetic basis for molecular analysis of leukemia, lymphoma, and solid tumors. In *Molecular Genetics in Cancer Diagnosis* (J. Cossman, ed.). Elsevier, New York, pp. 73-104.
472. Osgood, E. E. (1957). A unifying concept of the etiology of the leukemias, lymphomas, and cancers. *JNCI 18*:155–166.
473. Pierce, G. B., Nakane, P. K., and Mazurkiewicz, J. E. (1974). Natural history of malignant stem cells. In *Differentiation and Control of Malignancy of Tumor Cells* (W. Nakahara, T. Ono, T. Sugimura, and H. Sugano, eds.). University of Tokyo Press, Tokyo, pp. 453–469.
474. Lotem, J., and Sachs, L. (1974). Different blocks in the differentiation of myeloid leukemia cells. *Proc. Natl. Acad. Sci. USA 71*:3507–3511.
475. Potter, V. R. (1978). Phenotypic diversity in experimental hepatomas: The concept or partially blocked ontogeny. *Br. J. Cancer 38*:1–23.
476. Potter, V. R. (1988). On the road to the blocked ontogeny theory. *Adv. Oncol. 4*:3–8.

PART II
Animal and Viral Models for Chronic Myelogenous Leukemia

2

The Abelson Tyrosine Kinase in *Drosophila:* Application of Genetic Strategies to Understand Its Normal Function

F. Michael Hoffmann, Mark J. Henkemeyer, Randy L. Bennett, and Frank B. Gertler *University of Wisconsin-Madison, Madison, Wisconsin*

INTRODUCTION

The conservation of the Abelson tyrosine kinase throughout evolution is indicated by the high degree of amino acid sequence similarity between the mammalian Abelson protein and sequences found in three lower eukaryotes: *Drosophila melanogaster, Calliphora erythrocephala*, and *Caenorhabditis elegans* (1–3). This high degree of conservation over great evolutionary distances connotes that the Abelson tyrosine kinase may participate in essential cellular processes. Analysis of the *abl* tyrosine kinase in *Drosophila* and *Caenorhabditis* permits the application of genetic strategies to study the role of the tyrosine kinase in normal cellular functions. Additionally, through the identification of genes that interact genetically with the *abl* gene, proteins that serve as regulators or substrates of the *abl* tyrosine kinase activity can be identified. Identification of such proteins may provide important clues to the biochemical processes through which the oncogenic forms of the Abelson tyrosine kinase act in the genesis of leukemias.

The growing number of proto-oncogene homologs, growth factor receptors, and growth factors identified in *Drosophila* suggests that much of the biochemical machinery required for cellular proliferation and differentiation has been conserved through evolution. In addition to the *abl* gene, several other *Droso-*

phila genes have been identified by their strong sequence similarities to vertebrate proto-oncogenes, growth factor receptors, or growth factors (4,5). For example, *Drosophila* homologs have been identified for the *src, ras, int*-1, *raf, rel, ets*, and *myb* proto-oncogenes (6-20). *Drosophila* genes encoding proteins similar to the receptors for epidermal growth factor (EGF) and insulin have been identified (21-23). In addition, sequences similar to EGF and transforming growth factor β (TGF-β) have been identified in *Drosophila* (24,25). Evidence that *Drosophila* homologs have important roles during normal development comes from the growing number of mutations isolated in the *Drosophila* homologs. For example, mutations in the *Drosophila raf* homolog and the *Drosophila* EGF receptor homolog interfere with normal cell proliferation (Reference 17 and Shilo, personal communication). In contrast, several of the *Drosophila* homologs are required for the proper differentiation of cells but not for their proliferation. For example, the *Drosophila rel* homolog, *dorsal*, is required for the proper specification of ventral embryonic cells (18); the *Drosophila int*-1 homolog, *wingless*, is required to specify the correct developmental fate of the cells at the boundaries of the 14 metameric segments of the early embryo (26).

In this chapter, we focus on the structural and functional homologies between the *Drosophila* and mammalian Abelson tyrosine kinases and on the role of the *abl* tyrosine kinase during *Drosophila* development. Much of the information described is obtained by the analysis of mutant phenotypes and localization of the protein during development. We describe genetic strategies for identifying substrates and/or regulatory proteins of the *abl* tyrosine kinase. These approaches may provide us with reagents that could identify c-*abl* substrates in mammalian cells.

MOLECULAR IDENTIFICATION AND CHARACTERIZATION

Isolation of DNA Clones

A DNA probe from the Abelson murine leukemia virus was used to identify similar *Drosophila* sequences using cross-hybridization under low-stringency conditions (6). Partial sequence analysis indicated that one of the clones that hybridizer to both v-*abl* and v-*src* probes had a significantly greater sequence similarity to the *abl* tyrosine kinase than to the *src* tyrosine kinase (7). The *Drosophila* sequence identified with the heterologous probe was used to initiate a chromosomal walk to isolate adjacent DNA in the *Drosophila* genome. These genomic sequences were used to screen *Drosophila* cDNA libraries, and several independent cDNA clones were isolated. The gene structure and protein-encoding capacities of the *Drosophila abl* gene were deduced from the DNA sequence of genomic and cDNA clones (1). The *Drosophila* gene consists of 10 exons extending over 26 kilobases (kb) of DNA. Its structure resembles the mammalian c-*abl* genes in that a large intron of 14.5 kb separates the first exon from the second exon, the

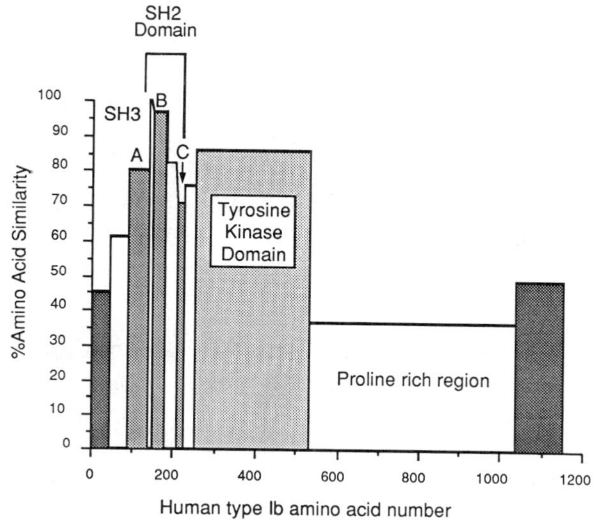

Figure 1 Percentage of similar amino acid residues between the human type 1b protein sequence (28) and the *Drosophila* protein sequence (1). Each boxed region represents a domain of the human c-*abl* protein. See text for descriptions of domains A, B, and C.

tyrosine kinase essential domain is divided among two exons in the 5′ half of the gene, and there is a large exon at the 3′ end encoding most of the carboxy-terminal domain of the protein. The exon-intron junctions, however, are not well conserved between the *Drosophila* and mammalian genes. In contrast, exon-intron junctions in the *Drosophila abl* gene and the *abl* sequences identified in *Calliphora* are conserved precisely (Durica, personal communication).

Comparison of Amino Acid Sequences in Specific Domains

The Amino Terminus

A large open reading frame spans all 10 exons and predicts a protein of 1521 amino acids (1). Computer-aided alignment of the predicted *Drosophila abl* amino acid sequence with the human c-*abl* sequence indicates several highly conserved regions of the protein (Figure 1). At the amino terminus, the *Drosophila* protein shows sequence similarity to the type 1b amino terminus of the human c-*abl* gene, one of the two forms of the human c-*abl* tyrosine kinase that differ in the 26 (type 1a) or 44 (type 1b) amino acids at the amino terminus (27,28). The *Drosophila* protein contains a glycine immediately after the initiating methionine, as do the human and murine type 1b proteins, and the *gag-abl* fusion protein from Abelson murine leukemia virus (27-29). The type 1a c-*abl* protein and the *bcr-abl* fusion protein found in chronic myelogenous leukemia (CML) cells do not have N-terminal glycines (30). These observations are of potential significance because the N-terminal glycine of v-*abl* is a site of myristylation, which is believed to aid in its association with the plasma membrane (31). Whether myristylation of the N-terminal glycine is required for the normal activity of the type 1b c-*abl* proteins is not known. Addition of myristic acid to the *src* tyrosine kinase is essential for the transforming activity of that oncoprotein (32,33).

The SH3 Domain

Sequence similarity of over 80% exists between the *Drosophila* and human c-*abl* SH3 domains (region A in Figure 1). The SH3 domain has recently been identified as a sequence that is highly conserved among cytoplasmic tyrosine kinases, with the exception of *fps-fes*, and is also found in the v-*crk* oncogene (34) and in the phosphatidylinositol-specific phospholipase C (35). It has been proposed that in the cytoplasmic tyrosine kinases this domain may serve as a site for protein-protein interactions that regulate tyrosine activity. This region of the mouse c-*abl* proto-oncogene was deleted in the transduction of the c-*abl* proto-oncogene to the Abelson murine leukemia virus. As the v-*abl* tyrosine kinase coded by the virus has altered catalytic properties (36,37), the removal of the SH3 domain during the transduction event may have led to the production of an unregulated oncogenic Abelson tyrosine kinase. Support for this hypothesis comes from the finding that small deletions and insertion mutations in this domain are sufficient to activate the c-*abl* tyrosine kinase as assayed by transformation of NIH 3T3 cells and lymphoid cells (Jackson and Baltimore, personal communication). Although the *bcr-abl* fusion protein of CML cells retains the SH3 sequences (30), juxtaposition of this domain to the *bcr* sequences may lead to conformational changes that also disrupt the normal functions of the SH3 domain.

The SH2 Domain

Adjacent to the SH3 domain is the SH2 domain. The sequence conservation between the *Drosophila* and human Abelson sequences in this domain is also great er than 80% (regions B and C in Figure 1). The SH2 domain was originally identified because of its conservation among all cytoplasmic tyrosine kinases (38). It contains two subdomains, B and C, also present in the v-*crk* oncogene and in the phosphatidylinositol-specific phospholipase C (34,35). Insertion mutations in the SH2 domain of v-*fps* disrupt its transforming ability but do not affect the catalytic activity of the tyrosine kinase domain when expressed in bacteria (38). The high degree of conservation between the *Drosophila* and human SH2 sequences suggests that the function of SH2 may be similar in *Drosophila* and humans.

The Kinase Catalytic Domain

Adjacent to the SH2 domain are the sequences required for the catalytic activity of the tyrosine kinase. There is over 80% amino acid sequence similarity between the *Drosophila* and human Abelson tyrosine kinases throughout this region. Two specific amino acids of the mammalian protein that are conserved are the lysine, which is involved in ATP binding, and the tyrosine, which serves as a major site for phosphorylation. This catalytic domain of the *Drosophila* protein exhibits tyrosine kinase activity when expressed in bacteria (1).

The remainder of the *Drosophila abl* protein, from amino acid 660 to 1521, is not highly related to the corresponding sequence of the human gene. There is some amino acid similarity through this region, but the alignment requires 28 gaps in the sequence. The carboxyl-terminal domain is also the least conserved region between the human and mouse c-*abl* proteins (28). The function of this domain is not known, although it is dispensable for transformation of fibroblasts by v-*abl* (39).

ISOLATION OF MUTATIONS IN *Drosophila abl*

Identification of *abl* Mutant Alleles

The chromosomal position of the *Drosophila abl* gene was located by in situ hybridization of ^{3}H-labeled DNA probes to a region of the third chromosome, designated 73B. The region is adjacent to a recessive eye color mutation called *scarlet*; several deletions of this chromosomal region had previously been isolated by screening mutagenized chromosomes for their failure to complement a *scarlet* mutation. *Drosophila abl* DNA probes were used to show that several of the *scarlet* chromosomal deletions removed the *abl* sequences in addition to the *scarlet* gene. The deletions removed 10–20 different genes in addition to the *abl* gene. The first step in the isolation of mutations in the *abl* gene was to isolate single gene mutations in each of the genes uncovered by these chromosomal deficiencies. At the time we were isolating these mutations, McKeown et al. were carrying out mutagenesis screens in the same region to obtain new alleles of the sex determination locus *transformer* (40). The combined screens of both laboratories produced alleles in 18 recessive lethal complementation groups in the portion of the chromosome uncovered by the deletions. These 18 recessive lethal complementation groups were ordered on the chromosome by their genetic complementation properties with a series of overlapping chromosomal deletions.

The chromosomal breakpoints of three of these deletions mapped to the DNA that contains the transcriptional unit of the *abl* gene (Figure 2) (41). Three independent alleles making up one of the recessive lethal complementation groups failed to complement these overlapping deletions that disrupted the *abl* transcriptional unit. These three mutant alleles were tentatively assigned as mutations in the *abl* gene on the basis of the coincidence of their genetic properties

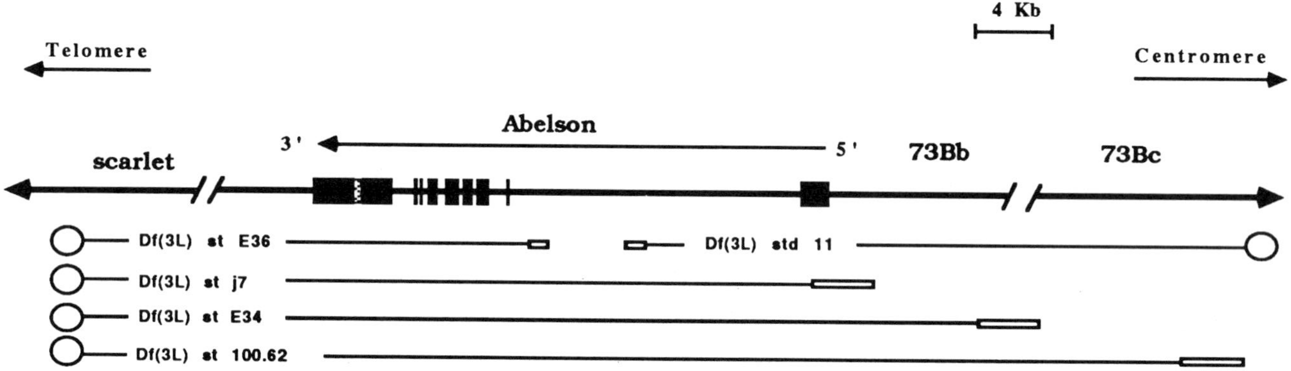

Figure 2 Molecular and genetic organization of the *Drosophila* Abelson homolog. The *abl* gene is located in a region on the left arm of the third chromosome designated 73B. The telomere is to the left, and the centromere is to the right. The Abelson transcription unit consists of 10 coding exons extending over 26 kb of genomic DNA. The Abelson gene is approximately 110 kb away from the eye color gene *scarlet*. Some chromosomal deletions that remove the *scarlet* gene are deleted for Abelson as well. Deletion breakpoints that have been mapped molecularly are indicated by boxes. In particular, Df(3L) stE36 is deleted for *abl* exons 2-10, and Df(3L) stj7 is deleted for the entire *abl* gene. Df(3L) stE34 removes all of *abl* and the next gene designated 73Bb. Df(3L) st100.62 removes *abl*, 73Bb and 73Bc. Another chromosomal deletion, Df(3L) std 11, removes DNA from the *abl* promoter, exon 1, and part of intron 1. 73Bc is also removed by Df(3L) std 11.

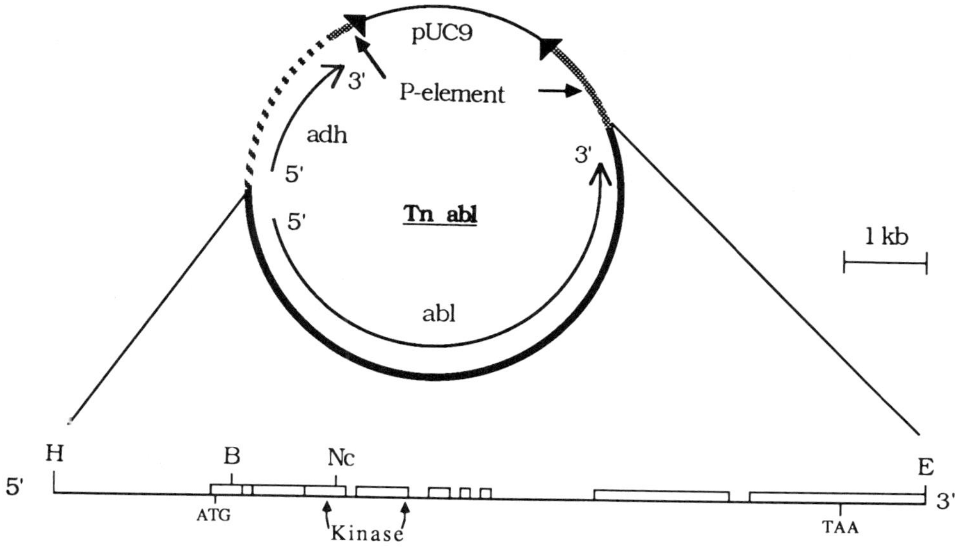

Figure 3 Map of the *Drosophila abl* transposon Tn*abl*. The P element vector pPA-1 was used to provide the P element terminal repeats, the *alcohol dehydrogenase (adh)* selectable marker gene, and the pUC9 bacterial plasmid sequences. The *abl* sequences were placed into pPA-1 by inserting three DNA fragments containing portions of the *Drosophila abl* gene into the vector (41). The orientations of the *abl* and *adh* genes are indicated. The *abl* exons are represented by boxes, and introns and untranscribed regions are represented by lines. ATG and TAA bracket the open reading frame. The location of the tyrosine kinase catalytic domain is indicated. Restriction sites used in the construction of the plasmid are shown (H, *Hind*III; B, *Bam*HI; N, *Nco*I; and E, *Eco*RI).

with the molecular evidence that the three chromosomal deficiencies disrupted the *abl* transcriptional unit.

Proof that the mutant alleles did indeed map to the *abl* gene was obtained by rescuing the mutant phenotypes of these alleles by reintroducing DNA containing the *abl* gene into the mutant flies (41). This was accomplished by inserting portions of genomic and cDNA clones from the *Drosophila abl* gene into a vector that included sequences from the *Drosophila* transposable element P (Figure 3). The P element sequences permit integration of the plasmid DNA into chromosomal DNA through the action of a P element transposase when introduced by microinjection into preblastoderm *Drosophila* embryos (42). Stable chromosomal insertions of the *abl* transposon, Tn*abl*, were recovered and mapped by genetic crosses and by in situ localization on polytene chromosomes.

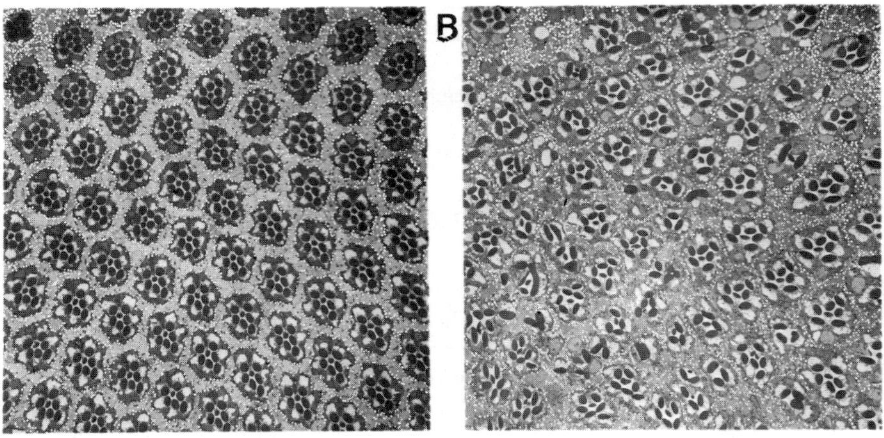

Figure 4 Electron micrographs of sections prepared from wild-type and *abl* mutant eyes. A trapezoidal cluster of eight retinal cells is present in each ommatidium of the wild-type eye (A). Only seven of the eight retinal cells (visualized by their electron-dense rhabdomere organelles) are observed in any one ommatidium. Note that the ommatidia form regular hexagonal arrays and that the trapezoidal clusters maintain the same orientation. The *abl* mutant eyes (B) exhibit a general disorganization of both the nexagonal arrays and the trapezoidal clusters. The ommatidia are often missing one or more of the eight retinal cells.

When tested with several different mutant *abl* alleles, one copy of Tn*abl* provided full rescue of all the *abl* mutant phenotypes. The significance of this result is twofold: it confirms the identification of the mutant alleles as *abl* mutations, and it indicated that Tn*abl* contains a functional *abl* gene.

The Mutant Phenotypes

The initial phenotype observed for *abl* mutant alleles was lethality late in development in the pupal case prior to emergence of the adult fly (41). Examination of the animals in the pupal case indicated that metamorphosis from the larval form to the adult fly was virtually complete. The only abnormality in the external structures of these dead animals was a roughening of the facets of the eye. Depending on which of the three mutant alleles was tested, 10–50% of the mutant flies escaped from the pupal lethality. The adult flies that emerged from the pupal case exhibited roughened eyes and were extremely weak, generally dying within the first couple of days after emergence from the pupal case; otherwise they were wild type in appearance. The flies and the animals were also functionally sterile in that they gave rise to no progeny, although both male and female gonads appeared structurally normal (41).

Further analysis of the roughened eye phenotype provided some cellular clues to the defects in these animals. Thin sections of the adult eye indicated that the regular architecture of retinal cells in the compound eye of the fly was severely disrupted. The wild type eye consists of 700 individual eyes, called ommatidia, arranged in a hexagonal array. The eight retinal cells within each ommatidium are organized in a trapezoidal pattern in which each of the eight cells can be uniquely identified (43). Examination of sections of adult eyes from *abl* mutant animals indicated that both the overall hexagonal array of the ommatidia and the trapezoidal array of retinal cells within each ommatidium were disrupted (Figure 4). Retinal cells were often absent from the clusters, suggesting a defect in the determination or viability of these neural cells. The failure of the developed animals to emerge from the pupal case, retinal defects, and the poor viability of animals that did emerge are all consistent with a role for the *abl* tyrosine kinase in neural cell differentiation. Defects in the adult central nervous system (CNS) assembled during metamorphosis could easily disrupt the coordinated neuromuscular activity necessary for the fully developed animal to escape from the pupal case. Studies on the localization of the *abl* protein provide further support for its role in *Drosophila* neural cell development (see below).

TEMPORAL AND SPATIAL REGULATION OF *abl* EXPRESSION

abl RNA During the *Drosophila* Life Cycle

Abelson transcripts are observed on Northern blots as multiple bands migrating with apparent molecular weights of 6.5-7.5 kb. The size heterogeneity is due to the use of several 3′ polyadenylation sites and alternative splicing of the last intron (44). When RNAs isolated from animals at different stages in development are examined, the highest levels of *abl* RNA are observed in unfertilized eggs and early embryos (References 44-46 and Rand and Hoffmann, unpublished). By analogy with other mRNAs in *Drosophila* oocytes, the *abl* mRNA is probably made in the germline-derived nurse cells in the ovaries and transported through cytoplasmic channels to the oocyte. Many mRNAs with critical roles in early *Drosophila* embryogenesis are provided to the oocyte by the nurse cells and stored there until embryogenesis begins. For example, RNA transcripts from some of the genes involved in the determination of anterior versus posterior and dorsal versus ventral positions in the embryo are synthesized neutrally and stored in the oocyte (47,48).

The genetic crosses that gave rise to the *abl* mutant animals described earlier utilized mothers that were heterozygous for an *abl* mutant allele. The oocytes derived from these mothers received *abl* mRNA from the wild-type *abl* gene; therefore functions of the *abl* protein early in development could be carried out by protein translated from this maternal mRNA. Since *abl* mutant flies die before giving rise to any progeny, we addressed the function of the *abl* maternal mRNA by inducing clones of *abl* mutant tissue in the germline of otherwise *abl* wild-type females. We did not observe defects in oogenesis, but the embryos derived from the *abl* null oocytes died during embryogenesis, indicating that maternal *abl* mRNA is required for early embryogenesis (Hoffmann, unpublished observations).

The level of the maternal *abl* RNA decreases in 2–4 and 4–6 h embryos. *De novo* zygotic expression of *abl* is first detected in 6–12-h embryos and persists through the remaining 12 h of embryogenesis. *abl* RNA is not detected in larval stages but increases in 24 h pupae. The level of *abl* RNA decreases in older pupae and reaches a low but detectable level in adult males and females. Adult females express the low-molecular-weight *abl* transcripts observed in unfertilized eggs, presumably from expression of the *abl* gene in the ovaries (Rand and Hoffmann, unpublished observations).

In Situ Localization of *abl* RNA in the Embryo

Northern blot analysis of RNA obtained from whole organisms indicates only when the RNA is expressed; it does not address whether the gene is expressed ubiquitously or is restricted to specific cells or tissues. Furthermore, at stages at which the RNA cannot be detected in the whole organism, the gene may be expressed in a minor subset of cells. To examine further when and where the *abl* gene is expressed, in situ hybridization analysis was performed on developmentally staged embryos (Henkemeyer and Hoffmann, unpublished observations).

During the first 2.5 h or embryogenesis, the embryo goes through 13 synchronous nuclear divisions followed by cellularization to form the cellular blastoderm. During the precellular stages, *abl* transcripts are detected uniformly in the embryo. Transcripts become localized to the band of cytoplasm between the yolk mass and the nuclei. When gastrulation begins, as indicated by the formation of the ventral furrow, *abl* transcripts are no longer detectable. *abl* transcripts are not detected during the period of embryogenesis when the major morphogenetic movements of gastrulation and segmentation take place. During this period there is limited cell division. Embryonic ectodermal cells undergo two to three rounds of cell division, mesodermal cells divide three times, and neuronal precursor cells divide approximately nine times (49). At about 8 h after fertilization the germ band begins to retract in a process known as germ band shortening, and the CNS cells begin to differentiate and extend axons (50). *abl* transcripts are once again detected at this stage along the developing ventral aspect of the embryo at the position of the ventral nerve cord and brain. RNA in situ analysis has not been done on animals at other stages of *Drosophila* development. The localization of *abl* transcripts to specific tissues and time periods in *Drosophila* embryogenesis suggests that expression of the *abl* tyrosine kinase is developmentally regulated. This conclusion is reinforced by localization studies of the *abl* protein using immunocytochemical staining of developing *Drosophila.*

Localization of *abl* Protein During Embryogenesis and Eye Morphogenesis

To gain the resolution required to determine unambiguously which tissues and cell types of the *abl* protein, we raised ant-*abl* antibodies that specifically detect the protein in *Drosophila*. We have localized *abl* protein expression during embryogenesis and eye morphogenesis using immunofluorescence and immunocytochemical techniques (Bennett and Hoffmann, unpublished observations).

The *abl* protein made from the maternal message is detected in all cells of the blastoderm with the anti-*abl* antibody, consistent with the RNA in sutu localization and genetic experiments showing that *abl* is required during early embryogenesis. It is not known how long this protein persists during embryogenesis.

The first neural processes appear at about 8 h after fertilization. It is in these cells, at this stage, that we detect tissue-specific expression of the *abl* protein in the embryo. In the CNS of the developing embryo the axon bundles form an orthogonal ladder consisting of two lateral bundles (the anterior and posterior commissures) within each segment (or neuromere) and longitudinal bundles (longitudinal connectives) that run within and between each neuromere. During CNS development the commissures form first, followed by the formation of the longitudinals. We first detect *abl* protein expression in the developing commissures and later in both the commissures and the longitudinal axon bundles. Later in development the level of *abl* protein in the commissures decreases, whereas the level in the longitudinal axon bundles remains constant. The *abl* protein is expressed in the CNS throughout the remainder of embryogenesis, localized in the axons, not in the cell bodies.

During the larval stages, distinct sheets of epithelial cells proliferate in structures called imaginal disks. Upon metamorphosis it is these cells that produce most of the external structures of the adult fly, including the head, thorax, wings, and legs. *abl* protein is detected only in the imaginal disks that produce the eyes. The eye imaginal disks begin to differentiate during the third larval instar, when a furrow, called the morphogenetic furrow, forms at the posterior end of the disk and moves toward the anterior end. Ahead of the furrow, cells are mitotically active and undifferentiated. Behind the morphogenetic furrow, the cells are organized into the clusters of differentiated cells that will make up the 700 ommatidia of the adult compound eye (43).

abl protein is not detected in the undifferentiated epithelial cells ahead of the furrow or in the cells immediately behind it, but it is expressed farther behind the furrow in the eight retinal cells that are incorporated into clusters, although they are not yet fully differentiated. In contrast to its location in the embryonic CNS, *abl* protein is present in both the cell bodies and the axons of the retinal cells. *abl* protein is detected in the retinal cells of eye disks during pupariation. We have not performed immunolocalization of the *abl* protein in pupae or adults, but the time of the peak *abl* RNA expression in pupae corresponds to the period during which the adult CNS differentiates (51). We anticipate that the *abl* protein is associated with the differentiation of the adult CNS at this time.

We were surprised to see *abl* protein restricted during development to differentiated non-proliferating neural cells of the *Drosophila* embryonic CNS and the eye. There is an increase in the level of c-*abl* RNA in 9-11 day embryos, a time in which organogenesis occurs (52). In adult mice, the c-*abl* RNA is expressed in all tissue types (27,53,54). The type 1b RNA is expressed at roughly constant levels in the mouse tissues tested, whereas the levels of type 1a RNA vary up to 10-fold between different mouse tissues (54).

The neural expression of the *Drosophila abl* protein is similar to the neural expression of the c-*src* tyrosine kinase during vertebrate development. In vertebrate development, there is 8- to 10-fold more c-*src* protein in neural cells from the brain and spinal cord than in fibroblasts (55). The neural c-*src* protein differs from the fibroblast c-*src* protein by insertion of six amino acids due to alternate RNA splicing in the nerve cells (56,57). Using immunolocalization, the c-*src* protein is found in developing neural cells during neural tube formation, neural differentiation in the cerebellum, and retinal cell differentiation (58-60). During neural tube formation c-*src* is expressed specifically in proliferating neural precursors but not in all proliferating cells of the germ layers. Later, the c-*src* protein is again expressed in the neural tissues of the CNS, where it accumulates in cells that are differentiating and nonproliferating. Like the embryonic *Drosophila abl* protein, the chicken c-*src* protein is localized to the neural process, not to the cell bodies (59). In addition to its expression in the neurons of the CNS, the chicken c-*src* protein accumulates in the developing retina (60). In this case, again like the eye disk *Drosophila abl* protein, c-*src* not only localizes in the axons but is also found in the cell bodies. We do not believe that the functions of the *Drosophila abl* protein in *Drosophila* neural development have been superseded by c-*src* protein in vertebrate neural development because both of the *Drosophila src* homologs also show neural expression in *Drosophila* (61,62).

It is possible that there is an association of the c-*abl* protein with vertebrate neural development that has been missed in the analysis of *abl* mRNA during mouse development. In an early study of c-*src* RNA expression (63), the correlation of c-*src* expression and neural (brain and retinal) differentiation was not seen; c-*src* mRNA was detected in several tissues and several stages of embrogenesis, but brain was among the tissues expressing low levels of c-*src* RNA. It will be interesting to see whether immunocytochemical analyses detect elevated expression of the vertebrate c-*abl* protein in specific cells at specific times in development.

CONSERVATION OF *abl* FUNCTION

Human c-*abl*-Fly *abl* Fusion Proteins Expressed in *Drosophila*

The protein encoded by the *Drosophila abl* homolog shows a high degree of sequence similarity to the mammalian c-*abl* tyrosine kinase catalytic domain and noncatalytic domains in the amino portion of the protein (described in Molecular Identification and Characterization). Two different proteins are produced by the human c-*abl* gene, type 1a and type 1b, which differ only in their amino-teminal 26 and 44 amino acids, respectively. Type 1b is most similar to *Drosophila* amino terminus in that it contains an N-terminal glycine and a putative myristylation signal sequence (28,64,65). Myristylation of the *abl* protein may play a crucial role in positioning the protein at cell membranes, near regulatory signals and substrates. To determine whether the two different human c-*abl* amino termini function in *Drosophila*, two chimeric human-fly *abl* genes, Tn1A and Tn1B, were made (Henkemeyer and Hoffmann, unpublished). The proteins encoded by Tn1A and Tn1B contain the human c-*abl* type 1a or type 1b amino termini, respectively, the human SH3 domain, and the human SH2 domain fused to the *Drosophila* tyrosine kinase catalytic domain and carboxy terminus. Transgenic flies containing insertions of transposons Tn1A or Tn1B were obtained using the method of P element-mediated germline transformation (42). Eight Tn1A and three Tn1B transgenic lines were recovered. Western blot analysis of total head proteins verified that the human-fly *abl* fusion proteins were expressed in both the Tn1A and Tn1B transgenic fly lines.

The fusion proteins expressed from Tn1A and Tn1B were tested for their ability to rescue *abl* mutant *Drosophila* to wild-type adults. The Tn1B fusion protein functioned as well as the wild-type *Drosophila abl* protein in rescuing *abl* mutant flies to normal adults. This result indicates that the SH3 and SH2 domains, if absolutely required for normal function of the *abl* tyrosine kinase, have been functionally conserved between humans and *Drosophila.* If the SH2 and SH3 domains function to interact with signals received by the cell to regulate the activity of the *abl* kinase, then this result indicates that the human SH2 and SH3 domains may be able to receive and respond to the appropriate signals during *Drosophila* development.

In contrast to Tn1B, Tn1A does not rescue *abl* mutant flies. Since the only difference between Tn1B and Tn1A lies in the extreme amino terminus, this result indicates that the type 1b, but not the type 1a human amino terminus can function in *Drosophila*. Experiments to determine whether the difference is related to myristylation are in progress.

Murine c-*abl* Type 1b Protein Expressed in *Drosophila*

The successful rescue of *abl* mutant *Drosophila* to wild-type adults with the fusion protein Tn1B led us to test whether a full-length mammalian c-*abl* protein could also function in *Drosophila* (Henkemeyer and Hoffmann, unpublished). A P element transposon (Tnc-*abl*) was constructed to express the full-length mouse c-*abl* type 1b protein in transgenic *Drosophila*. A total of five independent Tnc-*abl* germline transformants were obtained. Western blot analysis was used to measure the level of murine c-*abl* protein present in the five Tnc-*abl* lines. Tnc-*abl* transgenic lines that express high levels of c-*abl* protein do not rescue any of the *abl* mutant phenotypes. Since the full-length type 1b c-*abl* protein did not rescue the mutant phenotypes, in contrast to the Tn1B human-fly fusion protein, we believe the *Drosophila* and human catalytic domains may possess different biologic specificities. The implied difference in biologic specificities of the kinase domains is reinforced in the experiments described later. We have not ruled out, however, that the inability of the mouse c-*abl* protein to function in *Drosophila* is due to amino acids carboxy terminal to the kinase domain.

Transforming Activity of the *Drosophila abl* Tyrosine Kinase Domain

To further establish the functional homologies between the *Drosophila* and mammalian *abl* tyrosine kinases, we asked whether the *Drosophila abl* tyrosine kinase could be activated to a transforming oncoprotein. A v-*abl*-fly *abl* chimeric provirus, pvDabl, was constructed to express a fusion protein in which the *Drosophila abl* amino terminus and SH2 and SH3 domains are replaced with v-*abl gag* and SH2. A proviral vector that contains the wild-type *Drosophila abl* coding region (pDabl) was also constructed. To test the transforming activity of the viral-fly fusion protein and the wild-type *Drosophila abl* protein, pvDabl and pDabl were transfected onto NIH 3T3 fibroblasts. Cells transfected with pvDabl became transformed at 10% the efficiency of Abelson murine leukemia virus (A-MuLV provirus). The full-length *Drosophila abl* provirus clone, pDabl, did not cause transformation (Holland, Henkemeyer, Risser, and Hoffmann, unpublished observations). The results show that the *Drosophila abl* tyrosine kinase domain is activated to a transforming protein by the same amino-terminal substitution that activates the mammalian c-*abl* protein.

The v-*abl* tyrosine kinase is able to cause transformation of fibroblasts and lymphoid cells (66–68). The region of the protein responsible for lymphoid transformation appears to be in the tyrosine kinase catalytic domain (69). Experiments were carried out to determine whether the activated *Drosophila abl* tyrosine kinase also exhibits this lymphoid specificity. Virus pools from pvDabl-transformed fibroblasts were harvested and titered by measuring the transforming frequency upon infection of fresh NIH 3T3 fibroblasts. The virus stocks were then used to infect bone marrow cells in culture or for injection into newborn mice. The chimeric virus failed to transform the bone marrow cells in culture or to initiate luekemia in the mice (Holland, Henkemeyer, Risser, and Hoffmann, unpublished observation). The failure of the *Drosophila abl* kinase to transform lymphoid cells implies that the biologic specificities of *Drosophila* and mammalian *abl* kinase domains may have diverged.

A Transforming Viral-Fly *abl* Fusion Protein Expressed in *Drosophila*

Does an activated oncogene retain functions required for normal growth and development? The identification and characterization of *abl* mutations in *Drosophila* makes this question directly testable. A chimeric viral-fly *abl* transposon (Tnv-*abl*) whose translation product is identical to the transforming fusion protein encoded by pvDabl, described earlier, was constructed. One Tnv-*abl* germline transformant was recovered, and Western blot analysis of adult heads verified that the viral-fly fusion protein was expressed in the Tnv-*abl* transfenic fly line. In Tnv-*abl* transgenic *Drosophila*, expression of the viral-fly fusion protein caused no unusual domain phenotypes; however, in *Drosophila* mutant for the endogenous *abl* gene, the viral-fly fusion protein was able to rescue some *abl* mutant phenotypes (Henkemeyer and Hoffmann, unpublished). The rescue activity was reduced when compared with the wild-type *Drosophila abl* transposon Tn*abl*. Nevertheless, these results indicate that an *abl* tyrosine kinase that transformes mouse cells provides partial *abl* function during *Drosophila* development.

USING *Drosophila* GENETICS TO IDENTIFY SUBSTRATES FOR *abl*

Identification of a Gene That Is Haploinsufficient in an *abl* Mutant Background

Flies that are lacking wild-type *abl* produce die predominantly at late pupation, the only obvious external defect being roughened eyes. These phenotypes are caused by *abl* point mutations heterozygous with each other or with chromosomes that carry deletions that remove the *abl* gene. Some decisions cause more severe phenotypes when heterozygous with the point mutations (41). These mutant animals rarely make it to pupation, dying instead as young larvae or embryos. Along with removing part or all of the *abl* gene, all deletions that cause the more severe phenotype lack three other genes that map close to *abl*, lethal 73Bb, lethal 73Bc and *disabled* (*dab*). The animals with the severe phenotype are genetically null for the *abl* gene and hemizygous for the two nearby genes. We determined that one *dab* of these genes, *dab*, is required in two doses for the animal to reach pupation in an *abl*-deficient genetic background.

The observation that the number of copies of a specific gene, and hence the level of its gene product, may become critical in the absence of the *abl* tyrosine kinase suggested the following model. The action of the *abl* tyrosine kinase may be to modulate or to coordinate the levels of activity of several substrates. In the absence of the *abl* tyrosine kinase, the substrates function at a less than optimal level. The sum of these suboptimal activities leads to the phenotypic defects observed in the *abl* mutant animals. If we eliminate the *abl* gene and reduce the gene copy number of any one of the structural genes being regulated by *abl*, the phenotypic defects may be much more pronounced because there would be only half as much of the putative substrate functioning at a suboptimal level. In the presence of the *abl* tyrosine kinase, half the level of a specific substrate may be quite sufficient for its normal physiologic role, but the combinations of the absence of *abl* and the reduced level of the gene product could have synergistic effects. We refer to genes that are haploinsufficient dependent upon an *abl* mutant background as HDAs.

There is precedence for such gene dosage effects in *Drosophila*. A few *Drosophila* genes must be present in two copies to provide normal levels of function even in wild-type genetic backgrounds. One example of such a gene is *Ultrabithorax*, which is involved in determining segment identity during development (70). Another example of a gene required in two copies is the *decaptenaplegic* gene; it encodes a protein similar to TGF-β and is required in two copies for proper development of the head and tail regions of the embryo (71). The dosage sensitivity of some other *Drosophila* genes is exacerbated by the presence of other mutant genes in the genetic background. The *Notch* gene encodes a protein containing EGF-like repeats (24) and is required during embryogenesis for the determination of cells as epithelial rather than neural. One copy of *Notch* is sufficient for this embryonic function in a wild-type genetic background. If the animal is hemizygous for another gene, *Enhancer of split*, that is also involved in the epithelial versus neural decision, then one copy of the *Notch* gene is not sufficient for embryogenesis and the animal dies at this stage (72). The embryo can tolerate the loss of one normal copy of either the *Notch* gene or the *Enhancer of split* gene but is unable to develop with a single dose of each; thus, lowering the amount of one gene product sensitizes the animal to the dosage of the other.

In the case of *abl*, the *dab* gene located in the deletions that give the HDA phenotype may encode products that interact directly with or lie on the same pathway as *abl*. Further analysis of this phenomenon must address these questions: what is the molecular structure of *dab*? Is this a specific genetic interaction; that is, how many genes might cause the phenotypic shift in the manner observed in this situation?

Identification of a gene product whose level is critical in an *abl* mutant background is being accomplished by molecular cloning of the DNA from the chromosomal region affected by the deletions. Two deletions, stE34 and st100.62, most precisely define the chromosomal region 73Bc responsible for the HDA effect (Figure 2). Of deletions in the area, stE34 removes the most proximal DNA without showing the more severe phenotype when combined with a point mutation in *abl*. st100.62, which deletes DNA slightly more proximally that stE34, shows the more severe HDA phenotype. Hence, DNA responsible for the phenotypic shift must fall between the chromosomal breakpoints of the stE34 and st100.62 deletions. We have obtained cloned DNA spanning the 35 kb of DNA between the two breakpoints that must contain part of the *dab* gene. Northern blot analysis has revealed at least one candidate for the *dab* transcript. Preliminary results indicate that the *dab* transcript shows roughly the same spatial and temporal distribution as that of the *abl* m RNA. To prove that this transcript is indeed the HDA gene, we rescued the HDA phenotypic shoft by adding back a copy of the putative *dab* gene via P element-mediated germline transformation.

Analysis of animals that are completely lacking in both *abl* and *dab* has shown that these two genes play a critical role in the formation of the embryonic central nervous system (CNS) (69b). Double *abl,dab* mutants fail to form proper axonal connections. Furthermore, removal of both *abl* and *dab* activity appears to cause no perceptible defects in the overall proliferation of epidermal cells. The presence of one functional copy of either *abl* or *dab* allows for largely normal formation of the CNS. This defect in the double mutant is apparently specific to the CNS as the peripheral nervous system appears to be intact. These results suggest that there is some functional redundancy between *abl* and *dab.* Our genetic studies have allowed us to uncover a function for *abl* in the embryonic CNS that would otherwise have been masked by the function of *dab*.

Direct biochemical tests and structure analysis of the *dab* product will not be possible until its molecular cloning and characterization are completed. If such studies demonstrate that the *dab* gene encodes a substrate for *abl* then it might be possible to isolate the homologous gene from mammalian systems using molecular probes from *Drosophila.* As in the case of the yeast *ras* homologs, the *Drosophila* tryosine kinase may act in pathways that are unrelated to those of its mammalian counterpart (73). Even so, the analysis of potentially interacting genes, such as *dab*, may indicate conserved molecular interactions that are relevant for the mammalian c-*abl* tyrosine kinase, possibly at the level of conserved domains on potential kinase substrates.

Identification of Other HDA Loci by Mutagenesis Screens

We have begun to screen for mutations in *dab* gene and other gene(s) that show a dosage sensitivity in an *abl* mutant genetic background. Of 2500 mutagenized third chromosomes screened, four independent chromosomes showed the characteristic HDA phenotypic shift. This frequency of mutations is consistent with the presence of one or two genes on the third chromosome that can show the HDA effect. These four mutations fulfilled two other criteria that allowed them to be called HDAs: the mutated chromosomes caused the more severe prepupal lethal phenotype with two different *abl* point mutations, and the combination of the mutated chromosome and an *abl* point mutation is phenotypically wild type when a transposon containing the *abl* gene is introduced into the cross; that is, the prepupal lethality is dependent on an *abl* mutant genetic background. Analysis of the point mutations using deletions in the region shows that two of the four may be alleles of *dab*.

Recently, a mutagenic screen for suppressors of the *abl* mutant phenotype was undertaken (73b). Three independent mutations which compensate for the absence of *abl* have been isolated. Genetic analysis shows that all three mutations are in a single gene which we have called *enabled* (*ena*). Animals which are lacking in normal *abl* and heterozygous for an *ena* mutation are recovered as normal looking, fertile adults. Mutations in *ena* are also capable of compensating for the partial or complete loss of *dab*.

Using Specifically Altered *abl* Proteins to Select for Mutations in Interacting Proteins

Mutagenesis screens with *Drosophila* have identified genes whose products are likely to interact directly. For example, existing point mutations in a testis-specific β-tubulin gene were used in a mutagenesis screen to isolate a nontubulin gene, *haywire*, whose product may interact with β-tubulin protein in microtuble assembly (74). In establishing a biochemical pathway through which the *abl* tyrosine kinase responds and acts, it is important to isolate genes that directly interact with *abl*. It may be possible to increase the chances of isolating such genes by introducing specifically altered *abl* genes into *Drosophila* and performing mutagenesis screens similar to those already described. Regions of the *Drosophila* protein of particular interest are the putative regulatory SH2 and SH3 domains and the tyrosine kinase catalytic domain.

A potential strategy for creating useful specific alterations in the catalytic kinase domain of *abl* exists. As mentioned previously, although the *Drosophila* and mammalian kinase domains are very similar (77% identity and 87% similarity), it appears as though they are not functionally reciprocal. The viral-fly protein can transform fibroblasts but not lymphoid cells; the full-length murine c-*abl* protein could not rescue *abl* mutant flies. This lack of functional reciprocity could be due to codivergence of the *abl* tyrosine kinase with its substrates or the acquisition and loss of substrate during evolution. Regardless, we can use the inability of the murine c-*abl* protein to function in *Drosophila* to dissect the tyrosine kinase domain to map critical regions that may be involved in substrate recognition. By replacing specific regions of the *Drosophila* kinase domain with the corresponding regions from the mammalian kinase domain, chimeric kinase domains can be made and assayed for the rescue of *abl* mutant flies. In this manner it will be possible to define a critical region (or regions) in the kinase domain that may be involved in substrate recognition. Given the conservation of the kinase domains between *Drosophila* and mammals, such an approach could map this effect to a few critical amino acids. Upon defining the amino acid(s) that gives this effect, *Drosophila* lines expressing an *abl* tyrosine kinase with the specific amino acid change will be used to select for second site mutations, which allows the mutant kinase domain to rescue the *abl* mutant phenotypes. Such mutations may lie in biologically important substrates for the *Drosophila abl* tyrosine kinase activity. The cloning and characterization of these *Drosophila* genes would provide probes for the identification of similar sequences in mammalian DNA.

SUMMARY

Abelson tyrosine kinase sequences have been highly conserved through evolution. How can we make use of the presence of *abl* sequences in *Drosophila* to help us understand the role of the *abl* tyrosine kinase in CML? First, we can try to understand better the normal physiologic role of the *abl* tyrosine kinase in the terminal differentiation and/or function of *Drosophila* neural cells. Second, we can try to identify substrates and proteins that regulate the *abl* tyrosine kinase in *Drosophila* and use these to develop molecular probes for the corresponding molecules in human cells.

ACKNOWLEDGMENTS

Our work on the *Drosophila abl* gene has been supported by a grant (NP-483) from the American Cancer Society to Hoffmann. Additional support is provided by P30-CA07175 and T32-CA09135 from the NCI. We thank Bette Sheehan, David Gunn, and Dr. Jeff Ross for carefully reading the manuscript, and Kristen Adler for typing the manuscript.

REFERENCES

1. Henkemeyer, M. J., Bennett, R. L., Gertler, F. B., and Hoffmann, F. M. (1988). DNA sequence, structure, and tyrosine kinase activity of the *Drosophila melanogaster* Abelson proto-oncogene homolog. *Mol. Cell. Biol. 8*: 843–853.
2. Durica, D. S., Restrepo, M. A., Thomas, T. L., and Beckingham, K. (1987). Isolation and characterization of *abl* gene sequences in *Calliphora erythrocephala. Gene 59*:63–76.
3. Goodard, J. M., Weiland, J. J., and Capecchi, M. R. (1986). Isolation and characterization of *Caenorhabditis elegans* DNA sequences homologous to the v-*abl* oncogene. *Proc. Natl. Acad. Sci. USA 83*:2172–2176.

4. Shilo, B.-Z. (1987). Proto-oncogenes in *Drosophila melanogaster. Trends in Genet. 3*:69–72.
5. Hoffmann, F. M. (1989). Roles of *Drosophila* proto-oncogene and growth factor homologs during development of the fly. In *Current Topics in Microbiology, Biology, and Immunology* (P. Vogt, ed.). Springer-Verlag, Berlin.
6. Hoffman-Falk, H., Einat, P., Shilo, B.-Z., and Hoffmann, F. M. (1983). *Drosophila melanogaster* DNA clones homologous to vertebrate oncogenes: Evidence for a common ancestor to the *src* and *abl* cellular genes. *Cell 32*: 589–598.
7. Hoffmann, F. M., Fresco, L. D., Hoffman-Falk, H., and Shilo, B.-Z. (1983). Nucleotide sequences of the *Drosophila src* and *abl* homologs: Conservation and variability in the *src* family oncogenes. *Cell 35*:393–401.
8. Simon, M. A., Kornberg, T. B., and Bishop, J. M. (1983). Three loci related to the *src* oncogene and tyrosine-specific protein kinase activity in *Drosophila. Nature 302*:837–839.
9. Simon, M. A., Drees, B., Kornberg, T., and Bishop, J. M. (1985). The nucleotide sequence and the tissue-specific expression of *Drosophila* c-*src*. *Cell 42*:831–840.
10. Gregory, R. J., Kammermeyer, K. L., Vincent, W. S., III, and Wadsworth, S. G. (1987). Primary sequence and development expression of a novel *Drosophila melanogaster src* gene. *Mol. Cell. Biol. 7*:2119–2127.
11. Neuman-Silberg, F. S., Schejter, E., Hoffmann, F. M., and Shilo, B.-Z. (1984). The *Drosophila ras* oncogenes: Structure and nucleotide sequence. *Cell 37*:1027–1033.
12. Mozer, B., Marlor, R., Parkhurst, S., and Corces, V. (1985). Characterization and developmental expression of a *Drosophila ras* oncogenes, *Mol. Cell. Biol. 5*:885–889.
13. Brock, H. W. (1987). Sequence and genomic structure of *ras* homologues Dm*ras*85D and Dm*ras*64B of *Drosophila melanogaster. Gene 51*:129–137.
14. Rijsewijk, F., Schuermann, M., Wagenaar, E., Parren, P., Weigel, D., and Nusse, R. (1987). The *Drosophila* homolog of the mouse mammary oncogene *int*-1 is identical to the segment polarity gene *wingless. Cell 50*:649–657.
15. Baker, N. E. (1987). Molecular cloning of sequences from *wingless*, a segment polarity gene in *Drosophila*: The spatial distribution of a transcript in embryos. *EMBO J. 6*:1765–1773.
16. Mark, G. E., MacIntyre, R. J., Digan, M. E., Ambrosio, L., and Perrimon, N. (1987). *Drosophila melanogaster* homologs of the *raf* oncogene. *Mol. Cell. Biol. 7*:2134–2140.
17. Nishida, Y., Hata, M., Ayaki, T., Ryo, H., Yamagata, M., Shimizu, K., and Nishizuka, Y. (1988). Proliferation of both somatic and germ cells is affected in the *Drosophila* mutants of *raf* proto-oncogene. *EMBO J. 7*:775–781.
18. Steward, R. (1987). *Dorsal*, an embryonic polarity gene in *Drosophila*, is homologous to the vertebrate proto-oncogene, c-*rel*. *Science 238*:692–694.

19. Pribyl, L. J., Watson, D. K., McWilliams, M. J., Ascione, R., and Papas, T. S. (1988). The *Drosophila ets*-2 gene: Molecular structure, chromosomal localization, and developmental expression. *Dev. Biol. 127*:45–53.
20. Katzen, A. L., Kornberg, T. B., and Bishop, J. M. (1985). Isolation of the proto-oncogene c-*myb* from *D. melanogaster. Cell 41*:449–456.
21. Livneh, E., Glazer, L., Segel, D., Schlessinger, J., and Shilo, B.-Z. (1985). The *Drosophila* EGF receptor gene homolog: Conservation of both hormone binding and kinase domains. *Cell 40*:599–607.
22 Schejter, E. D., Segal, D., Glazer, L., and Shilo, B.-Z. (1986). Alternative 5′ exons and tissue-specific expression of the *Drosophila* EGF receptor homolog transcripts. *Cell 46*:1091–1101.
23. Petruzzelli, L., Herrera, R., Arenas-Garcia, R., Fernandez, R., Birnbaum, M. J., and Rosen, O. M. (1986). Isolation of a *Drosophila* genomic sequence homologous to the kinase domain of the human insulin receptor and detection of the phosphorylated *Drosophila* receptor with an anti-peptide antibody. *Proc. Natl. Acad. Sci. USA 83*:4710–4174.
24. Wharton, K. A., Johansen, K. M., Xu, T., and Artavanis-Tsakonas, S. (1985). Nucleotide sequence from the neurogenic locus *Notch* implies a gene product that shares homology with proteins containing EGF-like repeats. *Cell 43*:567–581.
25. Padgett, R. W., St. Johnston, R. D., and Gelbart, W. M. (1987). A transcript from a *Drosophila* pattern gene predicts a protein homologous to the transforming growth factor-β family. *Nature 325*:81–84.
26. Baker, N. E. (1988). Embryonic and imaginal requirements for *wingless*, a segment-polarity gene in *Drosophila. Dev. Biol. 125*:96–108.
27. Ben-Neriah, Y., Bernards, A., Paskind, M., Daley, G. Q., and Baltimore, D. (1986). Alternative 5′ exons in c-*abl* mRNA. *Cell 44*:577–586.
28. Shtivelman, E., Lifshitz, B., Gale, R. P., Roe, B. A., and Canaani, E. (1986). Alternative splicing of RNAs transcribed from the human *abl* gene and from the *bcr-abl* fused gene. *Cell 47*:277–284.
29. Reddy, E. P., Smith, M. J., and Srinivasan, A. (1983). Nucleotide sequence of Abelson murine leukemia virus genome: Structural similarity of its transforming gene product to other *onc* gene products with tyrosine-specific kinase activity. *Proc. Natl. Acad. Sci. USA 80*:3623–3627.
30. Mes-Masson, A.-M., McLaughlin, J., Daley, G. Q., Paskind, M., and Witte, O. N. (1986). Overlapping cDNA clones define the complete coding region for the p210$^{c\text{-}abl}$ gene product associated with chronic myelogenous leukemia cells containing the Philadelphia chromosome. *Proc. Natl. Acad. Sci. USA 83*:9768–9772.
31. Sefton, B. M., Trowbridge, I. S., Cooper, J. A., and Scolnick, E. M. (1982). The transforming proteins of Rous sarcoma virus, Harvey sarcoma virus and Abelson virus contain tightly bound lipid. *Cell 31*:465–474.
32. Cross, F. R., Garber, E. A., Pellman, D., and Hanafusa, H. (1984). A short sequence in the p60^{src} N terminus is required for p60^{src} myristylation and membrane association and for cell transformation. *Mol. Cell. Biol. 4*:1834–1842.

33. Kamps, M. P., Buss, J. E., and Sefton, B. M. (1985). Mutation of NH_2-terminal glycine of p60*src* prevents both myristolyation and morphological transformation. *Proc. Natl. Acad. Sci. USA 82*:4625–2628.
34. Mayer, B. J., Hamaguchi, M., and Hanafusa, H. (1988). A novel viral oncogene with structural similarity to phospholipase C. *Nature 332*:272–275.
35. Stahl, M. L., Ferenz, C. R., Kelleher, K. L., Kriz, R. W., and Knopf, J. L. (1988). Sequence similarity of phospholipase C with the non-catalytic region of *src*. *Nature 332*:269–272.
36. Davis, R. L., Konopka, J. B., and Witte, O. N. (1985). Activation of thec-*abl* oncogene by viral transduction or chromosomal translocation generates altered c-*abl* proteins with similar in vitro kinase properties. *Mol. Cell. Biol. 5*: 204–213.
37. Konopka, J. B., and Witte, O. N. (1985). Detection of c-*abl* tyrosine kinase activity in vitro permits direct comparison of normal and altered *abl* gene products. *Mol. Cell. Biol. 5*:3116–2123.
38. Sadowski, I., Stone, J. C., and Pawson, T. (1986). A noncatalytic domain conserved among cytoplasmic protein-tyrosine kinase modifies the kinase function and transforming activity of Fujinami sarcoma virus p130*gag-fps*. *Mol. Cell. Biol. 6*:4396–4408.
39. Prywes, R., Foulkes, J. G., and Baltimore, D. (1985). The minimum transforming region of v-*abl* is the segment encoding protein-tyrosine kinase. *J. Virol. 54*:114–122.
40. McKeown, M., Belote, J. M., and Baker, B. S. (1987). A molecular analysis of *transformer*, a gene in *Drosophila melanogaster* that controls female sexual differentiation. *Cell 48*:489–499.
41. Henkemeyer, M. J., Gertler, F. B., Goodwin, W., and Hoffmann, F. M. (1987). The *Drosophila* Abelson proto-oncogene homolog: Identification of mutant alleles that have pleiotropic effects late in development. *Cell 51*: 821–828.
42. Rubin, G. M., and Spradling, A. C. (1982). Genetic transformation of *Drosophila* with transposable element vectors. *Science 218*:348–353.
43. Tomlinson, A., and Ready, D. F. (1987). Neuronal differentiation in the *Drosophila ommatidium*. *Dev. Biol. 120*:366–376.
44. Telford, J., Burckhardt, J., Butler, B., and Pirrotta, V. (1985). Alternative processing and developmental control of the transcripts of *Drosophila abl* oncogene homologue. *EMBO J. 4*:2609–2615.
45. Lev, Z., Leibovitz, N., Segev, O., and Shilo, B.-Z. (1984). Expression of the *src* and *abl* cellular oncogenes during development of *Drosophila melanogaster*. *Mol. Cell. Biol. 4*:982–984.
46. Wadsworth, S. C., Madhavan, K., and Bilodeau-Wentworth, D. (1985). Maternal inheritance of transcripts from three *Drosophila src*-related genes. *Nucleic Acids Res. 13*:2153–2170.
47. Fronhöfer, H. G., and Nüsslein-Volhard, C. (1986). Organization of anterior pattern in the *Drosophila* embryo by the maternal gene *bicoid*. *Nature 324*: 120–125.

48. Santamaria, P., and Nüsslein-Volhard, C. (1983). Partial rescue of *dorsal*, a maternal effect mutation affecting the dorso-ventral pattern of the *Drosophila* embryo, by the injection of wild-type cytoplasm. *EMBO J. 2*:1695–1699.
49. Hartenstein, V., and Campos-Ortego, J. A. (1985). Fate-mapping in wild-type *Drosophila melanogaster*. I. The spatio-temporal pattern of embryonic cell divisions. *Roux's Arch Dev. Biol. 194*:181–195.
50. Campos-Ortega, J. A., and Hartenstein, V. (1985). *The Embryonic Development of* Drosophila Melanogaster. Springer-Verlag, Berlin, pp. 1–84 and 144–158.
51. Truman, J. W., and Bate, M. (1988). Spatial and temporal patterns of neurogenesis in the central nervous system of *Drosophila melanogaster*. *Dev. Biol. 125*:145–157.
52 Müller, R., Slamon, D. J., Tremblay, J. M., Cline, M. J., and Verma, I. M. (1982). Differential expression of cellular oncogenes during pre- and post-natal development of the mouse. *Nature 299*:640–644.
53. Wang, J. Y. J., and Baltimore, D. (1983). Cellular RNA homologous to the Abelson murine leukemia virus transforming gene: Expression and relationship to the viral sequence. *Mol. Cell. Biol. 3*:773–779.
54. Renshaw, M. W., Capozza, M. A., and Wang, J. Y. J. (1988). Differential expression of type-specific c-*abl* mRNAs in mouse tissues and cell lines. *Mol. Cell. Biol. 8*:4547–4551.
55. Cotton, P. C., and Brugge, J. S. (1983). Neural tissues express high levels of the cellular *src* gene product pp60$^{c\text{-}src}$. *Mol. Cell. Biol. 3*:1157–1162.
56. Martinez, R., Mathey-Prevot, B., Bernards, A., and Baltimore, D. (1987). Neuronal pp60$^{c\text{-}src}$ contains a six-amino acid insertion relative to its non-neuronal counterpart. *Science 237*:411–415.
57. Levy, J. B., Dorai, T., Wang, L.-H., and Brugge, J. S. (1987). The structurally distinct form of pp60$^{c\text{-}src}$ detected in neuronal cells is encoded by a unique c-*src* mRNA. *Mol. Cell. Biol. 7*:4142–4145.
58. Maness, P. F., Sorge, L. K., and Fults, D. W. (1986). An early developmental phase of pp60$^{c\text{-}src}$ expression in the neural ectoderm. *Dev. Biol. 117*:83–89.
59. Fults, D. W., Towle, A. C., Lauder, J. M., and Maness, P. F. (1985). pp60$^{c\text{-}src}$ in the developing cerebellum. *Mol. Cell. Biol. 5*:27–32.
60. Sorge, L. K., Levy, B. T., and Maness, P. F. (1984). pp60$^{c\text{-}src}$ is developmentally regulated in the neural retina. *Cell 36*:249–257.
61. Simon (1986). Studies of c-*src* function in *Drosophila*. Ph.D. dissertation, University of California, San Francisco.
62. Vincent, W. S., III, Gregory, R. J., and Wadsworth, S. C. (1988). Embryonic expression of a *Drosophila src* gene: Alternate forms of the protein are expressed in segmental stripes and in the nervous system (submitted for publication).
63. Gonda, T. J., Sheiness, D. K., and Bishop, J. M. (1982). Transcripts from the cellular homologs of retroviral oncogenes: Distribution among chicken tissues. *Mol. Cell. Biol. 2*:617–624.

64. Kaplan, J. M., Mardon, G., Bishop, J. M., and Varmus, H. E. (1988). The first seven amino acids encoded by the v-*src* oncogene act as a myristylation signal: Lysine 7 is a critical determinant. *Mol. Cell. Biol. 8*:2435–2441.
65. Buss, J. E., Der, C. J., and Solski, P. A. (1988). The six amino-terminal amino acids of $p60^{src}$ are sufficient to cause myristylation of $p21^{v\text{-}ras}$ *Mol. Cell. Biol. 8*:3960–3963.
66. Risser, R., Potter, M., and Rowe, W. P. (1978). Abelson virus-induced lymphomagenesis in mice. *J. Exp. Med. 148*:714–726.
67. Prywes, R., Foulkes, J. G., Rosenberg, N., and Baltimore, D. (1983). Sequences of the A-MuLV protein needed for fibroblast and lymphoid cell transformation. *Cell 34*:569–579.
68. Prywes, R., Hoag, J., Rosenberg, N., and Baltimore, D. (1985). Protein stabilization explains the *gag* requirement for transformation of lymphoid cells by Abelson murine leukemia virus. *J. Virol. 54*:123–132.
69. Mathey-Prevot, B., and Baltimore, D. (1988). Recombinants within the tyrosine kinase region of v-*abl* and v-*src* identify a v-*abl* segment that confers lymphoid specificity. *Mol. Cell. Biol. 8*:234–240.
69b. Gertler, F. B., Bennett, R. L., Clark, M. J., and Hoffmann, F. M. (1989). Drosphila *abl* tryosine kinase in embryonic CNS axons: a role in axonogenesis is revealed through dosage-sensitive interactions with *disabled. Cell 58*:103–113.
70. Lewis, E. B. (1978). A gene complex controlling segmentation in *Drosophila* embryo. *Genes Dev. 1*:868–879.
71. Irish, V. F., and Gelbart, W. M. (1987). The decapentaplegic gene is required for dorsal-ventral patterning of the *Drosophila* embryo. *Genes Dev. 1*:868–879.
72. Vassin, H., Vielmetter, J., and Campos-Ortega, J. A. (1985). Genetic interactions in early neurogenesis of *Drosophila melanogaster. J. Neurogent. 2*:291–308.
73. Robinson, L. C., Gibbs, J. B., Marshall, M. S., Sigal, I. D., and Tatchell, K. (1987). *cdc*25:a component of the *ras*-adenylate cyclase pathway in *Saccharomyces cerevisiae. Science 235*:1218–1221.
73b. Gertler, F.B., Doctor, J. S., and Hoffmann, F. M. (1990). Genetic Suppression of Mutations in the *Drosophila abl* Proto-oncogene. *Science* (in press).
74. Regan, C. L., and Fuller, M. T. (1988). Interacting genes that affect microtubule function: The *nc*2 allele of the *haywire* locus fails to complement mutations in the testis-specific β-tubulin gene of *Drosophila. Genes Dev. 2*: 82–92.

3

Organization and Expression of an *abl* Gene Homolog in *Calliphora erythrocephala*

David S. Durica *University of Oklahoma, Norman, Oklahoma*

INTRODUCTION

In mammals, rearrangements involving the N-terminal region of the c-*abl* locus are clearly associated with profound changes in the protein tyrosine kinase (PTK) activity of the encoded protein (see References 1-3 for review). These changes are observed as a result of either viral transduction or somatic mutation and are correlated in both instances to neoplastic transformation. Whether changes in the properties of the *abl* protein are effected through subunit interactions with other molecules, substrate specificity, or intracellular localization is still problematic, and the physiologic function of the c-*abl* gene and its products remains unclear. DNA sequences related to the mammalian PTK genes are highly conserved within metazoans, however, implying that homologs to the vertebrate genes may be performing related functions in invertebrate systems. This supposition in now being actively investigated (see References 4 and 5 for reviews). Characterizations of *abl* gene homologs have been reported for three invertebrates: the nematode *Caenorhabditis elegans* (6) and the dipterans *Drosophila melanogaster* (see Chapter 2) (7-13) and *Calliphora erythrocephala* (14), the subject of this review. The life cycles and culture requirements of these animals make them generally more tractable to studies of oogenesis and embryonic development than vertebrate systems and, clearly, more amenable to genetic manipulation and analysis. Thus interspecific comparisons to the vertebrate PTK gene families may reveal important structural and functional relationships between these sequences, which may also have relevance to the processes of gene duplication, divergence, and fixation.

Although *D. melanogaster* is an ideal organism for both classic and in vitro genetic analysis, its small size can frustrate biochemical characterizations, particularly tissue-specific biochemical isolations of macromolecules. We have therefore undertaken the approach of using a related but much larger fly to begin an examination of c-*abl* homolog function, in which the reproductive physiology of the organism is particularly amenable to a temporal biochemical analysis during oogenesis and ontogeny and whose gene organization and expression are also of interest in terms of gene evolution. Like *Drosophila, C. erythrocephala* is a higher dipteran, belonging to a family believed to have diverged from the drosophilid lineage approximately 100 million years ago (15). Oogenesis and embryogenesis are very similar in the two organisms (16–18). The mature oocytes of *C. erythrocephala*, however, are over an order of magnitude larger in volume than those of *D. melanogaster*, as measured by total RNA content (19,20). In addition, unlike in *D. melanogaster*, oogenesis can be easily synchronized (21). The females, which normally deposit their eggs on meat, do not begin follicular maturation until provided with the defined stimulus of meat feeding. Following this stimulus, a single follicle matures in each ovariole prior to the start of a new cycle of oogenesis. These events permit the simultaneous maturation of 100–200 identically staged follicles per female. This provides an experimental situation that is easily manipulated to produce large quantities of staged oocytes. The ability to synchronize egg laying further expedites biochemical studies during embryonic, larval, and pupal development, which occur on a time scale comparable to that of *D. melanogaster.* Like *Drosophila, C. erythrocephala* also possesses polytene chromosomes (22), facilitating the cytologic mapping of cloned genes.

ORGANIZATION OF *abl*-RELATED SEQUENCES IN THE *Calliphora* GENOME

The Ce*abl* Locus

As a first step in our analysis of *abl*-related sequences in the *C. erythrocephala* genome, a restriction fragment derived from the most conserved region of the *D. melanogaster abl* tyrosine kinase domain was tested for its ability to cross-hybridize with *C. erythrocephala* genomic DNA using Southern blot analysis. Under nonstringent hybridization conditions, these experiments detected between four and eight cross-hybridizing fragments, depending on the enzyme utilized and the strain of *C. erythrocephala* examined. Similar hybridization conditions were then employed to screen a *Calliphora* genomic recombinant DNA library, leading to the recovery of a single recombinant clone, designated Ce*abl*-1. To verify that Ce*abl*-1 was homologous to the *abl* kinase domain but not to unrelated *Drosophila* sequences present on the probe, a deoxyoligonucleotide corresponding to the *Drosophila abl* kinase domain was synthesized, and the regions of Ce*abl*-1 that cross-hybridized with this oligomer were mapped, subcloned, and sequenced (14). These studies confirmed that Ce*abl*-1 was indeed an *abl* proto-oncogene homolog and established the orientation of the transcription unit within the clone.

Once a homologous kinase domain in Ce*abl*-1 was identified, a 224 nt restriction fragment from this region was used to probe genomic Southern blots under stringent hybridization criteria, to assess *abl*-related gene copy number in the *Calliphora* genome. A example of such an experiment is shown in Figure 1A, where genomic DNA isolated from populations of three different strains of the organism are digested with a battery of different enzymes. Either one or two bands are observed, depending on the enzymes chosen for the digestion. On *Sal*I-*Eco*RI double digests, genomic DNA from two different populations of flies revealed a pair of hybridizing bands that migrated at 4.8 and 11 kb; a third strain showed only a single 11 kb band. The simplest interpretation of these data suggests that a single *abl* gene homolog is present in the *C. erythrocephala* genome and that the differences between the strains in banding patterns and signal intensity represent allelic polymorphism at this locus. This is further supported by Southern blot analysis of DNA samples isolated from individual progeny recovered from single pair matings, in which the hybridization patterns observed are consistent with the 4.8 and 11 kb fragments segregating as alleles.

Regions of Ce*abl*-1 were then used as a hybridization probe to screen genomic libraries, leading to the recovery of four additional clones (Ce*abl*-2, 3, 4, and 5) corresponding to the Ce*abl* locus. All these isolates contain either a 4.8 kb or 11 kb *Eco*RI-*Sal*I restriction fragment carrying the PTK domain, and restriction maps of two clones representative of these classes are presented in Figure 2. An inspection of the restriction map indicates that clones Ce*abl*-1 ("4.8 kb" class) and Ce*abl*-2 ("11 kb" class) share some common restriction sites, although they differ markedly in their overall organization. The two clones show restriction site polymorphisms at the extreme 5′ region of the inserts, although a sequence element that is highly repeated in the *Calliphora* genome is observed within a 3.7 kb *Sal*I-*Eco*RI restriction fragment in Ce*abl*-1 and a 2.0 kb *Hind*III restriction fragment in Ce*abl*-2 (Figure 2). Interestingly, this repetitive sequence is absent in the other clones (14). A 1.9 kb *Eco*RI-*Ava*I fragment (region A, Figure 2) is found in all clones, however, and sequence analysis (discussed later) has determined that the PTK domain spans this *Ava*I site. A 2.0 kb *Hind*III-*Eco*RI fragment located immediately 5′-ward of the PTK domain is observed in both Ce*abl*-1 and Ce*abl*-2 and is highly conserved at the nucleotide level in the area surrounding the *Eco*RI site (discussed later). The 3′ regions immediately downstream of the common *Ava*I site also cross-hybridize between these two clones (region B, Figure 2). The restriction maps for Ce*abl*-1 and Ce*abl*-2 again begin to diverge, however, downstream of the PTK domain, within the 3′ region of the gene. Southern blot analysis using probes derived from the last two coding exons (exon 9 and 10) of the *D. melanogaster abl* gene (13) hybridize at reduced strin-

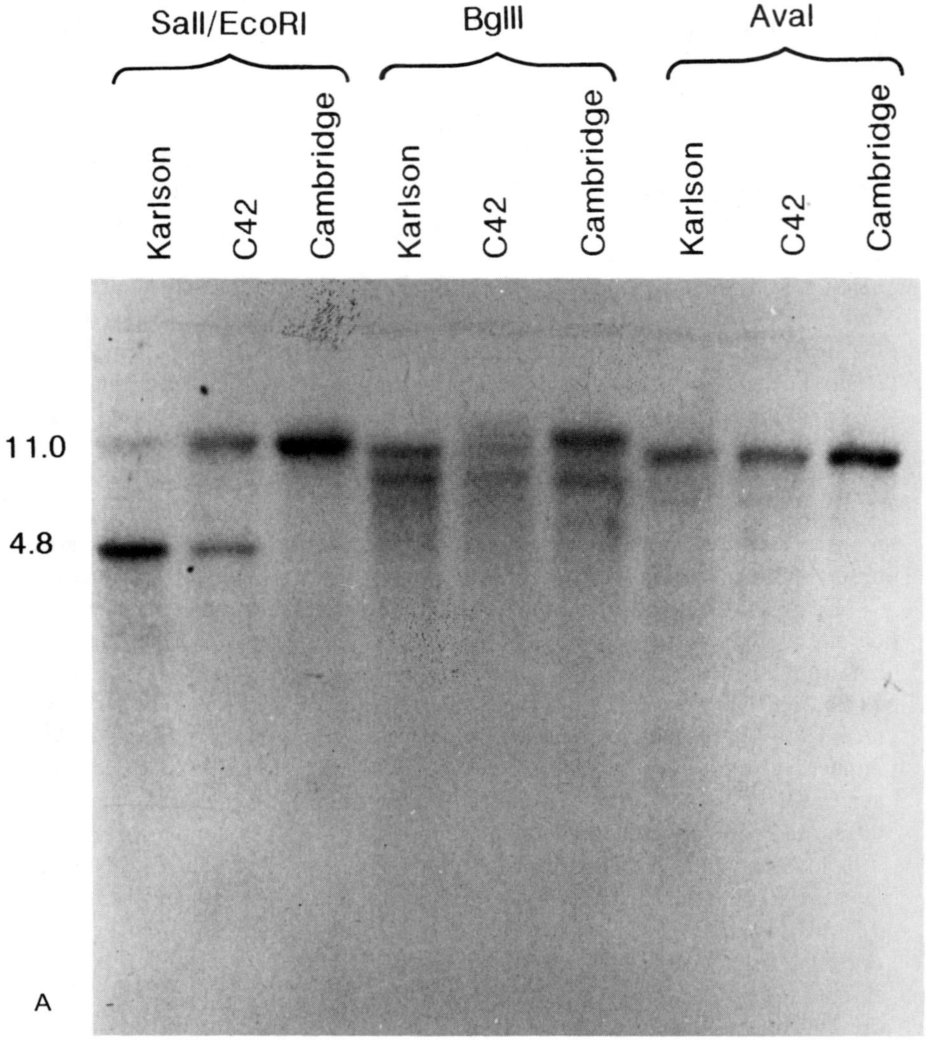

Figure 1 Representation of Ce*abl*-1 sequences in genomic DNA. Southern blots of *Eco*R1-*Sal*I- (lanes 1–3), *Bgl*II- (lanes 4–6), and *Ava*I- (lanes 7–9) digested genomic DNA, isolated from the Karlson (lanes 1, 4, and 7), C42 (lanes 2, 5, and 8), and Cambridge (lanes 3, 6, and 9) stocks were hybridized to (A) the 224 nt *Hpa*II-*Ava*II coding region fragment of Ce*abl*-1, radiolabeled by nick translation; and (B) the 4.8 kb *Eco*R1-*Sal*I fragment of Ce*abl*-1, radiolabeled by nick translation. (From Ref. 14.)

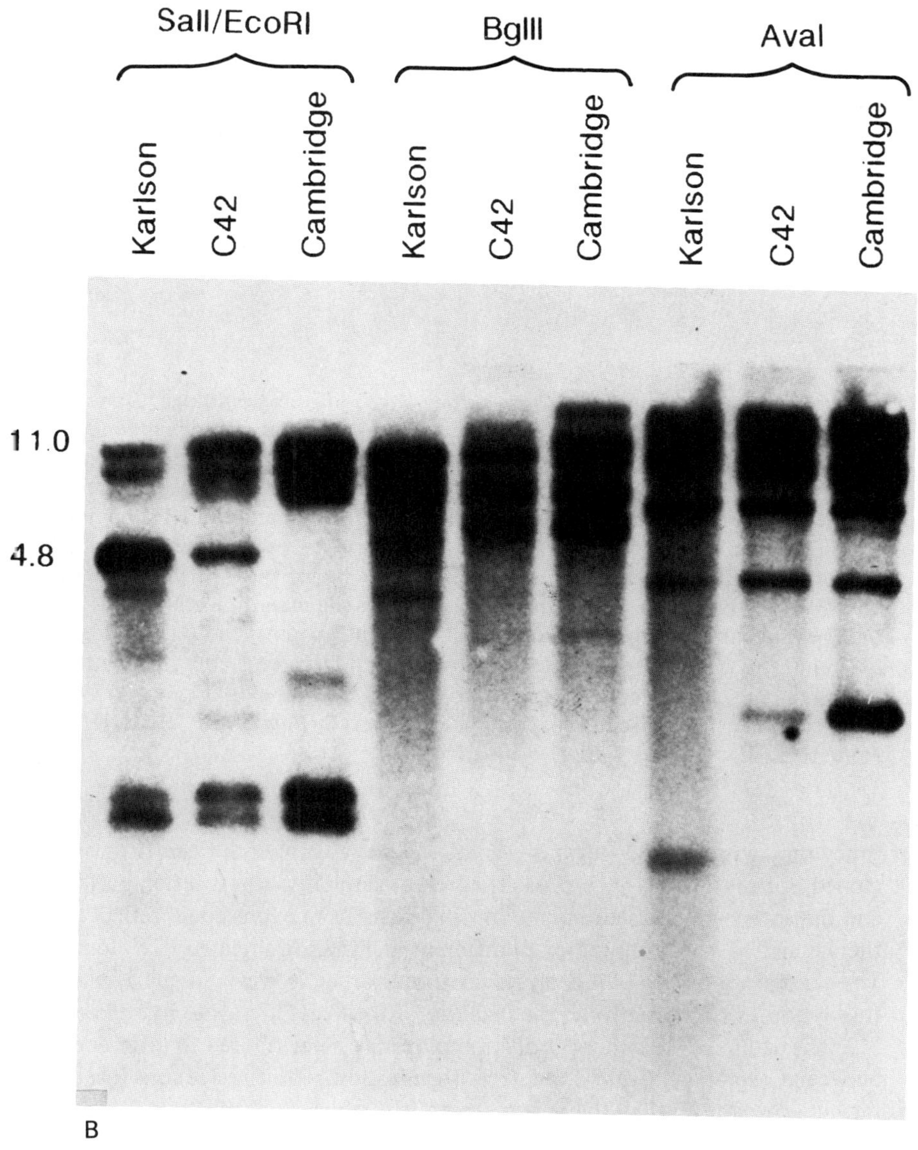

Figure 1 (continued)

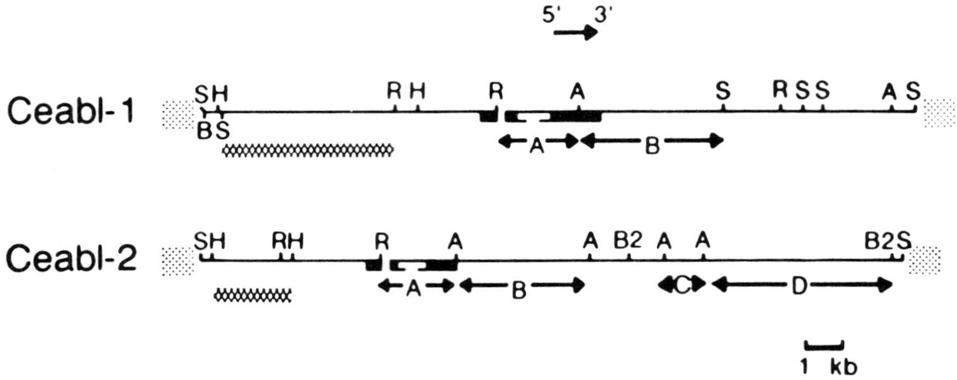

Figure 2 Restriction maps of *C. erythrocephala abl* gene homologs. Cloned regions of the *Calliphora* genome are indicated by solid lines, vector sequences by stippled blocks. The regions of the Ce*abl*-1 and Ce*abl*-2 clones that have been sequenced are indicated as a solid block below the map; as discussed in the text, this region corresponds to the N-terminus of the protein and the PTK domain. Coding sequences are indicated in black, intron sequences in white. A large 1 kb intron falls between the ATP binding site and the major tyrosine phosphorylation site (see Figure 3). The double arrows below the map indicate regions of the *Calliphora* gene that cross-hybridize with different exons of the *D. melanogaster abl* gene, and the checked bars indicate restriction fragments containing a repetitive sequence common to both the Ce*abl*-1 and Ce*abl*-2 clones (see text). Symbols for the enzymes used in mapping are A, *Ava*I; B, *Bam*HI; B2, *Bgl*II, H, *Hin*dIII; R, *Eco*RI, and S, *Sal*I.

gency only with Ce*abl*-2 (regions C and D, Figure 2), not with Ce*abl*-1 or other cloned isolates of the 4.8 kb class. The lack of similarity in restriction pattern and the absence of sequence homology in downstream exons could reflect that the 4.8 and 11 kb classes represent different loci sharing a related PTK domain. The genomic Southern blot analyses discussed earlier, however, argue against this hypothesis. Alternatively, the inability of the Ce*abl*-1 class to hybridize to 3′ exons of the *D. melanogaster abl* homolog may be attributed to differences between Ce*abl*-1 and Ce*abl*-2 in intron organization, with the 3′ exons located farther downstream than the region cloned in Ce*abl*-1. Such allele polymorphism due to variations in intron structure has been observed in other single copy genes in the Calliphoridae. Recent studies on the molecular cloning of the *topaz* gene in a related blowfly, *Lucilia cuprina,* indicate major restriction fragment polymorphisms between alleles due to differences in interspersed repetitive DNA located within introns (Elizur and Howell, personal communication, cited in Reference 21).

```
CAACATTCATTAAATGAATATTTGTTTTGATTTAAACAGACAGAAATTAGCCTAGACAAAAACACACTCACAGAT
                                        TERphelysglnthrgluileserleuasplysasnthrleuthrasp

                                                                     begin homology Dm.
                                                                   ▼ abl exon 3, aa. 130
TACTTTTATTACAAACATATTTTAATTGAATTTTATTTACTTTTTCCTATGATTTCAGAAGCTCTCTTGCAATCG
tyrphetyrtyrlyshisileleuileglupheTyrleuleupheproMETIleSerGluAlaLeuLeuGlnSer

                                        [thrargproleuphetrpargilealagluleuglnglnhis]
AGACCCCTGCCACATATACCAGCTGGTAGCTCACTACTAGGCGGTGTACCAGACACAGGCGACCTTTTGGGACAA
ArgProLeuProHisIleProAlaGlySerSerLeuLeuGlyGlyValProAspThrGlyAspLeuLeuGlyGln

                                                       restart homology, aa. 174 of
                                                       Drosophila abl
[glnaspser] [glyleuglyleuglnglyserserleugly]***▽                              [val]
AGTCAAGATGGCATTTCATTGCACACAACACAATCACATAGTCAGGGGGGACACAGTTCAACTACATCGGGGTTT
SerGlnAspGlyIleSerLeuHisThrThrGlnSerHisSerGlnGlyGlyHisSerSerThrThrSerGlyPhe

      begin homology, aa. 45 of murine c-abl type I cDNA
      ▼                                                                    A
GAGTCAGCCCACAGATGGACTTCCAAAGAAAATCTCTTAAGGCCTGGACCCGAAGAAGATGATCCACAGTTGTTT
GluSerAlaHisArgTrpThrSerLysGluAsnLeuLeuAlaProGlyProGluGluAspAspProGlnLeuPhe
         Ala      Asn                           ***     Ser    Asn      Asn

GTGGCTTTGTATGATTTTCAGGCGGGCGGAGAAAATCAGTTGAGCCTCAAGAAGGGTGAACAAGTACGCATATTA
ValAlaLeuTyrAspPheGlnAlaGlyGlyGluAsnGlnLeuSerLeuLysLysGlyGluGlnValArgIleLeu
                  Val    Ser   Asp   Thr       IleThr           LysLeu  Val

                                                                           v-abl
                     T                                                         ▼
TCGTACAACAAGTCAGGCGAATGGTGTGAGGCCCACTCCGATTCAGGCAATGTGGGCTGGGTGCCCTCAAATTAT
SerTyrAsnLysSerGlyGluTrpCysGluAlaHisSerAspSerGlyAsnValGlyTrpValProSerAsnTyr
Gly      HisAsn                          GlnThrLysAsn    Gln***

GTTACACCCCTG--EcoR1  site--AATTCCTTGGAAAAACATTCCTGGTATCATGGTCCCATATCGAGAAAT
ValThrProLeu                AsnSerLeuGluLysHisSerTrpTyrHisGlyProIleSerArgAsn
Ile      Val                                                           Val

GCGGCCGAATATCTATTAAGTTCGGGTATAAATGGTAGTTTCCTGGTAAGAGAAAGTGAAAGTTCACCAGGTCAA
AlaAlaGluTyrLeuLeuSerSerGlyIleAsnGlySerPheLeuValArgGluSerGluSerSerProGlyGln
      Gly
```

Figure 3 Comparative sequence analysis, Ce*abl*-1 and Ce*abl*-2, murine c-*abl*, and *D. melanogaster abl*. The nucleotide sequence of the *C. erythrocephala abl* homolog Ce*abl*-1 is presented and aligned with the amino acid sequences deduced for the 5′ coding region of the murine type I c-*abl* transcript and the *Drosophila abl* gene. Homology to the murine gene begins 45 amino acids into the murine primary sequence; for the *Drosophila* sequence, homology begins 130 amino acids into the *D. melanogaster abl* gene, as discussed in the text. Differences between the mouse and *Calliphora* proteins are indicated below the Ce*abl*-1 sequence; differences between the two dipteran proteins are indicated above the Ce*abl*-1 sequence. Over the region sequenced, the Ce*abl*-1 and Ce*abl*-2 genes encode identical proteins; nucleotide substitutions are indicated in italics.

```
                                                                    C
AGAAGTATTAGTTTAAGGTAAATACAATTTTTTGTAACTAAATTATTTTGAAATTAAAATTTAATTTCAATATTT
ArgSerIleSerLeuAr--------------------intron (71 nt)------------------------

      T
GTTTAAATTTTAGATATGAAGGACGTGTTTATCATTATCGAATATCTGAAGATCCCGATGGTAAAGTGTTTGTG
-------------gTyrGluGlyArgValTyrHisTyrArgIleSerGluAspProAspGlyLysValPheVal
                                              AsnThrAlaSer          LeuTyr

  [gln]
ACAGCCGAAGCCAAATTTAATACTCTCGCCGAATTGGTGCACCATCACAGTGTGCCACACGAGGGTCATGGACTG
ThrAlaGluAlaLysPheAsnThrLeuAlaGluLeuValHisHisHisSerValProHisGluGlyHisGlyLeu
SerSer   SerArg                                     ThrValAlaAsp******
                                                                    [←PTK
ATTACACCCCTCTTGTATCCAGCACCAAAGCAAAATAAACCAACAGTATTTCCTCTAAGTCCCGAACCCGATGAA
IleThrProLeuLeuTyrProAlaProLysGlnAsnLysProThrValPheProLeuSerProGluProAspGlu
      Thr   His                Arg               IleTyrGlyVal      AsnTyr   Lys

                        [met]           T
TGGGAAATTTGCCGCACTGATATTGTTATGAAACACAAACTGGGTGGTGGCCAATATGGTGAAGTTTATGAGGCG
TrpGluIleCysArgThrAspIleValMetLysHisLysLeuGlyGlyGlyGlnTyrGlyGluValTyrGluAla
      MetGlu            Thr                                                Gly
[val]
ATATGGAAACGTTATGGCAATACGGTTGCTGTTAAAACACTTAAAGAAGATACAATGGCCCTTAAGGATTTCCTT
IleTrpLysArgTyrGlyAsnThrValAlaValLYSThrLeuLysGluAspThrMetAlaLeuLysAspPheLeu
Val      Lys   SerLeu                                      GluValGluGlu

GAAGAGGCAGCCATTATGAAAGAAATGAAACATCCCAATTTAGTGCAACTAATTGGTAAGTAAAGACCAAAACTG
GluGluAlaAlaIleMetLysGluMetLysHisProAsnLeuValGlnLeuIleG---intron,~1.1 kb---
Lys         Val         Ile                         Leu

N(~700 nt)TTATTAATTTAAGTACTTTGAACAAATTAAATAATCTTGAACATATGAGCTAAAAATGTGAGGAA

AGAAGAGTGGTACCTGAAGTAGTTAACATTTGTTGAAAACCAATGAATTTGTTGTCATTGGAGGAATGTTGTTAA

                                              T  A
TTTTTGACAACTTGTACTGTAGTTAGATGTAATATTTAAGTAAGGTGTACTAAGGATTTTGATTTGCTCAATATT

                                             C             C
AACTCATTATTGTCCTGAAAAAGAGTTTTTTAAACTGACCACTAAAATGTTAACTTTATGTTTAATATTTCCTCT

C
TATTTTTATATTTCTTCCTTAGGTGTATGTACCCGTGAGCCACCATTCTATATAATCACTGAATTTATGTCTCAT
----------------------lyValCysThrArgGluProProPheTyrIleIleThrGluPheMetSerHis
                                                                     ThrTyr

GGCAATTTGTTGGATTTCCTGCGATCAGCCGGGCGTGAGACCCTCGATGCCGTAGCCCTGCTGTATATGGCAACG
GlyAsnLeuLeuAspPheLeuArgSerAlaGlyArgGluThrLeuAspAlaValAlaLeuLeuTyrMetAlaThr
                Tyr      GluCysAsn    GlnGluValSer      Val

                               [ser]
CAAATAGCGTCGGGCATGAGTTATTTGGAAGCTCGTAATTACATACATCGTGACTTGGCTGCCCGTAATTGTTTG
GlnIleAlaSerGlyMetSerTyrLeuGluAlaArgAsnTyrIleHisArgAspLeuAlaAlaArgAsnCysLeu
      Ser   Ala   Glu           LysLys   Phe
```

Figure 3 (continued)

```
GTGGGCGATAATAAATTGGTTAAAGTGGCCGATTTTGGTTTGGCTCGTCTGATGCGTGATGACACCTATACGGCA
ValGlyAspAsnLysLeuValLysValAlaAspPheGlyLeuAlaArgLeuMetArgAspAspThrTYRThrAla
      Glu   His                                  Ser           ThrGly

CATGCGGGCGCCAAGTTTCCCATCAAATGGACxxx  45 nt  xxCGGATGTGTGGGCGTTCGGTGTGCTGCTA
HisAlaGlyAlaLysPheProIleLysTrpThr                 AspValTrpAlaPheGlyValLeuLeu
                                    ala                   tyr         asp
TGGGAAATAGCCACGTATGGCATGTCGCCATATCCGGGCATCGATCTAACCGATGTTTTTCATAAATTGGAGAAA
TrpGluIleAlaThrTyrGlyMetSerProTyrProGlyIleAspLeuThrAspValPheHisLysLeuGluLys
                                                    SerGln    TyrGluLeu

                                                                          asp
GGTTATCGCATGGAAAGGCCACCGGGCTGTCCACCAGAAGTGTATGATTTAATGCGTCAATGTTGGCAATGGAAT
GlyTyrArgMetGluArgProProGlyCysProProGluValTyrAspLeuMetArgGlnCysTrpGlnTrpAsn
Asp                 Glu         GluLys        Glu         Ala

  thr                                                          intron, D.m. abl
            PTK→]                                                 ⬇
GCGGCGGATAGGCCCACATTTAAAAGCATACATCATGCTTTGGAACATATGTTTCAGGTGG
AlaAlaAspArgProThrPheLysSerIleHisHisAlaLeuGluHisMetPheGln
ProSer          Ser   AlaGlu        Gln    Phe    Thr
```

Figure 3 (continued)

Nucleotide sequence analysis of the Ce*abl*-1 and Ce*abl*-2 clones is also consistent with the assumption that these sequences represent alleles of the same chromosomal locus. The regions thus far determined bracket the *Eco*RI and *Ava*I sites that are common to both clones (Figures 2 and 3). In Figure 3, the nucleotide sequence of Ce*abl*-1 is given. Nucleotide substitutions that occur in Ce*abl*-2 are indicated above the Ce*abl*-1 sequence in italics. In this highly conserved region, the nucleotide sequences of Ce*abl*-1 and Ce*abl*-2 encode identical proteins and show only 0.6% mismatch; 10 substitutions between the clones are observed, with the majority occurring within presumed intervening sequence DNA.

The sequencing strategy for Ce*abl*-1 and Ce*abl*-2 has focused on the amino-terminal portion of the encoded protein and the PTK coding domain. In Figure 3, the deduced amino acid sequence for the Ce*abl* locus is given below the nucleotide sequence for Ce*abl*-1 and is compared to both the deduced murine type I sequence (23,24) and the sequence of the *D. melanogaster* protein (13). Amino acid identities between the mammalian sequence and the *Calliphora* sequence are indicated in bold type in the figure; highly conservative replacements are indicated in regular type, and other replacements are depicted in italics. The deduced primary sequence for the *Calliphora* protein allows four codon insertions relative to the mouse protein; to maintain optimal alignment, these sites are indicated by asterisks. Over the region sequenced, the open reading frame is interrupted at four positions by sequences containing canonical consensus splice junctions. Introns at precisely these positions are also observed in the *D. melanogaster abl* gene, although there is no similarity at the sequence level. The characterized intron-exon junctions within the PTK domain are not conserved when the mouse genomic sequences are compared to the two dipteran *abl* homologs (23,24). The *C. elegans abl* gene (6) also shows a different intron-exon organization. Within coding DNA, the *Drosophila* and *Calliphora abl* genes share only 68% homology at the nucleotide level, due primarily to third-base substitutions (14).

This locus clearly represents an *abl* PTK gene homolog sharing extremely strong similarity with the vertebrate c-*abl* genes (23–26) as well as with the *D. melanogaster abl* gene (13). The kinase domain (26) is enclosed by brackets in Figure 3. Within this region, eight conservative amino acid replacements (indicated above the sequence in enclosed boxes, Figure 3) distinguish the *Calliphora* sequence from the *D. melanogaster abl* protein. This represents 96.8% identity within the PTK domain (242 of 250 residues; a region of 14 amino acids within the kinase domain has not been completely determined and is excluded in this analysis). In comparison to the murine sequence, the *C. erythrocephala* protein shares 73% identity within this region. The most highly conserved features of the *abl* PTK domain are also conserved in the *Calliphora* sequence. These include the putative ATP binding site, sequences corresponding to the major site of autophosphorylation, and amino acids that have been observed to be invariant in comparisons between the vertebrate PTK genes (1-3).

Furthermore, the Ce*abl* locus shares sequence similarity upstream of the catalytic domain of murine *abl*, extending 73 codons 5′-ward of the segment of the murine gene transduced by Abelson murine leukemia virus. The human and mouse genes are known to encode variable 5′ exons (24,25) that are differentially spliced onto a common exon; homology between the Ce*abl* locus and the murine gene can be detected throughout most of the murine common exon. Similarity between the two sequences ends 17 codons upstream of the beginning of the common exon, corresponding to amino acid 45 of the murine *abl* type I cDNA (Figure 3). Beyond this point, there is no detectable positional similarity, although the murine type I protein (24), the homolog human type Ia protein (25), and the *Calliphora* protein contain a five amino acid stretch of hydroxylated amino acids. Between the kinase domain and the end of the detected homology, the predicted amino acid sequences are identical at 76.5% of the residues (140 of 183), and if conservative replacements are considered, this homology can be extended to 88.5% (162 of 183). Thus, the vertebrate and *Calliphora* primary amino acid sequences begin to diverge at approximately the region of the protein where variations in the N-terminus are detected intraspecifically due to differential processing of the vertebrate *abl* transcripts.

From primer extension studies, sequence analysis of cDNA clones, and tests of *abl* function in transgenic animals, a 5′ boundary to the *D. melanogaster abl* transcription unit has been localized (Reference 13 and Chapter 2). The deduced amino acid sequence for the N-terminus of this protein is considerably longer than that observed for the various vertebrate *abl* N-termini, with amino acid 45 in the murine type I *abl* protein and amino acid 63 of the murine type IV protein corresponding to amino acid 187 of the *Drosophila* protein. Similarly to the murine type IV and the human type Ib sequences, the deduced N-terminus of the *Drosophila* protein contains a potential site for myristylation (13). The transcription start point and N-terminal sequences of the *Drosophila* gene span three exons (13); amino acid 187 falls within the third exon, which begins at codon 130. The intron-exon junction corresponding to exon 3 is apparently conserved between the *Drosophila* and *Calliphora* genes (Figure 3). A consensus 3′ splice junction is present at this position in both Ce*abl*-1 and Ce*abl*-2, and the first 16 amino acids are identical between the two species. The sequence of the two *Calliphora* clones diverges radically from the published *Drosophila* sequence (13), however, over the next 30 codons. Over this region, the *Calliphora* sequence encodes an additional amino acid residue, and no similarity between the *Drosophila* and *Calliphora* primary sequences is obvious (Figure 3). Sequence homology then resumes at amino acid 174 of the *Drosophila* protein, and the two loci show only a single conservative change (gly →val at amino acid 182 of the *Drosophila* protein) until the beginning of the PTK domain. Although the divergence observed between the *Calliphora* and *Drosophila* sequence falls within a domain of the protein that shows distinct interspecific and intraspecific variability, the significance of this finding is at present unclear. Given the strong similarity observed on either side of the divergent region, a likely explanation for the incongruity is sequencing error. This region of the *D. melanogaster abl* gene is currently being re-examined (Hoffmann, personal communication).

On Southern blot analysis, neither the Ce*abl*-1 nor the Ce*abl*-2 clone contains sequences related to the first or second exons of the *Drosophila abl* gene, nor have these regions been observed to cross-hybridize with *Calliphora* genomic DNA. A detailed description of the 5′ region of the Ce*abl* locus therefore requires the recovery and analysis of cDNA clones to determine the extent of homology to vertebrate sequences and more accurately assess whether this locus contains multiple 5′ exons that can direct the synthesis of alternative mRNA species.

As discussed earlier, low stringency hybridization analysis suggested substantial divergence between the 3′ coding regions of the *Drosophila abl* gene and Ce*abl*-2. A 3200 nucleotide segment within the cross-hybridizing region has recently been determined (Robinson and Durica, unpublished), beginning at a *Bgl*II site with the 3′ region of Ce*abl*-2 (Figure 2). An amino acid sequence was deduced from the longest opening reading frames and consensus intron/exon junctions, then computer-aligned to the *Drosophila abl* protein. Alignment with the *Drosophila abl* protein begins within exon 9 and continues through the termination codon (13). The degree of similarity observed between the two dipteran genes in this region is much less than that observed for the PTK domain. The overall identity of the two encoded proteins within exon 9 and 10 is approximately 60% (compared to 97% within the PTK domain). Identities are strongest at the extreme carboxyl termini of the deduced proteins, while considerable divergence is observed surrounding the putative exon 9 and 10 boundaries. Allowing for maximum conservation of coding sequences, 18 gaps have been introduced into the alignment, ranging from 1 to 28 codons in length. Several of the gapped regions contain unbroken stretches of glutamine residues. Interspecific differences in polyglutamine tracts have been observed for the rat and human glucocorticoid receptors (27), while homopolymeric stretches of amino acids, including polyglutamine tracts, have also been reported in a number of developmentally regulated genes of *Drosophila* (28,29). The significance of these tracts in unknown. Searches of the unannotated GENBANK database using the 3′ Ce*abl*-2 sequence detected weak similarity between the extreme carboxyl-terminal region of Ce*abl* and the mouse c-*abl* gene, comparable to that observed between the *Drosophila* and human *abl* genes (13).

Additional *abl*-Related Sequences Within the *Calliphora* Genome

As discussed earlier, low-stringency hybridizations using a *Drosophila* PTK probe generated multiple cross-hybridizing bands on genomic Southern blots, which varied depending on the strain of fly used in the analysis. Similarly, when the 4.8 kb *Eco*RI-*Sal*I fragment of Ce*abl*-1 used as a hybridization probe, between five and eight strongly hybridizing fragments can be detected, depending on the enzyme used for digestion (Figure 1B). The restriction fragments characteristic of the Ce*abl* locus represent a subset of these bands. As revealed in Figure 1B, these cross-hybridizing sequences show population polymorphism between strains. To minimize the effects of population polymorphism, genomic Southern blots have also been performed on DNA isolated from single flies. On *Eco*RI + *Sal*I digests, four bands distinct from those associated with the Ce*abl* locus are normally observed, migrating at 9.5, 2.3, 1.7, and 1.6 kb. Of these, fragments migrating at 2.3 and 1.6 kb cross-hybridize to a *D. melanogaster abl* PTK domain probe. These results suggest that there are, at a minimum, two additional genes other than the Ce*abl* locus that share homology to the *D. melanogaster abl* PTK domain. In *D. melanogaster,* a number of genes have been characterized that fall within both the receptor class (30–32) and cytoplasmic class (33–35) of protein kinase homologs (reviewed in References 4 and 5). Using Southern blot analysis and in situ hybridization to polytene chromosomes, three loci cross-hybridize with v-*src* probes; the *abl* locus at band 73B of chromosome 3 (8) and the

Dsrc28C (34) and Dsrc (33) genes located at bands 28C and 64B of chromosomes 2 and 3, respectively. Comparisons between the Dsrc, Dsrc28C, and *abl* sequences indicates approximately 50% amino acid identity between the three encoded proteins within the PTK domain (34). Thus, Dsrc and Dsrc28C would be the most likely homologs to the cross-hybridizing sequences observed in the *C. erythrocephala* genome. We are currently attempting to examine the relationship of these sequences in the *C. erythrocephala* genome by in situ hybridization.

TRANSCRIPTION OF THE Ce*abl* LOCUS

Transcription of the *abl-src* Homologs of *D. melanogaster*

In *D. melanogaster,* Northern blot analysis of *abl*, Dsrc, and Dsrc28C gene transcripts indicates that the mRNAs of all three genes are actively transcribed during oogenesis, with the transcripts stored as maternal mRNA (10,11,33,34,36). Dsrc transcript localization during ontogeny has also been examined by in situ hybridization (33). Prior to 8.5 h of development, Dsrc transcripts appear uniformly distributed; thereafter, transcript accumulation becomes concentrated in presumptive neural structures and smooth muscle. Steady-state levels of Dsrc mRNA are low during late embryonic and larval development, accumulate in developing neural and presumptive visceral muscle in late larvae and early pupae, and are rare in adults, with the exception of ovarian tissue (33). RNA blot hybridizations indicate that the Dsrc28C gene, in addition to being expressed during oocyte development, is active during embryogenesis and in imaginal discs of third-instar larvae (34). Recently, the Dsrc28C protein has also been shown to accumulate in neuronal tissues during development and in imaginal cells (Wadsworth, personal communication).

Analysis of steady-state concentrations of *abl* mRNA indicates a biphasic developmental profile of transcript accumulation, in which mRNA levels are lowest during the larval stages (10,11,36). Northern blot analysis indicates that *abl* transcript levels are maximal in the egg, decline markedly following the rapid cleavage divisions of early embryogenesis, and remain low in larvae. They increase during early pupal development and again fall off in adults. Females have significantly higher mRNA levels than males, presumably owing to transcription during oogenesis (10,11,36). Using probes spanning the entire *abl* PTK domain and adjacent sequences, Northern blot analysis (10,11) has detected a broad band estimated between 7.5 and 5.5 kb; a discrete band at 3.0 kb has also been described (11). S_1 analysis indicates that the larger mRNA species is subject to tissue-specific differences in 3′ processing, including the alternative processing of a 3′ intron and multiple poly(A) addition sites (11). The origin of the 3.0 kb transcript is problematic; it has not been detected in all studies (10) and apparently does not hybridize at stringent criteria with probes derived from the most conserved region of *abl*, leading to the assumption that this region of the transcript is processed out of the 3.0 kb mENA (11). The size heterogeneity pattern of the large 7.5–5.5 kb mRNA changes during development, with maternal and early embryo transcripts containing a smaller mRNA class than transcripts from later stages (11).

Although measurements of overall *abl* transcript abundance correlate with stages of the *Drosophila* life cycle in which rapid cell proliferation is observed (10,11,36), recent genetic studies on the zygotic effects of *abl* mutations indicate transcription from this locus is not required for the proliferation of tissues responsible for adult structures (Reference 12 and Chapter 2). Although flies that are homozygous for recessive loss of function alleles of *abl* have reduced viability, typically dying prior to emerging from the pupal case, these pharate adults exhibit few phenotypic anomalies (12). Overt morphologic defects are limited to abnormalities of the retina, or, in combination with second-site mutations, disruptions in axonal organization of the central nervous system ((27) and Chapter 2). Thus *abl* gene transcription in the zygote, like D*src*, appears correlated with the differentiation of neural tissues. It should be emphasized that these zygotic effects do not address the question of *abl* gene function during early embryogenesis, since wild-type, maternally derived *abl* transcripts are present in mutant embryos.

Comparison of Ce*abl* Transcription to the *D. melanogaster abl* Locus

When *C. erythrocephala* oocyte poly(A)+ RNA is subjected to Northern blot analysis using a nick-translated 224 nt DNA probe derived from the Ce*abl* PTK domain, a distribution of at least four discrete mRNA transcript sizes, centering around ~6.5 kb, is observed (Figure 4). These size classes are approximately 10.5, 9, 6.5 and 4.4 kb, respectively. Since rehybridizing the same filters with an actin-coding region probe detects a single band (Figure 4), the heterogeneity of Ce*abl* transcripts does not appear to be due to generalized RNA degradation, suggesting that the variability results from differential processing. Steady-state concentrations of Ce*abl* transcripts have been estimated through their relative abundance in cDNA populations prepared from several stages of embryogenesis (de Valoir, Beckingham, and Durica, unpublished) and by Northern blot analysis (Voelker and Durica, unpublished). Transcripts begin to accumulate in immature oocytes and are stored as maternal mRNA. They are readily observed through at least eight hours of development, when the embryo is undergoing germ band shortening and abdominal segmentation (18), and are detectable until approximately 12–15 hours. As discussed previously, embryonic *Drosophila abl* transcripts begin to decrease in abundance much earlier, declining radically by gastrulation (3.4 hours). Ce*abl* transcript levels decline by 15 hours and remain low throughout the larval stage. A subset then reappears during pupal development,

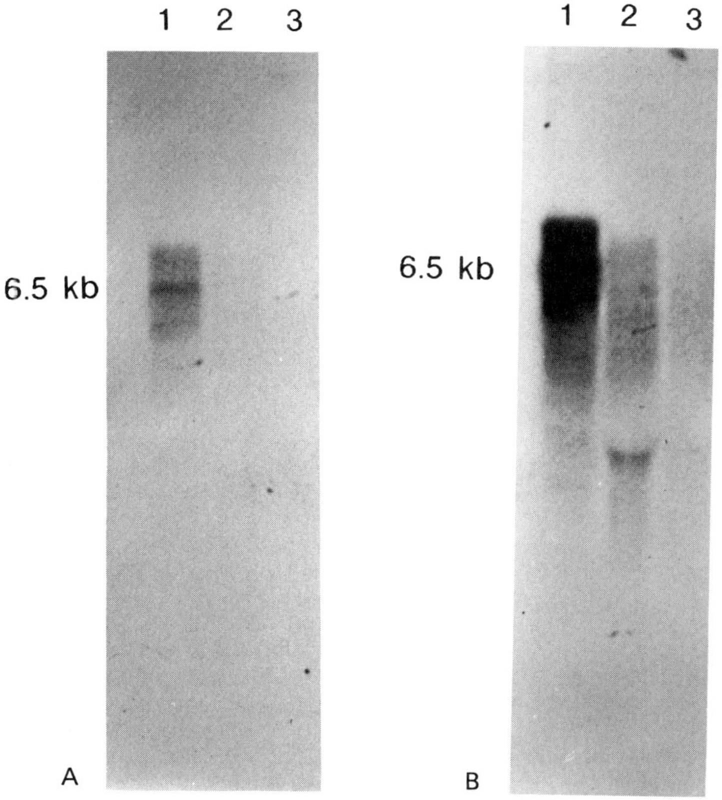

Figure 4 Localization of *abl* homologous RNA to mature oocytes. (A and B). Oocyte poly(A)+ RNA (5 μg) (lane 1) and 15 μg oocyte poly(A)– and total RNA (lanes 2 and 3, respectively) were glyoxylated, electrophoresed on 1.0% agarose gels, transferred to nitrocellulose, and hybridized to the 224 nt *Hpa*II-*Ava*II fragment of pCe*abl*1–4.8, which had been radiolabeled by nick translation. Following transfer and hybridization, the filter was autoradiographed for 4 h (A) and 18 h (B), respectively. (C) The filter used in A was washed to remove bound probe and then rehybridized to nick-translated plasmid DNA containing the entire *D. melanogaster* 88F actin gene. The autoradiograph represents a 96 h exposure. (From Ref. 14.)

where the two larger mRNA species (10.5 and 9 kb) are detected in isolated heads. Thus, Ce*abl* transcripts undergo developmental changes in abundance and size distribution pattern, apparently persist to later embryonic stages than *abl* transcripts in *Drosophila,* and show a pattern of expression in pupae consistent with transcription in neural tissue.

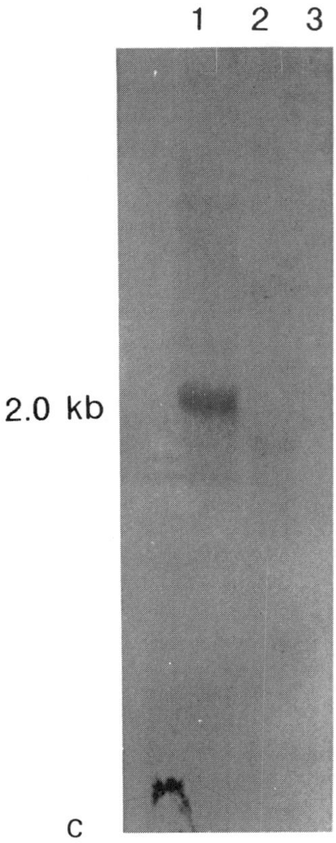

Figure 4 (continued)

Northern blot analysis using a coding region probe derived from sequences 3 of the PTK domain (region C, Figure 2) reveal the same transcript distribution as observed with the PTK probe. In preliminary experiments, antisense probes have also been synthesized which are complementary to a region 5′-ward of the PTK domain, corresponding to the beginning of the *D. melanogaster* exon 3 and the murine *c-abl* common exon. This region, which shows similarity to a domain found in a bovine phospholipase C gene (38) and the avian sarcoma virus CT10 *crk* oncogene (39), identified essentially the same transcript distribution as the aforementioned PTK and 3′ probes. Surprisingly, however, sense probes derived from a putative Ce*abl* intron located approximately 2 kb 5′-ward of this region (Figure 2) also hybridized to poly(A)+ mRNA (de Valoir, Beckingham, and

Durica, unpublished). Transcripts approximately 8 kb and 1.7 kb in size were observed in immature but not mature oocytes; the smaller 1.7 kb transcript was also detected in late pupa. This probe also cross-hybridizes with a 900 nt RNA in *D. melanogaster* adults. Whether the *Calliphora* transcripts are synthesized from intron sequences in the opposite orientation from the Ce*abl* gene, or whether this probe is detecting abundant transcripts from a related sequence elsewhere in the genome, is currently being investigated.

SUMMARY

We have begun to characterize the genomic organization and developmental expression of the *C. erythrocephala abl* gene homolog. We are currently in the process of mapping the boundaries of the Ce*abl* transcription unit, determining its nucleotide sequence, and recovering additional PTK homologs from the *Calliphora* genome. Implicit in these characterizations is an analysis of the structural relationships between these genes and homologs from other organisms.

Northern bot analysis has provided a rough developmental profile of Ce*abl* gene transcription. A higher resolution picture of the spatial and temporal pattern of expression of Ce*abl* transcripts and their resultant proteins will be monitored in situ through nucleic acid hybridization and immunocytochemistry. Information concerning the localization of these gene products is necessary to shed light on the ontologic role of these proteins and their conservation of function across taxonomic groups.

Finally, an analysis of Ce*abl* gene function can also be approached through surrogate genetic techniques. The use of chimeric genes and site-directed mutation to dissect critical domains within vertebrate proteins has developed into a valuable tool in the examination of oncogene activation and expression (40–42). The high level of structural conservation between the dipteran and vertebrate proteins implies conservation of enzymatic activity, but the physiologic significance of this conservation is not understood. Hybrid constructions can be generated, however, that permit tests for functional relatedness in transformation assays. Such constructions can be used to evaluate which regions of the protein may be involved in subcellular localization, substrate specificity, or regulation of kinase activity.

ACKNOWLEDGMENTS

I would like to thank Dr. James N. Thompson for a critical review of the manuscript. Support for this work has been provided by a grant (NP-592) from the American Cancer Society, and contract No. 3723 from the Oklahoma Center for the Advancement of Science and Technology.

REFERENCES

1. Hunter, T., and Cooper, J. A. (1986). Viral oncogenes and tyrosine phosphorylation. In *The Enzymes, Control by Phosphorylation*, Vol. XVII (P. D. Boyer and E. G. Krebs, eds.). Academic Press, New York, pp. 192–237.
2. Witte, O. (1986). Functions of the *abl* oncogene. *Cancer Surv. 5*:183–197.
3. Mes-Masson, A. M., and Witte, O. (1987). Role of the *abl* oncogene in chronic myelogenous leukemia. *Adv. Cancer Res. 49*:53–74.
4. Shilo, B.-Z. (1987). Proto-oncogenes in *Drosophila melanogaster. Trends Genet. 3*:69–72.
5. Hunter, T. (1987). A thousand and one protein kinases. *Cell 50*:823–829.
6. Goddard, J. M., Weiland, J. J., and Capecchi, M. R. (1986). Isolation and characterization of *Caenohabditis elegans* DNA sequences homologous to the v-*abl* oncogene. *Proc. Natl. Acad. Sci. USA 83*:2172–2176.
7. Simon, M. A., Kornberg, T. B., and Bishop, J. M. (1983). Three loci related to the *src* oncogene and tyrosine-specific protein kinase activity in *Drosophila. Nature 302*:837–839.
8. Hoffman-Falk, H., Einat, P., Shilo, B.-Z., and Hoffmann, F. M. (1983). Drosophila melanogaster DNA clones homologous to vertebrate oncogenes: Evidence for a common ancestor to *src* and *abl* cellular genes. *Cell 32*:589–598.
9. Hoffmann, F. M., Fresco, L. D., Hoffman-Falk, H., and Shilo, B.-Z. (1983). Nucleotide sequences of the Drosophila *src* and *abl* homologs: Conservation and variability in the *src* family oncogenes. *Cell 35*:393–401.
10. Lev, Z., Leibovitz, N., Segev, O., and Shilo, B.-Z. (1984). Expression of the *src* and *abl* cellular oncogenes during the development of *Drosophila melanogaster. Mol. Cell. Biol. 4*:982–984.
11. Telford, J., Burckhardt, J., Butler, B., and Pirrotta, V. (1985). Alternative processing and developmental control of the transcripts of the *Drosophila abl* oncogene homologue. *EMBO J. 4*:2609–2615.
12. Henkemeyer, M. J., Gertler, F. B., Goodman, W., and Hoffmann, F. M. (1987). The *Drosophila* Abelson proto-oncogene homologue: Identification of mutant alleles that have pleiotrophic effects late in development. *Cell 51*: 821–828.
13. Henkemeyer, M. J., Bennett, R. L., Gertler, F. B., and Hoffmann, F. M. (1988). DNA sequence, structure and tyrosine kinase activity of the *Drosophila melanogaster* Abelson proto-oncogene homolog. *Mol. Cell. Biol. 8*: 843–853.
14. Durica, D. S., Restrepo, M. A., Thomas, T. L., and Beckingham, K. (1987). Isolation and characterization of *abl* gene sequences in *Calliphora erythrocephala. Gene 59*:63–76.
15. Beverley, S. M., and Wilson, A. C. (1984). Molecular evolution in *Drosophila* and the higher diptera. A time scale for fly evolution. *J. Mol. Evol. 21*: 1–13.
16. Bier, K. (1963). Autoradiographische Untersuchungen über die Leistungen des Follikelepithels und der Nährzellen bei der Dotterbildung und Eiweissynthese im Fliegenovar. *Wilhelm Roux' Archiv. 154*:552–575.

17. Telfer, W. H. (1975). Development and physiology of the oocyte-nurse cell syncytium. *Anv. Insect Phys. 11*:223–319.
18. Van der Starre-Van der Molen, L. G. (1972). Embryogenesis of *Calliphora erythrocephala* Meigen. *Neth. J. Zool. 22*:119–182.
19. Kirchoff, C. (1981). Electrophoretic analysis of newly synthesized and stored maternal RNA during oogenesis of *Calliphora erythrocephala. Wilhelm Roux' Arch. 190*:331–338.
20. Anderson, K. V., and Lengyel, J. A. (1979). Rates of synthesis of major classes of RNA in *Drosophila* embryos. *Dev. Biol. 70*:217–231.
21. Rubacha, A., Tucker, M. A., de Valoir, T., Belikoff, E. J., and Beckingham, K. (1988). Oogenesis-specific genes of *Calliphora erythrocephala. Dev. Biol. 129*:449–463.
22. Ribbert, D. (1979). Chromomeres and puffing in experimentally induced polytene chromosomes of *Calliphora erythrocephala. Chromosoma 74*: 269–298.
23. Reddy, E. P., Smith, M. J., and Srinivasan, A. (1983). Abelson murine leukemia virus genome: Structural similarity of its transforming gene product to other *onc* gene products with tyrosine-specific kinase activity. *Proc. Natl. Acad. Sci. USA 80*:3623–3627.
24. Ben-Neriah, Y., Bernards, A., Paskind, M., Daley, G. Q., and Baltimore, D. (1986). Alternative 5′ exons in c-*abl* mRNA. *Cell 44*:577–586.
25. Shtivelman, E., Lifshitz, B., Gale, R. P., Roe, B. A., and Canaani, E. (1986). Alternative splicing of RNAs transcribed from the human *abl* gene and from the *bcr-abl* fused gene. *Cell 47*:277–284.
26. Bernards, A., Rubin, C. M., Westbrook, C. A., Paskind, M., and Baltimore, D. (1987). The first intron of the human c-*abl* gene is at least 200 kilobases long and is a target for translocations in chronic myelogenous leukemia. *Mol. Cell. Biol. 7*:3231–3236.
27. Miesfeld, R., Rusconi, S., Godowski, P. J., Maler, B. A., Okret, S., Wikström, A., Gustafsson, J., and Yamamoto, K. (1986). Genetic complementation of a glucocorticoid receptor deficiency by expression of cloned receptor cDNA. *Cell 46*:389–399.
28. Wharton, K. A., Yedvobnick, B., Finnerty, V. G., and Artavanis-Tsakanos, S. (1985) *opa*: a novel family of transcribed repeats shared by the *Notch* locus and other developmentally regulated loci in D. melanogaster. *Cell 40*: 55–62.
29. Poole, S. J., Kauvar, L. M., Drees, B., and Kornberg, T. (1985). The *engrailed* locus of Drosophila; structural analysis of an embryonic transcript. *Cell 40*:37–43.
30. Livneh, E., Glazer, L., Segal, D., Schlessinger, J., and Shilo, B.-Z. (1985). The *Drosophila* EGF receptor gene homolog: Conservation of both hormone binding and kinase domains. *Cell 40*:599–607.
31. Petruzelli, L., Herrera, R., Arenas-Garcia, R., Fernandez, R., Birnbaum, M. J., and Rosen, O. M. (1986). Isolation of a *Drosophila* genomic sequence homologous to the kinase domain of the human insulin receptor and detec-

tion of the phosphorylated *Drosophila* receptor with an anti-peptide antibody. *Proc. Natl. Acad. Sci. USA 83*:4710–4714.

32. Hafen, E., Basler, K., Edstroem, J.-E., and Rubin, G. M. (1987). *Sevenless,* a cell-specific homeotic gene of *Drosophila,* encodes a putative transmembrane receptor with a tyrosine kinase domain. *Science 236*:55–63.
33. Simon, M. A., Drees, B., Kornberg, T. B., and Bishop, J. M. (1985). The nucleotide sequence and tissue-specific expression of *Drosophila* c-*src*. *Cell 42*:831–840.
34. Gregory, R. J., Kammermeyer, K. L., Vincent, W. S., III, and Wadsworth, S. G. (1987). Primary sequence and developmental expression of a novel *Drosophila melanogaster* c-*src* gene. *Mol. Cell. Biol. 7*:2119–2127.
35. Mark, G. E., MacIntyre, R. J., Digan, M. E., Ambrosio, L., and Perrimon, N. (1987). *Drosophila melanogaster* homologs of the *raf* oncogene. *Mol. Cell. Biol. 7*:2134–2140.
36. Wadsworth, S. C., Madhavan, K., and Bilodeau-Wentworth, D. (1987). Maternal inheritance of transcripts from three *Drosophila src*-related genes. *Nucleic Acids Res. 13*:2153–2170.
37. Gertler, F. B., Bennett, R. L., Clark, M. J., and Hoffmann, F. M. (1989). Drosophila *abl* tyrosine kinase in embryonic CNS axons: a role in axonogenesis is revealed through dosage-sensitive interactions with *disabled. Cell 58*:103–113.
38. Stahl, M. L., Ferenz, C. R., Kelleher, K. L., Kriz, R. W., and Knopf, J. L. (1988). Sequence similarity of phospholipase C with the non-catalytic region of *scr. Nature 332*:269–272.
39. Mayer, B. J., Hamaguchi, M., and Hanafusa, H. (1988). A novel viral oncogene with structural similarity to phospholipase C. *Nature 332*:272–275.
40. Privalsky, M. L. (1987). Creation of a chimeric oncogene: Analysis of the biochemical and biological properties of a v-*erb*/*scr* fusion polypeptide. *J. Virol. 61*:1938–1948.
41. Mathey-Prevot, B., and Baltimore, D. (1988). Recombinants within the tyrosine kinase region of v-*abl* and c-*src* identify a v-*abl* segment that confers lymphoid specificity. *Mol. Cell. Biol. 8*:234–240.
42. Sadowski, I., Stone, J. C., and Pawson, T. (1986). A non-catalytic domain conserved among cytoplasmic protein-tyrosine kinases modifies the kinase function and transforming activity of Fujinami sarcoma virus $P130^{gag\text{-}fps}$ *Mol. Cell. Biol. 6*:4396–4408.

4
Viral Models for Understanding Chronic Myelogenous Leukemia

James A. McCubrey and Linda S. Steelman *East Carolina University, Greenville, North Carolina*

INTRODUCTION

Background

Chronic myelogenous leukemia (CML) is a human stem cell disorder associated with a consistent chromosomal abnormality. The translocated chromosome was identified initially by Nowell and Hungerford (1) and is referred to as the Philadelphia chromosome (Ph^1). A reciprocal translocation has occurred between chromosomes 9 and 22 (2). Some of the genes involved in the translocation have been identified as the proto-oncogene c-*abl* on chromosome 9 and the breakpoint cluster region (*bcr*) on chromosome 22 (3,4). This karyotypic abnormality is present in > 90% of patients with CML. The cellular and clinical aspects of CML have been reviewed recently (5-8), as has the molecular biology of the chromosomal translocation (9-12).

One of the results of the Ph^1 translocation is a chimeric gene product that contains genetic information from both the *bcr* and c-*abl* loci (13-16). This novel gene encodes a protein ($p210^{bcr\text{-}abl}$) that contains 5′ information from *bcr* and 3′ information from c-*abl* and, like the protein encoded by c-*abl* (p150), is a tyrosine-specific protein kinase (16). In addition, the *bcr-abl* gene may have regulatory regions that are different than those present in the c-*abl*. The tyrosine kinases encoded by *bcr-abl* and c-*abl* (p150), however, have similar distinct properties (17-20).

The *abl* gene was initially identified in the genome of Abelson murine leukemia virus (A-MuLV). Viral stocks of A-MuLV contain the replication competent helper virus, Moloney MuLV, and the transforming entity, A-MuLV. A-

MuLV arose by genetic recombination of Mo-MuLV and the cellular c-*abl* gene. v-*abl* contains sequences derived from the *gag* (group specific antigen) gene of the helper virus (Moloney MuLV, which was initially used to generate A-MuLV) and c-*abl* murine (References 21-28 and reviewed in References 11 and 12). Therefore, like *bcr-abl*, v-*abl* is a fusion gene distinct from c-*abl*. In addition, the v-*abl* gene is under the transcriptional control of the virally encoded long terminal repeat (LTR) sequences, which permits the v-*abl* gene to be constitutively expressed after A-MuLV infection. The v-*abl* and *bcr-abl* gene products are similar to the tyrosine kinase encoded by c-*abl* (murine and human); however, they may lack normal regulatory regions of the *abl* protein or of the c-*abl* gene that alter their cellular regulation.

Hematopoietic Cells and Growth Factors

CML is a clonal disease and has been characterized by the proliferation and accumulation of myeloid and some B lymphoid cells (5-8). Cytogenetic studies indicate that the Ph^1 translocation occurs in a hematopoietic stem cell (reviewed in Reference 5). The normal target stem cell for CML probably requires either granulocyte-macrophage colony-stimulating factor (GM-CSF) or interleukin-3 (IL-3) for proliferation and/or differentiation. Indeed, increased levels of GM-CSF and enhanced sensitivities to GM-CSF have been observed in cells isolated from patients with CML (reviewed in References 5, 7, and 9).

A consequence of the Ph^1 translocation may be an altered growth factor requirement that allows the transformed cell to grow in reduced quantities or in the absence of specific growth factors. The lack of continuous human hematopoietic growth factor-dependent cell lines that are not transformed has hampered research in determining the precise target cell(s) involved in the transformation process. The recent molecular cloning and insertion into expression vectors of human hematopoietic growth factors (29-31), it is hoped will enable investigators to isolate primitive growth factor-dependent human hematopoietic cell lines. These cell lines would be useful to determine the effects of the *bcr-abl* gene on cellular transformation and growth factor dependence.

Murine myeloid and lymphoid growth factor-dependent cell lines have been isolated that require IL-3 and in some cases GM-CSF for their continuous culture in vitro (32-35). These cell lines are nontumorigenic when injected into syngeneic mice, and spontaneous conversion to factor independence has not been observed in most cell lines. With continuous factor-dependent cell lines it must be remembered that karyotypic abnormalities have been observed in some of these cell lines (FDC-P1) (32) that may predispose their ability to be transformed. The murine factor-dependent cell lines are nonadherent and can be cultivated in either recombinant IL-3 or supernatants prepared from the myelomonocytic cell line WEHI-3B. They can be cultivated easily and inexpensively to large cell numbers ($> 10^9$) and retain their factor dependence.

Upon removal of ligand (IL-3), the cells enter the G_0 stage of the cell cycle and if IL-3 is withheld for more than 48 h the cells lose viability and eventually die. However, if IL-3 is added back to the culture after a 24 h interleukin deprivation, the G_0 cells re-enter the cell cycle with cell division occurring after 16–24 h (36). These cell lines have enabled investigators to study the mechanism(s) of growth factor-mediated signal transduction and to determine which oncogenes transform hematopoietic cells to growth factor independence. In addition, the consequences of transformation upon cellular differentiation have been investigated in these cell lines.

ABROGATION OF GROWTH FACTOR DEPENDENCE

A-MuLV

Many investigators have documented that factor-dependent cell lines can be transformed to factor independence after infection with A-MuLV (References 37–43 and Table 1). These studies have been performed with established myeloid (FDC-P1 and 33D C13) and lymphoid (Ba/F3 and FL5.12) as well as freshly isolated IL-3-dependent mast and myeloid cells. Approximately 0.1% of the A-MuLV-infected cells generate long-term factor-independent cell lines (40,41,43). The resulting factor-independent cell lines constitutively express the introduced v-*abl*-encoded tyrosine kinase, and upon injection into mice, tumors are observed in 100% of the mice with short latent periods (2–3 weeks). In addition, we have observed that factor-independent cell lines obtained after infection with either helper-free A-MuLV (A-MuLV ψ2) or A-MuLV (Mo-MuLV) are equally tumorigenic, indicating that viral spread and the presence of the helper virus is not necessary for either factor independence or tumorigenicity (43).

Recently, Kiperos and Wang (42) demonstrated that continuous expression of the v-*abl* gene was necessary for factor independence by infecting an IL-3-dependent cell line (FDC-P1) with a temperature-sensitive mutant of A-MuLV. At the permissive temperature, the cells were factor independent and expressed fourfold more v-*abl* tyrosine kinase than at the nonpermissive temperature. Moreover, the cells required IL-3 for growth at the nonpermissive temperature. The significance of these observations becomes more clear later in this review, when abrogation of factor dependence by other virally encoded oncogenes is discussed.

All the studies on abrogation of factor dependence after A-MuLV infection have indicated that a nonautocrine mechanism of transformation is involved. Growth of the A-MuLV transformants is density independent and is not inhibited by anti-IL-3 antibodies (37,38). None of the transformants have been observed to produce significant quantities of known lymphokines (IL-3 or GM-CSF) that would permit the growth of the factor-dependent parental cell lines. In addition, supernatants derived from the A-MuLV transformants have been

Table 1 Oncogenes That Do and Do Not Abrogate IL-3 Dependence

Oncogene	Oncogene product	Cell line	Tumorigenic	Reference
Oncogenes that abrogate IL-3 dependence				
v-*abl*	Tyrosine kinase	FDC-P1	+	37, 42, 43
		33D C13	+	41
		Ba/F3	ND[a]	40
		FL5.12	+	43
		Mast	+	38
		Myeloid	+	39
v-*src*	Tyrosine kinase	FDC-P1	ND	45
v-*fms*	Tyrosine kinase	FDC-P1	+	44
v-*erb-B*	Tyrosine kinase	33D C13	+	49
v-*myc*	DNA binding	FDC-P1	+	47
c-*myc*	DNA binding	FDC-P1	ND	48
GM-CSF	Growth factor	FDC-P1	+	53, 54
IL-3	Growth factor	FDC-P1	+	55
Oncogenes that do not abrogate factor dependence				
v-H-*ras*	GTP binding	Mast	ND	50
		FL5.12	ND	43
v-*mos*	Serine kinase	FL5.12	ND	43,47
v-*raf*	Serine kinase	FDC-P1	ND	47
v-*fos*	DNA binding	FDC-P1	ND	47
v-*fps*	Tyrosine kinase	Ba/F3	ND	40

[a]Not done.

examined for the presence of IL-1β, IL-2, and IL-4 and they have been routinely negative (43). Moreover, no mRNAs encoding IL-1β, IL-2, IL-3, IL-4, IL-6, GM-CSF, or M-CSF have been detected in the A-MuLV transformants (37,38,40,43). In addition, the genetic structure of many lymphokine genes (IL-1β, IL-2, IL-3, GM-CSF, M-CSF, IL-4, and IL-6) have been examined by conventional Southern blot analysis, and no differences have been detected between the parental cell lines and A-MuLV transformants (43).

The expression of IL-3 receptors was examined on IL-3-dependent and IL-3-independent cell lines. No difference in IL-3 receptor expression was detected between the A-MuLV factor-independent transformants and the parental cells.

These results suggest that neither the affinity nor the density of the IL-3 receptor changes after A-MuLV transformation.

Finally, when A-MuLV transformants were plated at low cell densities (0.2 cells per 96-well plate), no effect on the cloning efficiency was observed when exogenous rIL-2, rIL-3, rIL-4, rG-CSF, rGM-CSF, or rM-CSF was added (43). In summary, there is no evidence for an autocrine model in the abrogation of IL-3 dependence after infection with A-MuLV. The direct involvement of v-*abl* in abrogating factor dependence has been interpreted as a rôle of v-*abl* or a structurally similar protein in IL-3-mediated signal transduction.

v-*fms* and v-*src*

Recombinant neomycin^r (*neo*^{r}) retroviruses containing either v-*fms* or v-*src* transform the factor-dependent myeloid cell line FDC-P1 to factor independence by a nonautocrine mechanism (44,45). However, the cell lines were first selected for *neo*^{r} in the presence of IL-3 and then *neo*^{r} cells were then selected for factor independence. IL-3-independent subclones from the v-*src-neo*^{r} and v-*fms-neo*^{r} clones were obtained at a very low efficiency and after many weeks in culture. In addition, some of the v-*fms-neo*^{r} IL-3-independent clones contained multiple copies of the v-*fms* and neo^r genes. The v-*fms-neo*^{r} and v-*src-neo*^{r} IL-3-independent cell lines expressed either the v-*fms*- or v-*src*-encoded proteins, respectively. v-*src* is a tyrosine-specific protein kinase, and the v-*fms* gene product is similar in structure to the M-CSF (CSF-1) receptor and has an associated tyrosine kinase activity (46). There was no evidence for an autocrine mechanism of transformation in these studies as neither mRNA transcripts encoding nor supernatants containing IL-3 or GM-CSF were detected.

v-*src* has been shown to reduce but not totally relieve the factor dependence of the lymphoid IL-3-dependent cell line Ba/F3 (40). These cell lines were not selected for *neo*^{r}, and clones of v-*src*-infected cells grew very poorly; rapid proliferation was observed only after adding back limiting amounts of IL-3. Again there was no evidence for an autocrine mechanism of factor independence in these studies.

Recently we infected myeloid (FDC-P1) and lymphoid (FL5.12) IL-3-dependent cell lines with viruses containing either v-*src* or v-*fms* and directly selected for prolonged growth in the absence of IL-3 (43). Surprisingly, we recovered IL-3-independent cell lines that lacked either the v-*src* or v-*fms* provirus and did not express the oncogene-encoded proteins. The recovery of these cell lines was approximately 10- to 100-fold less frequent than the recovery of IL-3-independent cell lines after A-MuLV infection. Of four factor-independent cell lines obtained after infection with v-*src*, three had genetic rearrangements at the IL-3 locus and IL-3-specific growth factor was detected in supernatants prepared from these cell lines. Consistent with these observations, mRNA transcripts encoding IL-3 were detected in the IL-3-rearranged cell lines. These IL-3 rearranged cell lines had a significantly greater cloning efficiency in the presence of exogenously added IL-3 (26-fold) than did A-MuLV transformants (2.8-fold). Such results suggest that these cell lines were transformed by an autocrine mechanism. Moreover, the IL-3-rearranged cell lines formed tumors in 100% of the mice injected; however, a longer latency period (3–5 weeks) was observed than with the A-MuLV transformants (2–3 weeks).

The mechanism of abrogation of factor independence in the other IL-3-independent cell lines (four of seven lines not rearranged at the IL-3 locus) obtained after infection with either v-*src*- or v-*fms*-encoding retroviruses is not known. By conventional Southern blot analysis, they are not rearranged at the IL-1β, IL-2, IL-3, IL-4, IL-6, GM-CSF, or M-CSF loci, nor have mRNA transcripts encoding these proteins been detected in these cells. In addition, we have not detected any IL-1β, IL-2, IL-3, IL-4, or GM-CSF in supernatants prepared from these cultures. Moreover, these cells do not show any difference in cloning efficiency when rIL-2, IL-3, rIL-4, rG-CSF, rGM-CSF, or rM-CSF was added to the culture media. Upon injection into mice, each of these cell lines formed tumors in 67% of the mice, with longer latency periods (5–7 weeks) than those observed with either the A-MuLV-transformed or IL-3-rearanged cell lines. The mechanism of abrogation of factor-independence in these cell lines is currently under investigation, and it is possible that additional or unknown lymphokines or oncogenes have been activated by rearrangement in these cells.

v-*myc* and c-*myc*

IL-3-independent cell lines have been obtained after infection with v-*myc* directly (47) and recombinant viruses containing c-*myc* and *neo*^{r} (48). These experiments were performed with the established cell line FDC-P1. The results obtained with c-*myc* are similar to those described previously with either v-*fms-neo*^{r} or v-*src-neo*^{r} in that *neo*^{r} cells were selected first and then factor-independent cells were recovered at a low frequency after a long period in culture. Interestingly, the factor-independent cell lines isolated after infection with v-*myc* expressed only the introduced v-*myc*, not the endogenous c-*myc* (47). Unfortunately, the frequency of isolation of the IL-3-independent cell lines after infection with the v-*myc*-containing virus is not presented; therefore it is not known whether the IL-3-independent cell lines represent rare transformants.

v-*erb-B*

Recently it has been determined that the virally encoded v-*erb-B* oncogene transforms the 33D C13 cell line to factor independence and tumorigenicity (49). v-*erb-B* is an amino-terminal truncated form of the epidermal growth factor (EGF) receptor that has tyrosine kinase activity. In this study, cells were also transfected with the normal EGF receptor, and although these transfected cells utilized EGF for transduction of a mitogenic signal, they were not tumorigenic. Moreover, the EGF receptor was detected on the cell surface of the EGF receptor transformants, but v-*erb-B* was not detected on the cell surface of the v-*erb-B* transformants. The lines that constitutively expressed the v-*erb-B*-encoded tyrosine kinase were factor independent and tumorigenic.

Virally Encoded Oncogenes That Do Not Abrogate Factor Dependence

Infection of either myeloid or lymphoid IL-3-dependent cell lines with retroviruses containing v-*fps* (40), v-*fos* (46), v-*H-ras*, or v-*mos* (43,47,50) has not resulted in the isolation of factor-independent cell lines. However, Rein et al. (50) observed that continuous IL-3-dependent cultures were frequently isolated after Harvey murine sarcoma virus (H-MuSV) infection of freshly isolated myeloid cells. In addition, these H-MuSV cell lines remained IL-3 dependent even after long culture periods (greater than 2 years in culture). Vogt et al. (51,52) confirmed these results and also observed that in double-infection studies with v-*myc* and either v-H-ras or v-*abl*, IL-3-independent cell lines were recovered by an indirect mechanism. They observed that karyotypic abnormalities were associated with the conversion to factor independence. The initial v-*myc*-infected culture was diploid and factor dependent; however, the v-*abl* or v-*myc* factor-independent cultures ranged from triploid to octaploid. These karyotypic abnormalities were observed only after the cells went through a crisis period.

GM-CSF and IL-3

Retroviruses containing either the GM-CSF (53,54) or IL-3 genes (55) transform IL-3-dependent cells to factor independence. However, unlike most of the previously described studies with virally encoded oncogenes, these factor-independent cell lines are transformed by an autocrine mechanism since the cell lines produce the growth factors encoded by the growth factor genes contained in the retroviruses. Moreover, the growth of the transformed cell lines is inhibited if antibodies to the growth factors are included in the culture media. These autocrine factor-independent cell lines form tumors upon injection into mice.

Spontaneous Factor-Independent Cell Lines

Stocking et al. (56) observed that spontaneous factor-independent cell lines could be isolated from the IL-3-dependent cell line D35 at a frequency of (0.4-7×10^{-7}). Moreover, they observed that the factor-independent cell lines were rearranged at either the IL-3 or GM-CSF loci, and mRNAs encoding these genes were detected in these cells. This cell line was initially isolated after Friend spleen focus forming virus (Friend SFFV) infection of long-term marrow cultures from C3H/HeJ mice. The D35 cell line contains multiple copies of the Friend SFFV provirus and produces biologically active virus. The recovery of spontaneous factor-independent cell lines from the D35 line may be a result of the multiple Friend SFFV proviruses in this line. The other factor-dependent lines described in this review (FDC-P1, Ba/F3, and FL5.12) were not isolated after viral infection.

Summary of Factor Abrogation

Infection of long-term factor-dependent cell lines with A-MuLV and expression of the v-*abl*-encoded tyrosine kinase is the most efficient mechanism to render IL-3-dependent cells factor independent and tumorigenic. The experiments by Kiperos and Wang (42) indicate that continuous expression of the v-*abl* tyrosine kinase is necessary for factor-independent growth. These experiments with temperature-sensitive virus have not been done with other virally encoded oncogenes. Factor-independent cell lines isolated after infection with v-*fms*, v-*src*, or v-*myc* are recovered at 10- to 100-fold lower frequencies than after infection with A-MuLV and require longer periods of incubation to be recovered. Therefore, the role of the virally encoded oncogene (other than v-*abl*) in conferring factor independence is not clear. Most of these experiments have been performed with an established cell line (FDC-P1) that has been documented to contain chromosomal aberrations. This cell line may already have activated oncogenes or additional genes that render it sensitive to transformation.

Recently, Vogt et al. (51,52) have suggested that factor-independent cell lines are isolated by an indirect mechanism. After coinfection of freshly isolated IL-3-dependent myelocytes with v-*myc*- and either v-*H-ras*- or v-*abl*-containing retroviruses, factor-independent cell lines were recovered only after prolonged incubation periods. They have suggested that additional genetic changes (chromosomal aberrations) must occur in the cells for the factor-independent and transformed phenotypes to be manifested. In addition, Vogt et al. have indicated that not every A-MuLV- or v-*myc*-infected cell is capable of becoming factor independent. These observations may be similar to the progression observed from the chronic to the acute stages of CML. Additional chromosomal abnormalities are observed in the acute stages of CML when compared to the chronic stage. It may be possible to isolate v-*abl*-*neo*^{r}-infected cells that remain factor dependent. Selection for factor independence could then be performed, and the changes that occur during the conversion from factor-dependent to factor-independent growth could be monitored.

All the factor-independent cell lines isolated after infection with retroviruses that contain virally encoded oncogenes have arisen by a nonautocrine mechanism of transformation. Growth factors known to support the proliferation of the parental cell have not been observed in either supernatants or mRNA preparations prepared from the transformed cell lines. However, the parental cell lines can also be transformed by an autocrine mechanism of transformation. Autocrine transformed cells have been recovered after infection with retroviruses that contain growth factor genes and in cell lines in which rearrangements have occurred of the endogenous growth factor gene.

DIFFERENTIATION AND CELL SURFACE PHENOTYPE

Differentiation of IL-3-Dependent Cells

Rovera and colleagues (41) determined that the 33D C13 cell line (which was derived from normal mouse bone marrow and may represent a myeloblast) can be induced to terminal granulocytic differentiation in the presence of G-CSF. Differentiation occurred only when the cells were plated in the absence of IL-3. They also determined that the differentiated granulocytes were resistant to A-MuLV transformation (41). In addition, A-MuLV transforms 33D c13 when it is maintained in the presence of IL-3. However, once the cells are transformed to growth factor independence, they are no longer able to differentiate to mature granulocytes in the presence of G-CSF. Rovera and colleagues speculated that the same molecular mechanisms that interfered with the signal transmission pathway for IL-3-mediated growth may also affect the signal transmission pathway that leads to their differentiation (41).

Lymphoid IL-3-dependent cell lines represent the pro-B cell stage of differentiation (34,35,57). These cell lines are characterized by the lack of immunoglobulin (Ig) or T cell receptor (TcR) rearrangements and the presence of certain cell surface antigens that are expressed on early lymphoid and myeloid cells (34, 35). When lymphoid cell lines are cultured in the correct environment (absence of IL-3, presence of agar extract, concanavalin A supernatant, and feeder layer derived from stromal cells), the culture differentiates into polyclonal mature Ig-secreting B cells (35,58). The effect of A-MuLV on the differentiation of the pro-B cells into mature B cells in this culture system has not been reported.

Infection with A-MuLV does not result in rearrangement of the IG or TcR genes in the lymphoid cell line FL5.12, and we have not detected any differences between the parental and A-MuLV-transformed cell lines in the genetic structure or expression of the following oncogenes: c-*fms*, c-*fos*, c-*fps*, c-*myb*, c-*myc*, c-*raf*, c-*H-ras*, c-*K-ras*, and c-*src* (43).

Cell Surface Phenotype

An additional means to assess the biologic consequences of A-MuLV transformation of IL-3-dependent lymphoid and myeloid cells is to compare the cell surface phenotypes of parental and IL-3-independent cells. We (43) have examined the expression of genes that are detected at early stages of lymphoid and myeloid

Table 2 Cell Surface Phenotype of Factor-Independent Cell Lines[a]

	Cell line			
Cell surface antigen	FL5.12	FL-Abl	FDC-P1	FD-Abl
IL-2R	++	-	++	-
Mac-1	+	++	++	-
Mac-2	-	-	-	++
LFA-1	-	++	-	++
MHC class I	+	++	+	++

[a]No staining when compared with controls; +, mean fluorescence <20; ++, mean fluorescence >20.

differentiation. The phenotype of FL5.12, FDC-P1, and the A-MuLV-transformed cell lines are presented in Table 2. No differences in the expression of 12 of 17 cell surface antigens was detected between the parental and transformed cell lines [B220, MHC (major histocompatibility complex) class II, Thy1.2, Lyt-1, Mac-3, germinal center, LGP-200, MEL-14, AA4, GF1, Fc receptor, and transferrin receptor]. However, differences were detected in the expression of IL-2 receptor, Mac-1, Mac-2, LFA-1, and MHC class I between the parental and A-MuLV transformants.

The A-MuLV transformants were phenotypically different from the parental cell lines regardless of whether they were derived from FDC-P1 or FL5.12. A decrease in IL-2 receptor and increase in LFA-1 and MHC class I expression was observed on the cell surface of A-MuLV transformants compared to the parental cell lines. However, the expression of Mac-1 was not detectable on the cell surface of the parental lymphoid line, FL5.12, but it was detected on A-MuLV-transformed FL5.12 lines. Whereas Mac-1 was detectable on the myeloid parental line FDC-P1, it was not detected on the A-MuLV-transformed FDC-P1 lines. Moreover, Mac-2 was detected on the A-MuLV-transformed FDC-P1 lines, but it was not detected on the parental FDC-P1 line.

Poly(A)$^+$ RNA was isolated from the parental and transformed cell lines and examined for the expression of some of these genes. IL-2 receptor α-chain mRNA was readily detected in the parental cell lines but could not be detected in any of the A-MuLV transformants. In addition, two- to fivefold more MHC class I mRNA was detected in the A-MuLV transformants than in the parental cell lines. These results agree with the cell surface antigen expression patterns and indicate that the difference in antigen expression that we observed by fluorescence-activated cell sorting (FACS) analysis was not due to either masking or unmasking of antigen epitopes.

Although the functional consequences of these observations are unknown, they suggest a distinct pattern of gene expression is observed in the A-MuLV transformants from that observed in the parental lines. It is possible to monitor by both molecular biologic and cellular immunologic techniques the changes in gene expression that occur during the conversion of the parental IL-3-dependent cell to the fully transformed IL-3-independent cell. Moreover, the ability of the cells to differentiate after viral infection and respond to growth factors can be determined. These changes in gene expression and differentiation ability may be similar to those occurring from the initial transformation of a stem cell to the chronic and finally acute stages of CML.

SUMMARY

The similarities between v-*abl* and *bcr-abl* have been well documented (10,12) and indicate that studies of the A-MuLV transformation of myeloid cells may be beneficial in understanding CML. The ability to cultivate long-term growth factor-dependent myeloid and lymphoid cell lines that can be transformed by A-MuLV and other oncogene-containing retroviruses enables investigators to study the consequences of the introduction of an oncogene on gene expression and cellular phenotype. Moreover, the ability to monitor continuously the parental nontransformed cell is always available in these types of studies. Introduction of the recently cloned *bcr-abl* gene (59,60) into murine IL-3-dependent cell lines should provide interesting information concerning the role of *bcr-abl* in the transformation of myeloid and lymphoid cells. Moreover, the ability of the parental and transformed cell to differentiate in the presence of additional lymphokines once they have been transformed by an oncogene can be determined.

Recently, Vogt et al. (51,52) have determined that A-MuLV does not transform diploid myeloblasts by a direct mechanism and that the transformed (IL-3) independent cells contain karyotypic abnormalities. These observations may indicate that cellular transformation is more complex than inheritance and expression of a particular oncogene and may be similar to the karyotypic abnormalities that are observed during the transition from the chronic to the acute stage of CML.

NOTE ADDED IN PROOF

Since submission of this review, the *bcr-abl* gene has been shown to abrogate the growth factor dependency of IL-3 dependent cell lines (61,62).

REFERENCES

1. Nowell, P. C., and Hungerford, D. A. (1960). A minute chromosome in human chronic granulocytic leukemia. *Science 132*:1497–1501.

2. Rowley, J. D. (1973). A new consistent chromosome abnormality in chronic myelogenous leukemia identified by quinacrine fluorescence and Giemsa staining. *Nature 243*:290–291.
3. DeKlein, A. D., Van Kessel, A. G., Grosveld, G., Bartram, C. R., Hagemeijer, A., Bootsma, P., Spurr, N. K., Heisterkamp, N., Groffen, J., and Stephenson, J. R. (1982). A cellular oncogene is translocated to the Philadelphia chromosome in chronic myelocytic leukemia. *Nature 300*:765–767.
4. Heisterkamp, N., Stephenson, J. R., Groffen, J., Hansen, P. F., deKlein, A., Bartram, C. R., and Grosveld, G. (1983). Localization of the c-*abl* oncogene adjacent to a translocation break point in chronic myelocytic leukaemia. *Nature 306*:239–242.
5. Champlin, R. E., and Golde, D. W. (1985). Chronic myelogenous leukemia: Recent advances. *Blood 65*:1039–1047.
6. Sandberg, A. A., Gemmill, R. M., Hecht, B. K., and Hecht, F. (1986). The Philadelphia chromosome: A model of cancer and molecular cytogenetics. *Cancer Genet. Cytogenet. 21*:129–146.
7. Silver, R. T., and Gale, R. P. (1986). Chronic myeloid leukemia. *Am. J. Med. 80*:1137–1148.
8. Rosen, N., and Israel, M. A. (1987). Genetic abnormalities as biological tumor markers. *Semin. Oncol. 14*:213–331.
9. Dreazen, O., Canaani, E., and Gale, R. P. (1988). Molecular biology of chronic myelogenous leukemia. *Semin. Hematol. 25*:35–49.
10. Mes-Masson, A.-M., and Witte, O. N. (1987). Role of the *abl* oncogene in chronic myelogenous leukemia. *Adv. Cancer Res. 49*:53–73.
11. De Klein, A. (1987). Oncogene activation by chromosomal rearrangement in chronic myelocytic leukemia. *Mutat. Res. 186*:161–172.
12. Rosson, D., and Reddy, E. P. (1988). Activation of the *abl* oncogene and its involvement in chromosomal translocations in human leukemia. *Mutat. Res. 195*:231–243.
13. Gale, R. P., and Canaani, E. (1984). An 8-Kilobase *abl* RNA transcript in chronic myelogenous leukemia. *Proc. Natl. Acad. Sci. USA 81*:5648–5652.
14. Shtivelman, E., Lifshitz, B., Gale, R. P., and Canaani, E. (1985). Fused transcript of *abl* and *bcr* genes in chronic myelogenous leukemia. *Nature 315*:550–554.
15. Ben-Neriah, Y., Daley, G. O., Mes-Masson, A-M., Witte, O. N., and Baltimore, D. (1986). The chronic myelogenous leukemia-specific P210 protein in the product of the *bcr/abl* hybrid gene. *Science 233*:212–214.
16. Konopka, J. B., Watanabe, S. M., and Witte, O. N. (1984). An alteration of human c-*abl* protein in K562 leukemia cells unmasks associated tyrosine kinase activity. *Cell 37*:1035–1042.
17. Konopka, J. B., and Witte, O. N. (1985). Detection of an c-*abl* tyrosine kinase activity in vitro permits direct comparison of normal and altered *abl* gene products. *Mol. Cell. Biol. 5*:16–23.
18. Chan, L. C., Karhi, K. K., Rayter, S. I., Heisterkamp, N., Eridani, S., Powles, R., Lawler, S. D., Groffen, J., Foulkes, J. G., Greaves, M. F., and Wiede-

mann, L. M. (1987). A novel *abl* protein expressed in Philadelphia chromosome positive acute lymphoblastic leukemia. *Nature 325*:635–637.

19. Clark, S. S., McLaughlin, J., Crist, W. M., Champlin, R., and Witte, O. (1987). Unique forms of the *abl* tyrosine kinase distinguish Ph^1-positive CML from Ph^1-positive ALL. *Science 235*:85–88.
20. Kurzrock, R., Shtalrid, M., Romero, P., Kloetzer, W. S., Talpas, M., Trujillo, J. M., Blick, M., Beran, M., and Gutterman, J. U. (1987). A novel c-*abl* protein product in Philadelphia-positive acute lymphoblastic leukaemia. *Nature 325*:631–633.
21. Witte, O. N., Rosenberg, N., Paskind, M., Shields, A., and Baltimore, D. (1978). Identification of an Abelson murine leukemia virus-encoded protein present in transformed fibroblast and lymphoid cells. *Proc. Natl. Acad. Sci. USA 75*:2488–2492.
22. Witte, O. N., Dasqupta, A., and Baltimore, D. (1980). Abelson murine leukemia virus protein is phosphorylated in vitro to form phosphotyrosine. *Nature 283*:826–831.
23. Reynolds, F. H., Jr., Sacks, T. L., Deobagkar, D. N., and Stephenson, J. R. (1980). Cells nonproductively transformed by Abelson murine leukemia virus express a high molecular weight polyprotein containing structural and non-structural components. *Proc. Natl. Acad. Sci. USA 75*:3974–3978.
24. Reynolds, F. H., Jr., Van de Ven, W. J., and Stephenson, J. R. (1980). Abelson murine leukemia virus transformation defective mutants with impaired P120-associated protein kinase activity. *J. Virol. 36*:374–386.
25. Wang, J. Y., and Baltimore, D. (1983). Cellular RNA homologous to the Abelson murine leukemia virus transforming gene: Expression and relationship to the viral sequence. *Mol. Cell. Biol. 3*:773–779.
26. Reddy, E. P., Smith, M. J., and Srinivasan, A. (1983). Nucleotide sequence of Abelson murine leukemia virus genome: Structural similarity of its transforming gene product to other oncogene products with tyrosine-specific kinase activity. *Proc. Natl. Acad. Sci. USA 80*:3623–3627.
27. Prywes, R., Foulkes, J. G., Rosenberg, N., and Baltimore, D. (1983). Sequences of the A-MuLV protein needed for fibroblast and lymphoid cell transformation. *Cell 34*:569–579.
28. Oppi, C., Shore, S. K., and Reddy, E. P. (1987). Nucleotide sequence of testis-derived c-*abl* cDNAs: Implications for testis specific transcription and *abl* oncogene activation. *Proc. Natl. Acad. Sci. USA 84*:8200–8204.
29. Lee, F., Yokota, T., Otsuka, T., Gemmell, L., Larson, N., Luh, J., Arai, K., and Rennick, D. (1985). Isolation of cDNA for a human granulocyte-macrophage colony-stimulating factor by functional expression mammalian cells. *Proc. Natl. Acad. Sci. USA 82*:4360–4364.
30. Wong, G. G., Witek, J. S., Temple, P. A., Wilkens, K. M., Leary, A. C., Luxenberg, D. P., Jones, S. S., Brown, E. L., Kay, R. M., Orr, E. C., Shoemaker, C., Golde, D. W., Kaufmann, R. J., Hewick, R. M., Wang, E. A., and Clark, S. C. (1985). Human GM-CSF: Molecular cloning of the complementary DNA and purification of the natural and recombinant proteins. *Science 228*:810–815.

31. Yang, Y. C., Ciarletta, A. B., Temple, P. A., Chung, M. P., Kovacic, S., Witek-Giannotti, J. S., Leary, A. C., Kriz, R., Donahue, R. E., Wong, G. G., and Clark, S. C. (1986). Human IL-3 (Multi-CSF): Identification by expression cloning of a novel hematopoietic growth factor related to murine IL-3. *Cell 47*:3–10.
32. Dexter, T. M., Garland, J., Scott, D., Scolnick, E., and Metcalf, D. (1980). Growth of factor-dependent hemopoietic precursor cell lines. *J. Exp. Med. 152*:1036–1047.
33. Greenberger, J. S., Sakakeeny, M. A., Humpries, R. K., Eaves, C. J., and Eckner, R. J. (1983). Demonstration of permanent factor-dependent multipotential (erythroid/neutrophil/basophil) hemopoietic progenitor cell lines. *Proc. Natl. Acad. Sci. USA 80*:2931–2935.
34. Palacios, R., Henson, G., Steinmetz, M., and McKearn, J. P. (1984). Interleukin-3 supports growth of mouse pre-B cell clones in vitro. *Nature 309*: 126–131.
35. McKearn, J. P., McCubrey, J. A., and Fagg, B. (1985). Enrichment of hematopoietic precursor cells and cloning of multipotential B-lymphocyte precursors. *Proc. Natl. Acad. Sci. USA 82*:7414–7418.
36. London, L., and McKearn, J. P. (1987). Activation and growth of colony-stimulating factor-dependent cell lines is cell cycle stage dependent. *J. Exp. Med. 166*:1419–1435.
37. Cook, W. D., Metcalf, D., Nicola, N. A., Burgess, A. W., and Walker, F. (1985). Malignant transformation of a growth factor-dependent myeloid cell line by Abelson virus without evidence of an autocrine mechanism. *Cell 41*:677–683.
38. Pierce, J. H., Di Fiore, P. P., Aaronson, S. A., Potter, M., Pumphrey, J., Scott, A., and Ihle, J. N. (1985). Neoplastic transformation of mast cells by Abelson-MuLV abrogation of IL-3 dependence by a non-autocrine mechanism. *Cell 41*:685-693.
39. Oliff, A., Agranovsky, O., McKinney, M. D., Murty, V. V. S., and Bauchwitz, R. (1985). Friend murine leukemia virus-immortalized myeloid cells are converted into tumorigenic cell lines by Abelson leukemia virus. *Proc. Natl. Acad. Sci. USA 82*:3306–3310.
40. Mathey-Prevot, B., Nabel, G., Palacios, R., and Baltimore, D. (1986). Abelson virus abrogation of interleukin-3 dependence in a lymphoid cell line. *Mol. Cell. Biol. 6*:4133–4235.
41. Rovera, G., Valtieri, M., Mavilio, F., and Reddy, E. P. (1987). Effect of Abelson murine leukemia virus on granulocytic differentiation and interleukin-3 dependence of a murine progenitor cell line. *Oncogene 1*:29–35.
42. Kipreos, E. T., and Wang, J. Y. J. (1988). Reversible dependence on growth factor interleukin-3 myeloid cells expressing temperature sensitive v-*abl* oncogene. *Oncogene Res. 2*:29–35.
43. McCubrey, J. A., Holland, G., McKearn, J. P., and Risser, R. (1989). Abrogation of factor dependence in 2 IL-3-dependent cell lines can occur by 2 distinct mechanisms. *Oncogene Res. 4*:97–109.

44. Wheeler, E. F., Askew, D., May, S., Ihle, J. N., and Sherr, C. J. (1987). The v-*fms* oncogene induces factor independent growth and transformation of the interleukin-3-dependent myeloid cell line FDC-P1. *Mol. Cell. Biol. 7*:1637–1680.
45. Overell, R. W., Watson, J. D., Gallis, B., Weisser, K. E., Cosman, D., and Widmer, M. (1987). Nature and specificity of lymphokine independence induced by selectable retroviral vector expressing v-*src*. *Mol. Cell. Biol. 7*:3394–3401.
46. Scherr, C. J., Nettenmier, C. W., Sacca, R., Roussel, M. P., Look, A. T., and Stanley, E. R. (1985). The c-*fms* proto-oncogene product is related to the receptor for the mononuclear phagocyte growth factor CSF-1. *Cell 41*:665–676.
47. Rapp, U. R., Cleveland, J. L., Brightman, K., Scott, A., and Ihle, J. N. (1985). Abrogation of IL-3 and IL-2 dependence by recombinant murine retroviruses expressing v-*myc* oncogenes. *Nature 317*:434–438.
48. Dean, M., Cleveland, J. L., Rapp, U. R., and Ihle, J. N. (1987). Role of *myc* in the abrogation of IL-3-dependence of myeloid FDC-P1 cells. *Oncogene Res. 1*:279–296.
49. Pierce, J. H., Ruggiero, M., Fleming, T. P., DiFiore, P. P., Greenberger, J. S., Varticovski, L., Schlessinger, J., Rovera, G., and Aaronson, S. A. (1988). Signal transduction through the EGF receptor transfected in IL-3-dependent hematopoietic cells. *Science 239*:628–631.
50. Rein, A., Keller, J., Schultz, A. M., Holmes, K. L., Medicus, R., and Ihle, J. N. (1985). Infection of immune mast cells by Harvey sarcoma virus: Immortalization without loss of requirement for interleukin-3. *Mol. Cell. Biol. 5*:2257–2264.
51. Vogt, M., Lesley, J., Bogenberger, J., Volkman, J., and Haas, M. (1986). Coinfection with viruses carrying the v-*Ha-ras* and v-*myc* oncogenes leads to growth factor-independence of an indirect mechanism. *Mol. Cell. Biol. 6*:3345–3349.
52. Vogt, M., Lesley, J., Bogenberger, J. M., Haggblom, C., Swift, S., and Haas, M. (1987). The induction of growth factor-independence in murine myelocytes by oncogenes results in monoclonal cell lines and is correlated with cell crisis and karyotypic instability. *Oncogene Res. 2*:49–63.
53. Lang, R. A., Metcalf, D., Gough, N. M., Dunn, A. R., and Gonda, T. J. (1985). Expression of a hemopoietic growth factor cDNA in a factor-dependent cell line results in autonomous growth and tumorigenicity. *Cell 43*:531–542.
54. Laker, C., Stocking, C., Besgholz, U., Hess, N., DeLanarter, J. F., and Ostertag, W. (1987). Autocrine stimulation after transfer of the granulocyte/macrophage colony-stimulating factor gene and autonomous growth are distinct by interdependent steps in the oncogenic pathway. *Proc. Natl. Acad. Sci. USA 84*:8458–8462.
55. Campbell, H. D., Fung, M. C., Hapel, A. J., and Young, I. G. (1987). Cloning and expression of the murine interleukin-3 gene. In *Lymphokines*, Vol. 13, *Molecular Cloning and Analysis of Lymphokines* (D. R. Webb and D. V. Goeddel, eds.). Academic Press, Orlando, Florida, pp. 239–260.

56. Stocking, C., Loelinger, C., Kawai, M., Suciu, S., Gough, N., and Ostertag, W. (1988). Identification of genes involved in growth autonomy of hematopoietic cells by analysis of factor-indepencent mutants. *Cell 53*:869–879.
57. Palacios, R., and Steinmetz, M. (1985). IL-3-dependent mouse clones that express B-220 surface antigens, contain Ig genes in germline configuration, and generate B lymphocytes. *Cell 41*:727–734.
58. Kinashi, T., Inaba, K., Tsubata, T., Toshiro, K., Palacios, R., and Honjo, T. (1988). Differentiation of an interleukin-3-dependent precursor B-cell clone into immunoglobulin-producing cells in vitro. *Proc. Natl. Acad. Sci. USA 85*:4473–4477.
59. Mes-Masson, A.-M., McLaughlin, J., Daley, G., Paskind, M., and Witte, O. N. (1986). Overlapping cDNA clones define the complete coding region for the $P210^{c\text{-}abl}$ gene product associated with chronic myelogenous leukemia cells containing the Philadelphia chromosome. *Proc. Natl. Acad. Sci. USA 83*: 9769–9722.
60. McLaughlin, J., Chianese, E., and Witte, O. N. (1987). In vitro transformation of immature hematopoietic cells by the p210 *bcr/abl* oncogene product of the Philadelphia chromosome. *Proc. Natl. Acad. Sci. USA 84*:6558–6562.
61. Daley, G. Q., and Baltimore, D. (1988). Transformation of an interleukin-3 dependent hematopoietic cell line by the chronic myelogenous leukemia-specific p210 *bcr/abl* protein. *Proc. Natl. Acad. Sci. USA 85*: 9312-9316.
62. Hariharan, I. K., Adams, J. M., and Cory, S. (1988). *bcr/abl* oncogene renders myeloid cell line factor independent: potential autocrine mechanism in chronic myeloid leukemia. *Oncogene Research 3*:387–399.

5

The Abelson Leukemia Viral Oncogene

Scott K. Shore and E. Premkumar Reddy *The Wistar Insitute, Philadelphia, Pennsylvania*

INTRODUCTION

Abelson murine leukemia virus (A-MuLV) was isolated by Abelson and Rabstein in 1970 while they were studying the nature of tumors produced by Moloney murine leukemia virus (Mo-MuLV) in athymic mice. It was well established at that time that Mo-MuLV induced thymic leukemia in newborn mice, and these investigators were examining the nature of tumors that develop in mice that are depleted of the virus's natural target, the thymus. Chronic administration of prednisolone was known to induce and maintain an atrophied state in a murine thymus gland. It was into these mice that Abelson and Rabstein injected Mo-MuLV and examined the nature of the tumors that developed. In a study involving 163 mice, it was observed by these investigators that 131 of them developed leukemia despite induced atrophy of the thymus. Of the 131 mice that developed leukemia, in 19 this was found to be distinct from typical Mo-MuLV-induced disease. These 19 mice typically developed myeloid leukemias and lymphosarcomas. Of these 19, a single mouse developed an unusual invasive lymphosarcoma 65 days after Mo-MuLV inoculation (1,2). The animal exhibited multiple tumors of the lymph nodes with infiltration of the bone marrow, particularly into the cranium. The original tumor was transplanted, and filtered extracts of the original tumor or transplants of the tumor tissue were found to rapidly induce tumors in newborn and adult Balb/c mice (2-4). These tumors shared similar characteristics with the original tumor, including involvement of multiple bone marrow cavities, in some instances causing paraplegia. The thymus, on the other hand, never seemed to be affected by the virus or tumor cells.

This is contrary to the known effects of Mo-MuLV, which induces murine thymic lymphocytic leukemia (5,6). One of the distinctive features of the virus extract derived from this tumor was the very rapid induction of lymphosarcomas in newborn as well as adult Balb/c mice in which the latency was less than 2 weeks. This characteristic feature provided an early indication that this virus isolate could consist of an acute transforming virus. This isolate was named Abelson murine leukemia virus (A-MuLV).

Scher and Siegler were the first to show that the tumor extracts were also potent transformers of murine fibroblasts in vitro (7). By infecting cells at limiting dilutions they isolated a transformed cell line that did not produce an infectious virus. Infection of this nonproducer cell line with Mo-MuLV was found to rescue a transforming virus. Thus the identification of A-MuLV as a replication defective acute transforming retrovirus was made. Future work would identify A-MuLV was generated through the recombination of Mo-MuLV with the cellular *abl* gene. During this process the majority of Mo-MuLV was replaced, generating a fused genome between Mo-MuLV *gag* and c-*abl* sequences. The NIH 3T3 transformation assay developed by Scher and Siegler not only clarified the relationship between A-MuLV and Mo-MuLV but also provided a very convenient in vitro assay for the transforming component. This eliminated the need for the cumbersome tumor induction assay that was widely used before this study. The first nonproducer cell line that was isolated by Scher and Siegler was termed ANN-1 and was used extensively by later workers for the identification of protein products as well as molecular cloning experiments (7).

TRANSFORMATION BY A-MuLV

In Vivo

A-MuLV-induced leukemia has a very short latency period, involving lymphoblastic infiltration of the marrow, meninges, and lymph nodes, and shows no thymic association. First observed by Abelson and Rabstein (1), the neoplasm was unusual in its characteristics compared to other virally induced murine leukemias. The animals often showed deformities in the skull, for instance, as the proliferating cells spread rapidly to adjacent cranial structures. Although first diagnosed as a lymphoma (1,3), it was later determined that lymph node involvement was due to tumor infiltration (4). The tumor was thought to originate from immature lymphoid cells (1,3), specifically those in the bone marrow (4).

Although the initial isolation and characterization were performed in newborn Balb/c mice, they were extended to adult mice to determine if an age or strain specificity existed. Indeed, the Balb/c parent and its derivatives were the most sensitive strains across a variety of ages but other strains were resistant as adults (8). The presentation of Abelson disease is different in adults, in which cranial tumors are often absent and the mice have trouble walking with their hind legs, eventually becoming paralyzed (8,9). Autopsy revealed the proliferation of tumor cells in the lumbar vertebrae with invasion into the skeletal musculature (8). Crosses between the Balb/c and a resistant strain showed A-MuLV sensitivity to be a dominant trait, and this dominance was carried on two unique genes, termed *Av*-1 and *Av*-2, which were unlinked and had not previously been implicated in murine leukemogenesis (8,10). Although the presentation of the Abelson disease in adult and newborn mice appeared to be different, histologically the tumors were found to be identical, mostly consisting of lymphoid cells.

In addition to age, experimental conditions seem to play an important role in determining the target cell type transformed by A-MuLV. Adult Balb/c mice treated with pristane (2,6,10,14-tetramethylpentadecane) prior to A-MuLV injection were shown to present an increased spectrum of tumor types in addition to the typical Abelson lymphosarcoma (9). Other tumors that have been found to arise in pristane-primed mice include plasmacytomas, mastocytomas, and macrophage tumors (8,9,11,12). Occasionally a morphologic subset of lymphosarcomas, which have been termed ABLS tumors, was also observed (13). These tumors were later found to be myeloid in nature and devoid of integrated A-MuLV. Detailed examination indicated that these tumors are in fact induced by the helper Mo-MuLV, which integrated into the *myb* oncogene locus and transcriptionally activated this locus (14,15). The role of pristane in the induction of plasmacytomas in Balb/c mice is at present unclear. Pristane by itself is known to induce plasmacytomas in these mice with a latency period of 150-600 days, and the administration of A-MuLV appears to accelerate this process. Histologically, the plasmacytomas that develop in the virus-treated mice appear to be identical to those that arise from pristane treatment alone. However, virtually all the plasmacytomas that arise in mice treated with A-MuLV and pristane contain an integrated proviral genome of A-MuLV as well as a translocation involving the c-*myc* gene (16). The monocytic and macrophage tumors that arise in pristane-treated mice also have an integrated A-MuLV proviral genome, produce the virus-encoded protein products, and produce mast cell-specific or macrophage-specific proteins (11,12).

Although, typically, A-MuLV-injected mice do not show any signs of thymic leukemia, injection of this virus into the thymus of adult Balb/c and C57BL mice rapidly induces thymic leukemias (10,17-20). The tumors that arise clearly show T cell involvement as demonstrated by the presence of Thy-1 and Lyt-1 markers on primary tumor cells. When the tumor tissue was cultured and analyzed, they were found to be composed of a mixed population of T cell phenotypes, suggesting a primitive T lymphoid cell as the target of virus-induced transformation. It is interesting to note that the C57BL thymomas are also composed of cells positive for B220^{+} antigen, which is a pre-B cell marker, whereas B cells are not transformed following intravenous injection of virus into these mice (8,

19). Histologically, the A-MuLV-induced lymphosarcoma cell shows a large lobulated nucleus with sparse cytoplasm containing many free ribosomes. The cell is larger than a lymphoblast and has well-defined borders and an oval shape with a normal karyotype (3,4,21). The remarkably normal thymus gland in animals with Abelson disease suggested that cells other than T lymphocytes were involved. Induction of plasmacytomas in pristane-treated mice indicated that cells of B cell lineage may be the targets of this virus (9). The first evidence for this concept was provided by a study in which the surface markers in transplanted A-MuLV-induced tumors were examined (22). This study indicated that these tumor cells harbor surface immunoglobulin markers. When three of the lymphosarcomas induced by A-MuLV were established in culture and immunoglobulin synthesis in these cell lines was studied, it was found that these cell lines synthesized monomeric IgM molecules associated with the cell membrane (22). In one cell line IgG synthesis was also observed. The amount of immunoglobulin produced by these cells appeared to be very low, and often the synthesis was unstable (22). That A-MuLV transforms B cells was more clearly borne out in studies with in vitro transformed lymphoid cells.

In Vitro

A-MuLV appears to transform exclusively lymphoid cells in vivo, but it is capable of transforming both fibroblasts and lymphoid cells in vitro. A-MuLV is able to transform lymphoid cells derived from a variety of animal tissues (23–26). The initial in vitro transformation experiments were with murine splenocytes, which after infection caused tumors following transplantation in recipient pristane-primed mice (23,24). Donor and recipient cells were distinguished by chromosome markers, which established that the tumor cells were derived from the in vitro cultures that were exposed to the virus. A detailed understanding of the nature of the in vitro transformed cells comes from the studies carried out by Rosenberg and co-workers, who first established experimental conditions for the in vitro transformation of mouse fetal liver cells by A-MuLV (25). When mouse fetal liver cells were infected in vitro by A-MuLV, the cellular makeup of the culture changed over a period of 2 weeks, in which granulocytes appeared first and died in a few days; following this a new rapidly proliferating population of cells appeared that could be propagated indefinitely. These cells had surface markers for B cells or null cells, were able to form tumors following intraperitoneal injection into adult mice with or without pristane priming, and could be passaged indefinitely in the presence of β-mercaptoethanol. With the advent of a soft agar transformation system for lymphoid cells, it was possible to demonstrate that lymphoid cells derived from a variety of lymphoid tissues could be transformed by A-MuLV and that murine bone marrow cells showed transformation susceptibility (26). With optimal culture conditions in which β-mercaptoethanol was added to the culture medium, these investigators could obtain as many as 30 colonies per 10^6 cells. A comparison of transformation efficiency by the same virus stock of lymphoid versus NIH 3T3 cells indicated that in vitro A-MuLV was at least 100-fold more efficient in transforming fibroblasts compared to lymphocytes.

Specific studies on in vitro transformed lymphoid cells were undertaken by Rosenberg and coworkers to characterize and define the cell type being transformed by A-MuLV. A-MuLV-transformed bone marrow cultures were found to contain variety of phenotypes (24,27). Although the first reports suggested that the cells transformed in vitro by A-MuLV are null cells that did not synthesize appreciable amounts of Ig molecules (28), a more careful study by Siden et al. (29) indicated that culture conditions had a profound effect on the immunoglobulin synthesis by these cells. Culture conditions that reduced the growth rate of cells, such as reduced serum concentration in the medium or removal of β-mercaptoethanol from the medium, appeared to promote immunoglobulin synthesis by these cells. Under carefully controlled conditions, these investigators demonstrated that a majority of the in vitro transformed cell lines synthesize a μ chain but no detectable light chain (29). Aside from this μ-only phenotype, lines that make only light chain, both chains, or no immunoglobulin-related polypeptides have also been found (29–32). Cell types with no immunoglobulin synthesis appeared to contain terminal deoxynucleotidyltransferase activity, suggesting that they also are of lymphoid lineage (27). In the A-MuLV-infected fetal liver or placental cultures, besides the lymphoid transformants, colonies of erythroid cells have also been found to occur (33). Although these colonies could not be established as cell lines, the experiments nevertheless suggest that A-MuLV has the ability to alter growth in at least two different hematopoietic lineages. In early bone marrow cultures infected by A-MuLV, growth-restricted cells were observed when the culturing method included either a feeder layer or conditioned medium (34). Over a period of time with continued passage, a population of feeder-independent cells emerged that had a malignant phenotype and showed no demonstrable change in the transforming protein of the virus (35).

When the immunoglobulin gene structure in lymphoid cells transformed by A-MuLV in vitro was examined, it was found that only the heavy chain is rearranged (36). This further supported the idea that immature B cells are targets for A-MuLV transformation. Experiments utilizing the feeder method of marrow cultivation demonstrated that B cells at various stages of maturation are sensitive to A-MuLV transformation, and once transformed, they may continue to differentiate as determined by κ light-chain rearrangement and expression (37). When bone marrow cells that are continually stimulated by lipopolysaccharide (LPS) were transformed by A-MuLV, two novel types of membrane Ig-positive B cell lines were generated (38). One group was positive for membrane-bound IgM and

A-MuLV-encoded p160, suggesting that the transformation of mature B cells in vitro is possible under certain culture conditions. The second group of cells obtained in such cultures were positive for membrane IgG and secreted large amounts of immunoglobulin into the medium. However, these cells were negative for A-MuLV proviral genome and were nontumorigenic. The role of A-MuLV in the generation of this second group of cell lines is at present unclear, and immortalization of these cells could simply involve infection with helper Mo-MuLV.

Consistent with the Ig gene structure, A-MuLV-transformed cells express a number of B cell markers that include B220 antigen and the antigenic determinants recognized by monoclonal antibodies, such as BP-1, 6C3, AA4, and GF1 (39). These cells usually lack differentiation antigens associated with more differentiated B lymphocytes, such as Ia, ThB, and PC1, further supporting the notion that A-MuLV-transformed lymphoid cells are representatives of normal B cell precursors. Because of this unique property of A-MuLV to transform cells of B lymphocyte lineage, these cell lines served as valuable models for the study of early events in the immunodifferentiation of B lymphocytes (31,32,36).

A-MuLV MUTANTS

The plasticity of the A-MuLV genome is demonstrated by its ability to have sequences deleted and mutated. Initial studies on viral isolates showed a series of different protein products, all precipitated with anti-Abelson tumor sera (40,41). The sizes included the known 120 kD form along with species of 160, 100, and 90 kD. These findings suggested that much of the A-MuLV genome was unnecessary for transformation since all the recovered isolates were able to transform cells in vitro. Comparisons of the viral genomes suggested an internal deletion in p160 resulted in the formation of the p120 genome (42). The p100 and p90 strains appear to have arisen from the p120 strain as a result of frame shift mutations that result in premature termination of translation of the viral genome resulting in the synthesis of 100 and 90 kD proteins (42). The predominant feature in the generation of the new strains was the elimination of *abl*-specific sequences not essential for transformation, but transformation-defective (*td*) mutants were also identified (42–44). One of these, *p92td*, appeared to have arisen from p120 following an additional deletion of 700 bp and consequently did not possess the protein kinase activity inherent to the A-MuLV strains (42). *p92td*, although unable to autophosphorylate, is able to accept phosphates from an active donor, such as A-MuLV protein, in vitro; this lack of kinase activity therefore correlated with the inability of this strain to transform cells in vitro or in vivo (45). The p90 and p100 strains transform fibroblasts efficiently but appear less efficient in transforming lymphoid cells (44). Their protein products were shown to be weak protein kinases, unstable and synthesized in greater quantities than either p160 or p120. These mutants were poorly tumorigenic in vivo, and examination of the tumors induced by the p90 strain revealed that they now contained new variants (46). These variants fell into two categories: one appeared to be the regenerated p120 strain as a result of back mutation, and the others were smaller variants of p90. These latter viruses were weak transformers of lymphoid cells in vitro but were potent tumor inducers in vivo. Despite their weak transforming activity of lymphoid cells in vitro, they were potent transformers of fibroblasts, suggesting that transformation of these two cell types could be differentially affected by alterations in the viral genome (44,46). A series of *td* mutants were isolated from mink cells either by screening single infected mink cells or from spontaneous morphologic revertants of A-MuLV-infected mink cells (43). These revertants occur frequently during continued passage of these cells compared to murine and rat cells. *td* mutants could also be obtained from Fisher rat embryo (FRE) cells infected with A-MuLV, also by endpoint dilution (47). These mutants demonstrated a decreased kinase activity compared to the wild-type virus. Expression of p120 and p80 was present in FRE *td* mutant cells at levels similar to those found in wild-type virus-transformed cells, which was in contrast to the null expression levels found in the spontaneously reverted mink cells (43,47).

A-MuLV mutants have also been generated by mutagenesis of the wild-type virus. These temperature-sensitive (*ts*) mutants have been generated by chemical treatment (48), linker insertion (49), or site-directed mutagenesis (50). These mutants further demonstrated the need for a functional tyrosine kinase for NIH 3T3 transformation, as transformation is maintained only at the permissive temperature. Kipreos et al. (49) found two independent *ts* mutations to involve amino acid insertion within a 12 amino acid span in the kinase domain; amino acid mutations derived by Engelman and Rosenberg (50) were more 3′. None of the mutations affected the highly conserved regions of the kinase domain and are in regions known to be affected in other *ts* v-*src* mutants. When lymphoid cells infected by the *ts* mutant of Takemori et al. (48) were grown at a nonpermissive temperature, some of the cells showed the presence of surface IgG, suggesting that these cells resume the process of differentiation when A-MuLV gene product is inactive. At the same restrictive temperature infected NIH 3T3 cells were found to revert to a normal phenotype. Although the location of the lesion in the genome is unknown, the autokinase activity in these mutants was found to be 10- to 100-fold lower at the restrictive temperature (48).

A-MuLV PROTEIN

A 120 kD polypeptide was first identified immunologically in A-MuLV-transformed ANN-1 cells (51–53). The polypeptide was shown to share antigenic determinants with Mo-MuLV and contain sequences that were unrelated to the helper virus proteins. These latter sequences were shown to code for the transforming potential of the virus and were found to be homologous to a mouse cellular protein. The designation *abl* was given to these cell-derived sequences. The nature of the cell-derived information present in the p120 molecule was investigated using anti-A-MuLV-specific antisera by Witte et al. (54). For this they used an A-MuLV-transformed cell line termed L1, which when injected into C57L/J strain of mice was found to form tumors that subsequently regressed. This regression was accompanied by the appearance of antibodies in the mouse serum that cross-reacted with Mo-MuLV proteins as well as with p120. Following adsorption with Mo-MuLV proteins, sera that specifically cross-reacted with p120 were generated. These anti-A-MuLV tumor sera were later used in immunofluorescence studies that appeared to suggest that the p120 was expressed on the cell surface. A surface tumor antigen was also observed with anti-A-MuLV tumor sera raised in a different mouse strain (55). Later, studies with monoclonal anti-*abl* antibodies were unable to detect surface *abl* determinants. Only antibodies that react with p15 *gag* antigen were found to bind to the surface of A-MuLV-transformed cells (56). It is therefore likely that the original surface expression observed was due to detection of the determinants expressed by p15 *gag*.

Both p120 and p160 are associated in part with the membrane (54,56,57), and by analogy to Harvey murine sarcoma virus (H-MuSV) and Rous sarcoma virus (RSV), the addition of myristic acid to p15 glycine (amino acid 2) may be important in membrane association (58,59). The cellular localization of A-MuLV as determined by ^{35}S and ^{32}P labeling showed the existence of a difference in the distribution and kinase activity of the protein (60). The p120 molecule was found to be nonglycosylated; the p160 molecule appears to exist in both glycosylated and nonglycosylated forms (57). The presence of the carbohydrate prevents phosphorylation of the p160 but does segregate it exclusively to the membrane. The addition of carbohydrate was shown to occur in the *gag* leader sequences and plays no role in transformation (see A-MuLV Genome).

The discovery that the transforming protein of RSV possessed protein kinase activity raised the question of such an ability by A-MuLV (61). Witte et al. demonstrated that p120 is a tyrosine kinase, capable of both *cis*-acting autophosphorylation and *trans*-acting phosphorylation of exogenous substrates (62,63). The lack of transformation in A-MuLV mutants devoid of in vitro kinase activity strongly supported the idea that the kinase activity was essential for the transforming function of the virus. In vivo phosphotyrosine levels were found to be approximately 10 times higher in A-MuLV-transformed cells than in control uninfected cells, further strengthening this argument (64). The inherent kinase activity of A-MuLV was demonstrated following expression of cloned viral genome in *Escherichia coli* (65). This further allowed the localization of the enzymatically active viral domain (66). Peptide mapping showed that, in vitro and in vivo, phosphorylated proteins are not similar and that the phosphorylated region of A-MuLV in vitro maps to the *gag* and NH_2-terminal region (67). Although the substrate for A-MuLV is unknown, it shares with other tyrosine kinases the ability to phosphorylate a variety of cellular proteins (68,69). Analysis of proteins phosphorylated on tyrosine residues in transformed murine lymphocytes and fibroblasts by an antibody to phosphotyrosine revealed that different substrates are phosphorylated in different cell types (70).

A variety of anti-v-*abl* antibodies have been generated using a series of peptides as immunogens. These antipeptide antibodies have been used to map the regions of the protein necessary for kinase activity (71). These studies demonstrated that antibodies to a region that shares high homology with other tyrosine kinases (in the vicinity of autophosphorylated tyrosine) can block in vitro phosphorylation.

Immunoprecipitation of metabolically labeled proteins from normal murine thymus, spleen, and bone marrow with anti-A-MuLV tumor sera (54) revealed the presence of a 150 kD cross-reactive species (72). This normal cellular protein (NCP150) showed homology to A-MuLV when phosphorylated peptides were mapped, but NCP150 failed to demonstrate either the presence of phosphotyrosine or in vitro kinase activity (73). Altering the in vitro kinase assay conditions, Konopka and Witte (74) found that c-*abl* does possess an in vitro kinase activity and phosphotyrosine is present in c-*abl* protein phosphorylated in vitro. Since the level of expression of c-*abl* is lower than that of v-*abl* (73), the increased sensitivity of the improved in vitro kinase assay (74) was necessary for its identification. The A-MuLV and c-*abl* proteins differ in their sites of tyrosine phosphorylation in vitro; this can be attributed to the presence of *gag* in A-MuLV. In this regard, the in vitro phosphorylation of c-*abl* protein resembles the in vivo phosphorylation pattern of A-MuLV protein, with the same major site reacted (74). This is also the major site of tyrosine phosphorylation for other tyrosine kinases that share homology with A-MuLV (75).

A-MuLV GENOME

Molecular Cloning

Early studies with A-MuLV p120 strain showed that it contained 5′ and 3′ sequences common to Mo-MuLV and an insert that was homologous to a conserved cellular gene (76–79). A detailed structural analysis of the viral genome became possible with the advent of recombinant DNA techniques and the molecular cloning of both unintegrated and integrated forms of the viral genome (77, 78). Nucleotide sequence analysis of the proviral genome of p120 indeed showed that the proviral genome contained a long open reading frame encoding the p15, p12, and portions of p30 Mo-MuLV *gag* antigens at the 5′ end, which was fused in-frame to an open reading frame that was derived from mouse cellular sequences (Figure 1) (80). A protein made from this open reading frame would

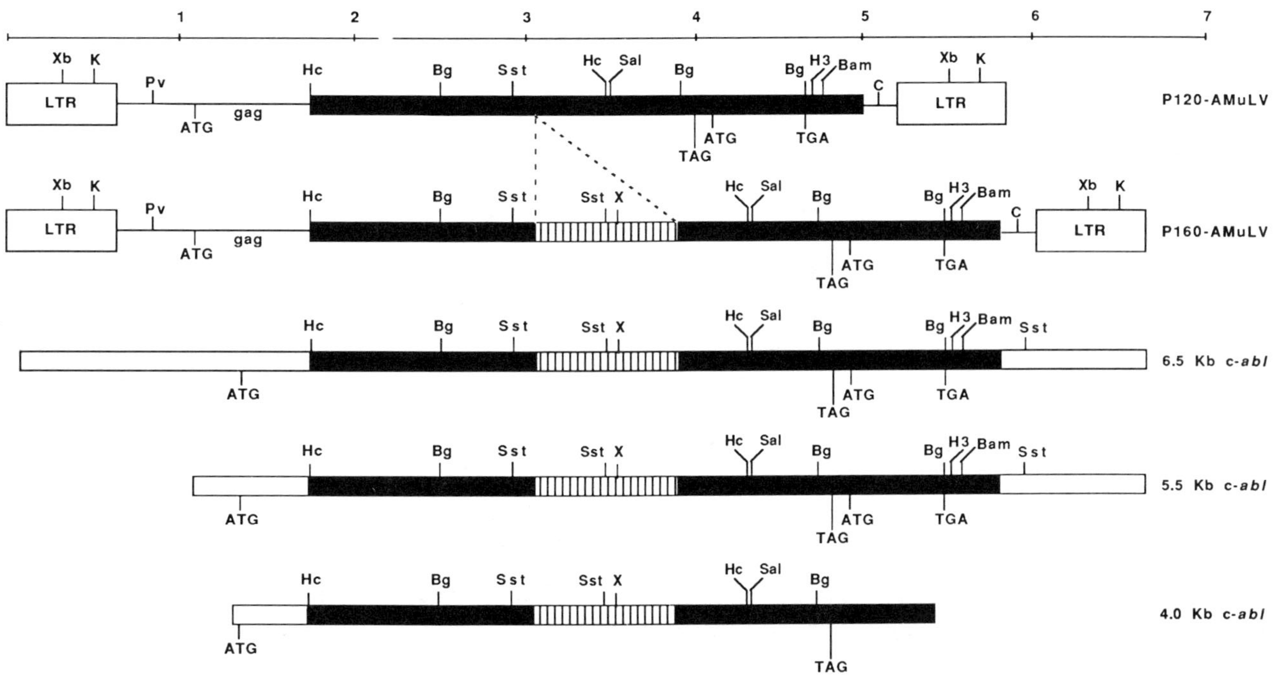

Figure 1 Comparison of murine c-*abl* and v-*abl* genomes. A-MuLV species p160 and p120 are compared with the two somatic c-*abl* mRNAs of 6.5 and 5.5 kb and the 4.0 kb transcript found in testis. The portion of c-*abl* incorporated into the virus is indicated by the block or bar areas.

contain 240 amino acids derived from the *gag* gene and 745 amino acids derived from the c-*abl* gene. A second open reading frame was present as well, downstream of the larger open reading frame, coding for a prospective 18 kD protein. It is unclear at this point whether this region codes for a functional protein. Comparison of the A-MuLV sequence to other tyrosine kinases revealed a highly homologous region, which suggested a common functional domain. Comparison of the nucleotide sequence of p120 strain to that of p160 revealed that the former strain was derived from the latter as a result of an in-frame deletion of 789 bp (Figure 1) (81,82). The recombination sites between the helper virus and the cellular sequences were identical, as was the presence of the 18 kD polypeptide open reading frame at the 3′ end (80,82). The 5′ recombination site is thought to involve a 4 bp homology between *gag* and c-*abl* (TACA), but no such homology was apparent at the 3′ end (83,84). The p120 strain was found to have undergone a point mutation in the *gag* gene leader sequences that prevents the synthesis of this leader sequence upstream of the start point of the p15 domain. This point mutation is absent in the p160 strain, which allows initiation of protein synthesis several amino acids upstream of the AUG codon used in the p120 strain. This stretch of extra sequence appears to contain a site that is glycosylated (80).

The presence of these two strains, p120 and p160, with identical Mo-MuLV recombination sites, suggests that they were the original viruses, with p120 derived from p160. This enables the various mutants to be categorized under the two progenitors according to an approximate genomic size of 5.5 or 6.3 kb. The similarity of transcript size suggested that the altered proteins are due to mutations that prematurely introduce stop codons. This in fact was found to be the case for p90, which has suffered the deletion of a single base G at position 2410, shifting the reading frame such that termination occurs 191 amino acids prematurely (82). Similar mutations seem to have generated the p100 strain, and thus these two strains represent naturally occurring mutants with a carboxy-terminal truncation of the transforming protein.

Molecular cloning and nucleotide sequence analysis of c-*abl* cDNA clones (83–85) allowed a detailed comparison of the viral and cellular genes and revealed that the v-*abl* gene product is a truncated version of the cellular gene (Figure 1). Thus, toward the amino-terminal end, 114 amino acids of the c-*abl* protein have been replaced by 240 amino acids derived from the viral *gag* gene. Although v-*abl* and c-*abl* share the same translation termination codon, the c-*abl* gene contains an extra 765 bp of noncoding sequences prior to the site of polyadenylation. The 5′ recombination site lies in the middle of the c-*abl* exon 3 (79,81), and the 3′ recombination site also appears to exist in the middle of an exon toward the 3′ end. A point mutation was observed at position 2545, resulting in the substitution of a glutamic acid residue in c-*abl* with lysine in p120 and p160 (80,82,84). By site-directed mutagenesis we have shown that this mutation is not involved in activating the transforming potential of p120 in fibroblasts (Shore, unpublished results).

Structural Requirements for Transformation by A-MuLV

Molecular cloning of the Abelson viral genome allowed site-directed mutagenesis, which helped to define the role played by some of the domains present in the viral genome. Thus, Srinivasan et al. used the in vitro transforming potential of the cloned DNA to map the promoter and enhancer regions of the viral long terminal repeats (LTRs) (86). In addition, the results from A-MuLV mutants clearly demonstrated that the entire genome is not essential for transformation. Digestion of cloned A-MuLV with restriction enzymes followed by calcium phosphate transfections showed that the 3′ portion of the virus up to the *Sal*I site in p120 (Figure 2C) or the *Pst*I site in p160 (Figure 2E) is not required for transformation (87,88). Regions of the 5′ genome were also found to be unnecessary for transformation, as shown by p160 focus formation following deletion of the majority of the *gag* sequences by digestion with *Bst*EII (Figure 2D) (88). The proximal 34 amino acids of p15 *gag* were found to be enough to function as the myristylation signal and allow A-MuLV transformation. However, insertional mutagenesis experiments with cloned p160 DNA showed that several mutants with insertions in the p15 and p12 *gag* regions exhibited a dramatically reduced transformation activity but insertions in the p30 *gag* sequences showed no effect (Figure 2A) (89). Rees-Jones and Goff (89) could not find any *abl* protein in most transformation-defective *gag*-mutated clones, even though the kinase activity of these proteins could be detected in a bacterial expression assay. The role of *gag* appears to be very complex and seems to involve subcellular compartmentalization as well as the stability and substrate specificity of the viral protein. Figure 2B shows an invariant region containing the kinase domain, which must be intact for transformation (87-90). In mutants made by the insertion of linkers that abolished transformation, the viral proteins were all shown to have lost their protein tyrosine kinase activity by bacterial expression experiments (89,90).

A surprising feature of A-MuLV is its lethal effect upon infection or transfection in certain fibroblasts (91). These cells upon continued culture revert to a flat phenotype or die. By creating a series of viral deletion mutants, the region responsible for this lethality was mapped to the 3′ end of the A-MuLV genome (92). Cloned p160 A-MuLV DNA, used in calcium phosphate transfections, has been reported to be a poor producer of transformed foci (93). Cotransfection with Mo-MuLV plasmid DNA was found to increase its transforming potential by 100-fold. The pMo-MuLV is thought to rescue A-MuLV from cells in which it may be toxic, allowing it to infect surrounding cells. Transfection of NIH 3T3 cells with cloned p120 A-MuLV, which was linearized by digestion with re-

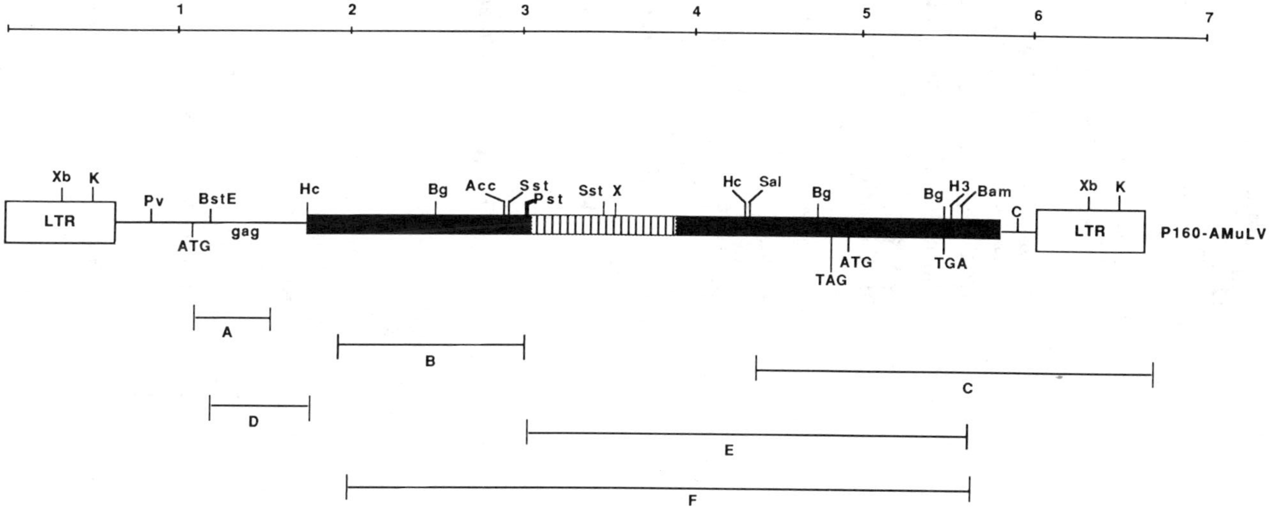

Figure 2 Domains of A-MuLV and their relationship to viral transformation. The viral p160 genome is shown with regions of biologic activity indicated by the lines underneath.

striction enzymes, produced a substantial level of focus formation as reported by Srinivasan et al. (87). Although the reason for this discrepancy is unclear, experiments in our laboratory have shown the critical importance of the carrier DNA. Our experiments show that when appropriate carrier DNA and transfection conditions were used, high transformation efficiencies could be achieved. It is clear, however, that cotransfection with pMo-MuLV increases pA-MuLV focus formation (93a).

The role of helper virus in lymphoid and fibroblast transformation was initially shown to be different in studies in which the virus was rescued from a nonproducer line by a variety of helper viruses (94). Every rescued A-MuLV virus was able to transform fibroblasts, but only strongly leukemogenic helpers were able to transform lymphoid cells. However, recent studies using a packaging cell line have shown that helper virus-free A-MuLV is efficient in bone marrow transformation in vitro as well as tumor induction in vivo, demonstrating that replication of the virus is not required (95). The role of *gag* is reported to be different in lymphoid and fibroblast transformation. In lymphoid transformation, viruses with deletions of *gag*, as in Figure 2D, and 3′ deletions from *Xho*I (Figure 2) were unable to transform bone marrow cells (88). Prywes et al. deleted smaller segments of A-MuLV *gag* and determined that only p15 *gag* sequences were necessary for lymphoid transformation (96). p15 appears to be involved in the stability of the A-MuLV protein product in lymphoid cells, and when these sequences were absent little or no accumulation of the steady-state level of protein that was necessary for transformation was observed (96).

The kinase domain also plays an important role in lymphoid transformation, as shown by Mathey-Prevot and Baltimore (97). By exchanging sequences that code for the protein kinase domain between v-*src* and v-*abl* genes (Figure 2F), they were able to confer the biologic activities of A-MuLV to a v-*src*-*v*-*abl* virus, termed v-SBL, which contained v-*abl* sequences at the 3′ end and v-*src* sequences at the 5′ end. On the other hand, the reciprocal construct, termed v-ARC, which contained v-*abl* sequences at the 5′ end and v-*src* sequences at the 3′ end, was found to be transformation defective, ostensibly due to a low kinase activity, in 3T3 cells and lymphoid cells. Although v-SBL could abrogate the IL-3 requirement of Ba/F3 cells, the v-ARC virus lacked such a capability. This delineates a region in A-MuLV that is unique from other related tyrosine kinases.

The minimum size of A-MuLV required for fibroblast and lymphoid transformation is also different. The smallest active A-MuLV construct in fibroblasts is inactive in lymphoid transformation (85). Some of this effect is due to missing *gag* sequences (96), but the carboxy end of A-MuLV may play a role as well. Truncated mutants of p120 have shown the requirement of the 3′ end for optimal lymphoid transformation (46). This reiterates the uniqueness of fibroblast versus lymphoid transformation by A-MuLV. The virus contains the sequences necessary for both, but it may be manipulated to favor one type over another.

A-MuLV-INDUCED ABROGATION OF FACTOR REQUIREMENTS

The observation by Whitlock and Witte (34) that A-MuLV-infected cells progress through a factor-dependent nontumorigenic state to a fully transformed malignant phenotype shows that A-MuLV has a pleiomorphic effect on the cell. A-MuLV may thus alter the growth requirements as well as the malignant status of cells. The possibility that these effects may be separated was suggested in experments that distinguished between A-MuLV mutants that transform lymphoid cells in vitro but not in vivo (46). The ability of A-MuLV to convert immortalized Friend murine leukemia virus (Fr-MuLV)-infected myeloid cells to fully malignant factor-inedependent cells demonstrates one property of A-MuLV function (98). Fr-MuLV-infected myeloid cells are factor-dependent nontumorigenic continuous cell lines that, when superinfected with A-MuLV, become IL-3 independent and capable of forming tumors in syngeneic mice. A-MuLV is capable of producing this type of immortalized cell on its own, and H-MuSV cannot mimic the effect of A-MuLV on the Fr-MuLV-immortalized cell lines. Using a *ts* A-MuLV mutant, the requirement for the functional kinase activity in rendering myeloid cells IL-3 independent has also been shown (99). The mechanism by which A-MuLV infection substitutes for IL-3 does not appear to be an autocrine mechanism (12,100). A-MuLV infection of both myeloid (100) and mast cells (12) relieves IL-3 dependence without affecting IL-3 release into the medium, IL-3 RNA transcription, or the number of IL-3 cell surface receptors. Similarly, A-MuLV is also able to produce factor independence in erythroid cells that are dependent on erythropoetin for growth and differentiation (101). Comparing the effects of A-MuLV and H-MuSV on erythroid cell transformation, Waneck et al. showed that both viruses infect the same target cells yet H-MuSV-infected cells remain erythropoetin dependent yet v-*abl* can substitute for or supersede the requirement for erythropoetin in A-MuLV-infected cells (101). As in the case of myeloid cells, A-MuLV alone is incapable of rendering a factor-independent continuous erythroid cell line. Not surprisingly, pre-B cells, the predominant target of A-MuLV transformation, also become IL-3 independent following A-MuLV infection (102). In vitro assays show that this is due to neither an autocrine mechanism nor activation of the c-*myc* gene. Another A-MuLV in vivo target, T cells, also become IL-2 independent by a nonautocrine mechanism (103). These studies show that there is a common A-MuLV-sensitive step in growth factor-induced signal transduction pathways in cells of different lineages.

Cells that become factor independent still show a responsiveness to the factor, demonstrating the integrity of the pathway, as seen in cells transformed by *ts* mutants (99). Studies on an IL-3-dependent stem cell 32D Cl3 by Rovera et al. (104) have shown that A-MuLV has an effect not only on growth factor dependence but also on the differentiation potential of hematopoietic cells. The 32D Cl3 cell line, which has been studied by these workers, requires IL-3 for growth, and in the presence of high concentrations of this growth factor, terminal differentiation of these cells is blocked. However, when removed from IL-3-containing medium and placed in a medium containing (G-CSF) they terminally differentiate in a period of 11-12 days and die. When these cells are transformed by A-MuLV, they become not only IL-3 independent but also resistant to (granulocyte colony-stimulating factor) G-CSF-induced terminal differentiation. When the cells are stimulated with G-CSF 12 h prior to infection, however, they become refractory to A-MuLV transformation and terminally differentiate. These experiments suggest that once the cells are committed to a differentiation pathway, A-MuLV has little or no effect on these pathways, but before such a commitment is made the viral infection results in an inability of the cell to enter these differentiation pathways.

SECONDARY EVENTS IN A-MuLV-INDUCED TRANSFORMATION

Several studies have also shown that in certain cells A-MuLV must cooperate with a second event for full transformation. Whitlock and Witte (34) first noted the progression of A-MuLV-infected cells as they move from factor dependence to a more fully malignant state. This was shown to occur over a period of passaging in vitro. The studies on growth factor abrogation have shown the necessity for secondary events as well. A-MuLV-induced IL-3 independence in myeloid cells cannot occur without the cells' first being immortalized by Fr-MuLV (98). In A-MuLV-infected erythroid cells, normal growth and differentiation proceed as the effects of erythropoetin are mimicked, yet the cells are neither immortalized nor tumorigenic (101). The nature of the second event is unclear, as some evidence suggests A-MuLV can initiate transformation (34,35) and other data show its involvement in progression (105). The cell type may play an important role in determining the action of A-MuLV and the necessity of specific secondary events. Secondary events that have been described are overexpression of c-*myc* (16) and *p53* (106), the release of transforming growth factor α (TGF-α) (107), and the need for functional epidermal growth factor (EGF) receptors (108).

Secondary events also appear to be involved in vivo. Grunwold et al. (109) have shown that the loss of the viral genome does not cause tumor regression, and Green et al. (110) found A-MuLV-induced tumors show clonal dominance, suggesting the outgrowth of only a few of the initially infected cells.

HZ2-FeSV: AN *abl*-CONTAINING FELINE RETROVIRUS

A feline retrovirus, Hardy-Zukerman 2 feline sarcoma virus (HZ2-FeSV), was later isolated from an adult male pet Siamese cat that had multiple spontaneous fibrosarcomas from which filtered extracts produced tumors when injected in a kitten (111). Infection of mink cells at limiting dilution yielded a nonproducer cell line from which HZ2-FeSV could be rescued by a variety of feline leukemia viruses (FeLV), showing it to be a replication-defective acute transforming retrovirus as well. This virus has transduced 439 amino acids of feline c-*abl* containing the tyrosine kinase region (112). The c-*abl* portion transduced extends farther upstream than the c-*abl* sequences present in A-MuLV. The 5′ recombination between FeLV *gag* and c-*abl* involves a six-base homology and occurs 25 amino acids downstream from the exon 2 splice acceptor site. The 3′ recombination occurs following the kinase region and fuses c-*abl* to 3′ FeLV *pol* sequences, eliminating approximately 800 carboxy-terminal amino acids of c-*abl*. The difference in tumor induction by these two *abl*-containing viruses, sarcoma by HZ2-FeSV versus lymphoid by A-MuLV, was shown to be due to the differences in the unique non-*abl* sequences, such as the LTRs and helper virus proteins (112).

ACKNOWLEDGMENTS

This work was supported by NIH grant numbers CA47937 and CA25875.

REFERENCES

1. Abelson, H. T., and Rabstein, L. S. (1970). Influence of prednisolone on Moloney leukemogenic virus in BALB/c mice. *Cancer Res. 30*:2208–2212.
2. Abelson, H. T., and Rabstein, L. S. (1970). Lymphosarcoma: Virus induced thymic-independent disease in mice. *Cancer Res. 30*:2213–2222.
3. Rabstein, L. S., Gazdar, A. F., Chopra, H. C., and Abelson, H. T. (1971). Early morphological changes associated with infection by a murine nonthymic lymphatic tumor virus. *JNCI 46*:481–491.
4. Siegler, R., Zajdel, S., and Lane, I. (1972). Pathogenesis of Abelson-virus induced murine leukemia. *JNCI 48*:189–218.
5. Moloney, J. B. (1960). Biological studies on a lymphoid-leukemia virus extracted from sarcoma 37. 1. Origin and introductory investigations. *JNCI 24*: 933–951.
6. Reddy, E. P., Dunn, C. Y., and Aaronson, S. A. (1980). Different lymphoid cell targets for transformation by replication-component Moloney and Rauscher mouse leukemia viruses. *Cell 19*:663–669.
7. Scher, C D., and Siegler, R. (1975). Direct transformation of 3T3 cells by Abelson murine leukemia virus. *Nature 253*:792–731.

8. Risser, R., Potter, M., and Rowe, W. P. (1978). Abelson virus-induced lymphomagenesis in mice. *J. Exp. Med. 148*:714–726.
9. Potter, M., Sklar, M. D., and Rowe, W. P. (1973). Rapid viral induction of plasmacytomas in pristane-primed BALB/c mice. *Science 182*:592–594.
10. Risser, R., Kachler, D., and Lamph, W. W. (1985). Different genes control the susceptibility of mice to Moloney or Abelson murine leukemia viruses. *J. Virol. 55*:547–553.
11. Pierce, J. H., DiFiore, P. P., Aaronson, S. A., Potter, M., Pumphrey, A., Scott, A., and Ihle, J. N. (1985). Neoplastic transformation of mast cells by Abelson-MuLV: Abrogation of IL-3 dependence by a non-autocrine mechanism. *Cell 41*:685–693.
12. Raschke, W. C., Baird, S., Ralph, P., and Nakoninz, I. (1978). Functional macrophage cell lines transformed by Abelson leukemia virus. *Cell 15*:261–267.
13. Potter, M., Reddy, E. P., and Wivel, N. A. (1975). Immunoglobulin production by lymphosarcomas induced by Abelson virus in mice. *Natl. Cancer Inst. Monogr. 48*:311–320.
14. Mushinski, J. F., Potter, M., Bauer, S. R., and Reddy, E. P. (1983). DNA rearrangement and altered RNA expression of the c-*myb* oncogene in mouse plasmacytoid lymphosarcomas. *Science 220*:795–798.
15. Shen-Ong, G. L. C., Potter, M., Mushinski, J. F., Lavu, S., and Reddy, E. P. (1984). Activation of the c-*myb* locus by viral insertional mutagenesis in plasmacytoid lymphosarcomas. *Science 226*:1077–1080.
16. Ohno, S., Migita, S., Weiner, F., Babonits, M., Klein, G., Mushinski, I. F., and Potter, M. (1984). Chromosomal translocations activating *myc* sequences and transduction of v-*abl* are critical events in the rapid induction of plasmacytomas by pristane and Abelson virus. *J. Exp. Med. 159*:1762–1777.
17. Cook, W. D., (1982). Rapid thymomas induced by Abelson murine leukemia virus. *Proc. Natl. Acad. Sci. USA 79*:2917–2921.
18. Scott, M. L., Davis, M. M., and Feinberg, M. B. (1986). Transformation of T-lymphoid cells by Abelson murine leukemia virus. *J. Virol. 59*:434–443.
19. Cook, W. D. (1985). Thymocyte subsets transformed by Abelson murine leukemia virus. *Mol. Cell Biol. 5*:390–397.
20. D'Andrea, E., Saggioro, D., Fleissner, E., and Chieco-Bianchi, L. (1987). Abelson murine leukemia virus-induced thymic lymphomas: Transformation of a primitive lymphoid precursor. *JNCI 79*:189–193.
21. Klein, G., Ohno, S., Rosenberg, N., Wiener, F., Spira, J., and Baltimore, D. (1980). Cytogenetic studies on Abelson-virus-induced mouse leukemias. *Int. J. Cancer 25*:805–811.
22. Premkumar, E., Potter, M., Singer, P. A., and Sklar, M. D. (1975). Synthesis, surface deposition and secretion of immunoglobulins by Abelson virus-transformed lumphosarcoma cell ines. *Cell 6*:149–159.
23. Sklar, M. D., White, B. J., and Rowe, W. P. (1974). Initiation of oncogenic transformation of mouse lymphocytes in vitro by Abelson leukemia virus. *Proc. Natl. Acad. Sci. USA 71*:4077–4081.

24. Raschke, W. C., Ralph, P., Watson, J., Sklar, M. D., and Cooh, H. (1975). Oncogenic transformation of murine lymphoid cells by in vitro infection with Abelson leukemia virus. *JNCI 54*:1249–1253.
25. Rosenberg, N., Baltimore, D., and Scher, C. D. (1975). In vitro transformation of lymphoid cells by Abelson murine leukemia virus. *Proc. Natl. Acad. Sci. USA 72*:1932–1936.
26. Rosenberg, N., and Baltimore, D. (1976). A quantitative assay for transformation of bone marrow cells by Abelson murine leukemia virus. *J. Exp. Med. 143*:1453–1463.
27. Silverstone, A. E., Rosenberg, N., Sato, V. L., Scheid, M. P., Boyse, E., and Baltimore, D. (1978). Correlating terminal deoxynucleotidyl transferase and cell surface markers in the pathway of lymphocyte autogeny. In *Differentiation of Normal and Neoplastic Hematopoietic Cells*, Vol. 2 (B. Clarkson, P. A. Marks, and J. E. Till, eds.). Cold Spring Harbor Laboratory, Cold Spring Harbor, New York, pp. 433–453.
28. Pratt, D. M., Strominger, J., Parkman, R., Kaplan, D., Schwaber, J., Rosenberg, N., and Scher, C. D. (1977). Abelson virus-transformed lymphocytes: Null cells that modulate H-2. *Cell 12*:683–690.
29. Siden, E. J., Baltimore, D., Clark, D., and Rosenberg, (1979). Immunoglobulin synthesis by lymphoid cells transformed in vitro by Abelson murine leukemia virus. *Cell 16*:389–396.
30. Boss, M., Greaves, M., and Teich, N. (1979). Abelson virus transformed hematopoietic cell lines with pre-B characteristics. *Nature 278*:551–553.
31. Alt, F. W., Rosenberg, N., Lewis, S., Thomas, E., and Baltimore, D. (1981). Organization and reorganization of immunoglobulin genes in A-MuLV-transformed cells: Rearrangement of heavy but not light chains. *Cell 27*: 381–390.
32. Lewis, S., Rosenberg, N., Alt, F., and Baltimore, D. (1982). Continuing gene rearrangement in an Abelson murine leukemic virus transformed cell line. *Cell 30*:807–816.
33. Waneck, G. L., and Rosenberg, N. (1981). Abelson leukemia virus induces lymphoid and erythroid colonies in infected fetal cell cultures. *Cell 26*: 79–89.
34. Whitlock, C. S., and Witte, O. N. (1981). Abelson-virus infected cells can exhibit restricted in vitro growth and low oncogenic potential. *J. Virol. 44*: 577–584.
35. Whitlock, C. S., Ziegler, S. F., and Witte, O. N. (1983). Progression of the transformed phenotype in clonal lines of Abelson virus-infected lymphocytes. *Mol. Cell. Biol. 3*:596–604.
36. Alt, F., Rosenberg, N., Casanova, R. J., Thomas, E. J., and Baltimore, D. (1982). Immunoglobulin heavy chain expression and class switching in a murine leukemia cell line. *Nature 296*:325–331.
37. Whitlock, C. A., Ziegler, S. F., Treiman, L. J., Stafford, J. I., and Witte, O. N. (1983). Differentiation of cloned populations of immature B cells after transformation with Abelson murine leukemia virus. *Cell 32*:903–911.

38. Serunian, L. A., and Rosenberg, N. (1986). Abelson virus potentiates long-term growth of mature B-lymphocytes. *Mol. Cell. Biol. 6*:183–194.
39. Risser, R. (1982). The pathogenesis of Abelson virus lymphomas of the mouse. *Biochim. Biophys. Acta 651*:213–244.
40. Rosenberg, N., Witte, O. N., and Baltimore, D. (1979). Characterization of Abelson murine leukemia virus isolated differing in p120 expression. *Cold Spring Harbor Symp. Quant. Biol. 44*:859–864.
41. Rosenberg, N., and Witte, O. N. (1980). Abelson murine leukemia virus mutants with alterations in the virus-specific p120 molecule. *J. Virol. 33*:340–348.
42. Goff, S. P., Witte, O. N., Gilboa, E., Rosenberg, N., and Baltimore, D. (1981). Genome structure of Abelson murine leukemia virus variants: Proviruses in fibroblasts and lymphoid cells. *J. Virol. 38*:460–468.
43. Sacks, T. L., Hershey, E. J., and Stephenson, J. R. (1979). Abelson murine leukemia virus-infected cell lines defective in transformation. *Virology 97*:231–240.
44. Rosenberg, N., Clark, D. R., and Witte, O. N. (1980). Abelson murine leukemia mutants deficient in kinase activity and lymphoid cell transformation. *J. Virol. 36*:766–774.
45. Witte, O. N., Goff, S., Rosenberg, N., and Baltimore, D. (1980). A transformation-defective mutant of Abelson murine leukemia virus lacks protein kinase activity. *Proc. Natl. Acad. Sci. USA 77*:4993–4997.
46. Murtagh, K., Skladany, G., Hoag, J., and Rosenberg, N. (1986). Abelson murine leukemia virus variants with increased oncogenic potential. *J. Virol. 60*:599–606.
47. Reynolds, F. J., Jr., Van de Ven, W. J., and Stephenson, J. R. (1980). Abelson murine leukemia virus transformed defective mutants with impaired p120-associated protein kinase activity. *J. Virol. 38*:374–386.
48. Takemori, T., Miyazoe, I., Shirasawa, T., Taniguchi, M., and Graf, T. (1987). A temperature-sensitive mutant of Abelson murine leukemia virus confers inducibility of IgM expression to transformed lymphoid cells. *EMBO J. 6*:951–956.
49. Kipreos, E. T., Lee, G. J., and Wang, J. Y. J. (1987). Isolation of temperature-sensitive tyrosine kinase mutants of v-*abl* oncogene by screening with antibodies for phosphotyrosine. *Proc. Natl. Acad. Sci. USA 84*:1345–1349.
50. Engleman, A., and Rosenberg, N. (1987). Isolation of temperature-sensitive Abelson virus mutants by site directed mutagenesis. *Proc. Natl. Acad. Sci. USA 84*:8021–8025.
51. Witte, O. N., Rosenberg, N., Paskind, M., Shields, A., and Baltimore, D. (1978). Identification of an Abelson murine leukemia virus-encoded protein present in transformed fibroblasts and lymphoid cells. *Proc. Natl. Acad. Sci. USA 75*:2488–2492.
52. van de Van, W. J. M., Reynolds, F. H., Nalewaik, R. P., and Stephenson, J. R. (1979). The nonstructural component of the Abelson murine leukemia virus polyprotein p120 is encoded by newly acquired genetic sequences. *J. Virol. 32*:1041–1045.

53. Reynolds, F. H., Jr., Sacks, T. L., Deobagkar, D. N., and Stephenson, J. R. (1980). Cells nonproductively transformed by Abelson murine leukemia virus express high molecular weight polyprotein containing structural and nonstructural components. *Proc. Natl. Acad. Sci. USA 75*:3974–3978.
54. Witte, O. N., Rosenberg, N., and Baltimore, D. (1979). Preparation of syngeneic tumor regressor serum reactive with the unique determinants of the Abelson MuLV encoded p120 protein at the cell surface. *J. Virol. 34*:776–784.
55. Risser, R., Stockert, E., and Old, L. J. (1978). Abelson-antigen. A viral tumor antigen that is also a differentiation antigen in Balb/c mice. *Proc. Natl. Acad. Sci. USA 75*:3918–3922.
56. Schiff-Maker, L., and Rosenberg, N. (1986). *Gag*-derived but not *abl*-derived determinants are exposed on the surface of Abelson virus-transformed cells. *Virology 154*:286–301.
57. Watanabe, S. M., Rosenberg, N., and Witte, O. N. (1984). A membrane associated, carbohydrate-modified form of the v-*abl* protein that cannot be phosphorylated in vivo or in vitro. *J. Virol. 51*:620–627.
58. Sefton, B. M., Trowbridge, I. S. Cooper, J. A., and Scolnick, E. M. (1982). The transforming proteins of Rous sarcoma virus, Harvey sarcoma virus, and Abelson virus contain tightly bound lipid. *Cell 31*:465–474.
59. Schultz, A., and Oroszlan, S. (1984). Myristilation of *gag-onc* fusion proteins in mammalian transforming retroviruses. *Virology 133*:431–437.
60. Boss, M. A., Dreyfus, G., and Baltimore, D. (1981). Localization of the Abelson murine leukemia virus protein in a detergent insoluble subsellular matrix: architecture of the protein. *J. Virol. 40*:472–481.
61. Collett, M. S., and Erikson, R. H. (1978). Protein kinase activity associated with the avian sarcoma virus *src* gene product. *Proc. Natl. Acad. Sci. USA 75*:2021–2024.
62. Witte, O. N., Sun, L., Rosenberg, N., and Baltimore, D. (1979). A *trans*-acting protein kinase identified in cells transformed by Abelson murine leukemia virus. *Cold Spring Harbor Symp. Quant. Biol. 44*:855–857.
63. Witte, O. N., Dasgupta, A., and Baltimore, D. (1980). Abelson murine leukemia virus protein is phosphorylated in vitro to form phosphotyrosine. *Nature 283*:826–831.
64. Sefton, B. M., Hunter, T., and Raschke, W. C. (1981). Evidence that the Abelson virus protein functions in vivo as a protein kinase that phosphorylates tyrosine. *Proc. Natl. Acad. Sci. USA 78*:1552–1556.
65. Wang, J. W. J., Queen, C., and Baltimore, D. (1985). Expression of an Abelson murine leukemia virus-encoded protein in *Escherichia coli* causes extensive phosphorylation of tyrosine residues. *J. Biol. Chem. 257*:13181–13184.
66. Wang, J. W. J., and Baltimore, D. (1985). Localization of tyrosine kinase-coding region in v-*abl* oncogene by the expression of v-*abl*-encoded proteins in bacteria. *J. Biol. Chem. 260*:64–71.
67. Witte, O. N., Ponticelli, A., Gifford, A., Baltimore, D., Rosenberg, N., and Elder, J. (1981). Phosphorylation of the Abelson murine leukemia virus transforming protein. *J. Virol. 39*:870–878.

68. Cooper, J. A., and Hunter, T. (1981). Four different classes of retroviruses induce phosphorylation of tyrosine present in similar proteins. *Mol. Cell. Biol. 1*:394–407.
69. Kamps, M. P., and Sefton, B. M. (1988). Most of the substrates of oncogenic viral tyrosine protein kinases can be phosphorylated by cellular tyrosine protein kinases in normal cells. *Oncogene Res. 3*:105–115.
70. Saggioro, D., Ferracini, R., DiRenzo, M. F., Naldini, L., Chieco-Bianchi, L., and Comoglio, P. M. (1986). Protein phosphorylation of tyrosine residues in v-abl transformed murine lymphocytes and fibroblasts. *Int. J. Cancer 37*: 623–628.
71. Konopka, J. B., Davis, R. L., Watanabe, S. M., Ponticelli, A. S., Schiff-Maker, L., Rosenberg, N., and Witte, O. N. (1984). Only site-directed antibodies reactive with the highly conserved *src*-homologous region of the v-*abl* protein neutralizes kinase activity. *J. Virol. 51*:223–232.
72. Witte, O. N., Rosenberg, N., and Baltimore, D. (1979). Identification of normal cellular protein cross-reactive to the major Abelson murine leukemia virus gene product. *Nature 281*:396–398.
73. Ponticelli, A. S., Whitlock, A., Rosenberg, N., and Witte, O. N. (1982). In vivo tyrosine phosphorylations of the Abelson virus transforming protein are absent in its normal cellular homolog. *Cell 29*:953–990.
74. Konopka, J. B., and Witte, O. N. (1985). Detection of a c-*abl* tyrosine kinase activity in vitro permits direct comparison of normal and altered *abl* gene products. *Mol. Cell. Biol. 5*:3116–3123.
75. Patschinsky, T., Hunter, T., Esch, F. S., Cooper, J. A., and Sefton, B. M. (1982). Analysis of the sequence of amino acids surrounding sites of tyrosine phosphorylation. *Proc. Natl. Acad. Sci. USA 79*:973–977.
76. Shields, A., Goff, S., Paskind, M., Otto, G., and Baltimore, D. (1979). Structure of the Abelson murine leukemia virus genome. *Cell 18*:955–962.
77. Goff, S. P., Gilboa, E., Witte, O. N., and Baltimore, D. (1980). Structure of the Abelson murine leukemia virus genome and the homologous cellular gene: Studies with cloned viral DNA. *Cell 22*:777–785.
78. Srinivasan, A., Reddy, E. P., and Aaronson, S. A. (1981). Abelson murine leukemia virus: Molecular cloning of infectious integrated proviral DNA. *Proc. Natl. Acad. Sci. USA 78*:2077–2081.
79. Hoffman, F. M., Fresco, L. D., Hoffman-Falk, H., and Shilo, B.-Z. (1983). Nucleotide sequence of the *Drosophila src* and *abl* homologs: Conservation and variability in the *src* family oncogene. *Cell 35*:393–401.
80. Reddy, E. P., Smith, M. J., and Srinivasan, A. (1983). Nucleotide sequence of Abelson murine leukemia virus genome: Structural similarity of its transforming gene product to other *onc* gene products with tyrosine-specific kinase activity. *Proc. Natl. Acad. Sci. USA 80*:3623–3627.
81. Latt, S. A., Goff, S. P., Tabin, C. J., Paskind, M., Wang, J. Y. J., and Baltimore, D. (1983). Cloning and analysis of reverse transcript P160 genomes of Abelson murine leukemia virus. *J. Virol. 45*:1195–1199.
82. Lee, R., Paskind, M., Wang, J. Y. J., and Baltimore, D. (1985). Abelson (P160) murine leukemia virus (Ab-MLV) *abl* gene. In *RNA Tumor Viruses*

(R. Weiss, N. Teich, H. Varmus, and J. Coffin, eds.). Cold Spring Harbor Laboratory, Cold Spring Harbor, New York, pp. 861–868.

83. Wang, J. Y. J., Ledley, F., Goff, S., Lee, R., Groner, Y., and Baltimore, D. (1984). The mouse c-*abl* locus: Molecular cloning and characterization. *Cell 36*:349–356.
84. Oppi, C., Shore, S. K., and Reddy, E. P. (1987). Nucleotide sequence analysis of testis-derived c-*abl* cDNAs: Implications for testis-specific transcription and *abl* oncogene activation. *Proc. Natl. Acad. Sic. USA 84*: 8200–8204.
85. Ben-Neriah, Y., Bernards, A., Paskind, M., Daley, G. Q., and Baltimore, D. (1986). Alternative 5′ exons in c-*abl* mRNA. *Cell 44*:577–586.
86. Srinivasan, A., Reddy, E. P., Dunn, C. Y., and Aaronson, S. A. (1984). Molecular dissection of transcriptional control elements within the long terminal repeat of the retrovirus. *Science 223*:286–289.
87. Srinivasan, A., Dunn, C. Y., Yuasa, Y., Devare, S. G., Reddy, E. P., and Aaronson, S. A. (1982). Abelson murine leukemia virus: Structural requirements for transforming gene function. *Proc. Natl. Acad. Sci. USA 79*: 5508–5512.
88. Prywes, R., Foulkes, J. G., Rosenberg, N., and Baltimore, D. (1983). Sequences of A-MuLV protein needed for fibroblast and lymphoid cell transformation. *Cell 34*:569–579.
89. Rees-Jones, R. W., and Goff, S. P. (1988). Insertional mutagenesis of the Abelson murine leukemia virus genome: Identification of mutants with altered kinase activity and defective transformation ability. *J. Virol. 62*: 978–986.
90. Prywes, R., Foulkes, J. G., and Baltimore, D. (1985). The minimum transforming region of v-*abl* is a segment encoding protein-tyrosine kinase. *J. Virol. 54*:114–112.
91. Ziegler, S. F., Whitlock, C. A., Goff, S. P., Gifford, A., and Witte, O. N. (1981). Lethal effect of the Abelson murine leukemia virus transforming gene product. *Cell 27*:477–486.
92. Watanabe, S. M., and Witte, O. N. (1983). Site-directed deletions of Abelson murine leukemia virus define 3′ sequences essential for transformation and lethality. *J. Virol. 45*:1028–1036.
93. Goff, S. P., Tabin, C. J., Wang, J., Weinberg, R., and Baltimore, D. (1982). Transfection of fibroblasts by cloned Abelson murine leukemia virus DNA recovery of transmissible virus by recombination with helper virus. *J. Virol. 41*:271–285.
93a. Shore, S. K. and Reddy, E. P. (1989). Transformation of NIH 373 cells by A-MuLV proviral DNA: effect of plasmid linearization and carrier DNA on transformation efficiency. *Oncogene. 4*:1411–1413.
94. Rosenberg, N., and Baltimore, D. (1978). The effect of helper virus on Abelson virus-induced transformation of lymphoid cells. *J. Exp. Med. 147*:1126–1141.
95. Green, P., Kaehler, D. A., and Risser, R. (1987). Cell transformation and

tumor induction by Abelson murine leukemia virus in the absence of helper virus. *Proc. Natl. Acad. Sci. USA 84*:5932–5936.

96. Prywes, R., Hoag, J., Rosenberg, N., and Baltimore, D. (1985). Protein stabilization explains the *gag* requirement for transformation of lymphoid cells by Abelson murine leukemia virus. *J. Virol. 54*:123–132.
97. Mathey-Prevot, B., and Baltimore, D. (1988). Recombinants within the tyrosine kinase region of v-*abl* and v-*src* identify a v-*abl* segment that confers lymphoid specificity. *Mol. Cell. Biol. 8*:234–240.
98. Oliff, A., Agranovsky, O., McKinney, M. D., Murty, V. V. V. S., and Bauchwitz, R. (1985). Friend murine leukemia virus-immortalized myeloid cells are converted into tumorigenic cell lines by Abelson virus. *Proc. Natl. Acad. Sci. USA 82*:3306–3310.
99. Kiproes, E. T., and Wang, J. Y. J. (1988). Reversible dependence on growth factor interleukin-3 in myeloid cells expressing temperature sensitive v-*abl* oncogene. *Oncogene Res. 2*:277–284.
100. Cook, W. D., Metcalf, D., Nicola, N. A., Burgess, A. W., and Walker, F. (1985). Malignant transformation of a growth factor-dependent myeloid cell line by Abelson virus without evidence of an autochrine mechanism. *Cell 41*:677–683.
101. Waneck, G. L., Keyes, L., and Rosenberg, N. (1986). Abelson virus drives the differentiation of Harvey virus-infected erythroid cells. *Cell 44*:337–344.
102. Mathey-Prevot, B., Nabel, G., Palacios, R., and Baltimore, D. (1986). Abelson virus abrogation of interleukin-3 dependence in a lymphoid cell line. *Mol. Cell. Biol. 6*:4133–4135.
103. Cook, W. D., Frazekas de St. Groth, B., Miller, J. F. A. P., McDonald, H. R., and Gabathuler, R. (1987). Abelson virus transformation of an interleukin 2-dependent antigen-specific T-cell line. *Mol. Cell. Biol. 7*:2631–2635.
104. Rovera, G., Valtieri, M., Mavilio, F., and Reddy, E. P. (1987). Effect of Abelson murine leukemia virus on granulocyte differentiation and IL-3 dependence of a murine progenitor cell line. *Oncogene 1*:29–35.
105. Saggioro, D., Zamarchi, R., D'Andrea, E., and Chieco-Bianchi, L. (1988). In vitro malignant progression of cells derived from Abelson leukemia virus-induced thymic lymphomas. *Br. J. Cancer 58*:152–157.
106. Wolf, D., Harris, N., and Rotter, V. (1984). Reconstitution of p53 expression in a nonproducer Ab-MuLV-transformed cell line by transfection of a functional p53 gene. *Cell 38*:119–126.
107. Twardzik, D., Todero, G. J., Marquardt, H., Reynolds, F. H., and Stephenson, J. R. (1982). Transformation induced by Abelson murine leukemia virus involves production of a polypeptide growth factor. *Science 216*:894–987.
108. Gebhardt, A., Bell, J. C., and Foulkes, J. G. (1986). Abelson transformed fibroblasts lacking the EGF receptor are not tumorigenic in nude mice. *EMBO J. 5*:2191–2195.

109. Grunwald, D. J., Dale, B., Dudley, J., Lamph, W. W., Sugden, B., Ozanne, B., and Risser, R. (1982). Loss of viral gene expression and retention of tumorigenicity by Abelson lymphoma cells. *J. Virol. 43*:92–102.
110. Green, P.L., Kachler, D. A., and Risser, R. (1987). Clonal dominance and progression in Abelson murine leukemia virus lymphomagenesis. *J. Virol. 61*:2192–2197.
111. Besmer, P., Hardy, W. S., Jr., Zuckerman, E. E., Bergold, P., Lederman, L., and Snyder, H. W. Jr. (1983). The Hardy-Zuckerman 2-FeSV, a new feline retrovirus with oncogene homology to Abelson MuLV. *Nature 303*: 825–828.
112. Bergold, P. J., Blumenthal, J. A., D'Andrea, E., Snyder, H. W., Lederman, L., Silverstone, A., Nguyen, H., and Besmer, P. (1987). Nucleic acid sequence and oncogenic properties of the HZ2 Feline sarcoma virus v-*abl* insert. *J. Virol. 61*:1193–1202.

PART III
Studies of the Structure of the Philadelphia Chromosome Translocation and the *bcr–abl* Gene in Chronic Myelogenous Leukemia

6

Philadelphia Chromosome Translocation

John Groffen, Christine Morris, and Nora Heisterkamp *Children's Hospital of Los Angeles, University of Southern California, Los Angeles, California*

INTRODUCTION

It is now well established that the oncogenes of RNA tumor viruses are derived from sequences in the genomes of host cells (for review, see Reference 1). The corresponding cellular sequences, termed "proto-oncogenes," are present in the human genome as normal cellular genes with normal cellular functions. Proto-oncogene amino acid sequences have been conserved throughout evolution, suggesting that they perform a critical role in normal cellular metabolism. Many of the oncogenes for which the normal cellular function has been unravelled to date appear to represent genes that encode either growth factors or growth factor membrane receptors. Cellular oncogenes have been associated with specific forms of human cancer and are believed to act individually or in concert. The interaction of oncogene-encoded proteins possibly accounts for the multistage nature of cancer. Oncogene changes associated with cancer generally embody qualitative or quantitative changes in the protein product encoded by an altered proto-oncogene, or normal oncogene expression in the wrong tissues or at the wrong stage of development. Our understanding of the cellular processes affected by the conversion of a proto-oncogene into a transforming oncogene is limited. A more complete understanding of these processes will be necessary to comprehend their role in tumorigenesis.

The Philadelphia chromosome (Ph^1) was the first specific karyotype marker found to characterize a particular human neoplastic disease, namely chronic myelocytic leukemia (CML) (2). It was believed to be present in the leukemic cells of about 92% of patients at diagnosis (3), but more recent research, described later, shows that nearer 99% of CML patients are Ph^1 positive. Chromosome banding techniques identified the Ph^1 as a deleted chromosome 22 (4,5), and revealed that the deleted part was translocated to the distal long arm of chromosome 9 (6). Thus, the Ph^1 was one product of a reciprocal chromosomal translocation, t(9;22)(q34;q11).

CML is a clonal myeloproliferative disorder arising from neoplastic transformation of a pluripotent stem cell and is characterized clinically by excessive growth of myeloid cells and their progenitors. Ph^1-positive leukemic cells have a growth advantage over normal bone marrow cells, and usually all nucleated cells in the bone marrow are Ph^1 positive at the time of diagnosis. Ph^1-negative normal cells persist, but their growth is apparently suppressed by the leukemic cells (7-9). The disease undergoes transformation to an aggressive leukemia on average 4 years after diagnosis. Ph^1-positive cells appear to lose their capacity to differentiate, and the accumulation of undifferentiated blast cells are directly or indirectly responsible for the invariably fatal outcome of this leukemia.

The cause of CML and the mechanisms that determine its progression are unknown at present. It is an acquired disease, but there are no clues to its etiology other than an increased risk in individuals exposed to ionizing radiation. During the last few years, molecular biologists have dissected the Ph^1 translocation and studied in detail the structure and expression of the affected genes. Their findings have significantly increased our understanding of the disease and form the basis of this review.

HUMAN *abl* AND CML

Characterization of Human *abl*

Cloning of the Abelson murine leukemia virus (A-MuLV)-genome enabled the construction of nucleic acid probes for the detection and isolation of homologous DNA from uninfected cells. Such studies showed that sequences highly homologous to the mouse v-*abl* oncogene occur at a single major chromosomal locus in the human. Hybridization of v-*abl* probes to human genomic DNA on Southern blots showed that the human *abl* proto-oncogene spans a region of at least 30 kilobases (kb) of genomic DNA (10).

Human DNA sequences homologous to v-*abl* were further characterized by hybridization of a cosmid library of human carcinoma DNA with a v-*abl* probe. Multiple cosmid clones were isolated and characterized by restriction enzyme mapping and hybridization with small individual regions of the v-*abl* oncogene (10). These experiments confirmed that human *abl* is a large gene with v-*abl* homologous sequences distributed discontinuously over a region of 32 kb. These sequences represent the entire v-*abl* human cellular homolog, are colinear with the viral v-*abl* transforming gene, and are dispersed over nine exons (10,11). The nucleic acid sequences of the regions encoding the tyrosine phosphorylation ac-

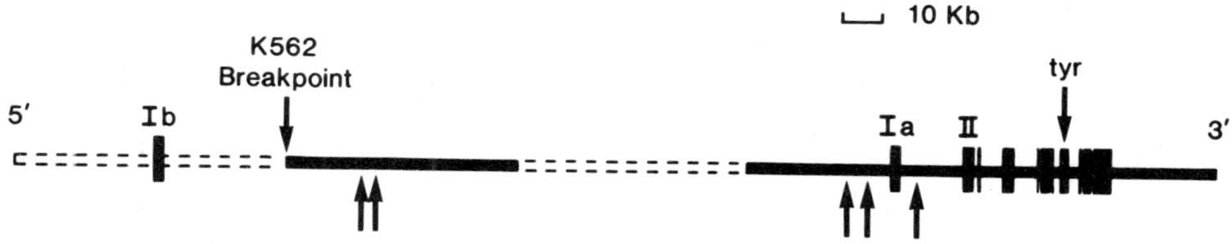

Figure 1 The human *abl* locus. The genomic DNA of the *abl* locus is represented by the horizontal line, with broken and solid lines indicating the regions uncloned and cloned to date. The position of the alternative exons Ib and Ia and the common exon II is indicated, as is the location of the exon containing the phosphotyrosine acceptor site (*tyr*). Arrows beneath the restriction map point to the position of the breakpoints on chromosome 9 in five CML patients; the position of the breakpoint in the CML cell line K562 is indicated above the map with an arrow.

ceptor sites of v-*abl* and human *abl* were determined (12,13). Extensive homology between this region of *abl* and the acceptor domains of the v-*src*, v-*yes*, and v-*fps-fes* family of viral oncogenes was found, as well as more distant relatedness to regions within the catalytic chain of the mammalian cyclic AMP-dependent protein kinase (12,13). These findings and the results of other comparative studies suggested that the normal cellular homologs of retroviral oncogenes with tyrosine-specific protein kinase activity were probably derived from a common progenitor and represented members of a diverse family of cellular protein kinases.

The human *abl* gene is related to v-*abl* sequences in much the same way that a mammalian gene is related to its mRNA. c-*abl* contains both exons and introns, but v-*abl* contains only the exon portion of the parental gene. This pattern is common to nearly all transduced oncogenes carried by retroviruses (1,14). However, whereas v-*abl* is approximately 3 kb in length (12,15,16), v-*abl* homologous mRNAs of 6 and 7 kb have been detected in human cells (17). The isolation of cDNAs corresponding to these mRNAs established the presence of three additional human *abl* exons designated exon II, and two alternative first exons, Ia and Ib (Figure 1) (11,18,19). All three are located 5′ to the v-*abl* homologous exons. Exon Ia is the most 5′ exon present within the 6 kb RNA species, and exon Ib represents the 5′ terminus of the 7 kb *abl* mRNA (18,19). Both mRNAs contain the first common exon, exon II.

Sequence analysis of exons Ia and Ib demonstrated that each encodes a different peptide (19). The two *abl* mRNAs initiate at different promoters and give rise to proteins that differ in their N-terminal. Similar alternative 5′ exons have been detected in the 5.3 and 6.5 kb mRNAs of mice (18). The coding regions of human exons Ia and Ib are conserved in their murine counterparts, strong evidence that the two *abl* proteins have distinct functions.

Alternative splicing, found in a number of DNA viruses (20) and in cellular genes, may function in the regulation of gene expression, determined by the promoter selected, or it may generate different proteins (21-26). The human *abl* gene has two distinct transcriptional promotors, and their coding regions begin within the two alternative first exons, Ia and Ib. Exon selection must therefore determine which of the two proteins is produced. To date, both *abl* mRNAs have been detected in approximately equal quantities in all tissues analyzed, suggesting that the two proteins are not expressed differentially (17,27). The low expression of *abl* in many tissues is reminiscent of the expression of some genes considered to have a "housekeeping" function, such as hypoxanthine phosphoribosyltransferase (HPRT). *abl*, like these genes, lacks TATA and CAAT boxes, and its two promoter regions are G + C rich and contain multiple GGGCGG repeats (28). This repeat was identified as the core within the consensus binding site of the Sp1 factor, which was found to regulate transcription in vitro (29).

The human *abl* locus is comparatively large: v-*abl* homologous exons alone are dispersed over a region of 32 kb. Exon Ia has been located 18 kb 5′ of exon III, the most 5′ v-*abl* homologous exon (11). Considerable stretches of DNA 5′ of this exon have been cloned, but none contained exon Ib (Figure 1) (References 19 and 30 and unpublished data). An intron greater than 100 kb in length appeared to separate exon Ib from the first common exon, exon II. Recent experiments using pulsed-field gel electrophoresis (PGFE) have now established that exon Ib is situated approximately 200 kb 5′ of exon II (Figure 1) (31). These data indicate that the *abl* locus has two unusual features. First, splicing must occur over very long distances. Second, when transcription initiates at exon Ib, exon Ia is spliced out and exon Ib is fused to exon II.

Experiments in vivo and in vitro argue strongly against a progressive scanning mechanism for splicing (32,33). Such a mechanism requires that splicing enzymes attach at one position and move along the RNA chain. Instead, normal and alternative splicing are thought to be determined by secondary structures within intervening sequences that juxtapose particular exons and exclude others. The current model proposes that regions of the RNA could be spliced in more than one way and assume different conformations, possibly stabilized by interaction with *trans*-acting factors, such as RNA or protein (34,35). How appropriately this model explains the different *abl* transcripts has yet to be established.

Relocation of *abl* DNA Sequences: A Direct Consequence of Chromosomal Translocation

The human *abl* gene was initially mapped to chromosome 9q using a combination of somatic cell hybrid and molecular techniques (36). This location was of interest because of the specific involvement of chromosome 9 in the t(9;22) characterizing CML, and for that reason the chromosomal location of *abl* in leukemic cells from patients with Ph^1-positive CML was investigated (37).

Hybrid cell lines were obtained by fusion of cells from mouse or Chinese hamster with leukocytes from different CML patients and from a normal donor. Each line contained a full complement of mouse or Chinese hamster chromosomes and a limited number of human chromosomes. DNA was isolated from those hybrids segregating the normal chromosomes 9 or 22 and from those segregating the rearranged derivatives of the Ph^1 translocation: $9q^+$ and $22q^-$, respectively. Subsequent Southern blot analysis using human *abl* and v-*abl* probes showed that the human *abl*-specific *Eco*R1 restriction fragments detected in control human placental DNA were present in DNA from the hybrid cell line containing chromosome 9 (10CB-23B), but not in the line containing the $9q^+$ chromosome (14CB-21A). Correspondingly, *abl*-specific fragments were not detected in the hybrid line that retained the normal chromosome 22 but were present in the two lines that contained the Ph^1 chromosome (1CB-17aNU and WESP-2A). This experiment established that in CML, the *abl* proto-oncogene is translocated from chromosome 9 to the Ph^1 chromosome as a direct consequence of the t(9;22). Moreover, this work localized the *abl* gene to band 9q34, and it provided the first conclusive evidence that the t(9;22) was a reciprocal translocation (37).

Above all, these results raised the possibility that the *abl* proto-oncogene is involved in the pathogenesis of Ph^1-positive CML. One would then expect that the breakpoint on chromosome 9 was either within or in close proximity to human *abl*. To investigate this possibility, high-molecular-weight DNA was isolated from spleen biopsy samples of three CML patients. The DNA was digested with *Bam*HI and subjected to Southern blot analysis. Extensive analysis with probes isolated from the v-*abl* homologous region of *abl* revealed no abnormalities or rearrangements in the DNA of these patients (38). A probe specific for the region 5′ of exon II also detected only germline fragments in normal human DNA and in DNA from two of the CML patients. However, in the DNA of the third patient (0319129), an abnormal restriction fragment was identified (Figure 2). The most likely explanation for this finding was that one allelic copy of DNA sequences immediately 5′ of the v-*abl* homologous sequences in this patient was normal, whereas the second was rearranged. Molecular cloning of the rearranged sequences confirmed this hypothesis: sequences in the 5′ region of the cloned fragment completely matched the *abl* locus on chromosome 9, whereas sequences more 3′ did not. A probe corresponding to these foreign 3′ sequences was isolated and hybridized to DNA extracted from several rodent-human somatic cell hybrids. Under stringent washing conditions, the 3′ probe hybridized to one fragment in normal human DNA, and it detected the same fragment in a somatic cell hybrid containing chromosome 22 as its only human component. The probe did not hybridize to rodent-human hybrids that contained human chromosome 9 (Figure 3) (38). Thus, the cloned rearranged *abl* fragment of one CML patient was chimeric and contained *abl* sequences from

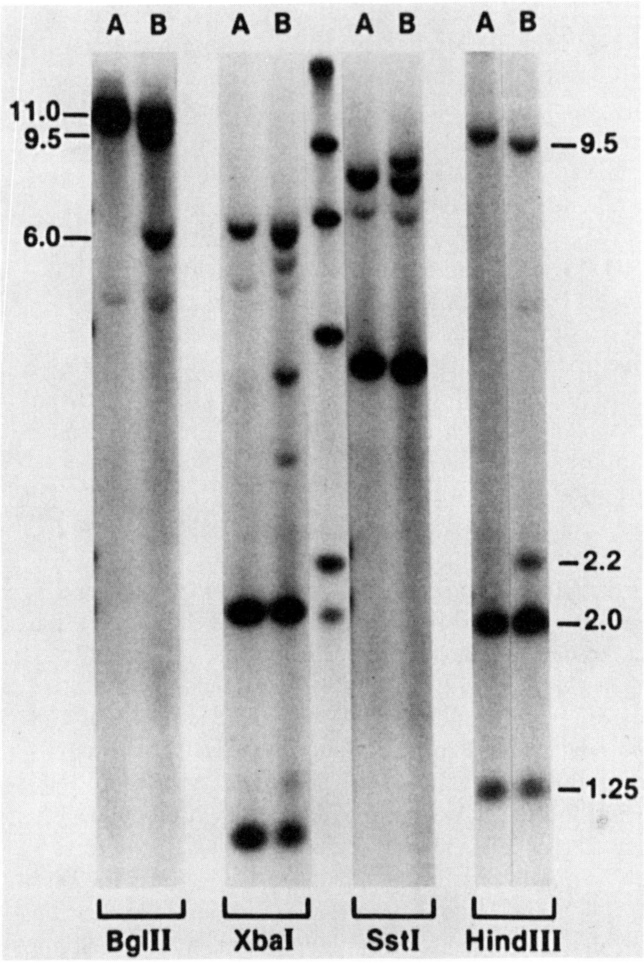

Figure 2 Restriction enzyme analysis of the DNA of CML patient 0319129. Restriction enzymes used and the molecular weights of the fragments in the *Bg*III and *Hind*III digestions are indicated. ^{32}P-labeled λ *Hind*III digestion fragments in the center of the figure served as a molecular weight marker for the *Xba*I and *Sst*I digestions. Southern blots were hybridized with a mixture of probes isolated from the region 5′ of exon II (see Figure 1). Control DNA of the cell line A673 is shown in lanes A; DNA of CML 03391929 is in lanes B. Abnormal band(s) are visible in all B lanes; the rearranged 6.0 kb *Bgl*II fragment was molecularly cloned.

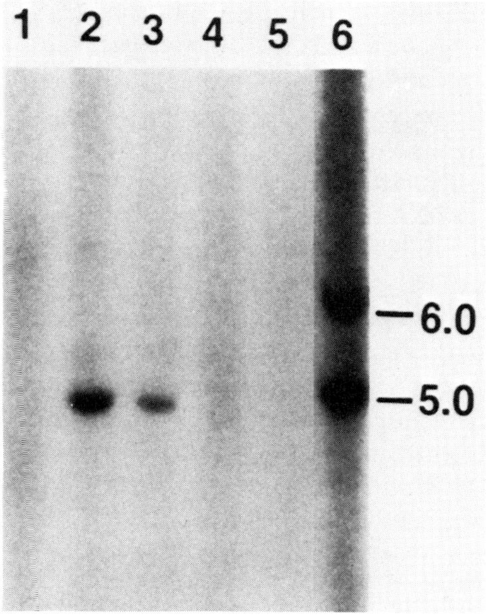

Figure 3 Chromosomal localization of the 3′ domain of the cloned breakpoint fragment. High-molecular-weight DNA was digested with *Bg*III, electrophoresed on an 0.75% agarose gel, blotted, and hybridized to a 1.2 HBg probe and included mouse (lane 1), A204 (lane 2), PgMe-25 Nu (chromosome 9, lane 4), WESP-2A (chromosome 22q-, lane 5), and CML patient 0319129 (lane 6).

chromosome 9 at its 5′ end and unknown sequences from chromosome 22 at its 3′ end.

Similar studies of leukemic DNA from other CML patients have confirmed the presence of breakpoints within the 5′ region of the *abl* gene (39-41). So far, all the breakpoints have been located at variable distances upstream (5′) of exon II, and all appear to be distributed more or less at random within this 5′ region of *abl* (Figure 1).

THE *bcr* GENE ON CHROMOSOME 22

Breakpoints Clustered Within a Limited Region, *bcr*, on the Ph[1] Chromosome

The cloning of a chimeric 9/22 breakpoint fragment from one patient enabled us to use the chromosome 22-specific sequences as a molecular probe. When hybridized to DNA isolated from the leukemic spleen of a second CML patient, abnormal restriction fragments were detected (39). This finding suggested that a breakpoint had occurred within the same limited stretch of chromosome 22 DNA as in the original patient from whom the probe was cloned. To investigate the possibility of "clustering" of CML breakpoints on chromosome 22, DNA was isolated from leukemic cells of 17 further patients with Ph^1-positive CML and subjected to Southern blot analysis using the chromosome 22-specific probe. All contained additional fragments that hybridized to this probe. In contrast, no additional fragments were detected in DNA from over 20 randomly selected non-CML subjects (39). Moreover, only germline fragments were detected in DNA isolated from cultured fibroblasts of Ph^1-positive CML patients, when DNA isolated from the leukemic cells of these patients clearly contained rearranged fragments. Based on these additional data (42), all Ph^1-positive CML patients appear to have a breakpoint in a very small region (approximately 5 kb) of chromosome 22 in their leukemic cells. We proposed the name breakpoint cluster region or *bcr* for this region (39). Recently the region was renamed M*bcr* for major breakpoint cluster region (43).

bcr Part of a Gene

It is obvious that the Philadelphia translocation has a profound influence on the cellular *abl* oncogene, resulting in the disruption of the linkage between the gene and sequences 5′ to it. Studies were done to determine the possible derivation of the sequences on chromosome 22 and how they were affected by the chromosomal break. One possibility was that *bcr* is a gene or part of a gene that had been disrupted as a consequence of the Ph^1 translocation.

Approximately 45 kb of chromosome 22 were cloned from a normal human cosmid library using a *bcr* probe (39). No homology was apparent between the restriction map of this region and that of human *sis*, an oncogene situated on chromosome 22 but translocated to chromosome 9 in the Ph^1 translocation (44, 45). Subsequent in situ hybridization studies indicated that *sis* was not located in the immediate proximity of the Ph^1 breakpoint (46). The immunoglobulin λ light-chain constant region (IGCL) and the Ph^1 chromosomal breakpoint have been localized to chromosome 22, band q11 (47–49). The analogy of *myc* and the Ig heavy-chain region (IGH) in the t(8;14) of Burkitt's lymphoma (50) suggested that *abl* is translocated into and activated by IGCL in CML. However, a IGCL probe showed no cross-homology with the sequences cloned from chromosome 22, nor did these sequences hybridize to a murine λ-variable region probe (Reference 39 and Heisterkamp et al., unpublished).

bcr was shown to contain protein-encoding sequences by using a probe that hybridized to sequences of a human fibroblast cDNA library. Several cDNA clones were subsequently isolated. The largest of these contained an insert of 2.2 kb and was characterized in detail by restriction enzyme mapping and sequence analysis (40). Northern blot analysis of a human fibroblast cell line and various

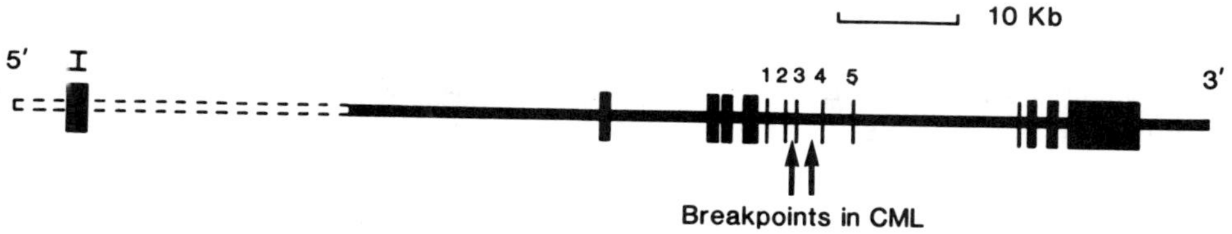

Figure 4 The human *bcr* locus. The solid horizontal line indicates the cloned genomic sequences of the *bcr* gene; the bracket line at 5′ represents genomic sequences not cloned to date, which separate the first *bcr* gene exon I from the main body of the *bcr* gene exons. The breakpoints in CML DNA are indicated with an arrow and are located in the introns between exons numbered 1–5 of the breakpoint cluster region.

tissues revealed mRNAs of 4.5 and 6.5 kb (40,51), which suggested that the cloned 2.2 kb cDNA was incomplete at its 5′ end and confirmed our hypothesis that this region of chromosome 22 encoded a gene, the *bcr* gene.

The orientation of the *bcr* gene on chromosome 22 was determined by preparing 5′ and 3′ probes from the cDNA, followed by hybridization to cosmids containing human chromosome 22 sequences. The 5′ end of the *bcr* gene lies toward the centromere of chromosome 22 and remains on the Ph^1 chromosome, whereas the 3′ end is translocated to chromosome 9 in the t(9;22) (40).

Computer programs were used to examine whether any homology could be detected between the *bcr* gene and oncogenes, growth factors, or other previously isolated proteins. No significant homology was found, and the *bcr* protein sequence yielded no clues to its cellular function or its possible role in CML. Recent analysis of the complete 5′ end of the 4.5 kb mRNA showed no significant homology with any other peptide sequences (52). Interestingly, stretches of nucleotides with a high GC content were found in the most 5′ region of the *bcr* gene. These regions are likely to display considerable secondary structure, a feature that has been associated with a reduction in the translational efficiency of eukaryotic mRNA, both in vitro and in vivo. The origin of the normal 6.5 kb *bcr* transcript also remains unclear. Probes isolated from different coding regions of the *bcr* gene hybridize to both transcripts, hence the 6.5 kb mRNA appears to contain most if not all of the sequences present in the 4.5 kb mRNA. The additional sequences in the 6.5 kb transcript may be located at its 5′ end, internally, or at its 3′ end. For example, the 6.5 kb *bcr* transcript may be generated by either a more distal polyadenylation signal or an alternative splice in the 3′ region.

Distribution of Breakpoints Within the *bcr* Gene

The isolation of *bcr* cDNA sequences allowed further characterization of the breakpoints on chromosome 22. The location of five *bcr* exons in the region affected by the Ph^1 translocation was determined (see Figure 4; the exons are numbered 1-5). These exons are relatively small and vary in size from 76 to 105 base pairs (40). This information enabled a more precise definition of the breakpoints in CML in terms of whether they occur in exon or intron regions. Six chimeric $9q^+$ and/or 22 q^- restriction enzyme fragments were sequenced across the breakpoint regions. The exact location of the breakpoints on chromosome 22 was determined by sequencing the corresponding normal chromosome 22 regions. None occurred within an exon, suggesting that breakpoints of the Ph^1 translocation only occur within introns of the *bcr* gene. Although the precise breakpoint on chromosome 22 differed for each CML patient, there was little variation in the number of *bcr* exons remaining on the Ph^1 chromosome. Four patients retained exon 2 and all sequences 5′ of it, whereas the DNA of the two remaining patients additionally retained exon 3 of the *bcr* gene on the Ph^1 chromosome (40).

EXPRESSION OF THE *bcr-abl* HYBRID GENE IN CML

A *bcr-abl* Hybrid mRNA

The significant molecular consequence of the Ph^1 translocation is relocation of the *abl* gene from chromosome 9 to chromosome 22, adjacent to and 3′ of the truncated *bcr* gene and in the same transcriptional orientation. The effect of the translocation on the expression of these genes was initially examined by isolating poly(A) RNA from the CML blast crisis cell line K562 (53) and control HeLa cells. A probe isolated from human *abl* exon III, the most 5′ v-*abl* homologous exon, detected mRNAs of 8.5, 7, and 6 kb in K562. The 7 and 6 kb mRNAs were also detected in RNA isolated from HeLa cells and represent transcripts from the normal, unrearranged *abl* allele on chromosome 9. The 8.5 kb *abl* mRNA, however, was unique to K562 (30,54). Subsequent studies showed that this abnormally large 8.5 kb *abl* mRNA was characteristic of leukemic cells from Ph^1-positive CML patients (51,55–57).

These data, in combination with the knowledge that the *abl* gene was disrupted by the Ph^1 translocation, led to the following hypothesis: the Ph^1 translocation causes head-to-tail fusion of *bcr* and *abl* genomic sequences, so generating a chimeric gene that is then transcribed into a chimeric *bcr-abl* mRNA. To test this hypothesis, two probes were isolated from the *bcr* cDNA: probe A, which corresponds to the 5′ region of the cDNA and ends in exon 2, and probe B, which starts in exon 5 and encompasses 3′ *bcr* cDNA sequences (see Figure 4). We reasoned that if the 8.5 kb *abl* mRNA were chimeric, it would hybridize to probe A, which contains *bcr* exons 5′ to the breakpoint, but not to probe B because 3′ exons of *bcr* have been translocated to the $9q^+$ chromosome. This reasoning proved correct (51) and confirmed that the abnormal 8.5 kb *abl* mRNA found in K562 was indeed chimeric and represented 5′ *bcr* sequences fused to *abl* sequences. Expression of the 8.5 kb *bcr-abl* chimeric mRNA was shown to correlate consistently with the presence of a Ph[1] chromosome in other cell lines and in blood cells from CML patients (51,56-58). It was not detected in normal tissue or in other types of leukemia (27,58,59).

The structure of the chimeric *bcr-abl* mRNA of K562 was examined in more detail by cloning the corresponding chimeric cDNA. As predicted from the genomic DNA organization, the cDNA encompassed all 5' *bcr* exons, including exon 3. The *bcr* sequence was then joined in frame to *abl* exon II (11,30). *abl* exon Ia was present on the Ph[1] chromosome in the genomic DNA of K562, but splicing had apparently deleted it from the mature chimeric mRNA. The CML cell line EM2 likewise has a chimeric mRNA, with *bcr* exon 3 joined to *abl* exon II (11). Almost all Ph[1]-positive CML cells studied contain the abnormal 8-8.5 kb transcript (51,57). However, two cases with an additional 9.0 kb transcript have been reported, indicating that other *bcr* and/or *abl* exons may be included (57).

Chimeric *bcr-abl* mRNA Translated

Using v-*abl* antisera, the normal cellular gene product of human *abl* was identified as a phosphoprotein with a molecular weight of 145,000 daltons (p145). The p145 *abl* protein does not exhibit tyrosine phosphorylation activity in vivo or in vitro (60), although under modified reaction conditions a relatively low in vitro kinase activity may be detected (61). This contrasts with the v-*abl* protein (160,000 daltons, p. 160), which has a high tyrosine-specific kinase activity in vitro (62) and is labeled on tyrosine in vivo (63). The enzyme activity of the v-*abl* protein is strongly correlated with its transforming ability (64). In the cell line K562, v-*abl* antisera precipitate two abnormally sized proteins, p210 and p190 (molecular weights 210,000 and 190,000 daltons), in addition to the normal protein, p145 (65,66). Unlike p145, p210 and p190 are phosphorylated in vivo and in vitro on tyrosine.

Abnormal p210 proteins with tyrosine kinase activity similar to that of p210 in K562 have been immunoprecipitated from phosphate-labeled CML cell lines EM2 and BV173. In addition, a p210 was identified in ^{32}P-labeled cells of three independent CML patients (67). These results established that the chimeric *bcr-abl* mRNA present in Ph[1]-positive CML cell lines and patient material is translated into a chimeric protein, p210 (Figure 5). The difference in molecular weight between p210 and the normal *abl* p145 is caused in part by the addition of a *bcr* moiety to the amino terminus of p145. This was confirmed when antisera specific for the segment of the *bcr* protein included in the *bcr-abl* protein immunoprecipitated the same abnormal protein, p210, as did *abl* antisera (68, 69).

The properties of human *bcr-abl* p210 and viral *gag-abl* p160 are similar, but the specific contribution of the *bcr* or *gag* moieties of these fusion proteins

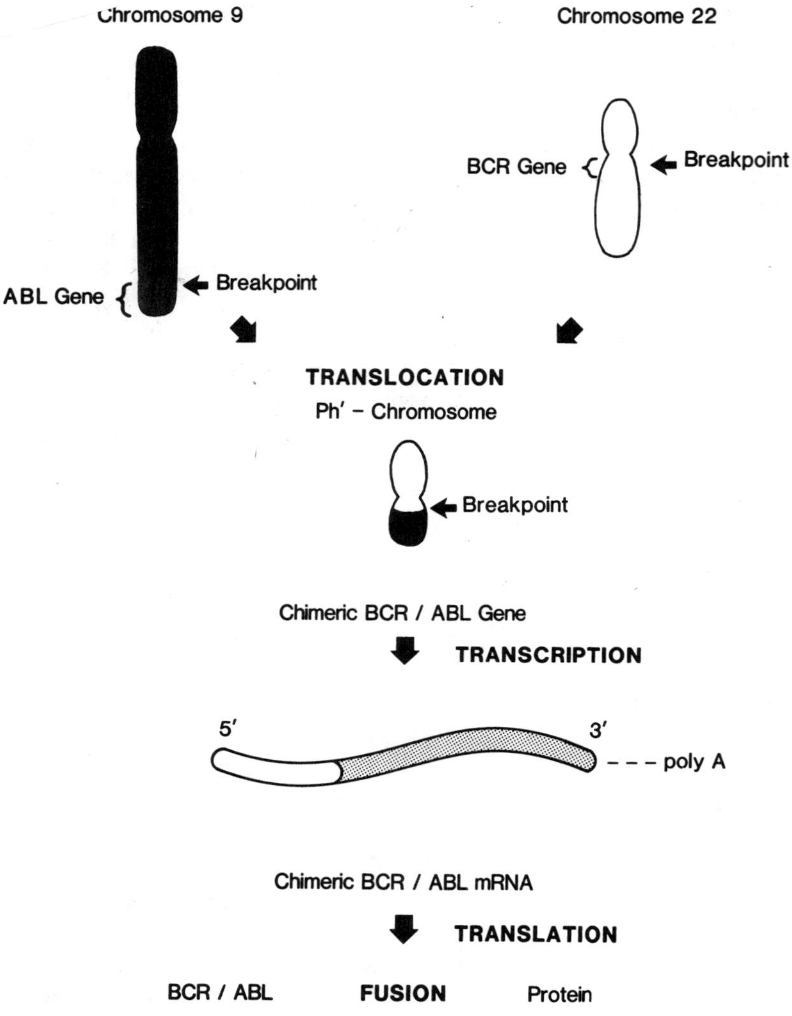

Figure 5 Schematic representation of the molecular genetic effects of the Ph[1] translocation in CML.

(apart from furnishing promoter sequences and a novel 5′ end) to the in vivo protein kinase activity is unclear. Interestingly, the normal *bcr* gene product is a phosphoprotein (p160) with an associated serine-threonine protein kinase activity, making it entirely dissimilar to *gag* (68). The *bcr* cDNA sequence has no homology with the conserved tyrosine-specific domain of the protein kinase family, and it is unlikely that the *bcr* gene product belongs to this group. p210 contains phosphothreonine and phosphoserine in addition to phosphotyrosine (68). Perhaps the *bcr-abl* p210 protein has both intrinsic tyrosine kinase (*abl*) and serine kinase (*bcr*) activities that interact with each other in some way. The normal cellular substrates of both the *bcr* and the *abl* proteins may also be affected by *bcr-abl* p210.

REARRANGEMENT OF *abl* IN VARIANT Ph^1 TRANSLOCATIONS

In most CML patients, the Ph^1 chromosome is one product of the translocation t(9;22)(q34;q11), which is known as the standard Ph^1 translocation. Variant Ph^1 translocations have been described in a small proportion (3–8%) of patients with CML (70–74). These variants involve chromosome 22 and some chromosome other than 9 (simple translocations) or one or more chromosome in addition to chromosomes 9 and 22 (complex translocations). Some CML patients also show a masked Ph^1 chromosome where part of another chromosome is attached to the long arm of chromosome 22. In all variant rearrangements, the breakpoint on chromosome 22 is within band q11, the same as in the standard t(9;22). The fate of the *abl* oncogene in these variants, particularly those that lack obvious involvement of chromosomes 9 or 22, was of prime interest.

By using somatic cell hybrid and chromosome in situ hybridization techniques, Bartram et al. first demonstrated translocation of *abl* from chromosome 9 to $22q^-$ in two patients with complex Ph^1 translocations: a t(1;9;22)(p32;q34;q11) and a t(9;11;22)(q34;q12;q11) (75). This was subsequently confirmed in three other patients who had complex translocations involving chromosomes 9 and 22 and a third chromosome (76). Despite the involvement of chromosomes other than 9 and 22 in these translocations, the *abl* gene was consistently relocated to the Ph^1 chromosome. This was not surprising if it is assumed that these complex translocations involve reciprocal chromosomal rearrangements. Indeed, before the application of molecular techniques, the existence of complex Ph^1 translocations was considered good evidence that the apposition of 9q34 and 22q11 was critical for the development of CML (77).

Simple variant Ph^1 translocations were initially characterized by an apparent lack of involvement of chromosome 9, and this posed a problem in determining a uniform model for the Ph^1 chromosome. Cytogenetically, the Ph^1 seemed to result from a reciprocal translocation between chromosome 22 and some chromosome other than 9. However, in situ hybridization and somatic cell hybrid studies have clearly shown that *abl* is translocated to chromosome 22q, indicating that the distal part of chromosome 9 also participates in these translocations (76,78-82). Hagemeijer et al. correctly concluded that simple variants do not exist and that all variant Ph^1 translocations are complex, involving at least three chromosomes (78).

The third kind of variant is rare and occurs when the Ph^1 is masked by material from another chromosome. Chromosome 9 was apparently not involved in some of these variants. In situ hybridization studies again demonstrated that *abl* sequences were translocated to the masked Ph^1 and were located interstitially at the breakpoint between chromosome 22, band q11, and the attached chromosomal material (76,82).

Molecular rearrangement of *bcr* has been demonstrated for complex, simple, and masked variants using Southern blot and in situ hybridization techniques (76,78,80-83). The common feature of all Ph^1 translocations, both standard and variant, is the movement of *abl* sequences from chromosome 9 next to the 5′ part of the *bcr* gene on chromosome 22.

Ph^1-NEGATIVE CML

Ph^1-positive CML is a relatively well defined clinical and hematologic entity (84, 85). However, about 10% of adult patients formerly diagnosed as CML lacked the Ph^1 chromosome: these patients were clinically and hematologically more varied (85). The subsequent establishment of precise criteria to diagnose myeloproliferative disorders (MPD) and myelodysplastic syndromes (MDS) (86,87) made it clear that Ph^1-negative CML as diagnosed in the past represented a heterogeneous group of disorders, most of which differed clinically and hematologically from those with Ph^1-positive CML (88,89). Of 47 patients retrospectively analyzed, only 1 patient was thought to have a disorder indistinguishable from Ph^1-positive CML and 31 were reclassified as one of the myelodysplastic syndromes, usually chronic myelomonocytic leukemia (CMML, 21 cases) (88, 89). It was suggested that Ph^1-negative CML does not exist as a separate entity (89), and this argument was strengthened by early molecular studies that showed that *abl* remained on chromosome 9 and that the *bcr* region was not rearranged in Ph^1-negative patients (39,55,75). However, molecular studies have subsequently shown that a few Ph^1-negative patients who are clinically and hematologically typical of Ph^1-positive CML have the same genomic changes as in Ph^1-positive CML. That is, *abl* sequences are transposed to chromosome 22q11 and inserted into the *bcr* region, resulting in fusion of 5′ *bcr* and *abl* sequences (Figure 6) (90-94). Some of these patients show cytogenetic changes that suggest they have complex translocations giving rise to masked Ph^1 chromosomes, but other patients show apparently normal karyotypes and the mechanism of their *bcr-abl* rearrangement has yet to be explained.

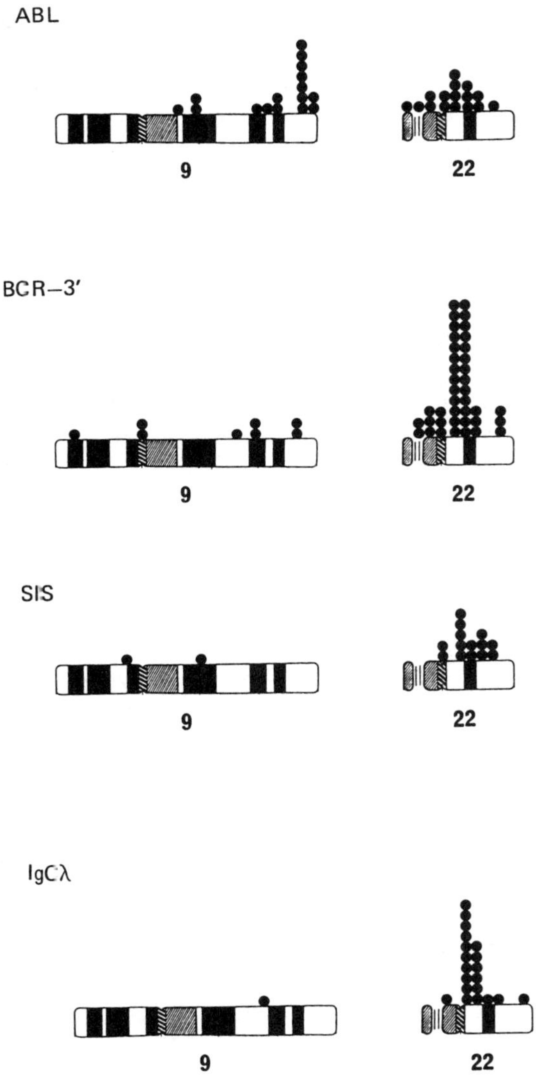

Figure 6 In situ hybridization of *abl, bcr*-3′, *sis*, and IGCλ probes to leukemic metaphase cells of a Ph[1]-negative patient. The regional distribution of labeled sites on chromosomes 9 and 22 is known. There was significant labeling of *abl* on chromosomes 9 and 22, but the other probes hybridized only to chromosome 22. A cytogenetically undetectable insertion of *abl* sequences from chromosome 9 to within the *bcr* gene was indicated, and this was supported by M*bcr* rearrangement on Southern blot analysis.

These studies show that correct diagnosis is critical when efforts are made to correlate clinical features with molecular changes in Ph^1-negative CML. Patients with true Ph^1-negative CML are rare, probably about 1% of all CML patients, but no accurate survey of their incidence has yet been made. Their prognosis appears to be the same as that for Ph^1-positive CML and contrasts with the poor prognosis of patients with chronic myelomonocytic leukemia (95).

Ph^1 TRANSLOCATION IN OTHER LEUKEMIAS

The Ph^1 chromosome has also been reported in malignant hematopoietic disorders other than CML, including different subtypes of acute leukemias for which no preceding chronic phase has been observed (96,97). It is found in the leukemic cells of 2-3% of patients presenting with acute myeloid leukemia (AML), and a similar incidence (2-6%) is reported for childhood acute lymphoblastic leukemia (ALL) (98-101). The Ph^1 chromosome is the most frequent chromosomal abnormality in adult ALL, with an incidence of 17-25% (102, 103). The clinical distinction between the blast crisis of CML and de novo Ph^1-positive acute leukemia is not always clear, and for many years these leukemias were considered manifestations of the same disease, CML, presenting in the lymphoid or myeloid blast phase (96,104,105). Reports of patients who present with Ph^1-positive ALL or AML but revert to CML following treatment provide a strong argument in favor of this view (96,104,105). In addition, lymphoid blast crisis, which affects about one-third of the CML patients, is clinically very similar to Ph^1-positive ALL. However, there are some inconsistencies. Often there are less than 100% Ph^1-positive cells in the bone marrow of ALL patients, and clinical remission is accompanied by elimination of the Ph^1 chromosome from the bone marrow cells (105,106).

The Ph^1 chromosome of acute leukemia results from a translocation between chromosomes 9 and 22, t(9;22)(q34;q11), and is cytogenetically indistinguishable from its counterpart in CML. Variant Ph^1 translocations occur with a frequency similar to that observed in CML, although some report an increased incidence among ALL patients (106,107). Discriminating at the molecular level between the Ph^1 chromosome of ALL and that of CML has been the subject of several recent investigations, with interesting results. Leukemic cells from Ph^1-positive ALL patients do not always show rearrangement of the 5.8 kb breakpoint cluster region characteristic of CML (107,108). Nonetheless, translocation of *abl* to chromosome 22 has been demonstrated in Ph^1-positive ALL, irrespective of the presence or absence of rearrangement in M*bcr*. Additional evidence for the involvement of *abl* was obtained using *abl* DNA probes and antisera (109, 110). An abnormally sized phosphoprotein with a molecular weight of 190,000 daltons (p190) was detected in three Ph^1-positive ALL patients who did not have a M*bcr* rearrangement, and this has been confirmed by others (111). Recent results indicate that the breakpoint on chromosome 22 in Ph[1]-positive, M*bcr*-negative ALL occurs within the *bcr* gene but that it is some distance upstream (5′) of the (major) breakpoint cluster region (112). These data suggest that, as in CML, a *bcr-abl* fusion protein is produced as a result of the t(9;22) in Ph[1]-positive ALL. It is also clear that apparently similar cytogenetic abnormalities do not necessarily yield identical genomic events. In some cases of Ph[1]-positive ALL, *abl* is fused with *bcr* in a manner indistinguishable from that found in Ph[1]-positive CML, and it has been suggested that these patients have presented in the acute phase of CML. In other cases, *abl* is joined to sequences farther upstream in *bcr*, and this group corresponds to patients who present with de novo ALL (107,110–112). The genetic mechanisms that determine the production of p190 versus p210 and how the two proteins influence the hematologic expression of the diseases in which they are found is at present unknown.

SUMMARY AND FUTURE DIRECTIONS

The Ph[1] chromosome was the first specific karyotypic abnormality associated with a particular neoplastic disease in the human. It is found in the leukemic cells of about 99% of patients with CML and usually represents one product of a reciprocal translocation, t(9;22)(q34;q11). For many years it was suspected that chromosomal abnormalities cause cancer by altering the expression of specific genes. Significant recent developments in our understanding of the molecular consequences of the Ph[1] translocation strengthen that assumption.

The Ph[1] translocation generates a hybrid gene consisting of 5′ regulatory, promoter, and exon sequences of the *bcr* gene on chromosome 22 fused to 3′ exons and polyadenylation-termination sequences of the *abl* proto-oncogene from chromosome 9. The breakpoints on chromosomes 9 and 22, the association of *abl* and *bcr*, and structural changes in these genes have a similar nature in all patients correctly diagnosed as CML, whether they have the standard Ph[1] translocation or complex, simple, or masked variant Ph[1] translocations, and even in some who have no cytogenetic evidence of t(9;22) and are karyotypically normal. A specific genomic lesion causing this leukemia is indicated.

The question remains whether the Ph[1] translocation is the prime transforming event in CML and is directly responsible for the uncontrolled proliferation exhibited by Ph[1]-positive stem cells. Fialkow has suggested that the pathogenesis of CML involves at least three steps, the first of which is the clonal proliferation of a pluripotential Ph[1]-negative stem cell (113). The evidence for this step came from glucose-6-phosphate dehydrogenase (G6PD) analysis of Ph[1]-negative transformed B cell lines established from a CML patient. Of these cell lines, 70% showed the same G6PD isoenzyme B as the Ph[1]-positive leukemic clone from that patient. Furthermore, chromosome aberrations were found in several lines with isoenzyme B but not in lines with isoenzyme A. The authors suggested that clonally derived karyotypically unstable Ph^1-negative cells were present in CML patients, and that these represented an early malignant clone, some cell(s) of which later acquired the Ph^1 chromosome and led to the development of full CML (114). Other evidence that the Ph^1 may not be the primary transforming event has come from rare patients who lacked the Ph^1 at diagnosis but subsequently acquired the abnormality at a later stage (115) or from patients who presented with Ph^1-positive CML but only had Ph^1-negative leukemic cells at acute transformation (116).

The mechanism by which the Ph^1 translocation occurs is unknown. It is probably a random event that comes to notice because of the selective proliferative advantage it confers on the hematopoietic stem cell. Evidence obtained to date suggests that the translocation is a random event. However, *Alu* sequences are frequently present in close proximity to the breakpoints (40,41), and these may enhance the probability of illegitimate homologous recombination. Recombination between *abl* and *bcr* must also clearly be favored by the extraordinarily large size of these genes, but only certain configurations allow the production of a functional protein that provides a selective growth advantage to the cell.

Circumstantial evidence indicates that the production of an active p210 must confer some selective advantage on cells expressing it. The attachment of a *bcr* moiety to the *abl* protein results in an elevated tyrosine kinase activity similar to the tyrosine kinase activity of v-*abl* and it is likely to have transforming potential. The specific involvement of the *bcr-abl* protein in leukemia can reasonably be attributed to the amino-terminal *bcr* sequences. No significant homology between *bcr* and A-MuLV *gag* sequences has been detected, and it appears that *bcr-abl* lacks the ability to transform NIH 3T3 cells whereas these cells are transformed efficiently by v-*abl* (117). However, the human *abl* part of the *bcr-abl* protein is highly homologous to v-*abl*, and it is anticipated that this region of human *abl* under the control of an appropriate promoter has the potential to transform NIH 3T3 cells.

The emphasis of research in Ph^1-positive leukemia is now shifting away from molecular cloning. It seems well established that fusion of *abl* and *bcr* genes plays a crucial role in the pathogenesis of CML and ALL. Future studies should address such questions as how the hybrid protein is involved in leukemia. Research aimed at investigating the normal function of *abl* and *bcr* may be important in efforts to understand their abnormal functioning in leukemia and to increase our understanding of the disease. Perhaps the development of *bcr-abl* transgenic mice wll result in an animal model for the study of CML that will provide some insight into the effects of the chimeric *bcr-abl* protein and the function of the normal *bcr* and *abl* gene products.

ACKNOWLEDGMENTS

We wish to thank all colleagues who provided data prior to publication. We would also like to thank Trish Rodriguez and Karen Betz for assistance in preparing the manuscript.

REFERENCES

1. Bishop, M. J. (1983). Cellular oncogenes and retroviruses. *Annu. Rev. Biochem. 52*:301.
2. Nowell, P. C., and Hungerford, O. A. (1960). A minute chromosome in human chronic granulocytic leukemia. *Science 132*:1497.
3. Rowley, J. D., and Testa, J. R. (1982). Chromosomal abnormalities in malignant haematologic diseases. *Adv. Cancer Res. 36*:103.
4. Caspersson, T., Gahrton, G., Lindsten, J., and Zech, L. (1970). Identification of the Philadelphia chromosome as a number 22 by quinicrine mustard fluorescence analysis. *Exp. Cell Res. 63*:238.
5. O'Riordan, M. L., Robinson, J. A., Buckton, K. E., and Evans, H. J. (1971). Distinguishing between the chromosomes involved in Down's syndrome (trisomy 21), and chronic myeloid leukemia (Ph^1) by fluorescence. *Nature 230*:167.
6. Rowley, J. D. (1973). A new consistent chromosomal abnormality in chronic myelogenous leukaemia identified by quinacrine fluorescence and Giemsa staining. *Nature 243*:290.
7. Dube, I. D., Gupta, C. M., Kalousek, D. K., and Eaves, A. C. (1984). Cytogenetic studies of early myeloid progenitor compartments in Ph^1-positive chronic myeloid leukemia (CML). *Br. J. Haematol. 56*:633.
8. Dube, I. D., Kalousek, D. K., Coulombel, L., Gupta, C. M., Eaves, C. J., and Eaves, A. C. (1984). Cytogenetic studies of early myeloid progenitor compartments in Ph^1-positive chronic myeloid leukemia. II. Long-term culture reveals the persistence of Ph^1-negative progenitors in treated as well as newly diagnosed patients. *Blood 63*:1172.
9. Frassoni, F., Repetto, M., Podesta, M., Piaggio, G., Raffo, M. R., Sessarago, M., Bacigalupo, A., and Marmont, A. M. (1986). Competitive survival/proliferation of normal and Ph^1-positive haemopoietic cells. *Br. J. Haematol. 63*:135.
10. Heisterkamp, N., Groffen, J., and Stephenson, J. R. (1985). The human v-*abl* cellular homologue. *J. Mol. Appl. Genet. 2*:57.
11. Shtivelman, E., Lifshitz, B., Gale, R. P., and Canaani, E. (1985). Fused transcript of *abl* and *bcr* genes in chronic myelogenous leukaemia. *Nature 315*:550.
12. Reddy, E., Smith, M., and Srinivasan, A. (1983). Nucleotide sequence of Abelson murine leukemia virus genome; structural similarity of its transforming gene product to other *onc* gene products with tyrosine-specific kinase activity. *Proc. Natl. Acad. Sci. USA 80*:3623.

13. Groffen, J., Heisterkamp, N., Reynolds, F. H., Jr., and Stephenson, J. R. (1983). Homology between phosphotyrosine acceptor site of human c-*abl* and viral oncogene products. *Nature 304*:364.
14. Goff, S. P. (1985). The Abelson murine leukemia virus oncogene (42115). *Proc. Soc. Exp. Biol. Med. 179*:403.
15. Goff, S. P., Gilboa, E., Witte, O. N., and Baltimore, D. (1980). Structure of the Abelson murine leukemia virus genome and the homologous cellular gene: Studies with cloned viral DNA. *Cell 22*:777.
16. Reddy, E., Smith, M., and Srinivasan, A. (1983). Correction. *Proc. Natl. Acad. Sci. USA 80*:7372.
17. Wang, J. Y. J., and Baltimore, D. (1983). Cellular RNA homologous to the Abelson murine leukemia virus transforming gene: Expression and relationship to the viral sequence. *Mol. Cell. Biol. 3*:773.
18. Ben-Neriah, Y., Bernards, A., Paskind, M., Daley, G. Q., and Baltimore, D. (1986). Alternative 5′ exons in c-*abl* mRNA. *Cell 44*:577.
19. Shtivelman, E., Lifshitz, B., Gale, R. P., Roe, B. A., and Canaani, E. (1986). Alternative splicing of RNAs transcribed from the human *abl* gene and from the *bcr-abl* gene. *Cell 47*:277.
20. Ziff, E. (1985). Splicing in adenovirus and other animal viruses. *Int. Rev. Cytol. 93*:327.
21. Benyajati, C., Spoerel, N., Haymerie, H., and Ashburner, M. (1983). The messenger RNA for alcohol dehydrogenase in *Drosophila melanogaster* differs in its 5′ end in different developmental stages. *Cell 33*:125.
22. Young, R. A., Hagenbuchle, O., and Schibler, U. (1981). A single mouse α-amylase gene specifies two different tissue-specific mRNAs. *Cell 23*:451.
23. Early, P., Rogers, J., Davis, M., Calame, K., Bond, M., Wall, R., and Hood, L. (1980). Two mRNAs can be produced from a single immunoglobulin gene by alternative RNA processing pathways. *Cell 20*:313.
24. Amara, S. G., Jonas, V., Rosenfeld, M. G., Ong, E. S., and Evans, R. M. (1982). Alternative RNA processing in calcitonin gene expression generates mRNAs coding different polypeptide products. *Nature 298*:240.
25. Rozek, C. E., and Davidson, N. (1983). *Drosophila* has one myosin heavy-chain gene with three developmentally regulated transcripts. *Cell 32*:23.
26. Basi, G. S., Boardman, M., and Storti, R. V. (1984). Alternative splicing of a *Drosophila* tropomyosin gene generates muscle tropomyosin isoforms with different carboxy-terminal ends. *Mol. Cell. Biol. 4*:2828.
27. Westin, E. H., Wong-Staal, F., Gelman, E. P., Dalla-Favera, R., Papas, T., Lautenberger, J. A., Eva, A., Reddy, E. P., Tronick, S. R., Aaronson, S. A., and Gallo, R. C. (1982). Expression of cellular homologue of retroviral oncogenes in human hematopoietic cells. *Proc. Natl. Acad. Sci. USA 79*: 2490.
28. Melton, D. W., McEwan, C., McKie, A. B., and Reid, A. M. (1986). Expression of the mouse HPRT gene: Deletional analysis of the promoter region of an X-chromosome linked housekeeping gene. *Cell 44*:319.
29. Dynan, W. S., Sazer, S., Tjian, R., and Schimke, R. (1986). Transcription factor Sp1 recognizes a DNA sequence in the mouse dihydrofolate reductase promoter. *Nature 319*:246.

30. Grosveld, G., Verwoerd, T., van Agthoven, T., de Klein, A., Ramachandran, K. L., Heisterkamp, N., Stam, K., and Groffen, J. (1986). The chronic myelocytic cell line K562 contains a breakpoint in *bcr* and produces a chimeric *bcr-abl* transcript. *Mol. Cell. Biol. 6*:607.
31. Westbrook, C. A., Rubin, C. M., Le Beau, M. M., Kaminer, L. S., Smith, S. D., Rowley, F. D., and Diaz, M. O. (1987). Molecular analysis of TCRB and ABL in a t(7;9)-containing cell line (SUP-T3) from a human T-cell leukemia. *Proc. Natl. Acad. Sci. USA 84*:251.
32. Kuhne, T., Wieringa, B., Weiser, J., and Weissmann, C. (1983). Evidence against a scanning model of RNA splicing. *EMBO J. 2*:727.
33. Solnick, D. (1985). Trans splicing of mRNA precursors. *Cell 42*:157.
34. Solnick, D. (1985). Alternative splicing caused by RNA secondary structure. *Cell 43*:667.
35. Breitbart, R. E., Nguyen, H. T., Medford, R. M., Destree, A. T., Mahdavi, V., and Nadal-Ginard, B. (1985). Intricate combinatorial patterns of exon splicing generate multiple regulated troponin T isoforms from a single gene. *Cell 41*:67.
36. Heisterkamp, N., Groffen, J., Stephenson, J. R., Spurr, N. K., Goodfellow, P. N., Solomon, E., Carrit, B., and Bodmer, W. F. (1982). Chromosomal localization of human cellular homologues of two viral oncogenes. *Nature 299*:747.
37. de Klein, A., Geurts van Kessel, A., Grosveld, G., Bartram, C. R., Hagemeijer, A., Bootsma, D., Spurr, N. K., Heisterkamp, N., Groffen, J., and Stephenson, J. R. (1982). A cellular oncogene is translocated to the Philadelphia chromosome in chronic myelocytic leukemia. *Nature 300*:765.
38. Heisterkamp, N., Stephenson, J. R., Groffen, J., Hansen, P. F., de Klein, A., Bartram, C. R., and Grosveld, G. (1983). Localization of the c-*abl* oncogene adjacent to a translocation breakpoint in chronic myelocytic leukemia. *Nature 306*:239.
39. Groffen, J., Stephenson, J. R., Heisterkamp, N., de Klein, A., Bartram, C. R., and Grosveld, C. (1984). Philadelphia chromosomal breakpoints are clustered within a limited region, *bcr*, on chromosome 22. *Cell 36*:93.
40. Heisterkamp, N., Stam, K., Groffen, J., de Klein, A., and Grosveld, G. (1985). Structural organization of the *bcr* gene and its role in the Ph^1 translocation. *Nature 314*:758.
41. De Klein, A., Van Agthoven, T., Groffen, C., Heisterkamp, N., Groffen, J., and Grosveld, G. (1986). Molecular analysis of both translocation products of a Philadelphia positive CML patient. *Nucleic Acids Res. 14*:7071.
42. Leibowitz, D., Schaefer-Rego, K., Popenoe, D. W., Maers, J. G., and Bank, A. (1985). Variable breakpoints on the Philadelphia chromosome in chronic myelogenous leukemia. *Blood 66*:243.
43. Groffen, J. (1987). Nomenclature proposal: UCLA symposium on chronic myeloid leukemia. *Annapolis Mol. USA* 1987.
44. Dalla-Favera, R., Gelman, E. P., Gallo, R. C., and Wong-Staal, F. (1981). A human oncogene homologous to the transforming gene (v-*sis*) of simian sarcoma virus. *Nature 292*:31.

45. Groffen, J., Heisterkamp, N., Stephenson, J. R., van Kessel, A., de Klein, A., Grosveld, G., and Bootsma, D. (1983). c-*sis* is translocated from chromosome 22 to chromosome 9 in chronic myelocytic leukemia. *J. Exp. Med. 158*:9.
46. Bartram, C. R., de Klein, A., Hagemeijer, A., Grosveld, G., Heisterkamp, N., and Groffen, J. (1984). Localization of the human c-*sis* oncogene in Ph^1-positive and Ph^1-negative chronic myelocytic leukemia by in situ hybridization. *Blood 223*.
47. McBride, O. W., Hieter, P. A., Hollis, G. F., Swan, D., Otey, M. C., and Leder, P. (1982). Chromosomal location of human kappa and lambda immunoglobulin light chain constant region genes. *J. Exp. Med. 155*:1480.
48. Yunis, J. J. (1983). The chromosomal basis of human neoplasia. *Science 221*:227.
49. Miller, J., Bothwell, A., and Storb, U. (1982). Physical linkage of the constant region genes for immunoglobulins I and III. *Proc. Natl. Acad. Sci. USA 78*:3829.
50. Battey, J., Moulding, C., Taub, R., Murphy, W., Stewart, T., Potter, H., Lenoir, G., and Leder, P. (1983). The human c-*myc* oncogene: Burkitt lymphoma. *Cell 34*:799.
51. Stam, K., Heisterkamp, N., Grosveld, G., de Klein, A., Verma, R. S., Coleman, M., Dosik, H., and Groffen, J. (1985). Evidence of new chimeric *bcr*-c-*abl* mRNA in patients with chronic myelocytic leukemia and the Philadelphia chromosome. *N. Engl. J. Med. 313*:1429.
52. Hariharan, I. K., and Adams, J. M. (1987). cDNA sequence for human *bcr*, the gene that translocates to the *abl* oncogene in chronic myeloid leukaemia. *EMBO J. 6*:115.
53. Lozzio, C. B., and Lozzio, B. B. (1975). Human chronic myelogenous leukemia cell line with positive Philadelphia chromosome. *Blood 45*:321.
54. Collins, S. J., and Groudine, M. T. (1983). Rearrangement and amplification of c-*abl* sequences in the human chronic myelogenous leukemia cell line K562. *Proc. Natl. Acad. Sci. USA 80*:4813.
55. Canaani, E., Gale, R. P., and Steiner-Saltz, D. (1984). Altered transcription of an oncogene in chronic myeloid leukemia. *Lancet 593*.
56. Collins, S. J., Kubbonishi, I., Myoshi, I., and Goudine, M. T. (1984). Altered transcription of the c-*abl* oncogene in K-562 and other chronic myelogenous leukemia cells. *Science 225*:72.
57. Gale, R. P., and Cannani, E. (1984). A novel 8 kb *abl* RNA transcript in chronic myelogenous leukemia. *Proc. Natl. Acad. Sci. USA 81*:5648.
58. Romero, P., Blick, M., Talpaz, M., Murphy, E., Hester, J., and Gutterman, J. (1986). C-*sis* and c-*abl* expression in chronic myelogenous leukemia and other hematologic malignancies.. *Blood 67*:839.
59. Gale, R. P., and Cannani, E. (1985). The molecular biology of chronic myelogenous leukaemia. *Br. J. Haematol. 60*:395.
60. Ponticelli, A. S., Whitlock, C. A., Rosenberg, N., and Witte, O. N. (1982). In vivo tyrosine phosphorylations of the Abelson virus transforming protein are absent in its normal cell homolog. *Cell 29*:953.

61. Konopka, J. B., and Witte, O. N. (1985). Detection of c-*abl* tyrosine kinase activity in vitro permits direct comparison of normal and altered *abl* gene products. *Mol. Cell. Biol. 5*:3116.
62. Witte, O., Dasgupta, A., and Baltimore, D. (1980). Abelson murine leukemia virus protein is phosphorylated in vitro to form phosphotyrosine. *Nature 283*:826.
63. Sefton, B. M., Hunter, T., and Raschke, W. C. (1981). Evidence that the Abelson virus protein functions in vivo as a protein kinase that phosphorylates tyrosine. *Proc. Natl. Acad. Sci. USA 78*:1552.
64. Rosenberg, N. E., Clark, D. R., and Witte, O. N. (1980). Abelson murine leukemia virus mutants deficient in kinase activity and lymphoid cell transformation. *J. Virol. 36*:766.
65. Davis, R. L., Konopka, J. B., and Witte, O. N. (1985). Activation of the c-*abl* oncogene by viral transduction or chromosomal translocation generates altered c-*abl* proteins with similar in vitro kinase properties. *Mol. Cell. Biol. 5*:204.
66. Konopka, J. B., Watanabe, S. M., and Witte, O. N. (1984). An alteration of the human c-*abl* protein in K562 leukemia cells unmasks associated tyrosine kinase activity. *Cell 37*:1035.
67. Konopka, J. B., Watanabe, S. M., Singer, J. W., Collins, S. J., and Witte, O. N. (1985). Cell lines and clinical isolated derived from Ph[1]-positive chronic myelogenous leukemia patients express c-*abl* proteins with a common structural alteration. *Proc. Natl. Acad. Sci. USA 82*:1810.
68. Stam, K., Heisterkamp, N., Reynolds, F. H., Jr., and Groffen, J. (1987). Evidence that the Ph[1] gene encodes a 160,000 dalton phosphoprotein with associated kinase activity. *Mol. Cell. Biol.* 1955.
69. Ben-Neriah, Y., Daley, G. Q., Mes-Masson, A.-M., Witte, O. N., and Baltimore, D. (1986). The chronic myelogenous leukemia specific p210 protein is the product of the *bcr/abl* hybrid gene. *Science 223*:212.
70. First International Workshop on Chromosomes in Leukemia, 1977 (1978). Chromosomes in Ph[1]-positive chronic granulocyte leukaemia. *Br. J. Haematol. 39*:505.
71. Sandberg, A. A. (19xx). Chromosomes and causation of human cancer and leukemia. XL. The Ph[1] and other translocations in CML. *Cancer 46*:2221–2226.
72. Oshimura, M.; Ohyashkik, K., Terada, H., Takaku, F., and Tonomura, A. (1982). Variant Ph[1] translocations in CML and their incidence, including two cases with sequential lymphoid and myeloid crisis. *Cancer Genet. Cytogenet. 5*:187.
73. Bernstein, R., Pinto, M. R., Wallace, C., Penfold, G., and Mendelow, B. (1984). The incidence, type and subsequent evolution of 14 variants Ph[1] translocations in 180 South African patients with Ph[1]-positive chronic myeloid leukemia. *Cancer Genet. Cytogenet. 12*:225.
74. Heim, S., Billstrom, R., Kristofferson, U., Mandahl, N., Strombeck, B., and Mitelman, F. (1985). Variant Ph[1] translocations in chronic myeloid leukemia. *Cancer Genet. Cytogenet. 18*:215.

75. Bartram, C. R., de Klein, A., Hagemeijer, A., van Agthoven, T., van Kessel, A. G., Bootsma, D., Grosveld, G., Ferguson-Smith, M. A., Davies, T., Stone, M., Heisterkamp, N., Stephenson, J. R., and Groffen, J. (1983). Translocation of c-*abl* oncogene correlates with the presence of a Philadelphia chromosome in chronic myelocytic leukemia. *Nature 306*:227.
76. Morris, C. M., Rosman, L., Archer, S. A., Cochrane, J. M., and Fitzgerald, P. H. (19xx). A cytogenetic and molecular analysis of five variant Ph^1 translocations in chronic myeloid leukemia. *Cancer Genet. Cytogenet.* in press.
77. Rowley, J. D. (1982). Identification of the constant chromosome regions involved in human hematologic malignant disease. *Science 216*:749.
78. Hagemeijer, A., Bartram, C. R., Smit, E. M. E., van Agthoven, A. J., and Bootsma, D. (1984). Is the chromosomal region 9q34 always involved in variants of the Ph^1 translocation? *Cancer Genet. Cytogenet. 13*:1.
79. Morris, C. M., and Fitzgerald, P. H. (1987). Complexity of an apparently simple variant Ph^1 translocation in chronic myeloid leukemia. *Leuk. Res. 11*:163.
80. Bartram, C. R., Anger, B., Carbonell, F., and Kleihauer, E. (1985). Involvement of chromosome 9 in variant Ph^1 translocation. *Leuk. Res. 9*:1133.
81. Mareni, C., Sessarago, M., Coviello, O. A., Origone, P., and Ajmar, F. (1986). Involvement of chromosomal region 9q34 in a case of variant Ph^1 translocation t(22;22). *Leuk. Res. 10*:1131.
82. Hagemeijer, A., de Klein, A., Godde-Salz, E., Turc-Carel, C., Smit, E. M. E., van Agthroven, A. J., and Grosveld, G. C. (1985). Translocation of c-*abl* to "masked" Ph^1 in chronic myeloid leukemia. *Cancer Genet. Cytogenet. 18*:95.
83. Alimena, G., Hagemeijer, A., Bakhuis, J., De Cula, M. R., Diverio, D., and Montefusco, E. (1987). Cytogenetic and molecular characterization of a masked Philadelphia chromosome in chronic myelocytic leukemia. *Cancer Genet. Cytogenet. 27*:21.
84. Galton, D. A. G. (1969). Chemotherapy of chronic myelocytic leukaemia. *Semin. Hematol. 6*:323.
85. Koeffler, H. P., and Golde, D. W. (1981). Chronic myelogenous leukemia—new concepts (first of two parts). *N. Engl. J. Med. 304*:1201.
86. Laszlo, J. (1975). Myeloproliferative disorders (MPD): Myelofibrosis, myelosclerosis, extramedullary hematopoiesis, undifferentiated MPD, and hemorrhagic thrombocythemia. *Semin. Hematol. 12*:409.
87. Bennett, J. M., Catovsky, D., Daniel, M. T., Flandrin, G., Galton, D. A. G., Gralnick, H. R., and Sultan, C. (19xx). The French-American-British (FAB) Cooperative Group. Proposals for the classification of the myelodysplastic syndromes. *Br. J. Haematol. 51*:189–199.
88. Pugh, W. C., Pearson, M., Vardiman, J. W., and Rowley, J. D. (1985). Philadelphia chromosome negative chronic myelogenous leukaemia: A morphological reassessment. *Br. J. Haematol. 60*:457.
89. Travis, L. B., Pierre, R. V., and DeWald, G. W. (1986). Ph^1-negative chronic granulocytic leukemia: A non-entity. *Am. J. Clin. Pathol. 85*:186.

90. Bartram, C. R., Kleihauer, E., de Klein, A., Grosveld, G., Teyssier, J. J., Heisterkamp, N., and Groffen, J. (1985). c-*abl* and *bcr* are rearranged in Ph[1]-negative CML patient. *EMBO J. 4*:683.
91. Morris, C. M., Reeve, A. E., Fitzgerald, P. H., Hollings, P. E., Beard, M. E. J., and Heaton, D. C. (1986). Genomic diversity correlates with clinical variation in Ph[1]-negative chronic myeloid leukemia. *Nature 330*: 281.
92. Ganeson, T. S., Rassool, F., Guo, A.-P., Th'ng, K. H., Dowding, C., Hibbins, J. A., Young, B. D., White, H., Kumaran, T. O., Galton, D. A. G., and Goldman, J. M. (1986). Rearrangements of the *bcr* gene in Philadelphia chromosome-negative chronic myeloid leukemia. *Blood 68*:957.
93. Kurzrock, R., Blick, M. B., Talpaz, M., Velasquez, W. S., Trujillo, J. M., Kouttab, N. M., Kloetzer, W. S., Arlinghaus, R. B., and Gutterman, J. U. (1986). Rearrangement in the breakpoint cluster region and the clinical course in Philadelphia-negative chronic myelogenous leukemia. *Ann. Intern. Med. 105*:673.
94. Wiedemann, L. M., Karhi, K. K., Shivji, M. K. K., Rayter, S. I., Pegram, S. M., Dowden, G., Bevan, D., Will, A., Galton, D. A. G., and Chan, L. C. (1988). The correlation of breakpoint cluster region rearrangement and P210 *phl/abl* expression with morphological analysis of Ph[1]-negative chronic myeloid leukemia and other myeloproliferative diseases. *Blood 71*: 349.
95. Fitzgerald, P. H., Beard, M. E. J., Morris, C. M., Heaton, D. C., and Reeve, A. E. (1987). Ph[1]-negative chronic myeloid leukaemia. *Br. J. Haematol. 66*:311.
96. Beard, M. E. J., Durrant, J., Catovsky, D., Wiltshaw, E., Amess, J. L., Brearley, R. L., Kirk, B., Wrigley, P. F. M., Janossy, G., Greaves, M. F., and Galton, D. A. G. (1976). Blast crisis of chronic myeloid leukaemia (CML). I. Presentation simulating acute lymphoid leukaemia (ALL). *Br. J. Haematol. 34*:167.
97. Oshimura, A., Sandberg, A. A. (1977). Chromosomes and causation of human cancer and leukemia. XXV. Significance of the Ph[1] (including unusual translocations) in various acute leukemias. *Cancer 40*:1149.
98. Sasaki, M., Kondo, K., and Tomiyasu, T. (1988). Cytogenetic characterization of ten cases of Ph[1]-positive acute myelogenous leukemia. *Cancer Genet. Cytogenet. 9*:119.
99. Yunis, J. J., Brunning, R. D., Howe, R. B., and Lobell, A. (1984). High-resolution chromosomes as an independent prognostic indicator in adult acute nonlymphocytic leukemia. *N. Engl. J. Med. 311*:812.
100. Chessells, J. M., Janossy, G., Lawler, S. D., Secker, and Walker, L. M. (1979). The Ph[1] chromosome in childhood leukemia. *Br. J. Haematol. 41*:25.
101. Priest, J. R., Robison, L. L., McKenna, R. W., Lindquist, L. L., Warkentin, P. L., LeBien, T. W., Wood, W. G., Kersey, J. H., Coccia, P. F., and Nesbit, M. E. (1980). Philadelphia chromosome positive childhood acute lymphoblastic leukemia. *Blood 56*:15.

102. Champlin, R. E., and Golde, D. W. (1985). Chronic myelogenous leukemia: Recent advances. *Blood 65*:1039.
103. Le Beau, M. M., and Rowley, J. D. (1984). Recurring chromosomal abnormalities in leukaemia and lymphoma. *Cancer Surveys 3*:371.
104. Catovsky, D. (1979). Ph[1] positive acute leukaemia and chronic granulocytic leukemia: One or two diseases. *Br. J. Haematol. 42*:493.
105. Sandberg, A. A., Kohno, S., Wake, N., and Minowada, J. (1980). Chromosomes and causation of human cancer and leukemia. XLII. Ph[1]-positive ALL: An entity within myeloproliferative disorders? *Cancer Genet. Cytogenet. 2*:145.
106. Rowley, J. D. (1980). Ph[1]-positive leukemia, including chronic myelogenous leukemia. *Clin. Haematol. 9*:55.
107. De Klein, A., Hagemeijer, A., Bartram, C. R., Houwen, R., Hoefsloot, L., Carbonell, F., Chan, L., Barnett, M., Greaves, M., Kleihauer, E., Heisterkamp, N., Groffen, J., and Grosveld, G. (1986). *bcr* rearrangement and translocations of the c-*abl* oncogene in Philadelphia positive acute lymphoblastic leukemia. *Blood 68*:1369.
108. Erikson, J., Griffin, C. A., Ar-Rushdi, A., Valtieri, M., Hoxie, J., Finan, J., Emanuel, B. S., Rovera, G., Nowell, P. C., and Croce, C. M. (1986). Heterogeneity of chromosome 22 breakpoints in Philadelphia positive (Ph^+) acute lymphocytic leukemia. *Proc. Natl. Acad. Sci. USA 83*:1807.
109. Chan, L. C., Karhi, K. K., Rayter, S. I., Heisterkamp, N., Eridani, S., Powles, R., Lawler, S. D., Groffen, J., Foulkes, J. G., Greaves, M. F., and Wiedemann, L. M. (1987). A novel *abl* protein expressed in Philadelphia chromosome positive acute lymphoblastic leukemia. *Nature 325*:635.
110. Kurzrock, R., Shtalrid, M., Romero, P., Kloetzer, W. S., Talpas, M., Trujillo, J. M., Blick, M., Beran, M., and Gutterman, J. U. (1987). A novel c-*abl* protein product in Philadelphia-positive acute lymphoblastic leukaemia. *Nature 335*:631.
111. Clark, S. S., Laughlin, J., Crist, W. M., Champlin, R., and Witte, O. N. (1987). Unique forms of the *abl* tyrosine kinase distinguish Ph[1]-positive CML from Ph[1]-positive ALL. *Science 235*:85.
112. Hermans, A., Heisterkamp, N., von Lindern, M., van Baal, S., Meijer, D., van der Plas, D., Wiedemann, L., Groffen, J., Bootsma, D., and Grosveld, G. (1987). Unique fusion of *bcr* and c-*abl* genes in Philadelphia chromosome positive acute lymphoblastic leukemia. *Cell 51*:33–40.
113. Fialkow, P. J. (1984). Clonal evolution of human myeloid leukemias. In *Genes and Cancer*, (J. M. Bishop, J. D. Rowley, and M. Greaves, eds.). Alan R. Liss, New York, pp. 2115.
114. Fialkow, P. J., Martini, P. J., Najfield, V., Penfold, G. K., Jacobson, R. J., and Hansen, J. A. (1981). Evidence for a multistep pathogenesis of chronic myelogenous leukemia. *Blood 58*:158.
115. Lisker, F., Casas, L., Mutchinick, O., Perez-Chavez, F., and Labardini, J. (1980). Late-appearing Philadelphia chromosome in two patients with chronic myelogenous leukemia. *Blood 56*:812.

116. Hagemeijer, A., Smit, E. M. E., Lowenberg, B., and Abels, J. (1979). Chronic myeloid leukemia with permanent disappearance of the Ph[1] chromosome and development of new clonal subpopulations. *Blood 53*:1.
117. Daley, G. Q., McLaughlin, J., Witte, O. N., and Baltimore, D. (1987). The CML specific P210 *bcr/abl* protein, unlike v-*abl*, does not transform NIH/3T3 fibroblasts, *Science 237*:532.

7
Variation of *BCR-ABL* Breakpoint and Its Relationship to Prognosis

David Leibowitz *Indiana University, Indianapolis, Indiana*

Patients with chronic myelogenous leukemia (CML) have chromosome 22 translocation breakpoints that fall within intervening sequences (introns) located within the *bcr* (1). A number of small exons of the *BCR* gene are located within the *bcr*, and the location of the chromosome 22 breakpoint within the *bcr* determines which of the small exons code for amino acids in the *BCR-ABL* fusion protein (Figure 1) (2,3).* Only the exons that remain on the Philadelphia (Ph[1]) chromosome are represented in the *BCR-ABL* fusion transcript and code for amino acids in the fusion protein (p210). The majority of patients have breakpoints located either between *bcr* exons 2 and 3 or between *bcr* exons 3 and 4. There are occasional patients with breakpoints located between *bcr* exons 1 and 2, and these patients do splice in-frame from the *BCR* sequence to the *ABL* sequence, generating a functional mRNA (4–6).

The p210 fusion protein has two common forms, which differ by the inclusion or exclusion of the 25 amino acids encoded by *bcr* exon 3. If the chromosome 22 breakpoint falls within the intron between *bcr* exon 2 and 3, exon 3 does not remain on the Ph[1] chromosome and the junction between the *BCR* and *ABL* sequences is from *bcr* exon 2 to *ABL* exon II (Figure 1). If the chromosome 22 breakpoint is located between *bcr* exons 3 and 4, exon 3 remains on the Ph[1] chromosome and the amino acids encoded by exon 3 appear in p210. There

---

**A note on nomenclature: ABL, BCR,* and *BCR-ABL* are the names of genes located on chromosome 9 and 11, and the Ph[1] chromosome respectively. "*bcr*" in lowercase letters refers to the 5.8 kb breakpoint cluster region which is located in the center of the *BCR* gene.

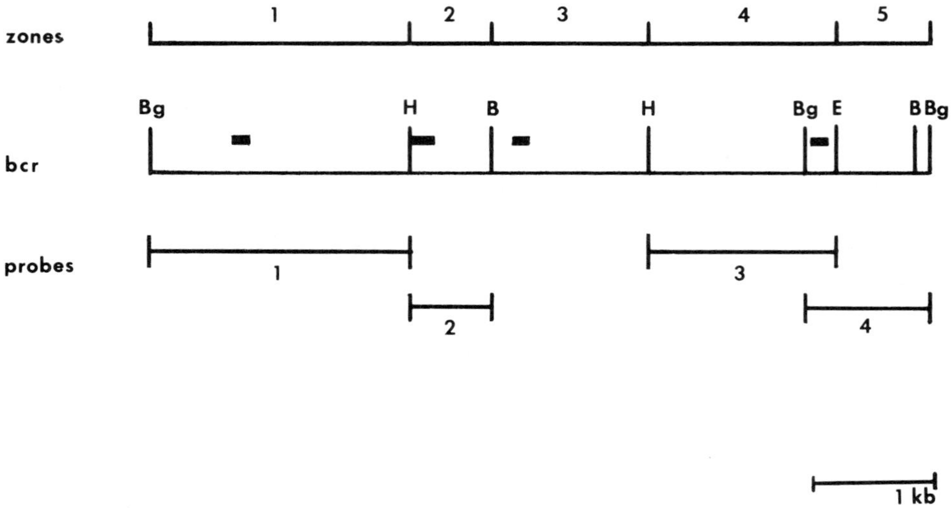

Figure 1 A schematic representation of the *bcr*. (*bcr,* middle line) Restriction sites within the 5.8 Kb *bcr*. The small solid rectangles indicate the coding exons of the *BCR* gene, which are located within the *bcr*. They are numbered 1-4 from left to right, respectively. (Probes, lower lines) The genomic fragments used in the initial breakpoint mapping study (4). (Zones, top line) The areas within the *bcr* defined by restriction mapping. Chromosome 22 translocation breakpoints for each patient were assigned to one of these zones. The majority of patients have breakpoints that fall within zone 2, 3, or 4. In the initial publication, breakpoints in zone 4 were referred to as "3′ breakpoints" and breakpoints in zone 1, 2, or 3 were referred to as "5′ breakpoints"; that is, the *Hind*III site between zones 3 and 4 serves as the divider for 5′ versus 3′ breakpoints.

are rare patients with breakpoints located farther 5′ who may not include *bcr* exon 2, and very rare patients lose *bcr* exon 1, and even one of the more 5′ exons, during the translocation (7,8).

What has emerged over the last couple of years is that there is a relationship between the location of the *bcr* breakpoint and the length of the chronic phase. The location of the breakpoint correlates with the length of the chronic phase, although the precise relationship and the clinical usefulness of the information are not yet fully understood. The initial study, from this laboratory, examined the location of the *bcr* breakpoint in 26 patients with CML, 9 in blast crisis and 17 in chronic phase (4).

The *bcr* was divided into an arbitrary set of zones, numbered 1-5, based upon the restriction map. Southern blotting and restriction mapping were performed on each of the patients. It was possible to determine which of the restriction zones contained the chromosome 22 translocation breakpoints for each of the patients (see Figure 1).

Separating the patients into chronic phase and blast crisis produced a striking result: virtually all the patients in blast crisis at the time the blood sample was collected had chromosome 22 breakpoints located toward the 3′ end of the *bcr* (zone 4 in Figure 1). The chronic-phase patients had breakpoints distributed randomly across the central portion of the *bcr* (zones 2, 3, and 4, Figure 1). The initial data also suggested that the patients with 3′ breakpoints had a shorter chronic phase than the patients with more 5′ breakpoints.

These data demonstrated a correlation between being in blast crisis, or progressing toward it, and having a chromosome 22 translocation breakpoint located in the 3′ portion of the *bcr*. A number of hypotheses could explain these data. (1) Patients with 3′ breakpoints had a shorter chronic phase than patients with 5′ breakpoints. In this case, if a population was sampled at a single point in time it could appear that there were a large number of blast crisis patients with 3′ breakpoints. (2) It was necessary to have a 3′ breakpoint to enter blast crisis. The initial set of data did not indicate which of these two hypotheses was most likely.

Although the patients in blast crisis with 3′ breakpoints each had a short chronic phase, the number of patients studied was not sufficient to prove that patients with 3′ breakpoints categorically had shorter chronic phases. One concern, which remains only partially answered, was how to account for the variability of when individual patients present to a physician and have a diagnosis established. The hypothesis that a 3′ breakpoint was required for progression into blast crisis was intellectually appealing but turned out to be incorrect. As the original group was followed and as additional patients were studied, it became clear that the patients with 5′ breakpoints did indeed progress into blast crisis and that their translocation breakpoint remained unchanged.

Following the initial observation, a number of laboratories have gathered data that show convincingly that patients with 3′ breakpoints have a shortened chronic phase in comparison to patients with a 5′ breakpoint. The hypothesis that all blast crisis patients had 3′ breakpoints was an artifact of the fact that the initial study essentially examined a group of patients at a fixed point in time. Since the patients with 3′ breakpoints had shorter chronic phases, at any one point there appeared to be a larger number of blast crisis patients with 3′ breakpoints. With a small sample size, a single observation could well include only patients with 3′ breakpoints who were in blast crisis.

A retrospective study by Eisenberg et al. examined 68 patients, including patients in chronic phase and blast crisis (5). This study showed a statistically significant difference between the length of the chronic phase for 5′ versus 3′ patients. The patients with 5′ breakpoints had roughly twice as long a period in chronic phase as compared to patients with 3′ breakpoints. The average chronic phase for patients with 5′ breakpoints was 50.6 months; for 3′ breakpoint patients the average was 30.2 months. This difference was statistically significant. These authors performed breakpoint mapping on eight patients during both the chronic phase and the terminal phase. Of these eight patients, six had 5′ breakpoints and two had 3′ breakpoints, and in all cases the breakpoint remained the same throughout the course of the disease.

Another study by Mills et al. included 22 patients, with prospective data on 3 patients (9). The study included samples from 12 patients in chronic phase and 7 patients in blast crisis and samples in both chronic and blase phase from 3 patients. There was no evidence for any change in the location of the breakpoint during the course of the disease. Duration of chronic phase to the point of study was determined for patients who were still in chronic phase, and the length of the antecedent chronic phase was taken for patients in blast crisis. The median length of chronic phase was 52 weeks for patients with 3′ breakpoints and 203 weeks for patients with 5′ breakpoints. This difference was statistically significant, so that in this study patients with 5′ breakpoints had, on the average, a chronic phase that was fourfold longer than in patients with 3′ breakpoints.

A group of investigators at M. D. Anderson retrospectively determined the *bcr* breakpoint location for 100 patients with CML (6). They found a statistically significant difference in the length of the chronic phase for patients with breakpoints in zone 3 compared to zone 4. The definition of zones for patients with 5′ breakpoints was slightly different than in other studies. Patients with breakpoints in zone 3 had an average chronic phase of 68 months, but patients with breakpoints in zone 4 had an average length of 43 months. This was statistically significant, with a $P = 0.04$. There was also a suggestion, although the result was not statistically significant, that patients in zone 1 combined with zone 2 had shorter chronic phases than the zone 3 patients.

These four studies provide strong evidence supporting the hypothesis that patients with breakpoints in zone 3 have a longer chronic phase than patients with breakpoints in zone 4. The implication is clearly that patients with breakpoints located 5′ to zone 4 have a longer chronic phase, and the only item that questions the more general conclusion is the suggestion of a slightly different result in the study by Shtalrid et al. (6). The Shtalrid study considered patients with breakpoints in zones 1 and 2 as a single group and suggested that these patients also have a shorter chronic phase in comparison to zone 3 patients. This difference lacked statistical significance, and additional studies will undoubtedly clarify the question.

An intriguing report from Dreazen et al. discussed a few unusual patients with abnormally long chronic-phase durations (10). These investigators were able to identify six patients with an unusually long chronic phase. Although all these patients are described as having *bcr* rearrangements, it was possible to localize the breakpoint to a zone of the *bcr* in only four of the patients. These four breakpoints were not clustered in a particular region of the *bcr*.

Although examining only a small number of patients, this study reinforces the point that the course of CML, like the course of other diseases, is not determined by any one factor. Whereas the location of the breakpoint within the *bcr* will help to project the relative length of the chronic phase, it is not the sole factor that determines the progression to blast crisis, and there are clearly patients in whom other as yet undescribed factors are of equal or greater importance.

Quite recently an additional retrospective series was published by Prezpiorka (11). The data as reported are incomplete: the unique method used for the restriction mapping precludes a meaningful interpretation of the data, either as a single study or in combination with the previously published studies. The reported information was generated by performing a double-restriction digest and then hybridizing the Southern blots with a single probe from the 3′ region of the *bcr*. The figures in the publication show a single abnormal band present in almost every patient's sample, which was interpreted in the text as indicating that the subjects had a Ph^1 chromosome translocation breakpoint lying in the 3′ portion of the *bcr*.

The other published studies have quite consistently confirmed a general principle of restriction mapping: if the breakpoint for a reciprocal translocation falls within the sequence included by the probe fragment itself, the blot demonstrates two abnormal bands, since the probe visualizes (hybridizes to) each of the resultant abnormal chromosomes, in addition to the remaining normal chromosome. Occasional patients fail to demonstrate two abnormal fragments, but the results from this laboratory and the other published series have detected two abnormal bands, representing each member of the reciprocal translocation, in at least 80% of the cases examined (4,5,12).

One cause for the appearance of only a single band is the frequent deletion of the chromosome 22 sequence during the translocation. This was initially described by identifying deletions large enough to be seen on Southern blots (13). Numerous other laboratories have subsequently confirmed the finding, both by Southern blotting and by DNA sequencing (5,6,9,14). This phenomenon can result in the appearance of a single band when only one probe is used for the restriction mapping. The appearance of a single abnormal band when using a 3′ *bcr* probe in patients who have undergone deletion of sequence within the *bcr* itself may only identify the $9q^+$ chromosome translocation breakpoint. The breakpoint from the Ph^1 chromosome could well lie farther 5′ within the *bcr*, which would not be detected without additional restriction mapping using a 5′ *bcr* probe. Only performing complete restriction mapping, as done in the previous series that use at least two hybridization probes, will provide the correct determination of the chromosome 22 translocation breakpoints of the Ph^1 chromosome as well as the $9q^+$ chromosome. The patients described in the Prezpiorka study must be re-examined with a 5′ *bcr* probe before the data are meaningful.

Considering the accumulated evidence, it seems well established that patients whose Ph^1 chromosome-chromosome 22 breakpoint falls within zone 3 have a longer chronic phase than patients whose breakpoint is located farther 3′ in the *bcr*. The magnitude of the difference is not precisely established, although it appears that patients with 5′ breakpoints have a chronic phase from two- to five-fold longer. There are clearly also patients whose course does not agree with this general condition: patients with 3′ breakpoints who have long chronic phases and some patients with 5′ breakpoints who have shorter chronic phases.

The manner in which time of presentation and diagnosis affects the observed length of the chronic phase remains a Gordian knot. A patient with an apparent short chronic phase could simply be an individual in whom the initial portion of the chronic phase was asymptomatic. The individual may not have presented to a physician, or the diagnosis may not have been apparent. Another question regards the effect of different treatments on the length of the chronic phase. The study from M. D. Anderson included a large proportion of patients who were treated with interferon. It is possible that patients treated with interferon behave differently from patients treated with other agents, potentially masking a difference between the groups previously identified. Further, it is conceivable that patients with 3′ breakpoints, with short chronic phases when treated with traditional regimens, have a particularly good response to treatment with interferon, masking the previously observed differences.

Questions regarding interferon in comparison to other treatment regimens should be answered by additional studies looking at larger numbers of patients. It is not as apparent how to resolve the question about time of presentation and severity of the chronic phase: there is no control population of normal people who can be screened for the Ph^1 chromosome. It is hoped that some information will settle out of studies with larger numbers of patients.

There is enough evidence to justify using this information as part of the data with which judgments and recommendations for patient care are made. Like other prognostic factors, *bcr* breakpoint location is not the sole determinant of the course of the disease. All other things being equal, it is reasonable to recommend that a patient with a 3′ breakpoint may appropriately undergo bone marrow transplantation at an earlier point within the chronic phase of CML than a patient with a 5′ breakpoint. If other prognostic factors suggest a less aggressive course, it is not appropriate to choose early marrow transplantation solely on the basis of *bcr* breakpoint location (15-17). A large prospective study correlating breakpoint location with prognosis is underway within Cancer and Leukemia Group B (CALGB).

A preliminary study done at the University of Minnesota reinforces this point. Examining a group of CML patients who had undergone bone marrow transplant, it appeared that patients who had 3′ breakpoints were more likely to relapse than patients with 5′ breakpoints. If this result is borne out by additional data, it may mean that patients with 3′ breakpoints, who have a more aggressive disease, may also require new treatment approaches.

Although *bcr* breakpoint location is one indicator of the course of CML, we do not understand how that effect is mediated. It may depend upon the presence or absence of *bcr* exon 3-encoded amino acids or upon the proportion of alternatively spliced products containing *bcr* exons 2 and 3. This may not provide a complete answer, and another possibility is that sequences within the *bcr* affect the regulation of *BCR-ABL* expression. When the mechanism by which breakpoint location exerts its effect is better understood, it should be possible to make better use of the information in estimating the clinical course of individual patients.

ACKNOWLEDGMENTS

Supported in part by funds from NIH, CA 44028. The author is the recipient of a Junior Faculty Research Award from the American Cancer Society.

REFERENCES

1. Goffen, J., Stephenson, J. R., Heisterkamp, N., deKlein, A., Bartram, C. R., and Grosveld, G. (1984). Philadelphia chromosomal breakpoints are clustered within a limited region, bcr, on chromosome 22. *Cell 36*:93-99.
2. Shtivelman, E., Lifshitz, B., Gale, R., and Canaani, E. (1985). Fused transcript of *abl* and *bcr* genes in chronic myelogenous leukaemia. *Nature 315*(13): 550.
3. Shtivelman, E., Lifshitz, B., Gale, R., Roe, B., and Canaani, E. (1986). Alternative splicing of RNAs transcribed from the human *abl* gene and from the *bcr-abl* fused gene. *Cell 47*:277-284.
4. Schaefer-Rego, K., Dudek, H., Popenoe, D., Arlin, Z., Mears, J. G., Bank, A., and Leibowitz, D. (1987). CML patients in blast crisis have breakpoints localized to a specific region of the *bcr*. *Blood 70*:448-455.
5. Eisenberg, A., Silver, R., Soper, L., Arlin, Z., Coleman, M., Bernhardt, B., and Benn, P. (1988). The location of breakpoints within the breakpoint cluster region (*bcr*) of chromosome 22 in chronic myeloid leukemia. *Leukemia 2*: 642-647.
6. Shtalrid, M., Talpaz, M., Kurzrock, R., Kantarjian, H., Trujillo, J., Gutterman, J., Yoffe, G., and Blick, M. (1988). Analysis of breakpoints within the *bcr* gene and their correlation with the clinical course of Philadelphia-positive chronic myelogenous leukemia. *Blood 72*:485-490.
7. Van Denderen, J., Hermans, A., Meeuwsen, T., Troelstra, C., Zegers, N., Boersma, W., Grosveld, G., and Van Ewijk, W. (1989). Antibody recognition of the tumor-specific *bcr-abl* joining region in chronic myeloid leukemia. *J. Exp. Med. 169*:87-98.

8. Timmons, M. T., and Witte, O. N. (1989). Structural characterization of the *bcr* gene product. *Oncogene 4*:559–567.
9. Mills, K. I., MacKenzie, E. D., and Birnie, G. D. (1988). The site of the breakpoint within the *bcr* is a prognostic factor in Philadephia-positive CML patients. *Blood 72*:1237–1241.
10. Dreazen, O., Berman, M., and Gale, R. P. (1988). Molecular abnormalities of *bcr* and c-*abl* in chronic myelogenous leukemia associated with a long chronic phase. *Blood 71*:797–799.
11. Przepiorka, D. (1988). Breakpoint zone of *bcr* in chronic myelogenous leukemia does not correlate with disease phase or prognosis. *Cancer Genet. Cytogenet. 36*:117–122.
12. Benn, P., Soper, L., Eisenberg, A., Silver, R. T., Coleman, M., Cacciapaglia, B., Bennett, L., Baird, M., Silverstein, M., Berger, C., and Bernhardt, B. (1987). Utility of molecular genetic analysis of *bcr* rearrangement in the diagnosis of chronic myeloid leukemia. *Can. Genet. Cytogenet. 29*:1–7.
13. Popenoe, D. W., Schaefer-Rego, K., Mears, J. G., Bank, A., and Leibowitz, D. (1986). Frequent and extensive deletion during the 9,22 translocation in CML. *Blood 68*:1123–1128.
14. de Klein, A., Hermans, A., Bootsma, D., Grosveld, G., Heisterkamp, N., Stam, K., and Groffen, J. (1986). The role of the Philadelphia translocation in chronic myelocytic leukemia. *Ann. Clin. Res. 18*:278–283.
15. Sokal, J. E., Baccarani, M., Tura, S., Fiacchini, M., Cervantes, F., Rozman, C., Gomez, G. A., Galton, D. A., Canellos, G. P., Braun, T. J., et al. (1985). Prognostic discrimination among younger patients with chronic granulocytic leukemia: Relevance to bone marrow transplantation. *Blood 66*:1352–1357.
16. Sokal, J. E., Cox, E. B., Baccarini, M., Tura, S., Gomez, G. A., Robertson, J. E., Tso, C. Y., Braun, T. J., Clarkson, B. D., Cervantes, F., et al. (1984). Prognostic discrimination in "good-risk" chronic granulocytic leukemia. *Blood 63*:789–799.
17. Sokal, J. E., Gomez, G. A., Baccarani, M., Tura, S., Clarkson, B. D., Cervantes, F., Rozman, C., Carbonell, F., Anger, B., Heimpel, H., Nissen, N. I., and Robertson, J. E. (1988). Prognostic significance of additional cytogenetic abnormalities at diagnosis of Philadelphia chromosome-positive chronic granulocytic leukemia. *Blood 72*:294–298.

8

bcr-abl RNA in Chronic Myelogenous Leukemia and Acute Lymphocytic Leukemia

Eli Canaani, Christophe Marcelle, and Elena Fainstein *The Weizmann Institute of Science, Rehovot, Israel*

Robert Peter Gale *University of California, Los Angeles, California*

Carlo Croce *The Wistar Institute, Philadelphia, Pennsylvania*

Miron Prokocimer *Tel-Aviv University, Petah Tikva, Israel*

Alain Berrebi *Kaplan Hospital, Rehovot, Israel*

INTRODUCTION

Chronic myelogenous leukemia (CML) is a myeloproliferative disorder in which the neoplastic transformation of a stem cell results in the proliferation and accumulation of myeloid cells and their progenitors. Clinically, the disease is divided into two phases, a chronic phase of 3-4 years' duration followed by an acute phase (blast crisis) of 3-6 months (for review, see Reference 1). In some patients, there is a transitional accelerated phase. During the chronic phase, the neoplastic clone represents the majority of the replicating myeloid cells. These cells mature normally and respond to normal myelopoietic regulatory factors. The principal abnormality during the chronic phase appears to be an increase in the stem cell compartment committed to myeloid differentiation. In the acute phase, in contrast, the leukemic cells lose their ability to differentiate and mature normally; response to regulatory factors of myelopoiesis is typically lost.

In 1960, Nowell and Hungerford described a minute G group chromosome in bone marrow cells from two patients with CML; they designated this the Philadelphia[1] or Ph[1] chromosome (2). Over the next several years the Ph[1] chromosome was found to be a constant feature of CML. As the concept of a genetic (DNA) basis of cancer evolved, the presence of a consistent chromosomal abnormality in human cancer assumed increasing importance. In 1970 Caspersson and co-workers demonstrated the Ph[1] chromosome to be a shortened chromosome 22, and in 1973 Rowley suggested it arose from a reciprocal translocation between chromosomes 9 and 22 designated t(9;22) (3). Cell synchronization and high-resolution banding technique have identified the chromosome breakpoints as t(9;22) (q34.1;q11.21) (4).

The Ph[1] chromosome is present in hematopoietic cells from 95% of individuals with CML (5–7). It is also rarely found in some patients with other types of leukemia, such as polycytlemia Vera, myelofibrosis, and refractory sideroblastic anemia. Approximately 5% of adults with acute myelogenous leukemia (AML) and up to 10% of children and 25% of adults with acute lymphocytic leukemia (ALL) have the Ph[1] chromosome (8). In most cases the Ph[1] chromosome detected in acute leukemia is cytogenetically idential to that detected in CML (4).

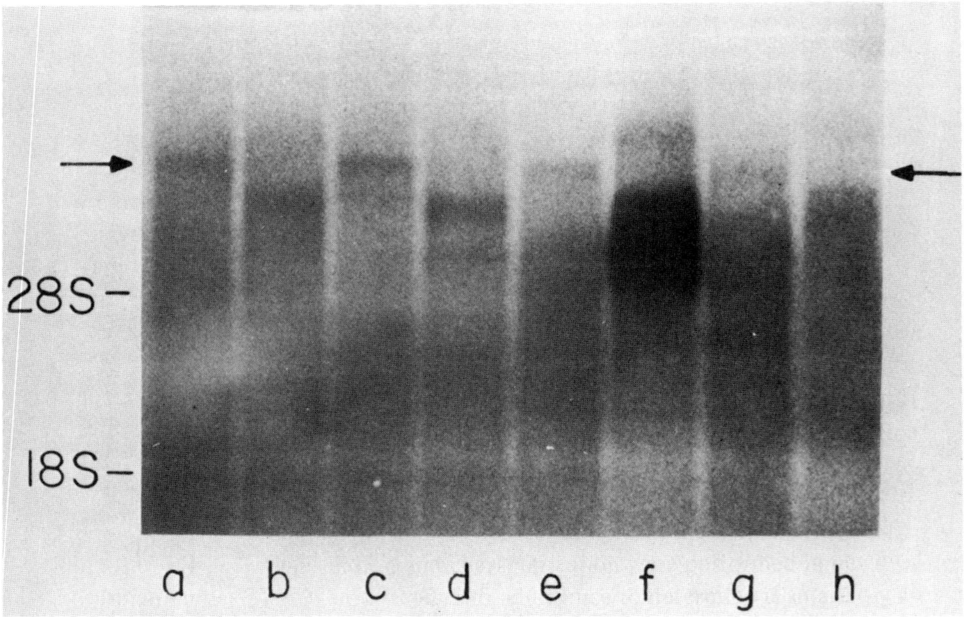

Figure 1 An 8.6 kb *abl* RNA in leukemic cells from CML patients. Northern blot analysis of RNAs from Ph[1]-positive and Ph[1]-negative cells. Arrow points to 8.6 kb transcript. Details detailed in text. (From Reference 12.)

A NOVEL *abl* RNA IN CML CELLS

The extreme specificity of chromosomal breakpoints in CML raised the possibility that the chromosomal aberration affected a gene(s), perhaps an oncogene(s), located at the breakpoint(s). The two oncogenes *abl* and *sis* were mapped near the breakpoints on chromosomes 9 and 22, respectively. Moreover, both genes were found to be included within the segments exchanged between these chromosomes (9,10). To study possible involvement of the two genes in CML we examined their transcription in leukemic cells of patients and in CML cell lines (11,12). We found that *sis* is not expressed and therefore is not involved in CML. In contrast, a novel 8.6 kb *abl* transcript was detected in essentially all CML samples analyzed. An example of this analysis is shown in Figure 1, demonstrating the new transcript in the leukemic cells from four CML patients (lanes b, d, f, and h) and its absence in HeLa cells, AMLs, and a Ph[1]-negative CML (lanes a, c, e, and g, respectively). The 8.6 kb *abl* RNA is detected in both chronic and acute phases of CML and is absent from Ph[1] chromosome-negative leukemias. The close association between this RNA and the Ph[1] chromosome implicated the *abl* gene in the t(9;22) translocation. This conclusion was supported by different types of studies conducted by others during 1983 and 1984. Thus, Heisterkamp et al. (13) cloned the t(9;22) breakpoint of one CML and showed that it resided 14 kbp upstream from the main body of the *abl* gene. In addition, the Witte and Arlinghaus groups (14,15) detected a novel *abl* protein of 210 kD in CML cell lines. To further study the nature of the 8.6 kb *abl* RNA we constructed cDNA libraries and cloned normal *abl* RNAs as well as the CML-specific *abl* RNA.

THE HUMAN *abl* GENE AND ITS TRANSCRIPTS

Using a probe derived from the Abelson leukemia viral genome, we initially cloned three overlapping normal *abl* cDNA clones. The cDNA spanned around 6 kb and was used to clone the *abl* locus (16). A region of around 50 kbp was cloned in five overlapping phages and mapped by hybridization to cDNA fragments (Figure 2). Hence, it was possible to identify 11 exons in the locus, of which the last (exon XI) included the 3′ two-thirds of the cDNA. This observation in conjunction with the results of the nucleotide sequencing analysis of the cDNA (see later) suggests that *abl* sequences downstream of the kinase region, which are all included in exon XI, carry a single function and were possibly derived during evolution from a separate ancestral gene.

Sequencing analysis of the genomic clone λ-15 and the 5′ terminus of the cDNA clone p18 showed that the last 226 nucleotides of the cDNA corresponded to *abl* exon I. This exon contains the first 26 amino acids of *abl* protein. Analysis of another clone, K8, showed that it shared sequences 3′ of the *Mst*II

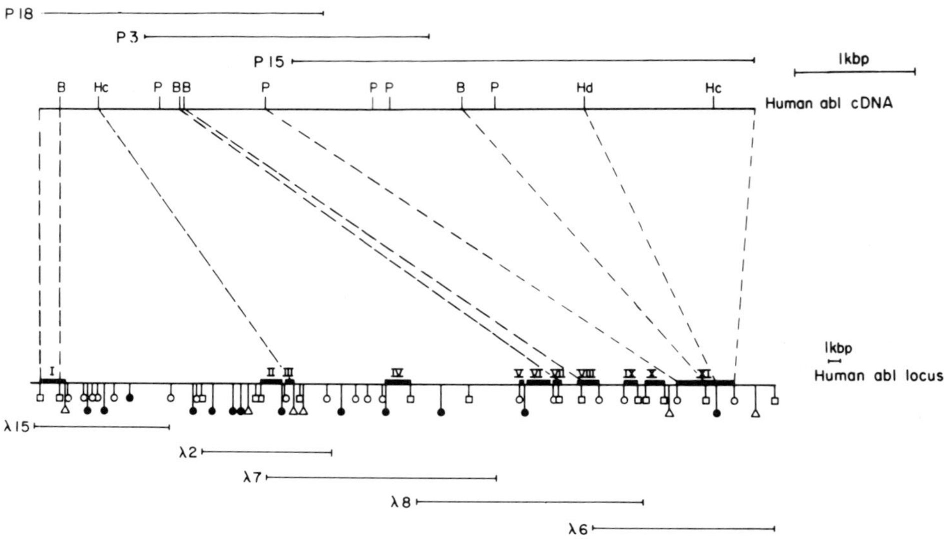

Figure 2 Physical maps of normal human *abl* cDNA and locus. Exons are depicted as dark boxes delineated between restriction sites bordering the hybridizable fragments. Restriction sites on cDNA are of *Bgl*III (B), *Hinc*II (Hc), *Pst*I (P), and *Hind*III (Hd). Sites on locus are *Bam*H1 (△), *Bg*III (□), *Hind*III (●), and *Eco*RI (○). (From Reference 16.)

site with p18 but diverged at a point 5′ of this site (Figure 3). The 1.25 kb new DNA fragment linked to *abl* exon II contains an open reading frame of 44 amino acids joined in phase to the open reading frame of exon II. The genomic region corresponding to the 1.25 kb fragment was cloned and designated exon Ib. The analogous sequence in clone p18 was designated exon Ia (17). Thus, the human *abl* gene contains two alternative first exons that code for different polypeptides. This results in the production of two normal *abl* proteins varying at their N-termini. The protein coded by exon Ib contains a part of the consensus signal for myristylation (18) and may therefore be anchored to the membrane through an N-terminal myristic acid. If this is the case, then the two *abl* proteins localize to two different subcellular compartments.

The two alternative first exons could give rise to the two normal *abl* transcripts. Indeed, radiolabeled probes specific to exons Ib and Ia hybridized to the 7 and 6 kb transcripts, respectively (Figure 4A). Thus, the 7 and 6 kb *abl* RNAs contain exons Ib and Ia, respectively. We next positioned the two alternative exons with respect to the body of the *abl* gene. Exon Ia corresponds to exon I, which we previously mapped at 19 kbp upstream of exon II (Figure 2). Exon Ib resides upstream of Ia. We performed chromosomal walking starting from the

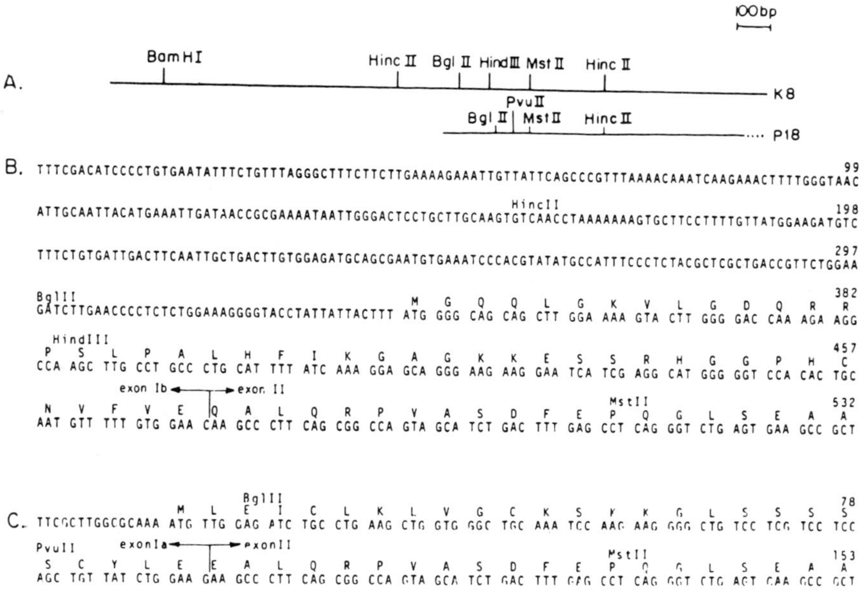

Figure 3 cDNA clones containing *abl* alternative first exons. Physical maps (A) and partial nucleotide sequences of *abl* cdna clones p18 (B) and K8(C). (From Reference 17.)

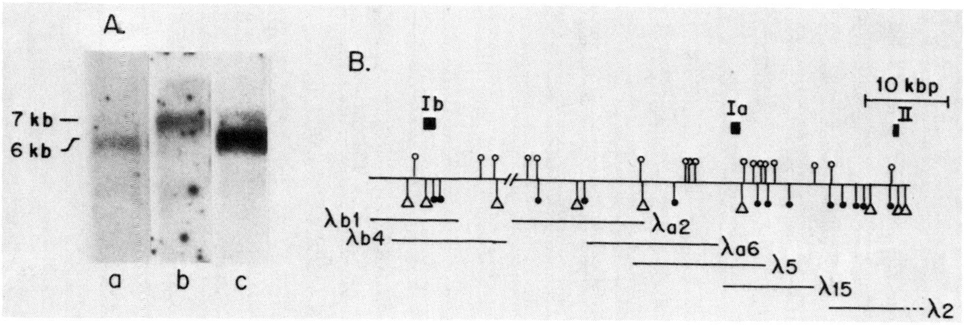

Figure 4 (A) Exons Ia and Ib are included in *abl* 6 and 7 kb mRNA, respectively. Northern blot hybridizations to probes specific to exons Ia, Ib, and VIII-XI (lanes a, b, and c, respectively). (B) Relative chromosomal locations of *abl* exons Ia, Ib, and II. (From Reference 17.)

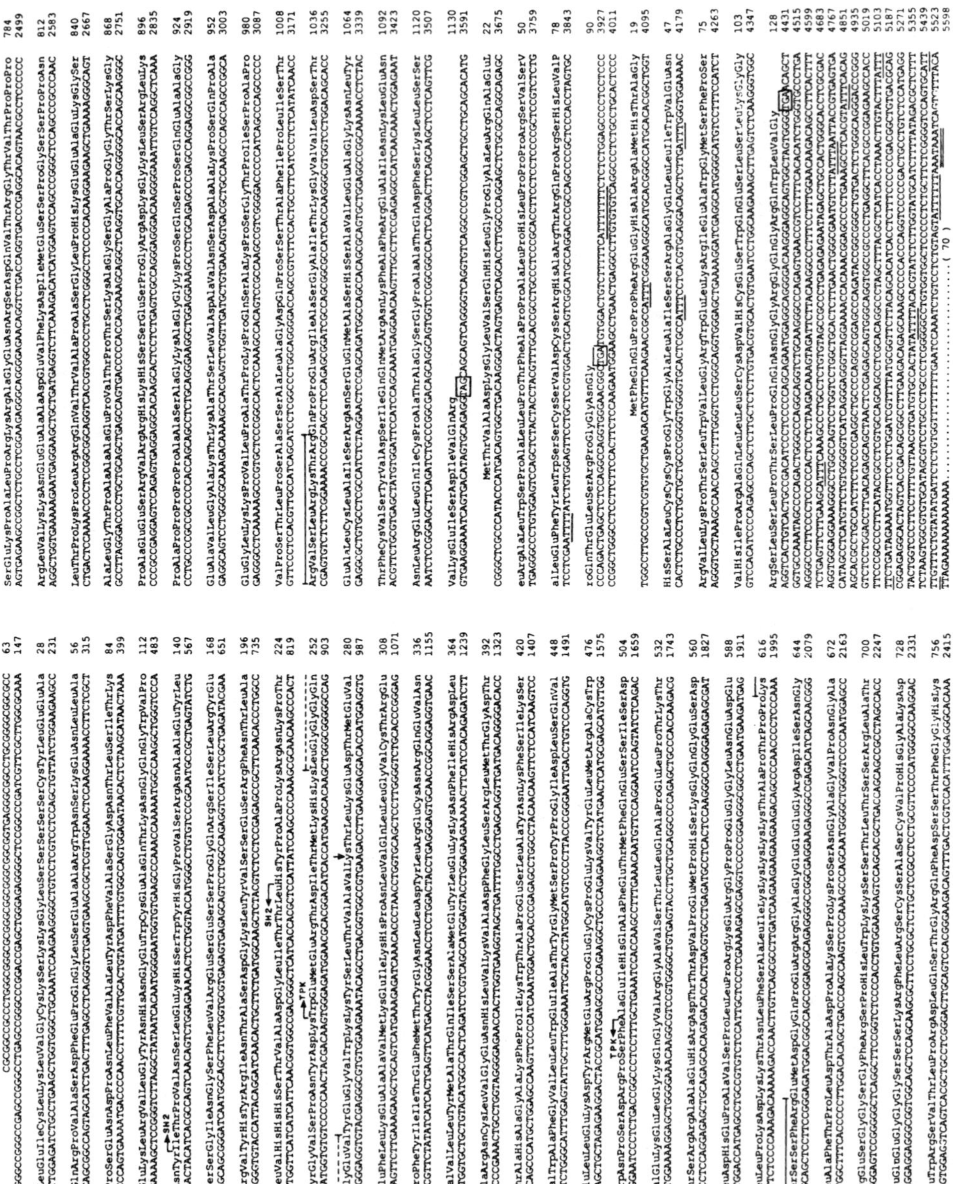
SH2
TPK

```
human c-abl MLEICLKLVGCKSKKGLSSSSSCYLEEALQRPVASDFEPQGLSEAARWNS 50
            ||||||||||||||||||||||||||||||||||||||||||||||||||
mouse c-abl MLEICLKLVGCKSKKGLSSSSSCYLEEALQRPVASDFEPQGLSEAARWNS 50

KENLLAGPSENDPNLFVALYDFVASGDNTLSITKGEKLRVLGYNHNGEWC 100
||||||||||||||||||||||||||||||||||||||||||||||||||
KENLLAGPSENDPNLFVALYDFVASGDNTLSITKGEKLRVLGYNHNGEWC 100

EAQTKNGQGWVPSNYITPVNSLEKHSWYHGPVSRNAAEYLLSSGINGSFL 150
||||||||||||||||||||||||||||||||||||||||||||||||||
EAQTKNGQGWVPSNYITPVNSLEKHSWYHGPVSRNAAEYLLSSGINGSFL 150

VRESESSPGQRSISLRYEGRVYHYRINTASDGKLYVSSESRFNTLAELVH 200
||||||||||||||||||||||||||||||||||||||||||||||||||
VRESESSPGQRSISLRYEGRVYHYRINTASDGKLYVSSESRFNTLAELVH 200

HHSTVADGLITTLHYPAPKRNKPTVYGVSPNYDKWEMERTDITMKHKLGG 250
||||||||||||||||||||||||*|||||||||||||||||||||||||
HHSTVADGLITTLHYPAPKRNKPTIYGVSPNYDKWEMERTDITMKHKLGG 250

GQYGEVYEGVWKKYSLTVAVKTLKEDTMEVEEFLKEAAVMKEIKHPNLVQ 300
||||||||||||||||||||||||||||||||||||||||||||||||||
GQYGEVYEGVWKKYSLTVAVKTLKEDTMEVEEFLKEAAVMKEIKHPNLVQ 300

LLGVCTREPPFYIITEFMTYGNLLDYLRECNRQEVNAVVLLYMATQISSA 350
|||||||||||||||||||||||||||||||||||*||||||||||||||
LLGVCTREPPFYIITEFMTYGNLLDYLRECNRQEVSAVVLLYMATQISSA 350

MEYLEKKNFIHRDLAARNCLVGENHLVKVADFGLSRLMTGDTYTAHAGAK 400
||||||||||||||||||||||||||||||||||||||||||||||||||
MEYLEKKNFIHRDLAARNCLVGENHLVKVADFGLSRLMTGDTYTAHAGAK 400

FPIKWTAPESLAYNKFSIKSDVWAFGVLLWEIATYGMSPYPGIDLSQVYE 450
||||||||||||||||||||||||||||||||||||||||||||||||||
FPIKWTAPESLAYNKFSIKSDVWAFGVLLWEIATYGMSPYPGIDLSQVYE 450

LLEKDYRMERPEGCPEKVYELMRACWQWNPSDRPSFAEIHQAFETMFQES 500
||||||||||||||||||||||||||||||||||||||||||||||||||
LLEKDYRMERPEGCPEKVYELMRACWQWNPSDRPSFAEIHQAFETMFQES 500

SISDEVEKELGKQGVRGAVSTLLQAPELPTKTRTSRRAAEHRDTTDVPEM 550
||||||||||||*|*||*****||||||||||||*|||||**|**|*||*
SISDEVEKELGKRGTRGGAGSMLQAPELPTKTRTCRRAAEQKDAPDTPEL 550

PHSKGQGESDPLDHEPAVSPLLPRKERGPPEGGLNEDERLLPKDKKTNLF 600
*|*||*||||*||*||||||||||||||||*|*|||||||||*|*|||||
LHTKGLGESDALDSEPAVSPLLPRKERGPPDGSLNEDERLLPRDRKTNLF 600

SALIKKKKKTAPTPPKRSSSFREMDGQPERRGAGEEEGRDISNGALAFTP 650
|||*|||||*||||||||||||||||||*||||*|***|***||**|*|*
SALLKKKKKMAPTPPKRSSSFREMDGQPDRRGASEDDSRELCNGPPALTS 650

LDTADPAKSPKPSNGAGVPNGALRESGGSGFRSPHLWKKSSTLTSSRLAT 700
*|*|*|*||||*||||||||||*||*|*|||||||*||||||||*||||*
.DAAGPTKSPKASNGAGVPNGAFREPGNSGFRSPHMWKKSSTLTGSRLAA 699

GEEEGGGSSSKRFLRSCSASCVPHGAKDTEWRSVTLPRDLQSTGRQFDSS 750
*|||*|*||||||||||||||*||||*|||||||||*|||*|*|*|||||
AEEESGMSSSKRFLRSCSASCMPHGARDTEWRSVTLDRDLPSAGKQFDSS 749

TFGGHKSEKPALPRKRAGENRSDQVTRGTVTPPPRLVKKNEEAADEVFKD 800
||||||||||||||||**|*||*||***|**|*|***|||||||*|*|||
TFGGHKSEKPALPRKRTSESRSEQVAKSTAMPLPGWLKKNEEAAEEGFKD 799

IMESSPGSSPPNLTPKPLRRQVTVAPASGLPHKEEAEKGSA..LGTPAAA 848
**|||||||||*||||*||||||**|*|||*||*||*||||***||||*|
T.ESSPGSSPPSLTPKLLRRQVTASPSSGLSHKKEATKGSASGMGTPATA 848

EPVTPTSKAGSGAPGGTSKGPAEESRVRRHKHSSESPGRDKGKLSRLKPA 898
||**|**|*******|*||***||*|||||||||||||||||*|**||||
EPAPPSNK......VGLSKASSEEMRVRRHKHSSESPGRDKGRLAKLKPA 892

PPPPPAASAGKAGGKPSQSPSQEAAGEAVLGAKTKATSL.VDAVNSDAAK 947
||||||***|||*|||*||||||*||||****|||*|||**||||*|**|
PPPPPACT.GKA.GKPAQSPSQE.AGEAGGPTKTKCTSLAMDAVNTDPTK 939

PSQPAEGLKKPVLPATPKPQS.AKPSGTPISPAPVPSTLPSASSALAGDQ 996
***|*|||*|||*|**|||||*|||*|||*||***|||*|**|**|||||
AGPPGEGLRKPVPPSVPKPQSTAKPPGTPTSPVSTPSTAPAPSP.LAGDQ 998

.PSSTAFIPLISTRVSLRKTRQPPERIASGAITKGVVLDSTEALCLAISR 1045
*|||*|||||||||||||||||||||||||*|||||||||||||||||||
QPSSAAFIPLISTRVSLRKTRQPPERIASGTITKGVVLDSTEALCLAISR 1038

NSEQMASHSAVLEAGKNLYTFCVSYVDSIQQMRNKFAFREAINKLENNLR 1095
||||||||||||||||||||||||||||||||||||||||||||||*|||
NSEQMASHSAVLEAGKNLYTFCVSYVDSIQQMRNKFAFREAINKLESNLR 1088

ELQICPATAGSGPAATQDFSKLLSSVKEISDIVQR 1130
|||||||||*|||||||||||||||||||||||*|
ELQICPATASSGPAATQDFSKLLSSVKEISDIVRR 1123
```

Figure 6 Comparison of human and mouse *abl* proteins. (Human sequence is from Fainstein, Gale, and Canaani, in preparation. Mouse sequence is from Reference 20.)

two exons but could not bridge the gap. The physical map of the cloned region is shown in Figure 4B, and from it we concluded that exon Ib resides more than 55 kbp upstream of exon II. More recently, using pulse-field gel electrophoresis, it was possible to determine that exon Ib lies at least 200 kbp upstream of exon II (19). This makes the *abl* gene one of the largest genes known. The ability of exons II and Ib to splice over 200 kbp seems remarkable. Moreover, the ability of exon II to splice to exons from far upstream, such as Ib or *bcr* exons (see later), is probably a significant factor in the pathogenesis of CML.

Figure 5 (continued) Complete nucleotide sequence of *abl* cDNA. Sequence contains exon Ia. AT motifs with a potential role in the instability of the RNA are underlined in the 3′ region. For other details see text. The sequence includes corrections to errors made in the partial sequence published in Reference 17. (Data are from Fainstein, Gale, and Canaani, in preparation.)

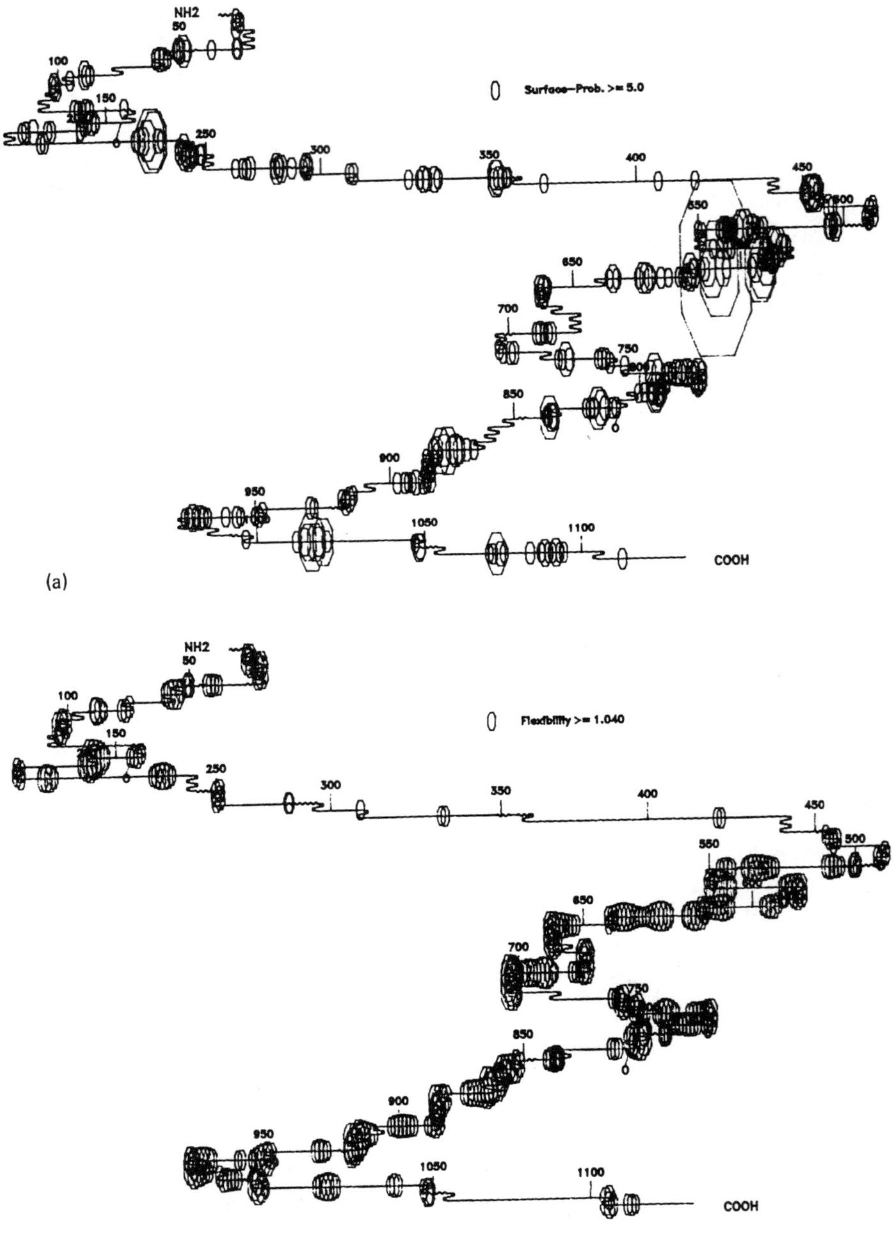

Figure 7 Chou-Fasman predictions of the surface probability (top) and flexibility (bottom) of *abl* protein. (Data are from Fainstein et al., in preparation.)

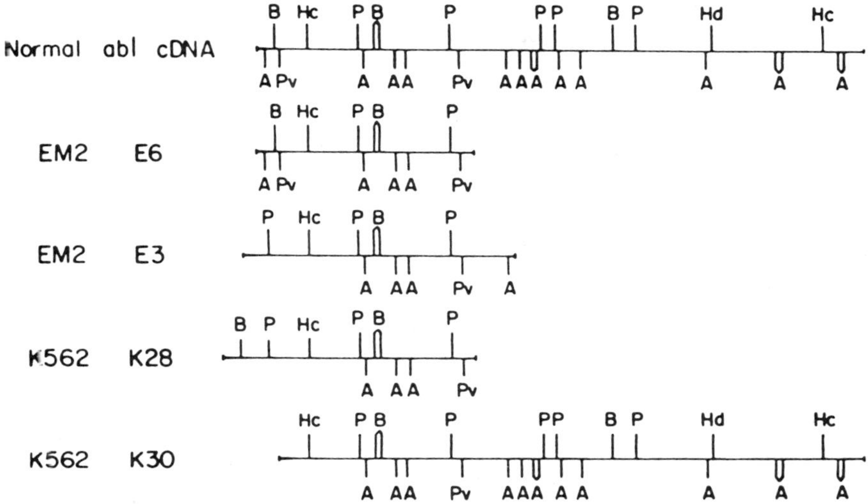

Figure 8 Comparison between maps of normal *abl* cDNA and *abl* cDNAs cloned from the K562 and EM2 lines. Restriction enzymes used included *Ava*I (A), *Bgl*II (B), *Pvu*II (Pv), *Hinc*II (Hc), *Pst*I (P), and *Hind*III (Hd). (From Reference 16.)

We have recently completed a sequence analysis of the normal *abl* cDNA (Fainstein, Gale, and Canaani, in preparation). The open reading frame coding for *abl* protein is preceded by a short 5′ untranslated sequence of 147 nucleotides (of exon Ia) and is followed by a long 3′ sequence of 2061 nucleotides (Figure 5). Within the 3′ sequence there are two open reading frames of 90 and 128 codons. Those are not homologous to the open reading frame at the 3′ region of mouse *abl* RNA (20). At present, there is no evidence that these open reading frames are translated in vivo. The 3′ region of *abl* cDNA contains multiple ATTT motifs that constitute part of the ATTTA consensus sequence thought to confer instability to mRNAs and, therefore, make them short-lived (21). The 3′ regions of human and mouse *abl* are 50% conserved. The *abl* protein is composed of 1130 amino acids and does not contain extended hydrophobic regions that could serve as transmembrane or signal peptides. The regions spanning amino acids 66-115 and 116-213 correspond to the SH3 and SH2 domains, respectively, which are conserved in cytoplasmic tyrosine kinases (22), phospholipase C (23), the GAP protein (24), and the *crk* oncogene (25). These domains have a regulatory role, and SH3 may interact with a cellular protein inhibitor. The tyrosine phosphorylating kinase (TPK) region spans amino acids 235–486 and includes the ATP binding site composed of the conserved nine amino acid peptide and lysine at positions 248-256 and 271, respectively. The major tyrosine residue phosphorylated in vitro (26) is in position 393. Two peptides containing suggested protein kinase C phosphorylation sites (27) span positions 616-622 and 1009-1016.

Comparison of the predicted amino acid sequence of the human protein with the analogous mouse species shows an overall homology of 86%. The two proteins are 99% homologous upstream and within of the kinase region. They share 73% homology downstream of the kinase region up to position 1000 and are 96% homologous within the C-terminal 130 amino acids (Figure 6). Remarkably, the same four domains of the protein are also apparent in plots of the surface probability and flexibility (Figure 7) drawn according to Chou-Fasman predictions (28). Thus, the region N-terminal to the kinase domain is highly conserved, flexible, and predicted to reside on the surface of the protein. The kinase domain and the C-terminus are highly conserved, rigid, and predicted to be embedded within the protein. Finally, the less conserved region between the kinase region and around position 1000 is flexible and exposed outside. This division of the protein into several domains predicts important and as yet unknown functions to the N and C termini.

CHARACTERIZATION OF THE CML-SPECIFIC *abl* RNA

To clone cDNA derived from the CML-specific 8.6 kb *abl* RNA we used RNA extracted from the cell lines K562 and EM2. The physical map of two *abl* cDNA clones from each library were compared with normal *abl* cDNA (Figure 8). Clone 6 has a map identical to the corresponding region on the normal cDNA, whereas clones E3, K28, and K30 share most restriction enzyme sites with normal *abl* cDNA but vary from the latter at the 5′ region. Thus, an constellation of sites for *Ava*I, *Bgl*III, and *Pvu*II enzymes present at the left end of the normal cDNA is missing from the three clones and is replaced in E3 and K28 with *Pst*I and *Hind*III sites. To analyze further the variance between normal *abl* cDNA and K562 and EM2 cDNAs, we sequenced the 5′ regions of K28 and E3 and compared them to the normal *abl* clone p18. The K28 and E3 sequences are identical to each other and diverge from normal *abl* cDNA 5′ to the first nucleotide of *abl* exon II (Figure 9); 3′ to this point the three sequences are identical. Thus, in K562 and EM2 *abl* the first exon was replaced with a new sequence. The inserted new DNA fragment is composed of an open reading frame that joins in phase the rest of *abl* open reading frame.

To test whether the K28 and E3 clones originated from the 8.6 kb CML specific *abl* RNA, we used the new DNA at the 5′ termini of these clones and hybridized it to RNAs from CML and non-CML lines. Indeed, the probe hybridized to the 8.6 kb transcript but not to the 7 and 6 kb normal species of *abl* RNA (16). Using the same probe we cloned the genomic DNA corresponding to it (16). Examination of the restriction enzymes map of this clone revealed that

```
             M   L   E   I   C   L   E   L   V   G   C   K   S   K   K   G   L   S   S   S
Normal      ATG TTG GAG ATC TGC CTG AAG CTG GTG GGC TGC AAA TCC AAG AAG GGG CTG TCC TCG TCC

             E   D   D   E   S   P   G   L   Y   G   F   L   N   V   I   V   H   S   A   T
K562        GAA GAT GAT GAC TCT CCG GGG CTC TAT GGG TTT CTG AAT GTC ATC GTC CAC TCA GCC ACT
EM2         --- --- --- --- --- --- --- --- --- --- --- --- --- --- --- --- --- --- --- ---
                                RNA junction
                                     point
                                       |
             S   S   C   Y   L   E   E   A   L   Q   R   P   V   A   S   D   F   E   P   Q
Normal      TCC AGC TGT TAT CTG GAA GAA GCC CTT CAG CGG CCA GTA GCA TCT GAC TTT GAG CCT CAG

             G   F   K   Q   S   S   K
K562        GGA TTT AAG CAG AGT TCA AAA --- --- --- --- --- --- --- --- --- --- --- --- ---
EM2         --- --- --- --- --- --- --- --- --- --- --- --- --- --- --- --- --- --- --- ---


             G   L   S   E   A   A   R   W   N   S   K   E
Normal      GGT CTG AGT GAA GCC GCT CGT TGG AAC TCC AAG GAA
K562        --- --- --- --- --- --- --- --- --- --- --- ---
EM2         --- --- --- --- --- --- --- --- --- --- --- ---
```

Figure 9 Nucleotide sequence of the region of divergence between normal and K562 and EM2 *abl* cDNAs. (From Reference 16.)

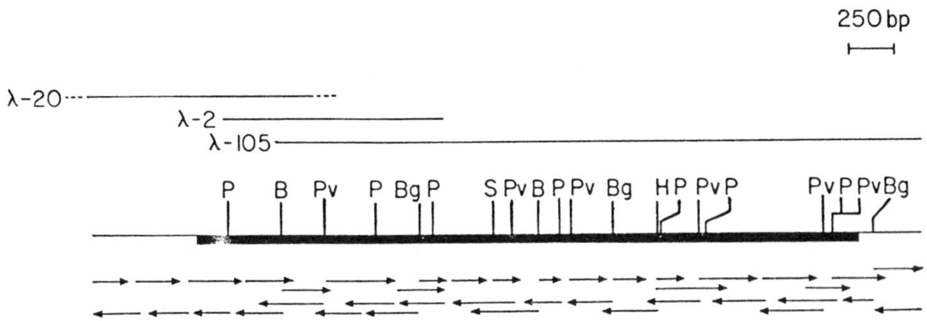


```
                                                                   GGGGGGAGGGTGG  -580

CGGCTCGATGGGGGAGCCGCCCCAGGGGGCCCCCCGCCCTGTGCCCACGGCGCGGCCCCTTTAAGGAGGCCCGCCTGGCTCCGC  -498

TCCATCGCGCATCGCGGCCGCCTCCCCCCGGCCCTCCCTTCCTGCGGCGCAGAGTGCGGGCCGGGCGGGAGTGCGGCGAGCCGGC  -413

TGGCTTAGCGTCCGAGGAGGCGGCGGCGGCGGCGGCAGCGGCGGCGGCGGGGCTGGTGGGGCGGTGCGGAAGCGAGAGGCGA  -328

GGAGCGCGCGGGCCGTGGCCAGAGTCTGGCGGCGGCCTGGCGGAGCGGAGAGCAGCGCCCGCGCCTCGCCGTGCGGAGGAGCCCC  -243

GCACACAATAGCGGCGCGCGCAGCCCGCGCCCTTCCCCCCGGCGCGCCCCGCCCCGCGCGCCGAGCGCCCCGCTCCGCCTCACCT  -158

GCCACCAGGGAGTGGGCGGGCATTGTTCGCCGCCGCCGCCGCCGCGCGGGGCCATGGGGGCCGCCCGGCGCCCGGGGCCGGGCCT  -73
                                                                            1
GGCGAGGCCGCCGCGCCGCCGCTGAGACGGGCCCCGCGCGCAGCCCGGCGGCGCAGGTAAGGCCGGCCGCGCCATGGTGGACCCG  12
                                                                   MetValAspPro  04

GTGGGCTTCGCGGAGGCGTGGAAGGCGCAGTTCCCGGACTCAGAGCCCCCGCGCATGGAGCTGCGCTCAGTGGGCGACATCGAG  96
ValGlyPheAlaGluAlaTrpLysAlaGlnPheProAspSerGluProProArgMetGluLeuArgSerValGlyAspIleGlu  32

CAGGAGCTGGAGCGCTGCAAGGCCTCCATTCGGCGCCTGGAGCAGGAGGTGAACCAGGAGCGCTTCCGCATGATCTACCTGCAG  180
GlnGluLeuGluArgCysLysAlaSerIleArgArgLeuGluGlnGluValAsnGlnGluArgPheArgMetIleTyrLeuGln  60

ACGTTGCTGGCCAAGGAAAAGAAGAGCTATGACCGGCAGCGATGGGGCTTCCGGCGCGCGGCGCAGGCCCCCGACGGCGCCTCC  264
ThrLeuLeuAlaLysGluLysLysSerTyrAspArgGlnArgTrpGlyPheArgArgAlaAlaGlnAlaProAspGlyAlaSer  88

GAGCCCCGAGCGTCCGCGTCGCGCCCGCAGCCAGCGCCCGCCGACGGAGCCGACCCGCCGCCCGCCGAGGAGCCCGAGGCCCGG  348
GluProArgAlaSerAlaSerArgProGlnProAlaProAlaAspGlyAlaAspProProProAlaGluGluProGluAlaArg  116

TTCCCCCGCGTGCAGCAGTGGAGCCACCAGCAGCGGGTGGGCGACCTCTTCCAGAAGCTGGCCAGCCAGCTGGGTGTGTACCGG  1776
PheProArgValGlnGlnTrpSerHisGlnGlnArgValGlyAspLeuPheGlnLysLeuAlaSerGlnLeuGlyValTyrArg  592

GCCTTCGTGGACAACTACGGAGTTGCCATGGAAATGGCTGAGAAGTGCTGTCAGGCCAATGCTCAGTTTGCAGAAATCTCCGAG  1860
AlaPheValAspAsnTyrGlyValAlaMetGluMetAlaGluLysCysCysGlnAlaAsnAlaGlnPheAlaGluIleSerGlu  620

AACCTGAGAGCCAGAAGCAACAAAGATGCCAAGGATCCAACGACCAAGAACTCTCTGGAAACTCTGCTCTACAAGCCTGTGGAC  1944
AsnLeuArgAlaArgSerAsnLysAspAlaLysAspProThrThrLysAsnSerLeuGluThrLeuLeuTyrLysProValAsp  648

CGTGTGACGAGGAGCACGCTGGTCCTCCATGACTTGCTGAAGCACACTCCTGCCAGCCACCCTGACCACCCCTTGCTGCAGGAC  2028
ArgValThrArgSerThrLeuValLeuHisAspLeuLeuLysHisThrProAlaSerHisProAspHisProLeuLeuGlnAsp  676

GCCCTCCGCATCTCACAGAACTTCCTGTCCAGCATCAATGAGGAGATCACACCCCGACGGCAGTCCATGACGGTGAAGAAGGGA  2112
AlaLeuArgIleSerGlnAsnPheLeuSerSerIleAsnGluGluIleThrProArgArgGlnSerMetThrValLysLysGly  704

GAGCACCGGCAGCTGCTGAAGGACAGCTTCATGGTGGAGCTGGTGGAGGGGGCCCGCAAGCTGCGGCACGTCTTCCTGTTCACC  2196
GluHisArgGlnLeuLeuLysAspSerPheMetValGluLeuValGluGlyAlaArgLysLeuArgHisValPheLeuPheThr  732

GACCTGCTTCTCTGCACCAAGCTCAAGAAGCAGAGCGGAGGCAAAACGCAGCAGTATGACTGCAAATGGTACATTCCGCTCACG  2280
AspLeuLeuLeuCysThrLysLeuLysLysGlnSerGlyGlyLysThrGlnGlnTyrAspCysLysTrpTyrIleProLeuThr  760

GATCTCAGCTTCCAGATGGTGGATGAACTGGAGGCAGTGCCCAACATCCCCCTGGTGCCCGATGAGGAGCTGGACGCTTTGAAG  2364
AspLeuSerPheGlnMetValAspGluLeuGluAlaValProAsnIleProLeuValProAspGluGluLeuAspAlaLeuLys  788

ATCAAGATCTCCCAGATCAAGAGTGACATCCAGAGAGAGAAGAGGGCGAACAAGGGCAGCAAGGCTACGGAGAGGCTGAAGAAG  2448
IleLysIleSerGlnIleLysSerAspIleGlnArgGluLysArgAlaAsnLysGlySerLysAlaThrGluArgLeuLysLys  816

AAGCTGTCGGAGCAGGAGTCACTGCTGCTGCTTATGTCTCCCAGCATGGCCTTCAGGGTGCACAGCCGCAACGGCAAGAGTTAC  2532
LysLeuSerGluGlnGluSerLeuLeuLeuLeuMetSerProSerMetAlaPheArgValHisSerArgAsnGlyLysSerTyr  844
```

CCCGACGGCGAGGGTTCTCCGGGTAAGGCCAGGCCCGGGACCGCCCGCAGGCCCGGGGCAGCCGCGTCGGGGGAACGGGACGAC 432
ProAspGlyGluGlySerProGlyLysAlaArgProGlyThrAlaArgArgProGlyAlaAlaAlaSerGlyGluArgAspAsp 144

CGGGGACCCCCCGCCAGCGTGGCGGCGCTCAGGTCCAACTTCGAGCGGATCCGGAAGGGCCATGGCCAGCCCGGGGCGGACGCC 516
ArgGlyProProAlaSerValAlaAlaLeuArgSerAsnPheGluArgIleArgLysGlyHisGlyGlnProGlyAlaAspAla 172

GAGAAGCCCTTCTACGTGAACGTCGAGTTTCACCACGAGCGCGGCCTGGTGAAGGTCAACGACAAAGAGGTGTCGGACCGCATC 600
GluLysProPheTyrValAsnValGluPheHisHisGluArgGlyLeuValLysValAsnAspLysGluValSerAspArgIle 200

AGCTCCCTTGGCAGCCAGGCCATGCAGATGGAGCGCAAAAAGTCCCAGCACGGCGCGGGCTCGAGCGTGGGGGATGCATCCAGG 684
SerSerLeuGlySerGlnAlaMetGlnMetGluArgLysLysSerGlnHisGlyAlaGlySerSerValGlyAspAlaSerArg 228

CCCCCTTACCGGGGACGCTCCTCGGAGAGCAGCTGCGGCGTCGACGGCGACTACGAGGACGCCGAGTTGAACCCCCGCTTCCTG 768
ProProTyrArgGlyArgSerSerGluSerSerCysGlyValAspGlyAspTyrGluAspAlaGluLeuAsnProArgPheLeu 256

AAGGACAACCTGATCGACGCCAATGGCGGTAGCAGGCCCCCTTGGCCGCCCCTGGAGTACCAGCCCTACCAGAGCATCTACGTC 852
LysAspAsnLeuIleAspAlaAsnGlyGlySerArgProProTrpProProLeuGluTyrGlnProTyrGlnSerIleTyrVal 284

GGGGGCATCATGGAAGGGGAGGGCAAGGGCCCGCTCCTGCGCAGCCAGAGCACCTCTGAGCAGGAGAAGCGCCTTACCTGGCCC 936
GlyGlyMetMetGluGlyGluGlyLysGlyProLeuLeuArgSerGlnSerThrSerGluGlnGluLysArgLeuThrTrpPro 312

CGCAGGTCCTACTCCCCCCGGAGTTTTGAGGATTGCGGAGGCGGCTATACCCCGGACTGCAGCTCCAATGAGAACCTCACCTCC 1020
ArgArgSerTyrSerProArgSerPheGluAspCysGlyGlyGlyTyrThrProAspCysSerSerAsnGluAsnLeuThrSer 340

AGCGAGGAGGACTTCTCCTCTGGCCAGTCCAGCCGCGTGTCCCCAAGCCCCACCACCTACCGCATGTTCCGGGACAAAAGCCGC 1104
SerGluGluAspPheSerSerGlyGlnSerSerArgValSerProSerProThrThrTyrArgMetPheArgAspLysSerArg 368

TCTCCCTCGCAGAACTCGCAACAGTCCTTCGACAGCAGCAGTCCCCCCACGCCGCAGTGCCATAAGCGGCACCGGCACTGCCCG 1188
SerProSerGlnAsnSerGlnGlnSerPheAspSerSerSerProProThrProGlnCysHisLysArgHisArgHisCysPro 396

GTTGTCGTGTCCGAGGCCACCATCGTGGGCGTCCGCAAGACCGGGCAGATCTGGCCCAACGATGACGAGGGCGCCTTCCATGGA 1272
ValValValSerGluAlaThrIleValGlyValArgLysThrGlyGlnIleTrpProAsnAspAspGluGlyAlaPheHisGly 424

GACGCAGATGGCTCGTTCGGAACACCACCTGGATACGGCTGCGCTGCAGACCGGGCAGAGGAGCAGCGCCGGCACCAAGATGGG 1356
AspAlaAspGlySerPheGlyThrProProGlyTyrGlyCysAlaAlaAspArgAlaGluGluGlnArgArgHisGlnAspGly 452

CTGCCCTACATTGATGACTCGCCCTCCTCATCGCCCCACCTCAGCAGCAAGGGCAGGGGCAGCCGGGATGCGCTGGTCTCGGGA 1440
LeuProTyrIleAspAspSerProSerSerSerProHisLeuSerSerLysGlyArgGlySerArgAspAlaLeuValSerGly 480

GCCCTGAAGTCCACTAAAGCGAGTGAGCTGGACTTGGAAAAGGGCTTGGAGATGAGAAAATGGGTCCTGTCGGGAATCCTGGCT 1524
AlaLeuLysSerThrLysAlaSerGluLeuAspLeuGluLysGlyLeuGluMetArgLysTrpValLeuSerGlyIleLeuAla 508

AGCGAGGAGACTTACCTGAGCCACCTGGAGGCACTGCTGCTGCCCATGAAGCCTTTGAAAGCCGCTGCCACCACCTCTCAGCCG 1608
SerGluGluThrTyrLeuSerHisLeuGluAlaLeuLeuLeuProMetLysProLeuLysAlaAlaAlaThrThrSerGlnPro 536

GTGCTGACGAGTCAGCAGATCGAGACCATCTTCTTCAAAGTGCCTGAGCTCTACGAGATCCACAAGGAGTCCTATGATGGGCTC 1692
ValLeuThrSerGlnGlnIleGluThrIlePhePheLysValProGluLeuTyrGluIleHisLysGluSerTyrAspGlyLeu 564

ACGTTCCTGATCTCCTCTGACTATGAGCGGGCTGAGTGGAGGGAGAACATCCGGGAGCAGCAGAAGAAGTGTTTCAGAAGCTTC 2616
ThrPheLeuIleSerSerAspTyrGluArgAlaGluTrpArgGluAsnIleArgGluGlnGlnLysLysCysPheArgSerPhe 872

TCCCTGACATCCGTGGAGCTGCAGATGCTGACCAACTCGTGTGTGAAACTCCAGACTGTCCACAGCATTCCGCTGACCATCAAT 2700
SerLeuThrSerValGluLeuGlnMetLeuThrAsnSerCysValLysLeuGlnThrValHisSerIleProLeuThrIleAsn 900

AAGGAAGATGATGAGTCTCCGGGGCTCTATGGGTTTCTGAATGTCATCGTCCACTCAGCCACTGGATTTAAGCAGAGTTCAAAT 2784
LysGluAspAspGluSerProGlyLeuTyrGlyPheLeuAsnValIleValHisSerAlaThrGlyPheLysGlnSerSerAsn 928

CTGTACTGCACCCTGGAGGTGGATTCCTTTGGGTATTTTGTGAATAAAGCAAAGACGCGCGTCTACAGGGACACAGCTGAGCCA 2868
LeuTyrCysThrLeuGluValAspSerPheGlyTyrPheValAsnLysAlaLysThrArgValTyrArgAspThrAlaGluPro 956

AACTGGAACGAGCTGGACCCGCAGGCCCTGCAGGACAGAGACTGGCAGCGCACCGTCATCGCCATGAATGGGATCGAAGTAAAG 2952
AsnTrpAsnGluLeuAspProGlnAlaLeuGlnAspArgAspTrpGlnArgThrValIleAlaMetAsnGlyIleGluValLys 984

CTCTCGGTCAAGTTCAACAGCAGGGAGTTCAGCTTGAAGAGGATGCCGTCCCGAAAACAGACAGGGGTCTTCGGAGTCAAGATT 3036
LeuSerValLysPheAsnSerArgGluPheSerLeuLysArgMetProSerArgLysGlnThrGlyValPheGlyValLysIle 1012

GCTGTGGTCACCAAGAGAGAGAGGTCCAAGGTGCCCTACATCGTGCGCCAGTGCGTGGAGGAGATCGAGCGCCGAGGCATGGAG 3120
AlaValValThrLysArgGluArgSerLysValProTyrIleValArgGlnCysValGluGluIleGluArgArgGlyMetGlu 1040

GAGGTGGGCATCTACCGCGTGTCCGGTGTGGCCACGGACATCCAGGCACTGAAGGCAGCCTTCGACGTCAATAACAAGGATGTG 3204
GluValGlyIleTyrArgValSerGlyValAlaThrAspIleGlnAlaLeuLysAlaAlaPheAspValAsnAsnLysAspVal 1068

TCGGTGATGATGAGCGAGATGGACGTGAACGCCATCGCAGGCACGCTGAAGCTGTACTTCCGTGAGCTGCCCGAGCCCCTCTTC 3288
SerValMetMetSerGluMetAspValAsnAlaIleAlaGlyThrLeuLysLeuTyrPheArgGluLeuProGluProLeuPhe 1096

ACTGACGAGTTCTACCCCAACTTCGCAGAGGGCATCGCTCTTTCAGACCCGGTTGCAAAGGAGAGCTGCATGCTCAACCTGCTG 3372
ThrAspGluPheTyrProAsnPheAlaGluGlyIleAlaLeuSerAspProValAlaLysGluSerCysMetLeuAsnLeuLeu 1124

CTGTCCCTGCCGGAGGCCAACCTGCTCACCTTCCTTTTCCTTCTGGACCACCTGAAAAGGGTGGCAGAGAAGGAGGCAGTCAAT 3456
LeuSerLeuProGluAlaAsnLeuLeuThrPheLeuPheLeuLeuAspHisLeuLysArgValAlaGluLysGluAlaValAsn 1152

AAGATGTCCCTGCACAACCTCGCCACGGTCTTTGGCCCCACGCTGCTCCGGCCCTCCGAGAAGGAGAGCAAGCTCCCTGCCAAC 3540
LysMetSerLeuHisAsnLeuAlaThrValPheGlyProThrLeuLeuArgProSerGluLysGluSerLysLeuProAlaAsn 1180

CCCAGCCAGCCTATCACCATGACTGACAGCTGGTCCTTGGAGGTCATGTCCCAGGTCCAGGTGCTGCTGTACTTCCTGCAGCTG 3624
ProSerGlnProIleThrMetThrAspSerTrpSerLeuGluValMetSerGlnValGlnValLeuLeuTyrPheLeuGlnLeu 1208

GAGGCCATCCCTGCCCCGGACAGCAAGAGACAGAGCATCCTGTTCTCCACCGAAGTCTAAAGGTCCCAGTCCATCTCCTGGAGG 3708
GluAlaIleProAlaProAspSerLysArgGlnSerIleLeuPheSerThrGluVal 1227

CAGACAGATGGCCTGGAAACCTCTGGCTAATCGGGCCATCCGTAGAGCGGGAACCTTCCTGAGGTGTCCTTGGGCCACCCCCAA 3792
GTGTTGGGCCATCTGCCAAGAGACAGCGACCCAAAGCCGAAGGACAGGTGGCCTGGGCAGATCTGCCCAGGTCTGGGAGCCCCA 3876
AGCTGGCCTCAGACTGTGGTTTTTTATGTGGCCACCCGAGGGCGCCCCAAGCCAGTTCATCTCGGAGTCCAGGCCTGACCCTGG 3960
CAGACACGGTGAAGCGACTCATTTTTATGAACTTAACTTAGAGTCTAAAAGATTTCTACTGGATCACTTGTCAAGATGCGCCCT 4044
CTCTGGGGAGAAGGGAACGTGACCGGATTCCCTCACTGTTGTATCTTGAATAAACGCTGCTGCTTCAAAAAAAA.....(80) 4111

Figure 10 Physical map and nucleotide sequence of *bcr* open reading frame (*orf*). λ-105 and λ-2 are cDNA clones, and λ-20 is an overlapping genomic clone. *orf* is indicated by the heavy line. P, *Pst*I; B, *Bam*HI; Pv, *Pvu*III; Bg, *Bgl*III; S, *Sac*I; and H, *Hind*III. The arrow at position -464 indicates the beginning of a *bcr-abl* cDNA clone (33). Underlined hexanucliotides are GC motifs, and underlined 18 bp sequences correspond to the inverted repeat. (From Reference 32.)

it is identical to the physical map of the breakpoint cluster region (*bcr*) reported previously by Groffen and his associates (29). This region is cleaved in the vast majority of CML patients so that sequences 5′ to the breakpoint remain on chromosome 22 and sequences 3′ to this site translocate to chromosome 9. Thus, we could conclude that the CML-specific 8.6 kb RNA is a fused transcript of *bcr* and *abl*. The fusion is through splicing of a 75 bp *bcr* exon to *abl* exon II. Subsequently, we isolated from other CML lines a transcript in which *abl* exon II is spliced to a different *bcr* exon (17). Heisterkamp et al. (30) termed these *bcr* exons 3 and 2, respectively, and showed that the chromosomal breaks in CMLs occur in the introns bound by *bcr* exons 2 and 3 or 3 and 4.

The results just described in conjunction with the results of others explain the involvement of *abl* and *bcr* in the t(9;22) aberration. As a result of the translocation the genes are juxtaposed on the Philadelphia chromosome in a head-to-tail configuration, with the *bcr* closer to the centromere. Transcription initiates at the *bcr* promoter, spans the truncated *bcr* gene, and extends into *abl* sequences. Although the breakpoints on chromosome 22 concentrate in a small area of several kilobasepairs within the *bcr* gene, they spread over the very large first intron of *abl* and can also occur at 3′ or 5′ of it (13,29). This results in the synthesis of primary transcripts of various lengths that can extend over hundreds of kilobasepairs. All these transcripts are spliced into an mRNA of 8.6 kbp composed of 3.3 and 5.3 kb of *bcr* and *abl* sequences, respectively. Depending on the location of the breakpoint within *bcr*, the mRNA includes or excludes *bcr* exon 3. The most important result of the events described here is the fusion of *bcr* and *abl* reading frames in phase and consequently the translation of the mRNA into a 210 kD fused protein containing 1104 *abl* amino acids and 902 or 927 amino acids of *bcr*. The protein has enhanced tyrosine kinase activity compared to the normal *abl* protein (31) and presumably triggers CML by substituting for *abl* in a signal transduction pathway. Perhaps the *bcr-abl* protein, unlike the normal species, cannot interact with a cellular regulator.

bcr NORMAL TRANSCRIPTS AND *bcr*-RELATED GENES

The *bcr* gene plays an important role in the pathogenesis of CML, but very little is known about it. We and others (32,33) have cloned and sequenced normal *bcr* cDNAs. Mes-Masson et al. characterized the *bcr* sequences within a *bcr-abl* cDNA cloned from K562 cells (34). Our sequence, which is derived from overlapping genomic and cDNA clones (32), is shown in Figure 10. The 5′ untranslated region is G + C rich (> 80%) and contains an inverted repeat of 18 nucleotides at positions -113 to -130 and -376 to -393. This repeat is likely to form a stem and loop structure, which could play a role in the regulation of translation of *bcr* mRNA. Three GC motifs located upstream and downstream of the 5′ terminus (position -464) of the longest cloned *bcr-abl* molecule (34) fit the

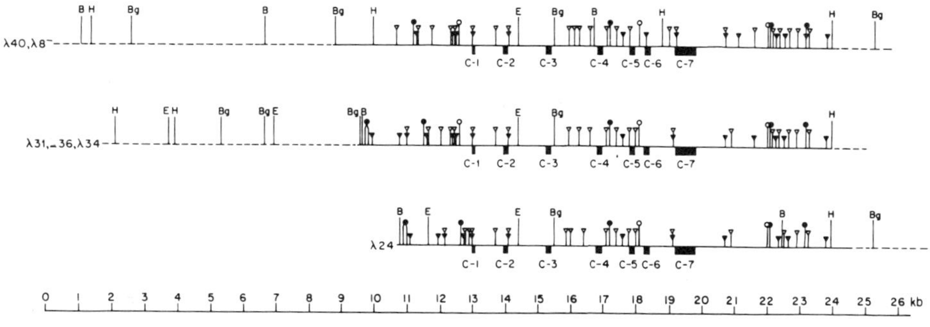

Figure 11 Physical maps of the 3′ region of the *bcr* gene (top line) and of two *bcr*-related genes. Exons C-1 to C-7 correspond to the last seven exons of the original *bcr* gene. H, E, Bg, and B correspond to sites for *Hind*III, *Eco*RI, *Bgl*II, and *Bam*HI, respectively; (○) *Sac*I; (●) *Hinc*II; (▽) *Pst*I; (▼) *Pvu*II. (From Reference 39.)

consensus sequence for interaction with the cellular transcription factor SP1 (35). No TATA or CAAT boxes were detected in this region. The *bcr* open reading frame contains 1227 codons. However, our cDNA clone λ-105 lacks a stretch of 44 codons beginning at amino acid 960. This stretch, which is present in cDNA VI-3 reported by others (30) and in the cDNA clone λ-105 we obtained, is all coded by a single exon, designated exon 5 (30). Thus, the larger *bcr* protein would contain 1271 amino acids. Inspection of the predicted amino acid sequence shows the constellation gly x gly xx gly at positions 164–169 followed by lys at position 190. This sequence roughly fits a consensus ATP binding site (36). Hydropathy analysis does not indicate a transmembrane region. This and the absence of gly at the N-terminus of the protein suggests that the *bcr* protein is not associated with the cell membrane. At present there is some controversy about the identity and number of normal *bcr* proteins. Species of 160 and 190 kD were described (37,38). Very recently, additional polypeptides of 135 kD (Amson et al., in preparation), as well as of other sizes (Li, Kloetzer, and Arlinghaus, in preparation), were also detected using polyclonal and monoclonal anti-*bcr* antibodies. Presumably, the different proteins are translated from several mRNA species transcribed from the single *bcr* gene.

By Northern blot analysis we identified two normal *bcr* transcripts of 7 and 4.5 kb (16,32). Both transcripts appear in all human cell lines examined, including those of hematopoietic origin (KG-1, SMS-SB, HL-60, Molt-4, Raji, and U937), fibroblastic (SV80 and Wish), epithelial (HeLa and A431), and neuronal origin (AS-32). In addition, both transcripts are found in embryos. A third species of 4 kb, which lacks sequences from the center of the cDNA, was detected in some preparations of KG-1 cells. All segments of *bcr* open reading frame as well as 5′ and 3′ untranslated sequences hybridized to both 7 and 4.5 kb RNA. Therefore we are able to determine neither the origin of the cDNA nor the origin of the additional 2.5 kb present within the 7 kb species. It is possible that the different *bcr* RNAs as well as the different *bcr* proteins are due to alternative splicing.

Using *bcr* cDNA as a probe to genomic blots we found that in addition to the original *bcr* gene, the human genome contains three truncated genes that apparently include the 3′ region but no other parts of the original *bcr* gene. Two of these genes were cloned and compared to the corresponding region from the original *bcr* gene (Figure 11). These two genes contain the last seven exons and six introns of *bcr* as well as some sequences upstream and downstream of it. The three *bcr*-related loci but not the original *bcr* gene hybridize with a *Bgl*III-*Ava*I fragment located at 9.6-9.8 kb of phage λ-36. This suggests that the three loci originated by translocation of the 3′ *bcr* region into the same locus on the human genome. The two cloned *bcr*-related genes show very high homology to the original *bcr* gene, and this may argue for functionality. However, our failure to detect transcripts containing solely 3′ *bcr* sequences in a variety of cell lines examined suggests that these *bcr*-related genes are inactive (32).

Applying somatic cell hybrids and in situ hybridization techniques, Croce et al. (39) and Budarf et al. (40) have recently mapped the *bcr*-related genes to the chromosome region 22q11 and determined their linear order and position with respect to Ewing's sarcoma and constitutional t(11;22) breakpoints and to the λ light-chain locus. Finally, Heisterkamp and Groffen (41) have now shown that the *bcr*-related sequences in two loci they cloned represent independent duplication and translocations into members of the gammaglutamyltranspeptidase gene family. This indicates that the *bcr* gene is susceptible to rearrangement events, not only at the central region involved in CML, but also at the 3′ domain of the gene and within the first *bcr* intron at the 5′ domain (see next section).

A NEW *bcr-abl* RNA AND PROTEIN IN ACUTE LYMPHOCYTIC LEUKEMIA

Around 10% of children and 25% of adults with acute lymphocytic leukemia have the Ph^1 chromosome. In approximately half these patients (42) the molecular abnormality varies from typical CML in that *abl* is translocated to chromosome 22, but the breakpoint on the latter is not within the central region of *bcr* and in one case was shown to be centromeric to it (43). Importantly, the leukemic cells of these patients contain a 190 kd *abl*-encoded protein kinase rather than the 210 kd protein typical of *bcr* (44–46).

We assumed that the 190 kd *abl* protein typical of Ph^1 chromosome-positive ALL is coded by a new chimeric *abl* mRNA. We therefore attempted to obtain a

A.

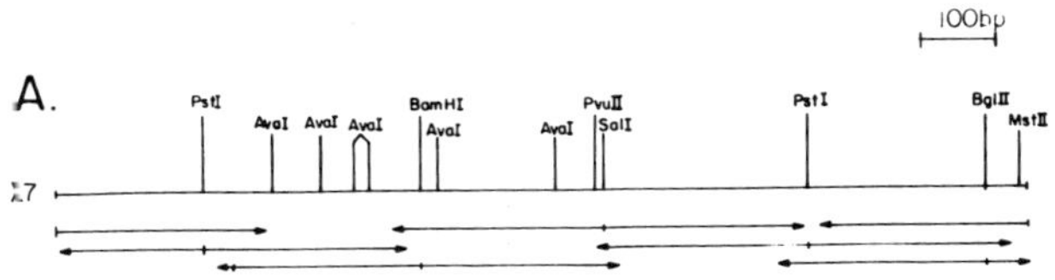

B.

```
                                                         GCCCCGCGCGCAGCCCCGGCGGCGCAGG   27
TAAGGCCGGCCGCGCCATGGTGGACCCGGTGGGCTTCGCGGAGGCGTGGAAGGCGCAGTTCCCGGACTCAGAGCCCCCG  106
CGCATGGAGCTGCGCTCAGTGGGCGACATCGAGCAGGAGCTGGAGCGCTGCAAGGCCTCCATTCGGCGCCTGGAGCAGG  185

                        Met Ile Tyr Leu Gln Thr Leu Leu Ala Lys Glu Lys Lys Ser   14
AGGTGAACTAGGAGCGCTTCCGC ATG ATC TAC CTG CAG ACG TTG CTG GCC AAG GAA AAG AAG AGC  250

Tyr Asp Arg Gln Arg Trp Gly Phe Arg Arg Ala Ala Gln Ala Pro Asp Gly Ala Ser Glu   34
TAT GAC CGG CAG CGA TGG GGC TTC CGG CGC GCG GCG CAG GCC CCC GAC GGC GCC TCC GAG  310

Pro Arg Ala Ser Ala Ser Arg Pro Gln Pro Ala Pro Ala Asp Gly Ala Asp Pro Pro Pro   54
CCC CGA GCG TCC GCG TCG CGC CCG CAG CCA GCG CCC GCC GAC GGA GCC GAC CCG CCG CCC  370

Ala Glu Glu Pro Glu Ala Arg Pro Asp Gly Glu Gly Ser Pro Gly Lys Ala Arg Pro Gly   74
GCC GAG GAG CCC GAG GCC CGG CCC GAC GGC GAG GGT TCT CCG GGT AAG GCC AGG CCC GGG  430

Thr Ala Arg Arg Pro Gly Ala Ala Ala Ser Gly Glu Arg Asp Asp Arg Gly Pro Pro Ala   94
ACC GCC CGC AGG CCC GGG GCA GCC GCG TCG GGG GAA CGG GAC GAC CGG GGA CCC CCC GCC  490

Ser Val Ala Ala Leu Arg Ser Asn Phe Glu Arg Ile Arg Lys Gly His Gly Gln Pro Gly  114
AGC GTG GCG GCG CTC AGG TCC AAC TTC GAG CGG ATC CGC AAG GGC CAT GGC CAG CCC GGG  550

Ala Asp Ala Glu Lys Pro Phe Tyr Val Asn Val Glu Phe His His Glu Arg Gly Leu Val  134
GCG GAC GCC GAG AAG CCC TTC TAC GTG AAC GTC GAG TTT CAC CAC GAG CGC GGC CTG GTG  610

Lys Val Asn Asp Lys Glu Val Ser Asp Arg Ile Ser Ser Leu Gly Ser Gln Ala Met Gln  154
AAG GTC AAC GAC AAA GAG GTG TCG GAC CGC ATC AGC TCC CTG GGC AGC CAG GCC ATG CAG  670

Met Glu Arg Lys Lys Ser Gln His Gly Ala Gly Ser Ser Val Gly Asp Ala Ser Arg Pro  174
ATG GAG CGC AAA AAG TCC CAG CAC GGC GCG GGC TCG AGC GTG GGG GAT GCA TCC AGG CCC  730

Pro Tyr Arg Gly Arg Ser Ser Glu Ser Ser Cys Gly Val Asp Gly Asp Tyr Glu Asp Ala  194
CCT TAC CGG GGA CGC TCC TCG GAG AGC AGC TGC GGC GTC GAC GGC GAC TAC GAG GAC GCC  790

Glu Leu Asn Pro Arg Phe Leu Lys Asp Asn Leu Ile Asp Ala Asn Gly Gly Ser Arg Pro  214
GAG TTG AAC CCC CGC TTC CTG AAG GAC AAC CTG ATC GAC GCC AAT GGC GGT AGC AGG CCC  850

Pro Trp Pro Pro Leu Glu Tyr Gln Pro Tyr Gln Ser Ile Tyr Val Gly Gly Met Met Glu  234
CCT TGG CCG CCC CTG GAG TAC CAG CCC TAC CAG AGC ATC TAC GTC GGG GGC ATG ATG GAA  910

Gly Glu Gly Lys Gly Pro Leu Leu Arg Ser Gln Ser Thr Ser Glu Gln Glu Lys Arg Leu  254
GGG GAG GGC AAG GGC CCG CTC CTG CGC AGC CAG AGC ACC TCT GAG CAG GAG AAG CGC CTT  970

Thr Trp Pro Arg Arg Ser Tyr Ser Pro Arg Ser Phe Glu Asp Cys Gly Gly Gly Tyr Thr  274
ACC TGG CCC CGC AGG TCC TAC TCC CCC CGG AGT TTT GAG GAT TGC GGA GGC GGC TAT ACC 1030

Pro Asp Cys Ser Ser Asn Glu Asn Leu Thr Ser Ser Glu Glu Asp Phe Ser Ser Gly Gln  294
CCG GAC TGC AGC TCC AAT GAG AAC CTC ACC TCC AGC GAG GAG GAC TTC TCC TCT GGC CAG 1090

Ser Ser Arg Val Ser Pro Ser Pro Thr Thr Tyr Arg Met Phe Arg Asp Lys Ser Arg Ser  314
TCC AGC CGC GTG TCC CCA AGC CCC ACC ACC TAC CGC ATG TTC CGG GAC AAA AGC CGC TCT 1150

Pro Ser Gln Asn Ser Gln Gln Ser Phe Asp Ser Ser Ser Pro Pro Thr Pro Gln Cys His  334
CCC TCG CAG AAC TCG CAA CAG TCC TTC GAC AGC AGC AGT CCC CCC ACG CCG CAG TGC CAT 1210

Lys Arg His Arg His Cys Pro Val Val Val Ser Glu Ala Thr Ile Val Gly Val Arg Lys  354
AAG CGG CAC CGG CAC TGC CCG GTT GTC GTG TCC GAG GCC ACC ATC GTG GGC GTC CGC AAG 1270

Thr Gly Gln Ile Trp Pro Asn Asp Gly Glu Gly Ala Phe His Gly Asp Ala Glu Ala Leu  374
ACC GGG CAG ATC TGG CCC AAC GAT GGC GAG GGC GCC TTC CAT GGA GAC GCA GAA GCC CTT 1330

Gln Arg Pro Val Ala Ser Asp Phe Gln Pro Gln                 bcr ⊥ abl            385
CAG CGG CCA GTA GCA TCT GAC TTT CAG CCT CAG GG                                  1365
```

C.

```
CAACGATGGCGAGGGCGCCTTCCATGGAGACGCAGGTGAGTTCCTCACGCCACGTGCGTGGCACACCTGCACGGGGA
                       bcr exon I ⊥ bcr intron I
```

Figure 12 (A) Physical map and (B) nucleotide sequence of cDNA clone obtained from RNA of ALL-1 cells. This clone had undergone a mutation at position 194 terminating there (box) the normal *bcr* open reading frame which starts at position 44 (arrow). (From Reference 47.)

cDNA copy of such RNA. From a cDNA library made with RNA of the ALL-1 cell line derived from a Ph[1] chromosome-positive ALL patient (43), we obtained several clones in which *abl* exon II was linked to a new sequence (47). The new sequence was found to correspond to the first exon of *bcr* (Figure 12). The identification of this new *bcr-abl* RNA junction in the ALL-1 cell line in which the central region of the *bcr* region is not rearranged, which lacks the 8.6 kb CML-specific *bcr-abl* RNA, suggested that in the Ph[1] chromosome of ALL-1 the breakpoint is in the 5′ region of *bcr*, probably within the first intron. The fused RNA should contain around 7 kb. Indeed, Hermans et al. (48) showed that in two Ph[1]-positive ALLs the breakpoints occurred in the first *bcr* intron. In further studies we used site-specific antibodies against different portions of the *bcr* polypeptide and showed that the p190 *abl* protein contains epitopes of *bcr* exon I but not of other *bcr* exons (47). This established that the cloned transcript encodes p210. It can be concluded that p190 results from the translocation of the tip of chromosome 9 into the first *bcr* intron and the consequent production of a 7 kb *bcr-abl* mRNA. Very recent studies suggest that breaks within the first intron tend to cluster in a small region of a 10 kbp adjacent to the second *bcr* exon (49).

p190 has been associated nearly exclusively with the acute leukemias ALL and AML. Two CML cases in whom p190 was detected (Grosveld, unpublished) constitute the only exception to his rule. This raises the possibility that the protein directly triggers acute leukemia. p210, on the other hand, is already detected in the chronic phase of CML (and presumably triggers this phase) and is also present in around half the cases of Ph[1]-positive ALL and AML (42,49). A possible interpretation of these observations is that the biologic properties and pathogenicity of the two proteins are different. p210 would enhance proliferation of myeloid stem cells, to be reflected in chronic-phase symptoms, and p190 would cause a malignant transformation of the affected cells. The association of p210 with acute leukemia could be explained as representing CMLs in which the chronic phase was very short and escaped detection or as CMLs that previously or subsequently to the t(9;22) translocation had undergone additional malignant mutations. An alternative interpretation postulates that p210 and p190 have similar biologic activity, but breaks in the central region of the *bcr* gene (resulting in production of p210) tend to occur in stem cells whose transformation leads to CML; other stem cells, whose transformation results in acute leukemia, suffer breaks either in the first intron or in the center of the *bcr* gene. Comparative analysis of the biologic activity of the two molecules in mice may shed some light on this issue.

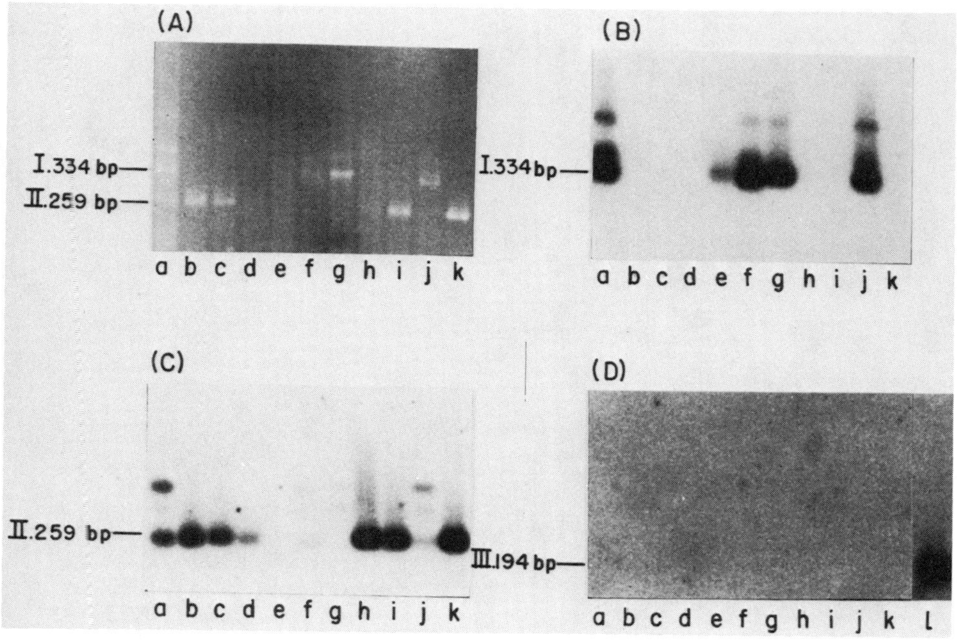

Figure 13 PCR analysis of RNA from CML patients. For details see text. (From Marcelle, Gale, Prokocimer, Berrebi and Canaani, in preparation.)

APPLICATION OF THE POLYMERASE CHAIN REACTION TO ANALYZE *bcr-abl* RNA IN PATIENTS

The realization that Ph[1] chromosome-positive leukemia patients synthesize one of three *bcr-abl* RNA junctions opened the way to detect and analyze such patients during different stages of their disease by applying the polymerase chain reaction (PCR). The chief advantage of this technique over genomic Southern blot analysis is its enormous sensitivity. Presumably, a small volume of peripheral blood should be sufficient for this analysis. Under optimal conditions this technique should detect leukemic cells mixed with large excess of normal cells (as is the situation with patients in remission or after bone marrow transplantation). In addition, this technique is clearly superior to the RNase protection method, which, because of incomplete digestion by the RNase, is highly unreliable in determination of the type of *bcr-abl* junction present in a given CML RNA (Hermans and Grosveld, unpublished; Canaani, unpublished).

The PCR method (50) is based on in vitro amplification of a DNA fragment of a known sequence. We have adapted the technique to use RNA as the starting template. Total cellular RNA is primed with an *abl* oligonucleotide and reverse

Table 1 *bcr-abl* Junctions in Ph¹-Positive Patients and Cell Lines

		Type of junction			
Ph¹-positive patients	No. of patients and cell lines	*bcr* 3-*abl* II	*bcr* 2-*abl* II	*bcr* 3-*abl*II plus *bcr* 2-*abl*II	*bcr* I-*abl* II
A. CML, chronic phase	13	5	8	0	0
B. CML, accelerated phase	3	0	2	1	0
C. CML, acute phase					
Myeloid	8	3	2	3	0
Lymphoid	6	0	6	0	0
Megakaryocytic	3	1	1	1	0
Erythroid	1	1	0	0	0
D. ALL	3	0	0	0	3

Source: From Marcelle, Gale, Prokocimer, Berrebi, and Canaani, in preparation.

transcribed. The cDNA is incubated with the same *abl* primer as well as with a *bcr* primer originating from exon I or 1 (the former is the first *bcr* exon, and the latter is designated according to Reference 29). Following 30-40 cycles of synthesis with the thermostable Taq 1 polymerase, the products are analyzed by agarose gel electrophoresis, blotting, and hybridization to oligonucleotide probes specific to one of the two CML junctions *bcr* exon 2-*abl* exon II and *bcr* exon 3-*abl* exon II or to the "ALL junction" *bcr* exon I-*abl* exon II. One such analysis is shown in Figure 13. RNA samples of several micrograms from 10 CML patients in acute phase were subjected to PCR amplification with CML (A, B, and C) or ALL (D) primers. The products were electrophoresed and detected by ultraviolet light (A) or by hybridization to probes specific for the 334 bp *bcr* 3-*abl* II junction (B), the 259 bp *bcr* 2-*abl* II junction (C), or the 194 bp *bcr* I-*abl* II junction (D). Samples a, e, f, g, and j contained the 334 bp CML junction. Samples a, b, c, d, f, h, i, j, and k contained the 259 bp CML junction. None of these samples showed the 194 bp ALL junction (a PCR product of a Ph^1-positive ALL RNA, shown in lane 1, served as a positive control). Several samples (a, f, and j) showed strong signals of *bcr* 3-*abl* II junction together with relatively small amounts (see Figure 13A) of the *bcr* 2-*abl* II junction. We interpret this result as evidence for alternative splicing. The 370 bp band is an artificial hybrid of the 334 and 259 bp DNA species. The identity of the hybridizable band of 570 bp apparent in some of the samples is at present not known. The result of the analysis to date (Marcelle et al., in preparation) is shown in Table 1. It is apparent that no CML patients contained the ALL type of RNA junction. Thus, transition to the acute phase of CML does not involve the synthesis of p190. It also appears that although chronic-phase patients and myeloid acute-phase patients can have either RNA junction species, patients with lymphocytic blast crisis tend to carry *bcr-abl* RNA with *bcr* 2-*abl* II junction.

REFERENCES

1. Champlin, R. E., and Golde, D. W. (1985). Chronic myelogenous leukemia: Recent advances. *Blood 65*:1039–1047.
2. Nowell, P. C., and Hungerford, D. A. (1960). A minute chromosome in human chronic granulocytic leukemia. *Science 132*:1497–1501.
3. Rowley, J. D. (1973). A new consistent chromosomal abnormality in chronic myelogenous leukemia identified by quinacrine fluorescence and Giemsa staining. *Nature 243*:145–147.
4. Parakash, O., and Yunis, J. J. (1984). High resolution chromosomes of t(9;22) positive leukemias. *Cancer Genet. Cytogenet. 11*:361–367.
5. Sandberg, A. A. (1980). Chromosomes and causation of human cancer and leukemia XL. The Ph^1 and other translocations in CML. *Cancer 46*:2221–2226.
6. Rowley, J. D., and Testa, J. R. (1982). Chromosomal abnormalities in malignant hematologic diseases. *Adv. Cancer Res. 36*:103–148.

7. Yunis, J. J. (1983). The chromosomal basis of human neoplasm. *Science 221*:227–236.
8. Third International Workshop on Chromosomes in Leukemia (1983). *Cancer Res. 43*:868–873.
9. de Klein, A., Geurtz van Kessel, A., Grosveld, G., Bartram, C. R., Hagemeijer, A., Bootsma, D., Spurr, N. K., Heisterkamp, N., Groffen, J., and Stephenson, J. R. (1982). A cellular oncogene (c-*abl*) is translocated to the Philadelphia chromosome in chronic myelocytic leukemia. *Nature 294*:765–767.
10. Groffen, J., Heisterkamp, N., Stephenson, J. R., Geurts van Kessel, A., de Klein, A., Grosveld, G., and Bootsma, G. (1983). c-*cis* translocated from chromosome 22 to chromosome 9 in chronic myelocytic leukemia. *J. Exp. Med. 158*:9–15.
11. Canaani, E., Gale, R. P., Steiner-Saltz, D., Berrebi, A., Aghai, E., and Januszewics, E. (1984). Altered transcription of an oncogene in chronic myeloid leukemia. *Lancet 1*:593–595.
12. Gale, R. P., and Canaani, E. (1984). An 8 kilobase *abl* transcript in chronic myelogenous leukemia. *Proc. Natl. Acad. Sci. USA 81*:5648–5652.
13. Heisterkamp, N., Stephenson, J. R., Groffen, J., Hansen, P. F., de Klein, A., Bartram, C. R., and Grosveld, G. (1983). Localization of the c-*abl* oncogene adjacent to a translocation point in chronic myelocytic leukemia. *Nature 306*:23999–242.
14. Konopka, J. B., Watanabe, S. M., and Witte, O. N. (1984). An alteration of the human c-*abl* protein in K562 leukemia cells unmasks associated tyrosine kinase activity cell. *Cell 37*:1035–1042.
15. Kloetzer, W., Kurzrock, R., Smith, L., Talpaz, M., Spiller, M., Gutterman, J., and Arlinghaus, R. (1985). The human cellular *abl* gene product in the chronic myelogenous leukemia cell line K562 has an associated tyrosine protein kinase activity. *Virology 140*:230–238.
16. Shtivelman, E., Lifshitz, B., Gale, R. P., and Canaani, E. (1985). Fused transcript of *abl* and *bcr* genes in chronic myelogenous leukemia. *Nature 315*: 550–554.
17. Shtivelman, E., Lifshitz, B., Gale, R. P., Roe, B. A., and Canaani, E. (1986). Alternative splicing of RNAs transcribed from the human *abl* gene and from the *bcr-abl* fused gene. *Cell 47*:277–284.
18. Magee, T., and Hanley, M. (1988). Sticky fingers and CAAX boxes. *Nature 335*:114–115.
19. Bernards, A., Rubin, C. M., Westbrook, C. A., Paskind, M., and Baltimore, D. (1987). The first intron of the human c-*abl* gene is at least 200 kilobases long and is a target for translocations in chronic myelogenous leukemia. *Mol. Cell. Biol. 7*:3231–3236.
20. Oppi, C., Shore, S. K., and Reddy, P. E. (1987). Nucleotide sequence of testis-derived c-*abl* cDNAs: Implications for testis-specific transcription and *abl* oncogene activation. *Proc. Natl. Acad. Sci. USA 84*:8200–8204.
21. Shaw, G., and Kamen, R. (1986). A conserved AU sequence from the 3′ untranslated region of GM-CSF mRNA mediates selective mRNA degradation. *Cell 46*:659–667.

22. Sadowski, I., Stone, J. C., and Pawson, T. (1986). A noncatalytic domain conserved among cytoplasmic protein tyrosine kinases modifies the kinase function and transforming activity of Fujinami sarcoma virus p130 *gag-fps*. *Mol. Cell. Biol. 6*:4396–4408.
23. Stahl, M. L., Ferenz, C. R., Kelleher, K. L., Kriz, R. W., and Knopf, J. L. (1988). Sequence similarity of phospholipase C with the non-catalytic region of *src*. *Nature 332*:269–272.
24. Vogel, U. S., Dixon, R. A. F., Schaber, M. D., Diehl, R. E., Marshall, M. S., Scolnick, E. M., Sigal, I. S., and Gibbs, J. B. (1988). Cloning of bovine GAP and its interaction with oncogenic *ras* p21. *Nature 335*:90–93.
25. Mayer, B. J., Hamaguchi, M., and Hanafusa, H. (1988). A novel viral oncogene with structural similarity to phospholipase C. *Nature 332*:272–275.
26. Konopka, J. B., and Witte, O. N. (1985). Detection of c-*abl* tyrosine kinase activity in vitro permits direct comparison of normal and altered *abl* gene products. *Mol. Cell. Biol. 5*:3116–3123.
27. Pendergast, A. M., Traugh, J. A., and Witte, O. N. (1987). Normal cellular and transformation-associated *abl* proteins share common sites for protein kinase C phosphorylation. *Mol. Cell. Biol. 7*:4280–4289.
28. Chou, P., and Fasman, G. D. (1978). Prediction of the secondary structure of the proteins from their amino acid sequence. *Adv. Enzymol. 47*:45–148.
29. Groffen, J., Stephenson, J. R., Heisterkamp, N., de Klein, A., Bartram, C. R., and Grosveld, G. (1984). Philadelphia chromosomal breakpoints are clustered within a limited region, bcr, on chromosome 22. *Cell 36*:93–99.
30. Heisterkamp, N., Stam, K., Groffen, J., de Klein, A., and Grosveld, G. (1985). Structural organization of the *bcr* gene and its role in the Ph^1 translocation. *Nature 315*:758–761.
31. Konopka, J. B., and Witte, O. N. (1985). Detection of c-*abl* tyrosine kinase activity in vitro permits direct comparison of normal and altered *abl* gene products. *Mol. Cell. Biol. 5*:3116–3123.
32. Lifshitz, B., Fainstein, E., Marcelle, C., Shtivelman, E., Amson, R., Gale, R. P., and Canaani, E. (1988). *bcr* genes and transcripts. *Oncogene 2*:113–117.
33. Hariharan, I. K., and Adams, J. M. (1987). cDNA sequence for human *bcr*, the gene that translocates to the *abl* oncogene in chronic myeloid leukemia. *EMBO J. 6*:115–119.
34. Mes-Masson, A. M., McLaughlin, J., Doley, G. Q., Paskind, M., and Witte, O. N. (1986). Overlapping cDNA clones define the complete coding region for the P210 c-*abl* gene product associated with CML cells containing the Philadelphia chromosome. *Proc. Natl. Acad. Sci. USA 83*:9768–9772.
35. Dynan, W. Z., Sazer, S., Tjian, R., and Schimke, R. (1986). Transcription factor SP1 recognizes a DNA sequence in the mouse dihydrofolate reductase promoter. *Nature 319*:246–248.
36. Kamps, M. P., Taylor, S. S., and Sefton, B. M. (1984). Direct evidence that oncogenic tyrosine kinases and cyclic AMP-dependent protein kinase have homologous ATP-binding sites. *Nature 310*:589–592.

37. Stam, K., Heisterkamp, N., Reynolds, F., and Groffen, J. (1987). Evidence that the *phl* gene encodes a 160,000 dalton phosphoprotein with associated kinase activity. *Mol. Cell. Biol. 7*:1955–1960.
38. Ben-Neriah, Y., Daley, G. Q., Mes-Masson, A. M., Witte, O. N., and Baltimore, D. (1986). The chronic myelogenous leukemia-specific P210 protein is the product of the *bcr-abl* hybrid gene. *Science 233*:212–214.
39. Croce, C. M., Huebner, K., Isobe, M., Fainstein, E., Lifshitz, B., Shtivelman, E., and Canaani, E. (1987). Mapping of four distinct *bcr*-related loci to chromosome region 22q11: Order of *bcr* loci relative to CML and ALL breakpoints. *Proc. Natl. Acad. Sci. USA 84*:7174–7178.
40. Budarf, M., Canaani, E., and Emanuel, B. S. (1988). Linear order of the four *bcl*-related loci in 22q11. *Genomics 3*:168–171.
41. Heisterkamp, N., and Groffen, J. (1988). Duplication of the *bcr* and gamma-glutamyl transpeptidase genes. *Nucleic Acids Res. 16*:8045–8056.
42. Dreazen, O., Canaani, E., and Gale, R. P. (1988). Molecular biology of chronic myelogenous leukemia. *Semin. Hematol. 25*:35–49.
43. Erikson, J., Griffin, C. A., Ar-Rushdi, A., Valtieri, M., Hoxie, J., Finan, J., Emanuel, B. S., Rovera, G., Nowell, P., and Croce, C. (1986). Heterogeneity of chromosome 22 breakpoint in Ph^1-positive acute lymphocytic leukemia. *Proc. Natl. Acad. Sci. USA 83*:1807–1811.
44. Clark, S. S., McLaughlin, J., Crist, W. M., Champlin, R., and Witte, O. N. (1987). Unique forms of the *abl* tyrosine kinase distinguish Ph^1-positive CML from Ph^1-positive ALL. *Science 235*:85–88.
45. Kurzrock, R., Shtalrid, M., Romero, P., Kloetzer, W. S., Talpas, M., Trujillo, J. M., Block, M., Beran, M., and Gutterman, J. U. (1987). A novel c-*abl* protein product in Philadelphia-positive acute lymphoblastic leukemia. *Nature 325*:631–635.
46. Chan, L. C., Karhi, K. K., Rayter, S. I., Heisterkamp, N., Eridani, S., Powles, R., Lawler, S. D., Groffen, J., Foulkes, J. G., Greaves, M. F., and Wiedemann, L. M. (1987). A novel *abl* protein expressed in Philadelphia chromosome positive acute lymphoblastic leukemia. *Nature 325*:635–637.
47. Fainstein, E., Marcelle, C., Rosner, A., Canaani, E., Gale, R. P., Dreazen, O., Smith, S. D., and Croce, C. M. (1987). A new fused transcript in Philadelphia chromosome positive acute lymphocytic leukemia. *Nature 330*:386–388.
48. Hermans, A., Heisterkamp, N., von Lindern, M., van Baal, S., Meijer, D., van der Plas, D., Wiedemann, L. M., Groffern, J., Bootsma, D., and Grosveld, G. (1987). Unique fusion of *bcr* and c-*abl* genes in Philadelphia chromosome positive acute lymphoblastic leukemia. *Cell 51*:33–40.
49. Chen, S. J., Chen, Z., Grousz, J. D., Hillion, J., d'Auriol, L., Flandrin, G., Larsen, C.-J., and Berger, R. (1988). Molecular cloning of a 5′ segment of the genomic *phl* gene defines a new breakpoint cluster region (*bcr* 2) in Philadelphia positive acute leukemias. *Leukemia 2*:634–641.
50. Saiki, R. K., Gelfand, D. H., Stoffel, S., Scharf, S. J., Higuchi, R., Horn, G. T., Mullis, K. B., and Erlich, H. A. (1988). Primer directed enzymatic amplification of DNA with a thrermostable DNA polymerase. *Science 239*: 487–491.

9

Detection of Chimeric *bcr-abl* mRNA and Minimal Residual Disease by Polymerase Chain Reaction

Ming-Sheng Lee and Sanford A. Stass *The University of Texas M. D. Anderson Cancer Center, Houston, Texas*

INTRODUCTION

Successful induction therapy has resulted in a high remission rate in patients with hematologic malignancies. However, disease recurrence remains a major problem. Relapse from clinically undetectable residual disease is the most likely mechanism. Detection of minimal residual disease remains extremely difficult. Several new techniques, such as flow cytometry (1) and Southern blot analysis (2,3), have been used to detect small populations of neoplastic cells in the remission samples. The sensitivity of these techniques is limited at the level of 1% of neoplastic cells (1,4). Patients in remission, however, may have residual neoplastic cells that are far below this level.

Recently we used the polymerase chain reaction (PCR) to preferentially amplify the hybrid DNA sequences of a chromosomal translocation, t(14;18), characteristic of follicular lymphoma. This technique detects the neoplastic cells carrying the t(14;18) in concentrations of $<1:100,000$ (5).

The major limitation of the PCR technique is that it can amplify only a short DNA segment (several hundred basepairs). It is feasible for the t(14;18) because the molecular breakpoints on both chromosomes occur within a limited region (6-8). However, this approach is not applicable to chromosomal translocations with variable breakpoints, such as the Philadelphia (Ph^1) chromosome in chronic myelogenous leukemia (CML).

The question of minimal residual disease is now important in CML since treatment has recently become more effective with the advent of recombinant human α-interferon therapy and allogeneic bone marrow transplant therapy. Such treatments have resulted in long-term cytogenetic remission in a significant number of CML patients (9,10). This success raises several important questions concerning the biology and clinical significance of minimal residual disease in Ph^1-positive CML. Do patients in long-term remission have minimal residual cells carrying Ph^1 chromosome? Does the presence of minimal residual cells carrying the Ph^1 chromosome indicate inevitable relapse? (That is, are Ph^1-positive cells in patients in long-term remission dormant, and when will they reactivate and start proliferating rapidly again?) Do patients with minimal residual cells carrying the Ph^1 chromosome require further therapy to prevent relapse?

The Ph^1 chromosome, t(9;22)(q34;q11), has been observed in more than 90% of patients with CML (11,12). Even though the breakpoints on chromosome 22q11 cluster within a small DNA segment designated *bcr* (13,14), the breakpoints on chromosome 9q34 occur at variable positions up to more than 100 kilobases (kb) 5′ to the second exon of the c-*abl* oncogene (15,16). Despite the variability of the molecular breakpoints at the DNA level, the fused *bcr-abl* gene is transcribed into two types of chimeric mRNA: one with *abl* exon II linked to *bcr* exon 2 (designated the L-6 junction), and the other one with *abl* exon II linked to *bcr* exon 3 (designated the K-28 junction) (17,18).

Taking advantage of these unique molecular characteristics of Ph^1-positive cells, we and other investigators have successfully modified the PCR technique to detect minimal residual disease in Ph^1-positive CML by using either S_1 nuclease protection or reverse transcriptase (19–23). This sensitive and specific assay provides us with a unique opportunity to explore the mechanism of disease recurrence in Ph^1-positive CML.

COMBINED METHOD OF S_1 NUCLEASE PROTECTION AND PCR

Two synthetic oligonucleotides of 99 bases (anti-K28 and anti-L6), 1 of 60 bases (MSL-60), and 5 of 12 bases [primer *bcr* ExII(+), primer *bcr* ExIII(+), primer *abl*(–), primer 18q21(+), and Primer J_H(–)] were used (Figure 1). The sequences of anti-K28 and anti-L6 were complementary to the K-28 junction and the L-6 junction of the chimeric *bcr-abl* mRNA, respectively. The sequence of MSL-60 was randomly selected except that the 12 bases of the 3′ end were complementary to the primer 18q21(+) and the bases of the 5′ end were identical to the primer J_H(–).

The S_1 protection reaction contained 5 μg total cellular RNA samples, 1 ng anti-K28, 1 ng anti-L6, and 1 ng MSL-60 and was performed as described (24). The S_1 nuclease-resistant hybrids were resuspended in a buffer containing 10

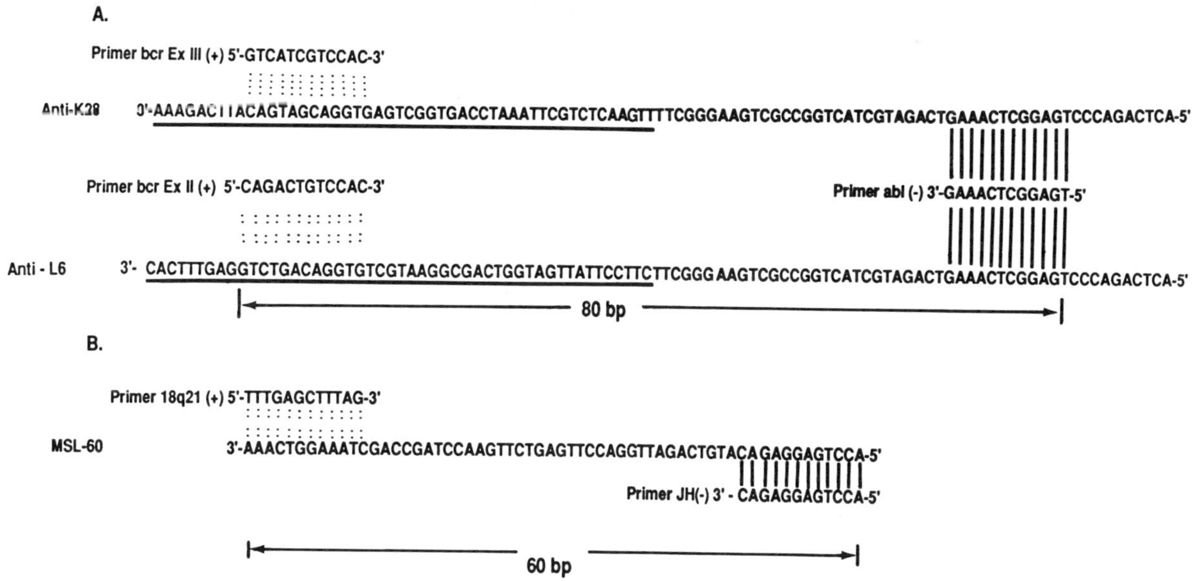

Figure 1 Sequence of the synthetic oligonucleotides used. (A) The sequences of the anti-K28 and anti-L6 oligomers are antisense to the K-28 and the L-6 mRNA junctions, respectively (11,12,15). Both antisense oligomers are 99 bases in which the 50 bases on the 5′ side are derived from the second exon of the *abl* gene and the 49 bases on the 3′ side (underlined) are derived from the second exon (for anti-L6) or the third exon (for anti-K28) of the *bcr* region. The sequences and locations of the corresponding primers relative to the antisense oligomers are specified [primers *bcr* ExII(+) and *abl*(−) for anti-L6; primers *bcr* ExIII(+) and *abl*(−) for anti-K28]. The complementary sequences are indicated by vertical dots, and the identical sequences are indicated by vertical lines. The predicted sequences amplified are 80 bp in size. (B) The sequence of the MSL-60 oligomer is shown along with its corresponding primers [18q21(+) and $J_H(-)$], which have been described (5). Except that the 12 bases of the 3′ end are complementary to the 18q21(+) primer (vertical dots) and the 12 bases of the 5′ end are identical to the $J_H(-)$ primer (vertical lines), the sequence of MSL-60 is randomly selected. Theoretically, it is not fully complementary to any RNA sequence.

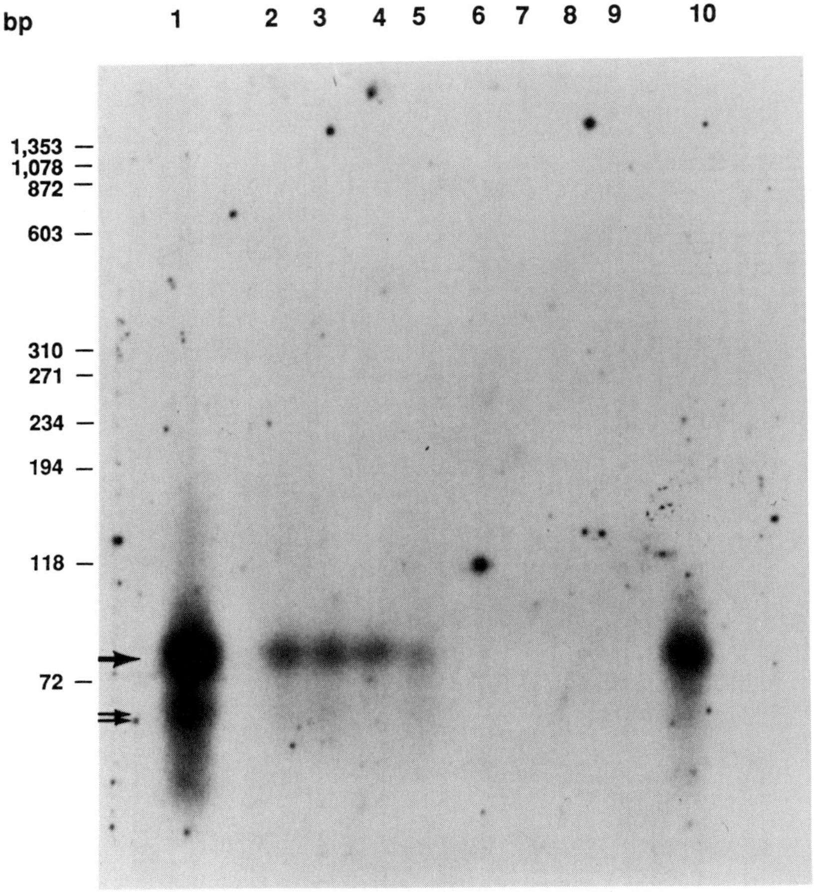

Figure 2 Southern blot analysis of the sequences that were protected from S_1 nuclease digestion and amplified by PCR. Lane 1: the pretreatment RNA sample from patient A was inadequately digested by S_1 nuclease and then PCR amplified for 25 cycles. Both 80 mers (horizontal arrow) and 60 mers (double horizontal arrows) were detected. Serial dilutions of this RNA sample with the normal RNA were subjected to adequate S_1 digestion and PCR amplification. Only the 80 mers were detected: 1:1 dilution at cycles 30 (lane 2) and 40 (lane 10). 1:100 at cycle 35 (lane 3), 1:5000 dilution at cycle 40 (lane 4), and 1:100,000 dilution at cycle 45 (lane 5). In contrast, neither the 80 mers nor the 60 mers were detected in the RNA samples from the lymph nodes involved by follicular lymphoma (lanes 6-9). The molecular weight markers were labeled on the left side of the figures.

mmol/L of Tris, pH 7.5, 50 mmol/L of NaCl, 10 mmol/L of $MgCl_2$, 1.5 mmol/L each of dNTP, 1 μmol/L of *bcr* ExII(+), 1 μmol/L of *bcr* ExIII(+), 1 μmol/L of *abl*(-), 1 μmol/L of 18q21(+), and 1 μmol of J_H(-). PCR was then performed as previously described (25). The PCR-amplified samples (5 μL) were then loaded to a 3% agarose minigel and subjected to electrophoresis (50 V) for 4 h or loaded to a 4% agarose gel and electrophoresis (50 V) for 16 h. The gel was then denatured, neutralized, and transferred to a nylon filter. The filter was prehybridized as described (21) and then hybridized with a mixture of ^{32}P end-labeled anti-K28, anti-L6, and MSL-60 (specific activity > 5 μCi/pmol) at 42°C for 18 h. The washing conditions and autoradiography were carried out as described (25).

To determine the sensitivity of the combined method of S_1 protection and PCR, we performed a mixing experiment. By means of the S_1 nuclease protection assay using radiolabeled anti-K28, anti-L6, and MSL-60, we could detect the presence of the chimeric *bcr-abl* transcripts in a sample containing 25 μg total cellular RNA from the K562 cell line. In samples with further dilutions, we could barely detect a faint and questionable band in the sample containing 2.5 μg total cellular RNA from the K562 cell line and 22.5 μg normal RNA. In contrast, we were able to detect a strong and convincing band representative of the chimeric *bcr-abl* transcripts in a sample containing 0.05 ng total cellular RNA from the K562 cell line and 5 μg normal RNA (i.e., a 1:100,000 dilution) by the combined method of S_1 nuclease protection and PCR (19).

To determine the specificity of this assay, we also analyzed four lymph node samples that were involved by follicular lymphoma. None of these samples showed *bcr* region rearrangement by Southern blot analysis. The RNA samples prepared from these lymph nodes were analyzed by our combined assay of S_1 nuclease protection and PCR. Even after 45 cycles of PCR amplification, no chimeric *bcr-abl* transcripts were detected in these samples, indicating that this assay was highly specific (Figure 2).

COMBINED METHOD OF REVERSE TRANSCRIPTION AND PCR (RT/PCR)

Two oligonucleotides of 16 bases were used as primers. Primer *bcr*(+), 5′-CAGACTGTCCACAGCA-3′, was derived from the sequence of the second exon of the *bcr* region. Primer *abl*(-), 3′-GACTGAAACTCGGAGT-5′, was complementary to the sequence of the second exon of the c-*abl* gene. In the presence of the L-6 junction of mRNA, cDNA fragments of 80 bp were expected to be amplified. In the presence of the K-28 junction mRNA, cDNA fragments of 155 bp were expected to be amplified.

Two oligonucleotides of 20 bases were used as probes to confirm that the amplified cDNA fragments indeed contained sequences representative of the L-6 and K-28 junction mRNAs. Probe L-6 (5′-AATAAGGAAGAAGCCCTTCA-3′)

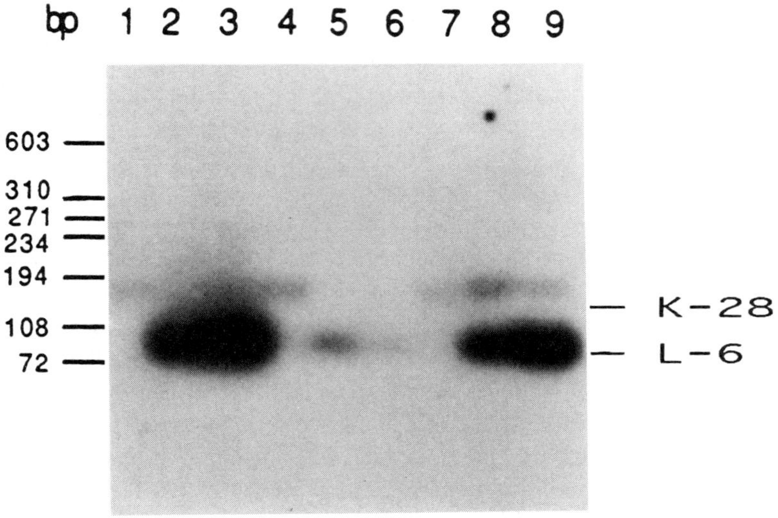

Figure 3 Southern blot analysis of the RT/PCR-amplified *bcr-abl* cDNAs in Ph^1-positive CML. After 60 cycles of RT/PCR amplification, cDNA fragments of the chimeric *bcr-abl* mRNAs were amplified in Ph^1-positive CML: a 80 bp band is detected in lanes 2, 3, 5, and 6; a 155 bp band is detected in lanes 1, 4, and 7; both bands of 155 and 80 bp are detected in lanes 8 and 9. Shown in lanes 1–7 are samples obtained in chronic phase. Shown in lanes 8 and 9 are samples in blast crisis.

and probe K-28 (5′-CAGAGTTCAAAAGCCCTTCA-3′) were derived from the sequences at the *bcr-abl* junctional region of the L-6 and K-28 mRNAs, respectively.

Samples of total cellular RNA (1-10 μg) were dispensed in 20 μL reverse transcription buffer containing 0.5 μg primer *abl*(-), 1 mM dNTPs (each of four), 20 units AMV reverse transcriptase (United States Biochemicals), and 20 units RNasin (Promega) and incubated at 42°C for 1 h. The sample was then suspended in 80 μL PCR buffer containing 0.5 μg primer *bcr*(+) and 2.5 units *Thermus aquaticus* DNA polymerase (Perkin-Elmer Cetus). PCR (denaturation of 94°C for 1 minute, annealing at 42-55°C for 1 minute, and extension at 72°C for 2 minutes) was then performed as described (26). PCR-amplified product (10 μL) was loaded onto a 2.5-3% agarose gel or 4% Nussieve agarose gel and size fractionated at 60 V for 5-6 h and then transferred to a nylon membrane. The membrane was then hybridized with a mixture of probes L-6 and K-28 that were 5′ end labeled with $[^{32}P]$-γ ATP. Washing was carried out with twofold SSPE-0.1% sodium dodecyl sulfate (SDS) at room temperature for 30 minutes and at 60°C for 15 minutes. Autoradiography was carried out against a single intensifying screen at -70°C for 4–16 h.

To study the feasibility and the specificity of the RT/PCR assay to detect the chimeric *bcr-abl* mRNAs in Ph[1]-positive CML, we selected 24 Ph[1]-positive CML samples with clonal *bcr* region rearrangement shown by Southern blot analysis and 6 lymphoma samples without *bcr* rearrangement. By means of the RT/PCR technique, we were able to amplify cDNA fragments of 155 bp (representative of the K-28 junction mRNA) and/or 80 bp (representative of the L-6 junction mRNA) in 24 of 24 CML samples with clonal *bcr* rearrangement: 9 had a band of 80 bp, 11 had a band of 155 bp, and 4 had two bands (155 and 80 bp). In contrast, none of the 6 lymphoma samples were amplifiable (Figure 3).

To determine the sensitivity of the RT/PCR assay, we performed a mixing experiment. Total cellular RNA samples prepared from two blood samples were used: one obtained from a patient in blastic phase of CML and the other from a normal individual. The CML sample was known to contain the L-6 junction mRNA. This sample was serially diluted with the normal sample (the total amounts of total cellular RNA used were 10 μg), and then RT/PCR was performed. After 60 cycles of amplification, we were able to detect the chimeric *bcr-abl* mRNA even when we loaded a sample equivalent to 0.1 ng of the original sample (20).

PATIENT STUDIES IN Ph[1]-POSITIVE CML: MINIMAL RESIDUAL DISEASE

Using the combined method of S_1 nuclease protection and PCR, we studied four blood samples obtained from four CML patients who had achieved complete hematologic remission from recombinant α-interferon therapy. While these four patients were in the chronic phase of disease, the blood samples obtained were shown to have Ph[1] chromosome by karyotyping and clonal *bcr* gene rearrangement by Southern blot analysis, but the chimeric *bcr-abl* transcripts were too low in abundance to be detected by using 25 μg of total cellular RNA and S_1 nuclease protection analysis. At the time of remission, karyotyping showed 100% diploid cells, Southern blot analysis showed no *bcr* gene rearrangement, and S_1 nuclease protection assay showed no chimeric *bcr-abl* transcripts. However, residual chimeric *bcr-abl* transcripts were detected in all four remission samples by our modified PCR technique.

Using the RT/PCR assay, we studied eight patients who had achieved complete remission for 6 months to 3 years after recombinant α-interferon therapy. Prior to treatment, six of these eight patients had the Ph[1] chromosome by karyotyping and *bcr* rearrangement by Southern blot analysis; the remaining two had clonal *bcr* rearrangement even though no Ph[1] chromosome could be detected by cytogenetic analysis. At the time of remission, all eight samples ap-

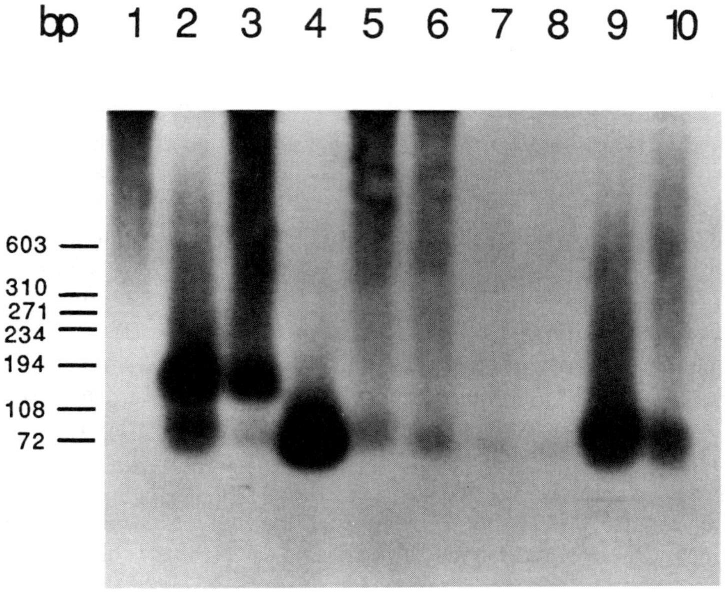

Figure 4 RT/PCR assay to detect minimal residual *bcr-abl* mRNAs in remission samples. RT/PCR was performed for 60 cycles in eight remission samples (lanes 2, 3, and 5–10). Lanes 4 and 5 were samples obtained from the same patient in different phases of disease: lane 4 was from chronic phase and lane 5 was in remission. Both bands of 155 and 80 bp are detected in lanes 2 and 3. A band of 80 bp is detected in lanes 4–10.

peared to be normal by means of routine blood counts, morphologic examination, karyotyping, and Southern blot analysis. However, minimal residual *bcr-abl* mRNAs were detected in all eight samples by the RT/PCR assay (Figure 4). Our findings suggest that interferon therapy suppresses the proliferation of Ph^1-positive clones; however, it does not completely eradicate the Ph^1-positive stem cells.

One advantage of the RT/PCR assay is the identification of the splicing pattern of the *bcr-abl* message. Using the RT/PCR assay, we studied whether a specific subtype of the *bcr-abl* mRNA junction was detected in samples with a specific chromosomal breakpoint on the *bcr* region. According to the patterns of *bcr* rearrangement by *Bgl*II and *Bam*HI digests, we identified the chromosomal breakpoint in the *bcr* region in 24 Ph^1-positive CML patients. It appears that there is a strong correlation between the chromosomal breakpoint in the *bcr* region and the specific *bcr-abl* mRNA junction expressed. Samples with the breakpoint 5′ to the *Bam*HI site of the second intron of the *bcr* region contained only the L-6 junction mRNA. When the breakpoint occurred at the more 3′ region, the majority of samples contained the K-28 junction, and intriguingly, a minority of them contained both L-6 and K-28 junctions even though only one clonal *bcr* rearrangement was shown by Southern blot analysis. There are two possible explanations for this observation. The first explanation is that there were two populations of Ph[1]-positive clones, one of which was too small to be detected by Southern blot analysis. The second possibility is that this is the result of alternative splicing as proposed by Shtivelman et al. We favor the second explanation, because in our study simultaneous expression of both mRNA junctions occurs exclusively in cases with the breakpoints falling within the more 3′ *bcr* region.

We then studied whether coexpression of two alternative *bcr-abl* mRNAs occurred more frequently in any particular phase of the disease. An interesting finding was that 2 of 21 samples studied in chronic phase versus 3 of 9 patients studied in blast crisis contained both the L-6 and K-28 junctions. This suggests alternative splicing is a rare event and occurs more frequently in blast crisis.

SUMMARY AND SIGNIFICANCE

It is now clear that PCR is a powerful molecular tool that allows the detection of minimal residual disease at a highly sensitive level. Furthermore, using such specific modifications as reverse transcriptase, one can definitively identify the two unique transcripts present in CML. Thus when one combines the sensitivity of PCR with the specificity for the disease (the *bcr-abl* transcripts) this methodology offers a specific detection system for minimal residual disease in CML. However, since we have so far detected these transcripts in patients who are cytogenetically and Southern blot negative and also have sustained remission, we do not know the long-term significance of PCR positivity. This is especially true in follicular lymphoma: some PCR-positive patients have been in clinical remission for longer than 10 years. Therefore, future studies must incorporate other parameters of cell growth and differentiation to determine the proliferative and biologic activities of the Ph[1]-positive cells as detected by PCR. One imminent possibility for determining the significance of using PCR technology is the investigation of whether the type of transcript present in CML relates to prognosis. In the final analysis PCR offers a tremendous opportunity for the biologic study of human neoplasia.

REFERENCES

1. Smith, B. R., Weinberg, D. S., Robert, N. J., Towle, M., Luther, E., Pinkus, G. S., and Ault, K. A. (1984). Circulating monoclonal B lymphocytes in non-Hodgkin's lymphoma. *N. Engl. J. Med. 311*:1476.

2. Hu, E., Trela, M., Thompson, J., Lowder, J., Horning, S., Levy, R., and Sklar, J. (1985). Detection of B-cell lymphoma in peripheral blood by DNA hybridization. *Lancet 2*:1092.
3. Wright, J. J., Poplack, D. G., Bakhshi, A., Reaman, G., Cole, D., Jensen, J. P., and Korsmeyer, S. J. (1987). Gene rearrangements as markers of clonal variations and minimal residual disease in acute lymphoblastic leukemia. *J. Clin. Oncol. 5*:735.
4. Cleary, M. L., Chao, J., Warnke, R., and Sklar, J. (1984). Immunoglobulin gene rearrangement as a diagnostic criterion of B-cell lymphoma. *Proc. Natl. Acad. Sci. USA 81*:593.
5. Lee, M. S., Chang, K. S., Cabanillas, F., Freireich, E. J., Trujillo, J. M., and Stass, S. A. (1987). Detection of minimal residual cells carrying the t(14;18) by DNA sequence amplification. *Science 237*:175.
6. Tsujimoto, Y., Gorham, J., Cossman, J., Jaffee, E., and Croce, C. M. (1985). The t(14;18) chromosome translocations involved in B-cell neoplasms result from mistakes in VDJ joining. *Science 229*:1390.
7. Cleary, M. L., Smith, S. D., and Sklar, J. (1986). Cloning and structural analysis of cDNAs for bcl-2 and a hybrid bcl-2/immunoglobulin transcript resulting from the t(14;18) translocation. *Cell 47*:19.
8. Bakhshi, A., Wright, J. J., Graninger, W., Seto, M., Owens, J., Cossman, J., Jensen, J. P., Goldman, P., and Korsmeyer, S. J. (1987). Mechanism of the t(14;18) chromosomal translocation: Structural analysis of both derivative 14 and 18 reciprocal partners. *Proc. Natl. Acad. Sci. USA 84*:2396.
9. Talpaz, M., Kantarjian, H. M., McCredie, K. B., Keating, M., Trujillo, J., and Gutterman, J. (1987). Clinical investigation of human alpha interferon in chronic myelogenous leukemia. *Blood 69*:1280.
10. Thomas, E. D., Clift, R. A., Fefer, A., Appelbaum, F. R., Beatty, P., Bensinger, W. I., Buckner, C. D., Cheever, M. A., Deeg, H. J., Doney, K., Flournoy, N., Greenberg, P., Hansen, J. A., Martin, P., McGuffin, R., Ramberg, R., Sanders, J. E., Singer, J., Stewart, P., Storb, R., Sullivan, K., Weiden, P. L., and Witherspoon, R. (1986). Marrow transplantation for the treatment of chronic myelogenous leukemia. *Ann. Intern. Med. 104*:155.
11. Rowley, J. D. (1973). A new consistent chromosomal abnormality in chronic myelogenous leukemia identified by quinacrine fluorescence and Giemsa staining. *Nature 243*:290.
12. Whang-Peng, J., Canellos, G. P., Carbone, P. P., and Tjio, J. H. (1968). Clinical implications of cytogenetic variants in chronic myelocytic leukemia (CML). *Blood 32*:755.
13. Groffen, J., Stephenson, J. R., Heisterkamp, N., de Klein, A., Bartram, C. R. and Grosveld, G. (1984). Philadelphia chromosomal breakpoints are clustered within a limited region, bcr, on chromosome 22. *Cell 36*:93.
14. Heisterkamp, N., Stam, K., Groffen, J., de Klein, A., and Grosveld, G. (1985). Structural organization of the bcr gene and its role in the Ph^1 translocation. *Nature 315*:758.

15. Heisterkamp, N., Stephenson, J. R., Groffen, J., Hansen, P. F., de Klein, A., Bartram, C. R., and Grosveld, G. (1983). Localization of the c-*abl* oncogene adjacent to a translocation breakpoint in chronic myelocytic leukemia. *Nature 306*:239.
16. Bernarde, A., Rubin, C. M., Westbrook, C. A., Paskind, M., and Baltimore, D. (1987). The first intron in the human c-*abl* gene is at least 200 kilobases long and is a target for translocation in chronic myelogenous leukemia. *Mol. Cell. Biol.* 7:3231.
17. Shtivelman, E., Lifshitz, B., Gale, R. P., Roe, B. A., and Canaani, E. (1986). Alternative splicing of RNAs transcribed from the human *abl* gene and from the *bcr/abl* fused gene. *Cell 47*:277.
18. Shtivelman, E., Gale, R. P., Dreazen, O., Berrebi, A., Zaizov, R., Kubonishi, I., Miyoshi, I., and Canaani, E. (1987). *bcr/abl* RNA in patients with chronic myelogenous leukemia. *Blood 69*:971.
19. Lee, M. S., Chang, K. S., Freireich, E. J., Kantarjian, H. M., Talpaz, M., Trujillo, J. M., and Stass, S. A. (1988). Detection of minimal residual *bcr/abl* transcripts by a modified polymerase chain reaction. *Blood 72*:893.
20. Lee, M. S., LeMaistre, A., Kantarjian, H. M., Talpaz, M., Freireich, E. J., Trujillo, J. M., and Stass, S. A. (1989). Detection of two alternative *bcr/abl* mRNAs and minimal residual disease in Philadelphia chromosome positive chronic myelogenic leukemia by polymerase chain reaction. *Blood 73*:2165.
21. Kawasaki, E. S., Clark, S. S., Coyne, M. Y., Smith, S. D., Champlin, R., Witte, O. N., and McCormick, F. P. (1988). Diagnosis of chronic myelogenous leukemia and acute leukemia by detection of leukemia-specific mRNA sequences amplified in vitro. *Proc. Natl. Acad. Sci. USA 85*:5689.
22. Hermans, A., Selleri, L., Gow, J., and Grosveld, G. C. (1988). Absence of alternative splicing in *bcr/abl* mRNA in chronic myeloid leukemia cell lines. *Blood 72*:2066.
23. Dobrovic, A., Trainor, K. J., and Morley, A. A. (1988). Detection of the molecular abnormality in chronic myeloid leukemia by use of the polymerase chain reaction. *Blood 72*:2063.
24. Berk, A. J., and Sharp, P. A. (1977). Sizing and mapping of early adenovirus mRNAs by electrophoresis of SI exonuclease-digested hybrids, *Cell 12*:721.
25. Saiki, R. K., Scharf, S., Faloona, F., Mullis, K. B., Horn, G. T., Erlich, M. A. and Arnheim, N. (1985). Enzymatic amplification of α-globulin genomic sequences and restriction site analysis for diagnosis of sickle cell anemia. *Science 230*:1350.
26. Saiki, R. K., Gelfand, D. H., Stoffel, S., Sharf, S. J., Higuchi, R., Horn, G. T., Mullis, K. B., and Erlich, H. A. (1988). Primer-directed enzymatic amplification of DNA with a thermostable DNA polymerase. *Science 239*: 487.

10

bcr-abl Structure and Expression in Chronic Myelogenous Leukemia Chronic Phase and Blast Phase

Steven J. Collins *Fred Hutchinson Cancer Research Center, Seattle, Washington*

INTRODUCTION

Chronic myelogenous leukemia (CML) is a clonal disorder involving a pluripotent stem cell from which granulocytes, erythrocytes, platelets, monocytes, macrophages, and B lymphocytes arise (1). A prominent feature of CML is the distinct clinical phase of the illness. The relatively benign chronic phase, characterized by hyperplasia of functionally mature granulocytes, inevitably progresses to the blast crisis phase in which immature blasts predominate and which usually proves lethal. There is considerable experimental and epidemiologic evidence indicating that the pathogenesis of malignancy is a multistage phenomenon, that cancer results not from a single mutation but from a series of mutations. The distinct clinical phases of CML together with the relative ease of obtaining leukemic patient samples at different stages of the disease combine to make CML one of the most important and widely studied examples in clinical medicine of this multistage pathogenesis of malignancy.

An important genetic event in the clonal development of CML involves the acquisition of the Philadelphia chromosome (Ph), which is present in over 90% of cases of CML. This aberrant chromosomal marker is generated by a reciprocal translocation between chromosomes 9 and 22 in which the c-*abl* oncogene is translocated from its usual position on the distal end of the q arm of chromosome 9 to a relatively restricted 5-6 kb region on chromosome 22, termed the breakpoint cluster region (*bcr*) (2,3). The breakpoint cluster region lies within the coding region of a relatively large (>50 kb of genomic sequences) gene that has been termed the *bcr* gene (4). The Philadelphia translocation generates a relatively large 8 kb *bcr-abl* fusion transcript (5-7) that codes for the aberrant *bcr-abl* fusion protein product (p210) that has been demonstrated in CML (8,9). The p210 *bcr-abl* fusion product has enhanced tyrosine kinase activity compared with the normal p145 c-*abl* product (8).

The presence of the aberrant *bcr-abl* fusion transcript coding for the p210 protein product in most cases of CML suggests that formation of the *bcr-abl* fusion gene is intimately involved in the pathogenesis of chronic-phase CML. What molecular events are involved in the evolution of CML from chronic phase to blast crisis? The acquisition of the *bcr-abl* fusion gene by itself cannot account for the progression of CML to blast crisis since many patients remain in stable chronic phase for years while harboring this aberrant fusion gene. Presumably other genetic events or mutations are involved in the progression of CML to blast crisis. In this chapter we review the molecular genetic events, particularly those involving the *bcr-abl* fusion gene, that may contribute to the progression of CML from chronic phase to blast crisis. The possible role of *bcr-abl* fusion gene copy number, of enhanced expression of the *bcr-abl* fusion transcript, and of mutations in other oncogenes including N-*ras* in the progression of CML from chronic phase to blast crisis are discussed.

COPY NUMBER OF THE *bcr-abl* FUSION GENE IN CHRONIC PHASE VERSUS BLAST CRISIS

Genomic Amplification of *bcr-abl* in CML

There are several examples in clinical medicine of an association between genomic amplification of certain oncogenes and the progression of particular malignancies. For example, in childhood neuroblastoma amplification and enhanced expression of the N-*myc* oncogene are associated with advanced disease and a significantly poorer prognosis (10). In small cell cancer of the lung genomic amplification of members of the *myc* family of oncogenes is associated with shortened survival (11). In human breast cancer there appears to be a statistically significant correlation between the presence of genomic amplification of the *neu* (also referred to as *HER*-2) oncogene and the time to relapse and overall patient survival (12).

This association between oncogene amplification and stage of disease for certain human malignancies raises the question of whether an analogous situation exists in CML; that is, is genomic amplification and enhanced expression of the aberrant *bcr-abl* fusion gene involved in the progression of CML from chronic phase to blast crisis? We have previously demonstrated that the K562 CML blast crisis cell line exhibits a four- to eightfold amplification and enhanced expression of the c-*abl* oncogene (13). Interestingly the immunoglobulin λ constant region locus is also amplified some four- to eightfold in this cell line, and in situ hybridization suggests that both the c-*abl* and immunoglobulin λ genes are tandemly amplified on an aberrant marker chromosome in K562 (14). These observations suggest that both the *bcr-abl* fusion gene and the immunoglobulin λ constant region locus reside on the same amplified unit in K562. This observation of genomic amplification of *bcr-abl* is interesting and suggests that this amplification may be related to the progression of the disease. Nevertheless, the genomic amplification of the *bcr-abl* fusion gene exhibited by the K562 cell line appears to be very unusual. We have performed Southern blot analysis of over 40 other CML samples (including over 20 blast crisis cells) but have not observed a similar degree of genomic amplification or found evidence of tandem amplification of the *bcr-abl* gene in any of these samples. In some CML blast crisis samples we have noted a two- to threefold amplification of a rearranged c-*abl* fragment (15, 16), but this degree of amplification is directly related to the number of Ph chromosomes per metaphase, suggesting that a single copy of the *bcr-abl* fusion gene rather than multiple copies was present on each of the multiple Ph chromosomes in these blast crisis patient samples.

Acquisition of Multiple Ph Chromosomes in CML

The evolution of CML from chronic phase to blast crisis is commonly associated with karyotypic changes, the most frequent of which is the development of two or more Ph chromosomes (17). This acquisition of multiple Ph chromosomes is noted in approximately 50% of blast crisis CML samples. Do the additional Ph chromosomes that frequently arise during the progression of CML from chronic phase to blast crisis result from a duplication of a pre-existing Ph, or do they result from a new 9;22 translocation event? This question can be addressed utilizing Southern blot analysis of genomic digests of CML samples probed with a *bcr* fragment. The breakpoint cluster region is an approximately 5-6 kb region on chromosome 22, which lies within the coding region of the *bcr* gene (3,4). In most cases of CML the breakpoint on the Ph lies within the *bcr* so that Southern blot analysis of CML DNA utilizing molecular probes within and flanking this region detects an aberrant rearranged fragment in addition to the normal chromosome 22 germline *bcr* fragment (3). Moreover, there is variation in the location of the chromosome 9 and 22 breakpoints in individual Philadelphia chromosomes such that the size of the rearranged *bcr* fragment varies from sample to sample. Thus a restriction endonuclease analysis of CML genomic DNA utilizing *bcr* probes provides a means of "fingerprinting" individual Ph chromosomes. In samples with more than one Ph chromosome, a second rearranged *bcr* fragment is noted on a Southern blot analysis if this second Ph arose from a second independent 9;22 translocation. However, in all six CML samples harboring multiple

Ph chromosomes that we have analyzed to date, we have noted only a single rearranged *bcr* fragment, suggesting that the new Ph chromosomes arose from a duplication (or triplication) of the initial Ph rather than from an independent translocation event (15). This analysis, however, was limited to analyzing breakpoints in the breakpoint cluster region itself and does not completely rule out a second independent Ph translocation. For example, in a significant number of cases of Ph-positive acute lymphoblastic leukemia, the chromosome 22 breakpoint lies within the *bcr* gene farther upstream from the breakpoint cluster region itself (18). Breaks in this region would not be detected with the usual breakpoint cluster region probes. Conceivably a second Ph chromosome involving a chromosome 22 break farther upstream in the *bcr* could arise during the progression of CML from chronic phase to blast crisis and probes farther upstream in the *bcr* gene would be necessary to detect such breaks.

Studies we have performed on a patient with CML who presented in lymphoid blast crisis with three Ph chromosomes per metaphase provide some insight into the relationship between the acquisition of multiple Ph chromosomes and the evolution of CML to blast crisis (16). At clinical presentation, in this patient's peripheral blood there were a significant number of terminally differentiating granulocytes in addition to the lymphoid blast crisis cells, and this allowed ready separation of chronic-phase granulocytes from the lymphoid blasts. A Southern blot analysis readily distinguished these lymphoid blast crisis cells from the terminally differentiating granulocytes, since only the blasts exhibited a rearrangement of the immunoglobulin heavy-chain J_H locus. In addition, Southern blot analysis of the patient blasts utilizing a 5′ c-*abl* probe revealed a rearranged c-*abl* fragment as well as the expected germline c-*abl* fragment. This rearranged c-*abl* fragment was amplified in the blasts, most likely reflecting the presence of the multiple Ph chromosomes per metaphase. Thus by comparing the intensity of hybridization of the amplified, rearranged c-*abl* fragment to the germline c-*abl* fragment the number of Ph chromosomes that each isolated cell population harbors could be estimated. We isolated blast crisis cells from this patient at the time of initial presentation and at the time of relapse. We also isolated terminally differentiated granulocytes at initial presentation and during a chemotherapy-induced partial "remission" when the peripheral blood blast population fell below 5%. We then performed Southern blot analysis on each of these samples to see which exhibited amplification of the rearranged c-*abl* fragment. If one of the major genetic events that distinguishes the lymphoid blast crisis cells from the terminally differentiated chronic-phase granulocytes is the development of multiple Ph chromosomes with concomitant amplification of the rearranged c-*abl* fragment, then one would predict that the terminally differentiated granulocytes would not display amplification of the rearranged c-*abl* fragment (i.e., precursors of these granulocytes display a single Ph). However, we were somewhat surprised to note that this was clearly not the case since the

Southern blot analysis indicated that the c-*abl* fragment was amplified to a similar degree in both the lymphoid blast crisis and granulocyte cell populations (16). In this particular patient it can be concluded that the development of multiple Ph chromosomes per se was not the sole genetic event leading to blast crisis suggesting that there are other genetic factors besides multiple Ph chromosomes that distinguish blast crisis from chronic-phase cells.

EXPRESSION OF THE *bcr-abl* FUSION TRANSCRIPT, CHRONIC PHASE VERSUS BLAST CRISIS

Patterns of Expression of the Normal *bcr* Gene

The evolution of CML from chronic phase to blast crisis may be related to the level of expression of the *bcr-abl* fusion gene. That is, the progression of CML to blast crisis may involve enhanced expression of the aberrant *bcr-abl* fusion transcript and p210 protein product. As noted earlier, tandem amplification of the *bcr-abl* fusion gene is rare in CML and acquisition of multiple Ph chromosomes occurs in no more than 50% of cases. Nevertheless, the *bcr-abl* fusion gene copy number may be only one determinant of *bcr-abl* gene expression. What other factors may be involved in controlling expression of the *bcr-abl* fusion transcript? Since the 5′ end of this aberrant transcript consists of *bcr* sequences (4,7) and since the important regulatory sequences of most genes are generally at the 5′ end, it is probable that the normal *bcr* gene and the *bcr-abl* fusion gene share the same 5′ regulatory sequences. This suggests that factors regulating normal *bcr* gene expression may also be involved in regulating expression of the aberrant *bcr-abl* hybrid transcript. Thus we have studied the patterns of expression of the normal *bcr* gene in an attempt to gain greater insight into the transcriptional control of the aberrant CML *bcr-abl* hybrid gene (19). We were particularly interested in determining whether there was preferential *bcr* expression in hematopoietic versus nonhematopoietic cells; whether there was a differential expression of the *bcr* gene in myeloid versus erythroid cells or T cells versus B cells; and whether *bcr* expression was different in resting versus actively proliferating cells.

We cloned a 3 kb *bcr*-specific cDNA clone from an HL-60 cDNA library and noted by Northern blot hybridization the presence of two *bcr* transcripts 7 and 4.5 kb in size in virtually all human cell types examined (19). Specifically we demonstrated approximately equal amounts of these *bcr* transcripts in a wide variety of different human cells. These included cultured hematopoietic cells of T lymphoid (Jurkatt), B lymphoid (Daudi), myeloid (HL-60 and KG-1), and erythroid (HEL) lineages; cultured skin and bone marrow fibroblasts; HL-60 cells terminally differentiated to mature granulocytes with retinoic acid and to macrophagelike cells with TPA; and both resting and actively proliferating peripheral blood lymphocytes. There did not appear to be preferential *bcr* expression in one human cell type versus another or in actively proliferating versus nonproliferating cells. Moreover we found the *bcr* gene to be evolutionarily conserved, and we identified distinct *bcr*-related fragments in Southern blots of mouse and chick DNA. In chick tissue we noted *bcr* transcripts approximately 6 and 4 kb in size. The highest levels of these transcripts were noted in chick brain, but low, barely detectable levels were noted in chick liver. Chick testes were unusual in exhibiting a truncated, approximately 1 kb *bcr*-related message. The widespread expression of the *bcr* gene as well as its evolutionary conservation suggests that this gene may play an important "housekeeping" role in normal cell physiology. Nevertheless the function of this gene product is at present unknown. The *bcr* 4.5 kb cDNA has been cloned and sequenced, and the deduced amino acid sequences have been compared by computer search with other known protein sequences without revealing any homologous proteins (20).

Expression of *bcr* and *bcr-abl* in CML

We also examined the expression of the normal untranslocated chromosome 22 *bcr* gene in various fresh Ph-positive CML patient samples and in CML blast crisis cell lines. As expected the *bcr* probe identified the aberrant 8 kb *bcr-abl* fusion mRNA that is transcribed from the Ph chromosome and that is also identified by the c-*abl* probe. Moreover, all the CML samples exhibited the normal 7 and 4.5 kb *bcr* transcripts (19). These latter transcripts most likely originate from the *bcr* gene on the normal intact chromosome 22 in these CML cells. Thus there appears to be no allelic exclusion of *bcr* transcription in these CML samples, and this is consistent with the suggestion that the *bcr* gene product may provide an essential cellular function.

We noted by a quantitative slot blot analysis that the relative amounts of Ph chromosome *bcr-abl* hybrid transcripts and normal chromosome 22 *bcr* transcripts were similar within individual CML samples (19). That is, those samples exhibiting relatively high amounts of the *bcr-abl* hybrid transcript also exhibited high amounts of the normal *bcr* transcript. Conversely, those samples exhibiting low amounts of the hybrid transcript also exhibited low amounts of the normal *bcr* transcript. A notable exception to this observation is demonstrated by the CML blast crisis cell line K562, which exhibits relatively large amounts of the *bcr-abl* fusion transcript but relatively small amounts of the normal *bcr* transcript (19). As noted earlier, K562 is exceptional among these CML samples in demonstrating an approximately four- to eightfold genomic amplification of the translocated c-*abl* oncogene. This coordinate expression of the normal *bcr* and the *bcr-abl* fusion transcripts in CML could be explained by the presence of cellular factors that interact with specific regulatory sequences common to both the normal chromosome 22 *bcr* gene and the Ph chromosome *bcr-abl* fusion gene. Thus nuclear factors regulating transcription from the 5′ region of the normal *bcr* gene may also regulate transcription of the *bcr-abl* fusion gene. This would result in approximately equal transcription of *bcr* and *bcr-abl* genes within a given CML sample. The specific nature of such *trans*-activating nuclear factors and the *cis*-acting regulatory sequences of the *bcr* gene with which they may interact are at present unknown.

bcr-abl Expression in Chronic Phase Versus Blast Crisis

We previously noted by Northern blot and dot blot analysis that CML blast crisis cell lines, including K562, EM2 (21), and KCL-22 (22), display enhanced expression of the *bcr-abl* fusion transcript when compared with chronic-phase CML cells (6). By Southern blot analysis we noted that this enhanced RNA expression is present in these cell lines in the absence of genomic amplification of the *bcr-abl* fusion gene (6). These observations suggest that increased expression of the aberrant *bcr-abl* fusion transcript may be critical to the progression of CML from chronic phase to blast crisis. Moreover, this enhanced expression may not be absolutely dependent on the presence of genomic amplification of *bcr-abl* or of the acquisition of multiple Ph chromosomes. To determine the relationship between enhanced expression of the *bcr-abl* fusion transcript and the progression of CML, we quantitated the relative levels of this hybrid transcript in blast crisis versus chronic-phase CML cells (23).

For this study we utilized poly (A) + RNA extracted from the peripheral blood leukocytes of patients with CML in both chronic phase and blast crisis. Patients were considered in chronic phase when peripheral blood indicated a leukocytosis of mostly mature polymorphonuclear leukocytes with fewer than 5% blasts. Patients were considered in blast crisis if the peripheral blood smear revealed greater than 15% blasts. Most blast crisis patients in this study had greater than 50% blasts in the peripheral blood. The blast cell population was further enriched on a Ficoll gradient, and in all cases the leukocyte fraction from blast crisis patients consisted of greater than 70% blasts prior to RNA and DNA extraction.

We probed Northern blots of poly (A) + RNA extracted from these patient samples with a v-*abl* probe that readily identifies the aberrant 8 kb *bcr-abl* fusion transcript originating from the Ph chromosome as well as the normal 7 and 6 kb c-*abl* mRNA that are transcribed from the untranslocated c-*abl* gene on chromosome 9. All these CML samples, both chronic phase and blast crisis, exhibited detectable levels of the *bcr-abl* fusion transcript. In virtually all these individual CML blast crisis samples a comparison of hybridization intensity of these three *abl* transcripts indicated that the aberrant 8 kb *bcr-abl* fusion transcript is the predominant *abl*-related message. Nevertheless we found considerable variation in the amount of this aberrant transcript from sample to sample, with approximately 50% of the blast crisis patients exhibiting relatively high amounts of this aberrant transcript but in the remaining samples the level of the *bcr-abl* transcript was comparable to the relatively low levels exhibited by chronic-phase CML samples (23). Relatively high levels of the *bcr-abl* fusion transcript were noted only in blast crisis samples. We have not to date observed a chronic-phase patient who exhibits relatively high levels of *abl*-related RNA.

Some of the patient blast crisis CML cells exhibit levels of the aberrant *bcr-abl* fusion transcript comparable to the K562 blast crisis cell line, which has amplified the c-*abl* oncogene four- to eightfold. However, although some of these high-expressing blast crisis samples displayed multiple Ph chromosomes per metaphase; others harbored a single Ph chromosome and did not demonstrate evidence of genomic amplification of c-*abl* by Southern blot analysis (23). Therefore, as is the case with certain cultured CML blast crisis cell lines noted earlier, mechanisms other than increased copy number of the *bcr-abl* fusion gene must be involved in the enhanced expression of the *bcr-abl* transcript in certain fresh patient blast crisis samples. Perhaps these mechanisms involve activation of specific *trans*-activating nuclear factors interacting with the *cis* regulatory sequences of the *bcr-abl* fusion gene (as well as the normal *bcr* gene), as discussed earlier.

Another study quantitating expression of the *bcr-abl* transcript in CML chronic-phase versus blast crisis cells, which utilized an S_1 nuclease analysis of steady-state mRNA, also demonstrated no consistent relationship between enhanced expression of the *bcr-abl* hybrid transcript and the blast crisis phase of CML (24).

It should be emphasized that these studies, which indicate no consistent correlation between expression of *bcr-abl* and the stage of CML, have involved a quantitation of the level of *bcr-abl* mRNA rather than the level or activity of the p210 *bcr-abl* fusion product itself. There may not necessarily be a direct relationship between the amount of *bcr-abl* mRNA transcript and the tyrosine kinase activity of the p210 *bcr-abl* fusion product. For instance, during the evolution of CML from chronic phase to blast crisis mutations within the *bcr-abl* fusion gene may arise that markedly increase the efficiency of translation of the *bcr-abl* transcript such that for a given amount of *bcr-abl* mRNA there may be a significant increase in the amount of the *bcr-abl* fusion product. Alternatively certain enzymes may be involved in regulating the activity of the p210 *bcr-abl* fusion product. An alteration in the activity of such enzymes may increase the tyrosine kinase activity of a given amount of p210 in CML cells and may lead to progressive disease. These are merely speculations, however, and will remain so until the physiologic role of both the normal c-*abl* product and the aberrant p210 *bcr-abl* fusion product are better clarified.

Other subtle changes may occur in the expression of the *bcr-abl* fusion gene during the evolution of CML to blast crisis. For example, the junction point of the *bcr-abl* fusion transcript in virtually all patients with Ph-positive CML consists of either *bcr* exon 2 or *bcr* exon 3 fused with the beginning of c-*abl* exon

II (24,25). Some recent studies suggest that CML patients with breakpoints in the 3′ end of the breakpoint cluster region exhibit more aggressive disease than those with more 5′ breakpoints (26). Patient CML samples exhibiting breaks in the 3′ end of the breakpoint cluster region generally have *bcr* exon 3 fused to c-*abl*; patients with more 5′ breakpoints have *bcr* exon 2 fused to c-*abl*. In some CML cells with 3′ breakpoints there is alternative splicing such that both *bcr* exon 2 and *bcr* exon 3 fusion transcripts are expressed in the same sample (24, 25). A possibility consistent with these observations is that the inclusion of *bcr* exon 3 within the fusion transcript may be related to more aggressive disease. Perhaps in patients exhibiting both fusion transcripts the *bcr* exon 3 transcript becomes the predominant transcript as the disease evolves from chronic phase to blast crisis. Again this is hypothetical and has not been experimentally confirmed.

ALTERATION ON OTHER ONCOGENES IN CML BLAST CRISIS

An Alteration in c-*myc* in a CML Blast Crisis Patient

The studies already discussed have concentrated on the changes occurring in the structure and expression of the *bcr-abl* fusion gene during the evolution of CML from chronic phase to blast crisis. Nevertheless there may be genetic events other than those involving the *bcr-abl* fusion gene that may lead to the progression of CML. Such genetic events could involve other specific oncogenes. For example, in a CML patient with promyelocytic blast crisis, genomic amplification of the c-*myc* oncogene was demonstrated in the patient blasts but not in the chronic-phase cells (27). This genomic c-*myc* amplification in this particular patient may be an unusual event since we have not observed a similar amplification of c-*myc* in any of our blast crisis samples. Nevertheless this observation points out the possible involvement of oncogenes other than *bcr-abl* in the evolution of blast crisis.

N-*ras* Point Mutations in CML

A likely candidate cellular oncogene that may be involved in the progression of CML to blast crisis is the N-*ras* proto-oncogene. Point mutations of members of the *ras* family of oncogenes have been described in approximately 10–20% of a wide variety of human malignancies (28). Acute myeloid leukemia (AML) cells exhibit a relatively high incidence of such point mutations, with some 25–50% of AML samples harboring single point mutations in the N-*ras* proto-oncogene at codons 12, 13, or 61 (29–33). The reason that AML cells exhibit selective point mutations in N-*ras* as opposed to other members of the *ras* proto-oncogene family is at present unknown but suggests that certain cellular oncogenes are preferentially activated in malignancies of a particular differentiative lineage. Indeed there are distinct hematopoietic lineage similarities between AML and CML. For example, some cases of AML, like CML, involve transformation of a multipotent hematopoietic stem cell (34). Moreover, the phenotype and clinical behavior of myeloid blast crisis CML closely resembles the phenotype of AML. Given these similarities the question arises of whether the incidence of N-*ras* point mutations in CML blast crisis approaches the relatively high incidence of N-*ras* point mutations that have been observed in AML and whether the acquisition of such point mutations is associated with the evolution of CML chronic phase to blast crisis.

We have directly addressed this question by surveying a series of CML chronic-phase and blast crisis samples to determine the incidence of N-*ras* point mutations at codons 12, 13, or 59-63 in these leukemic cells. For this survey we utilized a technique that involves the direct sequencing of N-*ras* genomic fragments that have been amplified in vitro utilizing the polymerase chain reaction (PCR) (35). This is an extremely powerful technique that requires relatively small amounts of genomic DNA, can accommodate a relatively large number of samples, and can document *ras* point mutations much more rapidly and efficiently than the laborious NIH 3T3 transforming assay that was initially utilized to identify the presence of *ras* point mutations in human tumor DNA (36,37).

We analyzed 41 fresh CML samples and 3 CML blast crisis cell lines. A Southern blot analysis of these samples utilizing specific 3′ and 5′ probes lying within the breakpoint cluster region indicated that 42 of 44 of these samples exhibited *bcr* rearrangements. The two negative samples were both Ph chromosome positive and may harbor breakpoints farther upstream within the *bcr* gene (18). The CML samples included 23 patients in chronic phase and 18 in blast crisis, as well as the 3 blast crisis cell lines. Using the PCR we successfully amplified and gel purified the appropriate N-*ras* genomic fragments in all 44 samples. Direct DNA sequencing of these fragments indicated, somewhat surprisingly, that none of them harbored point mutations in N-*ras* codons 12, 13, or 59-63.

Why are N-*ras* point mutations so infrequent in Ph-positive CML cells and relatively frequent in AML? Presumably, mutations of cellular oncogenes are maintained in malignant cells because they convey a selective proliferative advantage over cells not harboring such mutations. Both the c-*abl* and N-*ras* gene products are known to be associated with the cell membrane, and both may be involved in regulating signal transduction pathways that are triggered by specific proliferative signals. The generation of the *bcr-abl* fusion protein or the acquisition of N-*ras* point mutations in a hematopoietic stem cell may somehow alter a proliferation signal transduction pathway to favor proliferation. If both c-*abl* and N-*ras* are involved in the same or a similar proliferative signal transduction pathway(s) and if a mutation in either one of these proto-oncogenes can significantly alter this regulatory pathway to favor proliferation, then an activating point mutation arising in N-*ras* may not offer a significant proliferative advantage to a cell that already harbors an activated *bcr-abl* fusion gene. This may explain the rarity of demonstrable N-*ras* point mutations in Ph-positive CML cells. This explanation is hypothetical, however, and will remain so until there is a clearer understanding of the normal physiologic function of the c-*abl* and N-*ras* proto-oncogenes, as well as the relationship of this function to proliferative signal transduction in hematopoietic cells.

SUMMARY

Heterogeneity in CML Blast Crisis

We have attempted to determine the molecular events involved in the progression of CML from chronic phase to blast crisis. Unlike chronic-phase CML, in which virtually all patients display a common genetic alteration (i.e., the Philadelphia translocation), the development of blast crisis CML appears to be associated with heterogeneity in such molecular alterations. Thus some blast crisis samples exhibit genomic amplification of the *bcr-abl* fusion gene but others do not; some blast crisis samples display enhanced expression of the *bcr-abl* fusion transcript but others do not. Moreover, it will not be surprising if future studies indicate heterogeneity in the different types of oncogenes that may be altered in the evolution of CML from chronic phase to blast crisis. This heterogeneity in the genetic alterations that may be involved in the progression of CML may reflect the phenotypic heterogeneity generally found in CML blasts from patient to patient. In contrast to chronic-phase CML, which almost uniformly presents as granulocytic hyperplasia, there is considerable phenotypic variation in CML blast crisis, with some patient blasts exhibiting predominantly myeloid phenotype and others demonstrating lymphoid, erythroid, or megakaryocytic characteristics (38). This heterogeneity most likely reflects the transformation of the pluripotent stem cell that characterizes chronic-phase CML (1). Thus the genetic events that occur in chronic-phase CML cells and lead to the evolution of lymphoid blast crisis may differ from those genetic events leading to myeloid, erythroid, or megakaryocytic blast crisis. In contrast to chronic-phase CML, there may not be a common genetic alteration that occurs in the progression of CML to blast crisis.

Questions for the Future

Chronic myelogenous leukemia has historically served as a model for studying the relationship between the acquisition of a specific genetic mutation (i.e., the Ph chromosome translocation) and the clonal development and progression of malignancy. The recent identification of both the c-*abl* and *bcr* genes as intimately involved in the Ph translocation represents a major advance in our understanding of the molecular pathogenesis of this disorder. Nevertheless there remain numerous questions to be addressed concerning the relationship of this specific chromosomal translocation to the pathogenesis of CML. What is the physiologic role of the c-*abl* proto-oncogene, and how is this role disrupted in the *bcr-abl* fusion gene product? What is the normal cellular function of the *bcr* gene? Why are certain regions within the *bcr* gene particularly prone to breakage and fusion with c-*abl*? Why does the *bcr-abl* fusion gene manifest itself predominantly in the neoplastic hematopoietic stem cells of CML rather than in other types of human malignancies? What are the additional genetic events that occur in CML as the disease evolves from chronic phase to blast crisis? These are fundamental questions, and none will be easy to answer. Nevertheless the insight gained in the next several years in addressing these questions not only should increase our knowledge of the pathogenesis of CML but will undoubtedly be relevant to understanding the development and progression of other human malignancies as well.

REFERENCES

1. Fialkow, P., Jacobson, R., and Papayannopoulou, T. (1977). Chronic myelocytic leukemia: Clonal origin in a stem cell common to the granulocytic, erythrocyte, platelet and monocyte/macrophage. *Am. J. Med. 63*:125–131.
2. de Klein, A., Guerts van Kessel, A., Grosveld, G., Bartram, C., Hagemeijer, A., Bootsma, D., Spurr, N., Heisterkamp, N., Groffen, J., and Stephenson, J. (1982). A cellular oncogene is translocated to the Philadelphia chromosome in chronic myelocytic leukemia. *Nature 300*:765–767.
3. Groffen, J., Stephenson, J., Heisterkamp, N., de Klein, A., Bartram, C., and Grosveld, G. (1984). Philadelphia chromosomal breakpoints are clustered within a limited region, *bcr*, on chromosome 22. *Cell 36*:93–99.
4. Heisterkamp, N., Stam, J., Groffen, A., de Klein, A., and Grosveld, G. (1985). Structural organization of the *bcr* gene and its role in the Ph translocation. *Nature 315*:758–761.
5. Canaani, E., Gale, R., Steiner-Saltz, D., Berrebi, A., Aghai, E., and Januszewicz, E. (1984). Altered transcription of an oncogene in chronic myelocytic leukemia. *Lancet 1*:593–595.
6. Collins, S., Kubonishi, I., Miyoshi, I., and Groudine, M. (1984). Altered transcription of the c-*abl* oncogene in K-562 and other chronic myelogenous leukemia cells. *Science 225*:72–75.
7. Shtivelman, E., Lifshitz, B., Gale, R., and Canaani, E. (1985). Fused transcripts of *abl* and *bcr* genes in chronic myelogenous leukemia. *Nature 315*: 758–761.
8. Konopka, J., Watanabe, S., and Witte, O. (1984). An alteration of the human c-*abl* protein in K-562 leukemia cells unmasks associated tyrosine kinase activity. *Cell 37*:1035–1042.
9. Kloetzer, W., Kurzrock, R., Smith, L., Talpaz, M., Spiller, M., Gutterman, J., and Arlinghaus, R. (1985). The human cellular *abl* gene product in the chron-

ic myelogenous leukemia cell line K562 has an associated tyrosine protein kinase activity. *Virology 140*:230–238.

10. Brodeur, G., Seeger, R., Schwab, M., Varmus, H., and Bishop, J. (1984). Amplification of N-*myc* in untreated human neuroblastoma correlates with advanced disease stage. *Science 224*:1121–1124.
11. Johnson, B., Ihde, D., Makuch, R., Gazdar, A., Carney, D., Oie, H., Russell, E., Nau, M., and Minna, J. (1987). *myc* family oncogene amplification in tumor cell lines established from small cell lung cancer patients and its relationship to clinical status and course. *J. Clin. Invest. 79*:1629–1634.
12. Slamon, D., Clark, G., Wong, S., Levin, W., Ullrich, A., and McGuire, W. (1987). Human breast cancer: Correlation of relapse and survival with amplification of the *HER-2/neu* oncogene. *Science 235*:177–182.
13. Collins, S., and Groudine, M. (1983). Rearrangement and amplification of c-*abl* sequences in the human chronic myelogenous leukemia cell line K-562. *Proc. Natl. Acad. Sci. USA 80*:4813–4817.
14. Selden, J., Emanuel, B., Wang, E., Cannizzaro, L., Palumbo, A., Erikson, J., Nowell, P., Rovera, G., and Croce, C. (1983). Amplified C lambda and c-*abl* genes are on the same marker chromosome in K562 cells. *Proc. Natl. Acad. Sci. USA 80*:7289–7292.
15. Collins, S. (1986). Breakpoints on chromosomes 9 and 22 in Philadelphia chromosome positive CML: Amplification of rearranged c-*abl* oncogenes in CML blast crisis. *J. Clin. Invest. 78*:1392–1396.
16. Collins, S., and Groudine, M. (1987). Chronic myelogenous leukemia: Amplification of a rearranged c-*abl* oncogene in both chronic phase and blast crisis. *Blood 69*:893–898.
17. Sandberg, A. (1980). The cytogenetics of CML: Chronic phase and blast crisis. *Cancer Genet. Cytogenet. 217*:217–230.
18. Hermans, A., Heisterkamp, N., von Lindern, M., van Baal, S., Meijer, D., van der Plas, D., Wiedemann, L., Groffen, J., Bootsma, D., and Grosveld, G. (1987). Unique fusion of *bcr* and c-*abl* genes in Philadelphia chromosome positive acute lymphoblastic leukemia. *Cell 51*:33–40.
19. Collins, S., Coleman, H., and Groudine, M. (1987). Expression of *bcr* and *bcr-abl* fusion transcripts in normal and leukemic cells. *Mol. Cell. Biol. 7*: 2870–2876.
20. Hariharan, I., and Adams, J. (1987). cDNA sequence for human *bcr*, the gene that translocates to the *abl* oncogene in chronic myeloid leukemia. *EMBO J. 6*:115–119.
21. Keating, A., Raskind, W., and Singer, J. (1983). Two new Ph positive myeloid cell lines. *UCLA Symp. Mol. Cell. Biol. 11*:513–520.
22. Kubonishi, I., and Miyoshi, I. (1983). Establishment of a Ph chromosome positive cell line from chronic myelogenous leukemia in blast crisis. *Int. J. Cell Cloning 1*:105–117.
23. Andrews, D. F., and Collins, S. (1987). Heterogeneity in expression of the *bcr-abl* fusion transcript in CML blast crisis. *Leukemia 1*:718–724.
24. Shtivelman, E., Gale, R., Dreazen, O., Berribi, R., Zaizov, R., Kubonishi, I., Miyoshi, I., and Canaani, E. (1987). *bcr-abl* RNA in patients with chronic myelogenous leukemia. *Blood 69*:971–973.

25. Shtivelman, E., Lifshitz, B., Gale, R., Roe, B., and Canaani, E. (1986). Alternative splicing of RNAs transcribed from the human *abl* gene and from the *bcr-abl* fused gene. *Cell 47*:277–284.
26. Schaefer,-Rego, K., Dudek, H., Popenoe, D., Arlin, Z., Mears, G., Bank, A., and Leibowitz, D. (1987). CML patients in blast crisis have breakpoints localized to a specific region of the BCR. *Blood 70*:448–455.
27. McCarthy, D., Rassool, F., Goldman, J., Graham, S., and Birnie, G. (1984). Genomic alterations involving the c-*myc* protooncogene locus during the evolution of a case of chronic granulocytic leukemia. *Lancet 1*:1362–1365.
28. Varmus, H. (1984). The molecular genetics of cellular oncogenes. *Annu. Rev. Genet. 18*:560–585.
29. Bos, J., Marshall, C., Verlaan-de Vries, M., Veeneman, G., van der Eb, A., van Boom, J., Janssen, J., and Steenvoorden, A. (1985). Amino-acid substitutions at codon 13 of the N-*ras* oncogene in human acute myeloid leukemia. *Nature 315*:726–730.
30. Gambke, C., Hall, A., and Moroni, C. (1985). Activation of an N-*ras* gene in acute myeloblastic leukemia through somatic mutation in the first exon. *Proc. Natl. Acad. Sci. USA 82*:879–883.
31. Bos, J., Verlaan-de Vries, M., van der Eb, A., Janssen, K., Delwel, R., Lowenberg, B., and Colly, L. (1987). Mutations in N-*ras* predominate in acute myeloid leukemia. *Blood 69*:1237–1242.
32. Needleman, S., Kraus, M., Srivastava, S., Levine, P., and Aaronson, S. (1986). High frequency of N-*ras* activation in acute myelogenous leukemia. *Blood 67*:735–758.
33. Farr, C., Saiki, R., Erlich, H., McCormick, F., and Marshall, C. (1988). Analysis of *ras* gene mutations in acute myeloid leukemia by polymerase chain reaction and oligonucleotide probes. *Proc. Natl. Acad. Sci. USA 85*: 1629–1633.
34. Fialkow, P., Singer, J., Raskind, W., Adamson, J., Jacobson, R., Bernstein, I., Dow, L., Najfeld, V., and Veith, R. (1987). Clonal development, stem cell differentiation, and clinical remission in acute nonlymphocytic leukemia. *N. Engl. J. Med. 317*:468–473.
35. Collins, S. (1988). Direct sequencing of amplified genomic fragments documents N-*ras* point mutations in myeloid leukemia. *Oncogene Res. 3*:117–123.
36. Tabin, C., Bradley, S., Bargmann, C., Weinberg, R., Papageorge, A., Scolnick, E., Dhar, R., Lowy, D., and Chang, E. (1982). Mechanism of activation of a human oncogene. *Nature 300*:143–149.
37. Reddy, E., Reynolds, R., Santos, E., and Barbacid, M. (1982). A point mutation is responsible for the acquisition of transforming properties by the T24 human bladder carcinoma oncogene. *Nature 300*:149–155.
38. Griffin, J., Todd, R., Ritz, J., et al. (1983). Differentiation patterns in the blastic phase of chronic myeloid leukemia. *Blood 61*:85–91.

11

Analysis of the Philadelphia Chromosome by Pulsed-Field Gel Electrophoresis

Carol A. Westbrook *University of Chicago, Chicago, Illinois*

INTRODUCTION

The ability to reproducibly generate and electrophoretically separate very large restriction fragments—from fifty to several thousand kilobases of DNA—has had a major impact on the physical mapping of complex genomes. These long-range restriction mapping methods, collectively referred to here as pulsed-field gel electrophoresis (PFGE), have been used to analyze the genomes of such diverse organisms as yeast, malarial parasites, and *Escherichia coli*, as well as to map subchromosomal regions in the eukaryotic genome, such as the HLA complex. PFGE has provided a great deal of information about the structure of the human *abl* and *bcr* genes and the *bcr-abl* fusion gene found on the Philadelphia (Ph^1) chromosome. The use of PFGE for this purpose provides a model for its eventual use in the diagnosis and management of malignancies associated with other consistently occurring chromosomal abnormalities.

GENERAL PRINCIPLES OF PFGE

Technical Aspects and Equipment

The separation of DNA fragments by size in agarose gels is an important step in Southern hybridization analysis. Standard agarose gel electrophoresis is well suited to the analysis of DNA fragments produced by digestion with the commonly used, commercially available restriction enzymes, which are generally in the 1-20 kilobase (kb) range. For example, the "*bcr* rearrangement test" involves digestion of DNA with such enzymes as *Bam*HI, *Bgl*II, and *Hind*III, electrophoretic separation on agarose gels, and hybridization to probes from the *bcr* region of chromosome 22. The expected germline fragments, as well as the rearranged fragments that are diagnostic of CML, are usually in the 3-20 kb size range and are easily distinguished by this method.

Southern hybridization methods cannot be used to survey large regions of the genome because the upper limit of resolution for agarose gel electrophoresis is about 20 kb. DNA fragments larger than this run at about the same mobility and thus fail to separate by size. The newly developed pulsed-field gel techniques rely on alternating electrical fields that retard the movement of extremely large DNA fragments in a manner that is proportional to length. Resolution in the 50-1000 kb range is routine, with separations of up to 7000 kb under appropriate experimental conditions. Methods for alternating the current vary with the type of apparatus. Orthogonal-field alternating gel electrophoresis (OFAGE) (1,2) and controu clamped homogeneous electrical field electrophoresis (CHEF) (3) rely on arrays of electrodes that produce currents that vary diagonally across the gel. Field inversion gel electrophoresis (FIGE) (4) periodically reverses the polarity of a uniform field. Transverse alternating gel electrophoresis (TAFE) (5) varies the current at angles to the plane of a vertical gel. Newer techniques are continuously being described, although all are substantially equivalent. The type of apparatus used is dictated by such considerations as the size of gel, the ease of use, and the particular parameters being investigated.

Enzymes

Long-range mapping requires two elements: the ability to separate large DNA fragments and the ability to produce these fragments. For most applications, large DNA fragments for PFGE are produced the same way as are small DNA fragments for Southern hybridization: by restriction endonucleases. The generation of larger fragments requires enzymes that have fewer recognition sites within the genome. Enzymes commonly used for restriction mapping cleave DNA at recognition sequences that are 6 basepairs (bp) in length; for example, *Eco*RI recognizes GAATTC. Enzymes with 8 bp specificities produce much larger fragments than those with 6 bp specificity; the only two such enzymes currently available are *Not*I (GCGGGCCGC) and *Sfi*I (GGCCN$_5$GGCC). However, there are restriction endonucleases with 6 bp specificity that produce fragments in the range suitable for PFGE analysis because they have fewer recognition sites within the human genome than would be expected by chance alone, since the distribution of nucleotides within the genome is not random. For example, the G + C content of the human genome is 41%, so enzymes whose recognitions sequences are G + C rich cleave less frequently than those that are A + T rich. Furthermore, the sequence CpG itself is fivefold rarer than would be predicted from the G + C content, which may be a consequence of the hypermutability of 5mCpG, a methylated sequence that occurs extensively in human DNA (6). The rarity of CpG means that restriction endonuclease recognition sites that contain CpG, such as ACGCGT (*Mlu*I), are especially rare. In fact, many *Mlu*I recognition sites are methylated at C, and *Mlu*I does not cleave when its recognition site is methylated (7). This methylation results in even larger restriction fragments than predicted by sequence alone. In addition to *Not*I, *Sfi*I, and *Mlu*I, other enzymes that have been shown to be useful for long-range mapping include *Nru*I (TCGCGA), *Pvu*I (CGATCG), *Rsr*II (CGGWCCG), *Sac*II (CCGCGG), *Bss*HII (GCGCGC), and *Eag*I (CGGCCG).

All these enzymes except *Sfi*I contain methylatable CpGs, and one must be cautious when interpreting the results of PFGE analysis because heterogeneity of methylation can lead to variability in restriction fragment size. Our general experience in the analysis of the *abl* and *bcr* genes in blood cells and cell lines derived from leukemic cells is that most sites are either fully methylated or fully unmethylated in all cells, unambiguously producing a single germline restriction fragment (except for rare polymorphisms). We have found that our restriction maps of *bcr* and *abl* are quite consistent from sample to sample. However, our limited experience also suggests that methylation patterns may differ among tissues. This may be of particular importance when analyzing interspecies somatic cell hybrids or when comparing tumor cell DNA to skin fibroblast DNA of the same individual. Also of note is that methylation patterns are not propagated in cloned DNAs; thus, the identification of a *Not*I or *Mlu*I site within a phage clone of human DNA, or within a DNA sequence, does not unambiguously place the site on the restriction map because it may be uncleavable in the cell being analyzed. This caution does not hold for *Sfi*I, which appears to be unaffected by methylation (7).

Until recently, the commercial availability, purity, and consistency of restriction endonucleases for PFGE analysis have been limited. Trace nuclease contamination, inapparent on standard Southern analysis, is magnified when large fragments are analyzed and has been a common source of difficulty for our studies. Enzyme activity, which is usually tested on DNA in solution, is difficult to standardize in agarose and is another source of inconsistent results. Fortunately, as the demand for PFGE enzymes increases, the enzyme manufacturers are more cognizant of these problems, and high-quality enzymes have become more readily available within the last few years.

Preparation of DNA

Extremely high molecular weight, virtually intact chromosomal DNA is required for PFGE. DNA in solution is not suitable for these studies because shearing during handling reduces its size below that of the restriction fragments to be analyzed

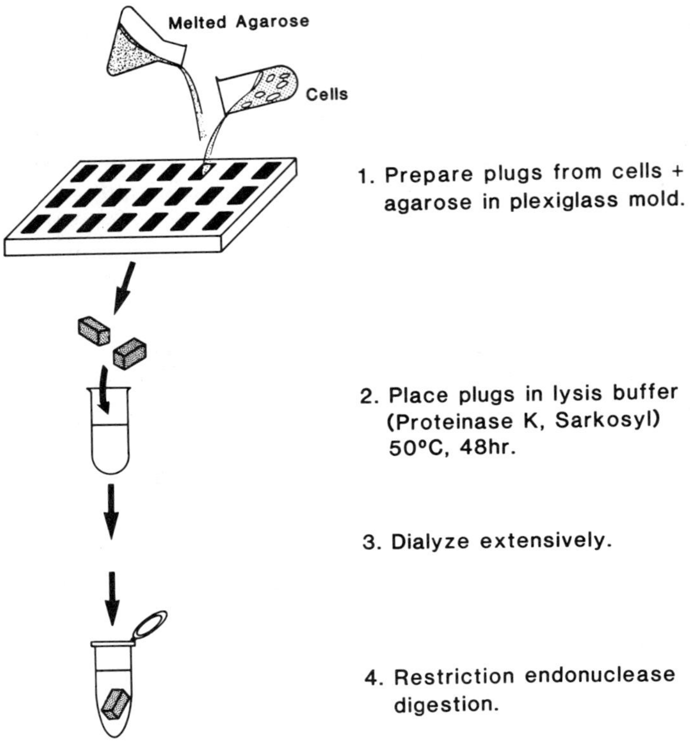

Figure 1 Preparation of high-molecular-weight DNA in agarose plugs for PFGE. Patient cells or cell lines are suspended in culture medium or saline at a concentration of 3.2 million viable cells per mL and mixed with an equal volume of 1% low-gelling temperature agarose in 100 mM NaCl and 0.5 M EDTA at 42°C. The warm agarose-cell mixture is dispensed into 50 μL aliquots each containing 1.6 million cells, or approximately 10 μg DNA, and allowed to set at 4°C. The hardened agarose plugs are placed in a solution containing 1% *n*-lauryl sarcosine, 1 mg/mL of proteinase K, 100 mM NaCl, and 0.5 M EDTA at 50°C for 48 h to lyse the cells and purify the DNA. The plugs are then dialyzed by several changes of TE buffer and stored at 4°C until ready to use. Restriction enzyme digests are carried out directly on the plugs.

and greatly decreases the signal strength. To circumvent this problem, DNA is handled in solid phase during the entire procedure. Very high molecular weight DNA is prepared by embedding viable cells or nuclei in agarose and directly lysing the cells and purifying the DNA in the agarose plugs; enzyme digestion and electrophoresis are performed directly on the agarose plugs, which contain approximately 10 μg DNA. Our protocol for the preparation of agarose plugs, which is based on a procedure devised by Schwartz and Cantor (1), is shown in Figure 1. Using this method, virtually 100% recovery of cellular DNA is obtained making it possible to analyze samples containing small numbers of cells. We find that the agarose plugs keep indefinitely if stored under sterile conditions at refrigerator temperatures, and they can be used for routine Southern analysis as well as for PFGE analysis.

The most important factor in obtaining good-quality DNA is that the starting materials—cell lines or patient cells—are viable at the start of preparation. Thus it is difficult to use frozen cells for preparation of agarose plugs, although cells frozen for viability in dimethylsulfoxide (DMSO) can be used if properly thawed and carefully handled. Occasionally we have had difficulty obtaining adequate plugs from fibroblast cell lines; in these cases preparing isolated nuclei is sometimes helpful, as demonstrated by Yang et al. (8). To ensure uniform amounts of DNA between samples, we routinely do viability counts in trypan blue and prepare our plugs based on the number of viable cells, rather than on the total cell count.

MAPPING THE *abl* GENE

The first long-range map of the *abl* locus (9) was the result of a study of the SUP-T3 cell line, which contained a translocation between chromosomes 7 and 9, t(7;9)(q36;q34). We hypothesized that *abl* was activated by this translocation because the chromosome 9 breakpoint was in the same band as the *abl* gene (band 9q34), and we wanted to examine the genomic region surrounding *abl* for evidence of rearrangement. Using probes kindly supplied by Groffen from within the *abl* common exons, that is, the regions of the gene homologous to v-*abl* and from an unknown distance 5′ of the *abl* common exons that had been cloned from chronic myelogenous leukemia (CML) breakpoints, we prepared a restriction map of this region of the genome. This map was constructed solely on the basis of cross-hybridization of probes to common restriction fragments. The project was unsuccessful in locating the t(7;9) breakpoint; however, it did provide us with a restriction map of 525 kb surrounding the *abl* gene. Although it was suspected that CML translocation breakpoints lie some distance from the v-*abl* homologous regions of the gene, we were quite surprised to find that at least one of our probes was over 200 kb away. Because of the variability in the position of translocation breakpoints and the long distances involved, it was unclear whether the *abl* gene was consistently disrupted in the t(9;22) of CML.

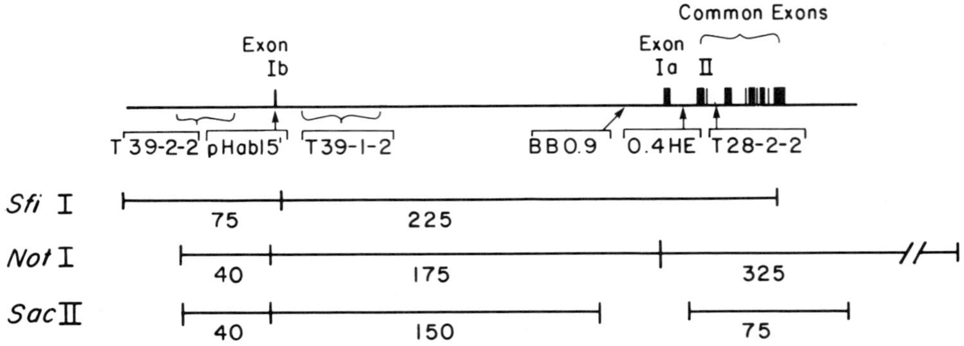

Figure 2 Long-range map of the *abl* locus. The upper line shows the structure of the *abl* gene roughly to scale; the exons are depicted as dark boxes above the line and are labeled according to the convention in Reference 11. The probes used for mapping are indicated by arrows when the precise location is known or by brackets when it has been estimated. The probes are described in References 9, 12, and 15. The bottom lines show the position of the cleavage sites for the indicated restriction enzyme and the sizes of restriction fragments in kilobases.

The participation of *abl* in these translocations became much clearer as more was learned about the unique structure of this gene. Ben Neriah et al. showed that several types of mRNA were transcribed from the murine *abl* gene, which differed in their 5′ terminal sequences, and suggested that they consisted of alternative 5′ exons added onto a set of common 3′ exons (10). Shtivelman et al. (11) reported similar results for the human *abl* gene and located one of these exons (exon Ia) 19 kb upstream of the common exons. The human Ib exon was also cloned but appeared to be even farther away, as it could not be demonstrated within 35 kb upstream of exon Ia. In collaboration with Bernards and Baltimore, we then placed these exons onto the long-range map of the *abl* locus that we obtained during the studies of SUP-T3 (12).

The more complete map of the *abl* gene that resulted from this collaboration is shown in Figure 2. The positions of several *Not*I, *Sfi*I, and *Sac*II sites were verified by direct sequencing as well as by enzymatic cleavage (as noted earlier, *Not*I and *Sac*II sites contain CpGs and are uncleavable if methylated). Several interesting features were immediately apparent upon inspection of this map. First was the size of *abl*; at 230 kb, it was the largest mammalian gene that had been identified at the time. The primary reason for the large size of this gene was the presence of the large first intron, requiring an unprecedented 200 kb splice to produce the type Ib mRNA. Since that time, of course, several very large genes whose transcription requires long-range splicing have been identified. It is noteworthy that at least two of these genes that contain very large introns, *bcr* and *bcl2*, have been shown to participate in chromosomal translocations (Reference 13 and this chapter). Another interesting feature of the *abl* map is the clustering of restriction sites for the rare cutting enzymes *Sac*II, *Sfi*I, and *Not*I, particularly in the vicinity of the promoter regions upstream of exons Ia and Ib. This clustering is no doubt due to the high G + C content of these regions and identifies these promoters as "HTF" islands. HTF islands are described as G + C-rich areas of the genome that usually occur upstream of coding sequences and are thought to play a role in transcriptional regulation (14). In this regard, one can speculate that the *Not*I/*Sac*II cluster 50 kb upstream of exon Ib also identifies an HTF island and that previously unidentified coding sequences may be nearby. It is noteworthy that the *Not*I site upstream of exon Ia is sometimes cleavable (and presumably methylated) when it is translocated to the Ph[1]; we have speculated that this methylation may influence transcription of the normal type Ia *abl* message (15).

The presence of the very large intron contained within the *abl* gene remains a puzzle. It seems remarkably inefficient for the cell to transcribe the entire 230 kb gene to splice a 7 kb mRNA; transcription of an RNA this size has been estimated to take over 2 h to complete (12). Apparently the first common *abl* exon has the ability to accept donor splices from far upstream, which may explain some of the specificity of the *bcr* region as a partner for *abl* on the Ph[1] chromosome, since most CML translocations occur within this large intron. There is also some evidence that the large *abl* intron contains additional coding sequences. Grosveld et al. have observed splicing of *bcr* exons to a sequence within this intron in K562 cells (16). Whether additional *abl* elements are present, either within this intron or upstream of exon Ib, remains to be seen. The reasons for the unique structure of the *abl* gene will become apparent as the function of the *abl* gene and the biology of the c-*abl* protein are better understood.

THE STRUCTURE OF THE *bcr-abl* GENE ON THE PHILADELPHIA CHROMOSOME

The Ph[1] in CML

The availability of a detailed map of *abl* gave us the ability to use PFGE to determine how this gene is involved in the translocations that give rise to the Philadelphia chromosome. For our initial analysis, we studied the BV173 cell line, derived from a patient in blast crisis of CML (15). We chose this cell line because, unlike the more commonly used CML cell line K562, BV173 has a clearly recognizable Ph[1] chromosome (actually it had three copies of the Ph[1]); also, our analysis of the rearranged *abl* gene was simplified because there is no normal *abl* homolog in these cells, which do not contain an intact chromosome 9.

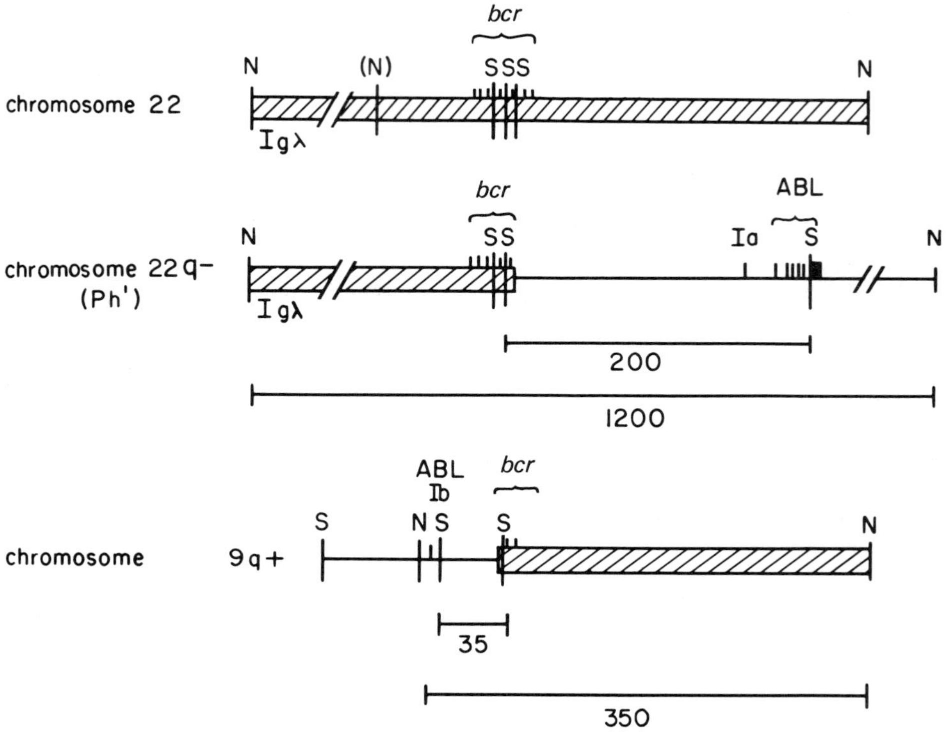

Figure 3A Schematic representation of the *bcr* and *abl* genes in the BV173 cell line. (A) The normal chromosome 22, the $22q^-$ chromosome, and the $9q^+$ chromosome are depicted; there is no normal chromosome 9 in this cell line. Sequences derived from chromosome 22 are shown as hatched lines, those from chromosome 9 as solid lines. The *bcr* and *abl* exons are depicted schematically as solid bars above the lines, and the restriction enzyme sites are shown for *Sfi*I (S) and *Not*I (N). The polymorphic *Not*I site is shown in parentheses. The rearranged *Not*I and *Sfi*I restriction fragments are shown, and the sizes are given in kilobases. (Based on Reference 15.) (B) Rearranged bands in the BV173 cell line. DNA was prepared from lymphoid leukemia cell lines with normal chromosomes 22 [lane 1, RS (4;11); lane 2, ML-2] and from BV173 cells (lane 3). Each lane contains approximately 10 μg DNA, digested with *Not*I and hybridized to the indicated probes. The sizes of the germline (G) and rearranged (R) restriction fragments are given in kilobases. The gel was prepared using the TAFE system (Beckman, Inc.) according to methods described in References 5 and 28.

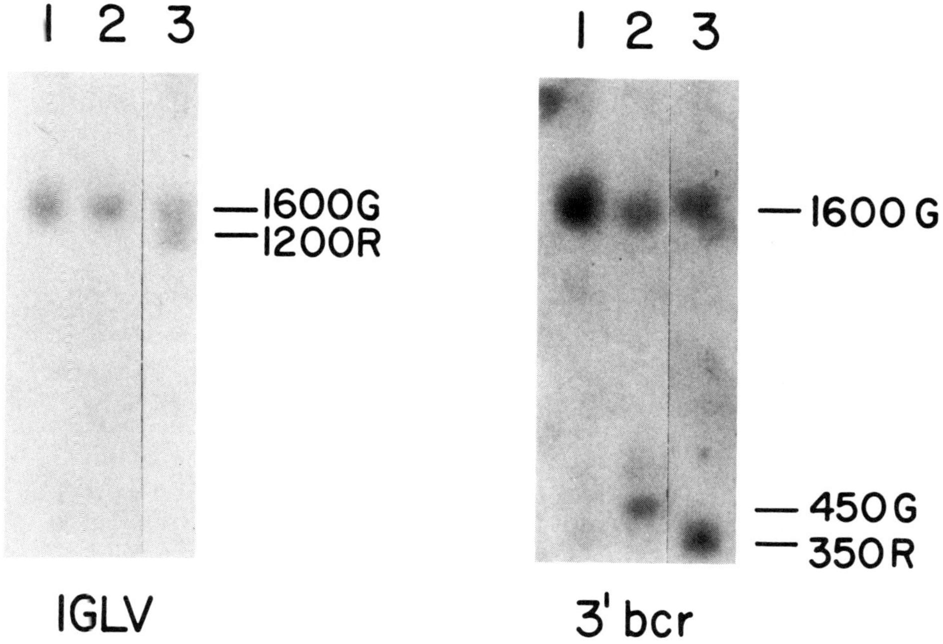

Figure 3B (continued)

Using a series of *abl* and *bcr* probes, as well as probes from the immunoglobulin λ gene, we prepared a final map of this translocation, which is shown in Figure 3. We were able to demonstrate the presence on the Ph^1 of the *bcr-abl* fusion gene, as well as a transcriptionally active, reciprocal 5′ *abl*-3′ *bcr* gene on the $9q^+$ chromosome. These fusion genes were easily demonstrable as rearranged restriction fragments on PFGE gels, similar to the standard "*bcr* rearrangement" but on a 10-fold larger scale. We have confirmed the utility of this approach by direct analysis of cells from several CML patients (Westbrook and Rubin, unpublished observations). We have also found that it is usually possible to determine the precise location of the breakpoint within the *abl* gene by the size of the rearranged *Sfi*I restriction fragments, since the location of the *Sfi*I sites was known for both the *bcr* and *abl* genes.

It is clear that most CML breakpoints lie within the large first *abl* intron, the majority of these within the 175 kb region between exons Ib and Ia. Several breakpoints have also been documented to occur within the 20 kb region between exons Ia and the first common exon (17,18). Although we have never done a systematic study, we believe that this distribution is consistent with a random occurrence of breakpoints and reflects the fact that the 175 kb region between Ib and Ia presents a 10-fold larger target for breakage than the 20 kb region between Ia and the first common exon.

One of the most interesting and unexpected findings in our study of BV173 was the demonstration of physical linkage of the *bcr* gene to the immunoglobulin λ locus. By analysis of somatic cell hybrids, it was previously shown that the λ genes were proximal to *bcr* on the long or q arm of chromosome 22 and that the immunoglobulin λ variable region genes (*IGL V*) were proximal to the immunoglobulin λ constant region genes (*IGLC*) but the physical distances separating these genes was unknown (19). When studying cell lines with normal chromosomes 22, we had observed hybridization of probes from the λ genes to a very large, approximately 1600 kb *Not*I restriction fragment that appeared to be the same size as that to which the *bcr* probes hybridized. We could not verify that both probes actually bound to the same germline fragment rather than to different fragments that happened fortuitously to be the same size. The analysis of the BV173 cell line, however, showed that *IGLC, bcr*, and *abl* genes all hybridized to the 1300 kb *rearranged* restriction fragment that contained the translocation breakpoint, thus demonstrating physical linkage of these genes on the Ph^1 chromosome (15,20). A similar linkage was observed for *IGLC* and *abl* in the SUP-B13 cell line (Westbrook and Rubin, unpublished observations). Furthermore, we also found cross-hybridization of the rearranged bands in BV173 to the probe U266 λV (21), which recognizes an *IGL V* class, as demonstrated in Figure 3B. Thus, there is linkage within 1300 kb of *IGL V* and *IGLC* to the *bcr-abl* fusion gene on the Ph^1, suggesting that *IGL V, IGLC*, and *bcr* are also linked on the normal chromosome 22.

The linkage of *IGLC* and *bcr* is not straightforward, however; in some samples, the *bcr* probes hybridize to a 450 kb band that does not hybridize to *IGLC* or *IGL V* probes. We have interpreted this to mean that there is a polymorphic *Not*I site between the immunoglobulin λ and the *bcr* genes (20). If this is the case, we would expect to see a smaller, 1200 kb *Not*I fragment hybridizing to the λ genes, but we have never observed a smaller fragment. There are several explanations for this discrepancy. It is possible that *IGLC* and *bcr* are much farther apart in the germline state, and the observed linkage on the Ph^1 may be unique to the particular cell lines studied, resulting from deletion of intervening sequences. Alternatively, the 450 kb *Not*I band may be accompanied by deletion of the λ genes. This is a particularly intriguing hypothesis, because we have only seen the 450 kb *bcr* band in lymphoid cell lines or lymphoid leukemias. Finally, the putative 1200 kb *IGLC* band may not be well resolved from the 1600 kb *IGLC* band under usual running conditions. Clearly, a more detailed study of the physical distances within the λ genes and their linkage to the *bcr* region is warranted.

The Ph^1 Chromosome in ALL

Molecular studies distinguished two subtypes of Ph^1-positive ALL, those with *bcr* rearrangements similar to those seen in CML and those characterized by the absence of a *bcr* rearrangement. The long-range restriction maps of the *abl* and *bcr* loci provided the means to investigate this latter group of patients, the "*bcr*-negative" subgroup of Ph^1-positive acute lymphoblastic leukemia (ALL), to determine the chromosomal localization of translocation breakpoints. Using PFGE, we were able to demonstrate in the SUP-B13 cell line, derived from a patient with *bcr*-negative Ph^1-positive ALL, that the breakpoint occurred within the same area in which CML breakpoints occur and suggested that an *abl* fusion gene may result from this translocation (22,23).

The role of the *bcr* gene was much more difficult to analyze. Studies by Erikson et al. (24) and de Klein et al. (25) using somatic cell hybrid analysis and/or in situ chromosomal hybridization showed that probes from the *bcr* translocate to chromosome 9 but the *IGLC* genes remain on chromosome 22 in several cases of *bcr*-negative Ph^1-positive ALL, demonstrating that the breakpoint lies between these two regions. Such a translocation would interrupt the linkage of *IGLC* to *bcr*, so we reasoned that we could detect the chromosome 22 translocation breakpoint using PFGE analysis. Studies of the SUP-B13 cell line showed a 350 kb rearranged *Not*I fragment with the *bcr* probe; this rearranged band represented the 9q$^+$ chromosome. The size of this band allowed us to estimate that the breakpoint occurred 50–250 kb upstream of *bcr* (20,22). Later, more precise mapping of the *abl* breakpoint in these cells to within 10 kb of a *Not*I site showed that the translocation occurred about 40–50 kb upstream of the *bcr* (23).

Probes from within the *abl* second intron enabled us to clone the translocation breakpoint in the SUP-B13 cell line (23). At that time, studies by Hermans et al. (26) had shown that the Ph^1 in *bcr*-negative ALL resulted in a fusion of the most 5′ exon of the *bcr* gene with the *abl* gene. We verified this assumption for the SUP-B13 cell line by showing that a probe for the first, most 5′ exon of the *bcr* gene (as distinguished from exon 1 of the *bcr*) did not hybridize to the 350 kb rearranged *Not*I band representing the 9q$^+$ chromosome but instead recognized a new fragment that also contained sequences from within the *abl* common exons and was derived from the Ph^1 chromosome. As expected, then, the translocation interrupted the *bcr* gene in the large first intron. These studies also enabled us to estimate that the maximum distance of the first *bcr* exon from the *bcr* was 150 kb, since both probes hybridize to the same 450 kb germline *Not*I restriction fragment and *bcr* itself is about 300 kb from the 3′ *Not*I site (see Figure 3). It will not be possible to be more precise about the size of this intron until the location of the restriction sites is known or the entire region is cloned and mapped.

Table 1 Sizes of *Not*I Restriction Fragments (in Kilobases) Determined by PFGE Analysis of Cells from Patients with Ph[1]-Positive ALL[a]

Patient	*bcr* rearrangement	3′ *bcr*		pHabl-5′		pAEB-2.3	
		G	R	G	R	G	R
1	+	1600	375	175	375	1600	1600
2	–	450	400	175	400	450	130
3	+	450	335	175	335	450	310
4	–	1600	470	174	470	1600	470
5	–	450	350	175	350	450	350
6	–	450	460	175	460	450	460
7	–	450	380	175	380	450	380

[a], G, germline fragment sizes; R, rearranged fragment sizes. In column 2, + indicates the presence of a *bcr* rearrangement, – indicates the *bcr* is not rearranged.
Source: Based on Hooberman et al. (28).

PFGE ANALYSIS AS A DIAGNOSTIC TOOL

The chromosome 22 breakpoint in Ph[1]-positive, *bcr*-negative ALL, which we cloned from the SUP-B13 cells, is very close to that cloned by van der Feltz et al. (26) (Wiedemann, personal communication) and lies in a region shown to contain breakpoints for in several other cases (27). Other translocations have not been identified, and it is clear that there is no localized "breakpoint cluster region" in ALL as there is in CML. We therefore investigated a group of patients with Ph[1]-positive ALL to determine if the translocation breakpoints in all cases of *bcr*-negative Ph[1]-positive ALL occur within the *bcr* gene and if we could reliably detect them by means of PFGE (28).

We obtained leukemic cells from seven cases of Ph[1]-positive ALL and prepared DNA in agarose plugs; two cases had *bcr* rearrangements, and the rest were *bcr* negative. The DNA was digested with *Not*I, separated by TAFE electrophoresis, and hybridized to *bcr* and *abl* probes. Table 1 shows a summary of our results. It is clear that all patients had rearrangements detected with these probes; in each case the rearranged band seen with the 3′-*bcr* probe also hybridized to the pHabl5′ probe, which is specific for *abl* exon Ib, therefore recognizing the $9q^+$ chromosome. Rearrangements with pHab15′ showed that the breakpoint occurred within the *abl* first intron. In some cases, the pA-EB2.3 probe (23) from the upstream regions of the *bcr* gene (cloned from the SUP-B13 breakpoint) recognized different fragments than the *bcr* probe, showing that the translocation occurred between the two probes. From the sizes of the rearranged fragments and with reference to our *abl* and *bcr* maps, we concluded that the breakpoints in all cases occurred either within the *bcr* gene or no more than 100 kb 5′

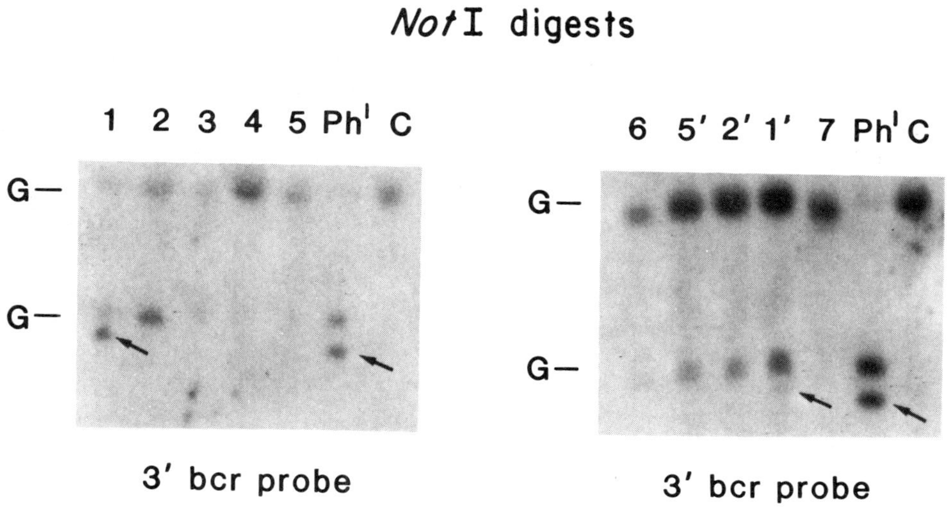

Figure 4 PFGE analysis of cells from patients with ALL for rearrangements within the *bcr* gene. DNA was prepared from cells obtained from seven patients with ALL at the diagnosis of leukemia (labeled 1–7); in three cases, remission samples were obtained from the same patients, labeled 5′, 2′, and 1′. DNA was also prepared from the SUP-B13 cells, a control for Ph^1-positive ALL with a known 350 kb rearranged band labeled Ph^1, and from RS(4;11), a cell line with normal chromosomes 9 and 22, labeled C. The DNA was digested with *Not*I, electrophoresed using the TAFE system (Beckman, Inc.), transferred to GeneScreen Plus membrane, and hybridized to the 3′ *bcr* probe according to our standard laboratory procedures (15,20,28). The positions of the germline fragments that contain the *bcr* gene are shown by G; the sizes are 1600 and 450 kb. Rearranged bands are shown by arrows. Note the expected 350 kb rearranged restriction fragment in the SUP-B13 cells. A 400 kb rearranged band is seen in the samples from patient 1, which is prominent in the diagnosis sample (labeled 1) and is only faintly seen during remission (labeled 1′).

of it. This study provides supportive evidence that, despite the variability in location of translocation breakpoints on chromosome 9 and 22, cases of Ph^1-positive ALL that are *bcr* negative all have the same molecular structure, a fusion of the most 5′ *bcr* exon with the *abl* common exons. Based on this limited series, we believe that PFGE analysis of *Not*I-digested DNA, hybridized sequentially to a *bcr* and an *abl* probe, is as useful for the diagnosis of the Ph^1 in ALL as Scuthern blot analysis for *bcr* rearrangement is for the diagnosis of CML.

We are currently exploring the utility of PFGE gels for the diagnosis of the Ph^1 in ALL. From a practical point of view, the sample quality requirements are about the same as those for cytogenetics or for RNA extraction; what is required is a sample with a high proportion of viable leukemic cells. We have found that we can easily and reproducibly prepare DNA in agarose plugs from fresh leukemic cells and can satisfactorily handle specimens that are several days old or have been shipped on ice across the country. An example, in Figure 4, shows a typical result from a series of samples from unselected patients with ALL, revealing rearrangement of a *Not*I fragment in the *bcr* gene in one patient. Whether this method will be useful for the management of patients with ALL remains to be seen. Certainly, PFGE is a research tool that is available now only in specialized laboratories, and the identification of the subtype of the Ph^1 may be more easily done by cytogenetics in combination with a standard *bcr* test or by a polymerase chain reaction method. Nonetheless, the experience gained with the use of PFGE for the analysis of the Ph^1 chromosome will eventually be applicable to the analysis of chromosomal abnormalities in other malignancies as their genetic basis is better understood. The PFGE method extends the horizons of the molecular analysis of leukemias.

ACKNOWLEDGMENTS

I am indebted to L. Wiedemann, C. Rubin, A. Hooberman, and J. Rowley for allowing the citation of unpublished data; to T. J. Vasicek for providing the U266 λV probe; and to C. M. Rubin and A. L. Hooberman for critical reading of this manuscript.

REFERENCES

1. Schwartz, D. C., and Cantor, C. R. (1984). Separation of yeast chromosome-sized DNAs by pulsed field gradient gel electrophoresis. *Cell 73*:67–75.
2. Carle, G. F., and Olson, M. V. (1986). Separation of chromosomal DNA moleculars from yeast by orthogonal-field gel electrophoresis. *Nucleic Acids. Res. 14*:5647–5664.
3. Chu, G., Vollrath, D., and Davis, R. W. (1986). Separation of large DNA molecules by contour-clamped homogeneous electric fields. *Science 234*: 1582–1585.
4. Carle, G. F., Frank, M., and Olson, M. V. (1986). Electrophoretic separations of large DNA molecules by periodic inversion of the electric field. *Science 232*:65–68.
5. Gardiner, K., Laas, W., and Patterson, D. (1986). Fractionation of large mammalian DNA restriction fragments using vertical pulsed-field gradient electrophoresis. *Somatic Cell. Mol. Genet. 12*:185–195.
6. Bird, A. (1980). DNA methylation and the frequency of CpG in animal DNA. *Nucleic Acids. Res. 8*:1499–1504.
7. Nelson, M., and McClelland, M. (1987). The effect of site-specific methylation on restriction-modification enzymes. *Nucleic Acids. Res. 15*:R219–R230.

8. Yang, Y.-C., Kovacic, S., Kriz, R., Wolf, S., Clark, S. C., Wellems, T. E., Nienhuis, A., and Epstein, N. (1988). The human genes for GM-CSF and IL 3 are closely linked in tandem on chromosome 5. *Blood 71*:958–961.
9. Westbrook, C. A., Rubin, C. M., Le Beau, M. M., Kaminer, L. S., Smith, S. D., Rowley, J. D., and Diaz, M. O. (1987). Molecular analysis of TCRB and ABL in a t(7;9)-containing cell line (SUP-T3) from a human T-cell leukemia. *Proc. Natl. Acad. Sci. USA 84*:251–255.
10. Ben-Neriah, A. J., Bernards, A., Paskind, M., Daley, G. Q., and Baltimore, D. (1986). Alternative 5′ exons in c-*abl* mRNA. *Cell 44*:577–586.
11. Shtivelman, E., Lifshitz, B., Gale, R. P., Roe, B. A., and Canaani, E. (1986). Alternative splicing of RNAs transcribed from the human *abl* gene and from the *bcr-abl* fused gene. *Cell 47*:277–284.
12. Bernards, A., Rubin, C. M., Westbrook, C. A., Paskind, M., and Baltimore, D. (1987). The first intron in the human c-*abl* gene is at least 200 kilobases long and is a target for translocations in chronic myelogenous leukemia. *Mol. Cell. Biol. 7*:3231–3236.
13. Weiss, L. M., Warnke, R. A., Sklar, J., andCleary, M. L. (1987). Molecular analysis of the t(14;18) chromosomal translocation in malignant lymphomas. *N. Engl. J. Med. 317*:1185–1189.
14. Brid, A. P. (1986). CpG-rich islands and the function of DNA methylation. *Nature 321*:209–213.
15. Westbrook, C. A., Rubin, C. M., Carrino, J. J., Le Beau, M. M., Bernards, A., and Rowley, J. D. (1988). Long-range mapping of the Philadelphia chromosome by pulsed-field gel electrophoresis. *Blood 71*:697–702.
16. Grosveld, G., Verwoerd, T., van Agthoven, T., de Klein, A., Ramachandran, K. L., Heisterkamp, N., Stam, E., and Groffen, J. (1986). The chronic myelocytic leukemia cell line K562 contains a breakpoint in *bcr* and produces a chimeric *bcr*/c-*abl* transcript. *Mol. Cell. Biol. 6*:607–616.
17. Heisterkamp, N., Stephenson, J. R., Groffen, J., Hansen, P. F., de Klein, A., Bartram, C. R., and Grosveld, G. (1983). Localization of the c-*abl* oncogene adjacent to a translocation break point in chronic myelocytic leukaemia. *Nature 306*:239–242.
18. Leibowitz, D., Schaefer-Rego, K., Popenoe, D. W., Mears, J. G., and Bank, A. (1985). Variable breakpoints on the Philadelphia chromosome in chronic myelogenous leukemia. *Blood 66*:243–245.
19. Emanuel, B. S., Selden, J. R., Wang, E., Nowell, P. C., and Croce, C. M. (1984). In situ hybridization and translocation breakpoint mapping. I. Nonidentical 22q11 breakpoint for the t(9;22) of CMl and the t(8;22) of Burkitt's lymphoma. *Cytogenet. Cell Genet. 38*:127–131.
20. Rubin, C. M., Westbrook, C. A., Smith, S. D., Hooberman, A. L., Colwick, A. L., Geiger, T. A., Steele, M. M., and Rowley, J. D. (1987). Philadelphia chromosome-positive acute lymphoblastic leukemia: Detection of a DNA rearrangement 50–250 kilobases proximal to BCR. In *Recent Advances in Leukemia and Lymphoma* (D. Golde and R. Gale, eds.). Alan R. Liss, New York, pp. 125–131.

21. Vasicek, T. J., and Leder, P. (1988). The structure of the human lambda complex (manuscript in preparation).
22. Rubin, C. M., Le Beaux, M. M., Smith, S. D., Rowley, J. D., and Westbrook, C. A. (1986). Philadelphia chromosome-positive acute lymphoblastic leukemia: DNA rearrangements on chromosomes 9 and 22 identified using pulsed field gel electrophoresis. *Blood 68*:264a.
23. Rubin, C. M., Carrino, J. J., Dickler, M. N., Leibowitz, D., Smith, S. D., and Westbrook, C. A. (1988). Heterogeneity of genomic fusion of *bcr* and *abl* in Philadelphia chromosome-positive acute lymphoblastic leukemia. *Proc. Natl. Acad. Sci. USA 85*:2795–2799.
24. Erikson, J., Griffin, C. A., Ar-Rushdi, A., Valtieri, M., Hoxie, J., Finan, J., Emanuel, B. S., Rovera, G., Nowell, P. C., and Croce, C. M. (1986). Heterogeneity of chromosome 22 breakpoint in Philadelphia-positive (Ph+) acute lymphocytic leukemia. *Proc. Natl. Acad. Sci. USA 83*:1807–1811.
25. de Klein, A., Hagemeijer, A., Bartram, C. R., Houwen, R., Hoesfloot, L., Carbonell, F., Chan, L., Barnett, M. L., Greaves, M., Kleihauer, E., Heisterkamp, N., Groffen, J., and Grosveld, G. (1986). *bcr* rearrangement and translocation of the *abl* oncogene in Philadelphia positive acute lymphoblastic leukemia. *Blood 68*:1369–1375.
26. van der Feltz, M. J. M., Shivji, M. K. K., Grosveld, G., and Wiedemann, L. M. (1988). Characterization of the translocation breakpoint in a patient with Philadelphia positive, *bcr* negative acute lymphoblastic leukaemia. *Oncogenes 3*:215–219.
27. Hermans, A., Heisterkamp, N., von Lindern, M., van Baal, S., Meijer, D., van der Plas, D., Wiedemann, L. M., Groffen, J., Bootsma, D., and Grosveld, G. (1987). Unique fusion of the *bcr* and c-*abl* genes in Philadelphia chromosome positive acute lymphoblastic leukemia. *Cell 51*:33–40.
28. Hooberman, A. H., Rubin, C. M., Barton, K. P., and Westbrook, C. A. Detection of the Philadelphia chromosome in acute lymphoblastic leukemia by pulsed-field gel electrophoresis (submitted for publication).

12
bcr and *bcr-abl* Proteins in Human Chronic Myelogenous Leukemia Cells

Ralph B. Arlinghaus and Wanjun Li *The University of Texas M. D. Anderson Cancer Center, Houston, Texas*

INTRODUCTION

Studies of RNA tumor viruses have led to the discovery of more than 20 proto-oncogenes (1), many coding for proteins that function in growth and differentiation pathways. The viral *abl* oncogene of the Abelson murine leukemia virus (A-MuLV), a fragment of the mouse c-*abl* proto-oncogene (2), is a member of the tyrosine protein kinase family (3) and is expressed as a 120 kD protein termed $p120^{gag\text{-}abl}$ (4). It is believed that the tyrosine kinase activity of the v-*abl* protein is important to the tumorigenicity and transforming activity of A-MuLV (5).

More than 90% of chronic myelogenous leukemia (CML) patients possess a nonrandom chromosomal aberration known as the Philadelphia chromosome (Ph^1) (6,7), which usually results from a reciprocal translocation of chromosomes 9 and 22. As a result, a truncated *abl* gene from chromosome 9 becomes fused to a 5.8 kilobase (kb) DNA segment on chromosome 22 called the breakpoint cluster region (*bcr*) (8,9). A hybrid *bcr-abl* transcript, estimated to be 8.5 kb, is detected in Ph^1-positive CML cells in addition to the normal 6 and 7 kb *abl* transcripts (10–12). The product of the fused *bcr* and *abl* genes is a 210 kD protein termed $p210^{bcr\text{-}abl}$, with an associated protein kinase activity (13–15). Like $p120^{gag\text{-}abl}$ of A-MuLV in virus induced pre-B cell malignancy, $p210^{bcr\text{-}abl}$ is believed to be a key factor in the process that leads to leukemia.

The scope of this review includes discussion of our recent work concerning *bcr* proteins and the *bcr-abl* protein of CML, their association with a 53 kD protein, and the regulation of *bcr-abl* expression by tumor promoters.

SITE-DIRECTED POLYCLONAL AND MONOCLONAL ANTIBODIES

Antibodies have been extremely useful to cell biologists for probing the structure, cellular location, and function of various intracellular proteins. Site-directed antibodies provide sophisticated tools for investigating these properties. This technology allows one to prepare highly specific antibodies to gene products that have never before been detected. Using this technology in 1984, we began our study of the gene products encoded by *bcr, abl*, and *bcr-abl* genes. Initially, antibodies were prepared against peptides predicted from the A-MuLV *abl* (v-*abl*) sequence. These included rabbit antibodies to peptides from v-*abl* residues 260-283 and 389-403. Both antibodies specifically detected $p210^{gag\text{-}abl}$, the tumor-causing protein encoded by the A-MuLV. However, only one of these antibodies was able to detect $p210^{bcr\text{-}abl}$ expressed in K562 cells, a cell line derived from a patient in the acute phase of Ph[1]-positive CML (16). It is note-

Table 1 Anti-*bcr* and *abl* Peptide Antibodies

Antibody	Region	Sequences	PK assay[a]
Rabbit antiserum			
R92	*bcr* 103–114	D G A D P P P A E E P E	+
R145	*bcr* 137–152	A A S G E R D D R G P P A S V A	+
R157	*bcr* 181–194	E F H H E R G L V K V N D K E	+
R156	*bcr* 298–310	R S Q S T S E Q E K R L T C	+
R72	*bcr* 417–426	D G E G A F H G D A	+
R705	*bcr* 683–699	N F L S S I N E E I T P R R O S M	+
R709	*bcr* 738–753	T K L K K Q S G G K T Q Q Y D C	+
R715	*bcr* 871–885	F S L T S V E L Q M L T N S C	+
R435	*bcr* 898–911	T I N K E D D E S P G L Y G	+
R476	v-*abl* 51–64	K E N L L A G P S E N D P N	+
R499	*abl* 389–403	D E V E K E L G K R G T R G G	+
Mouse monoclonal antibody			
P5C	*bcr* 898–911	T I N K E D D E S P G L Y G	+
P6D	*abl* 51–64	K E N L L A G P S E N D P N	+

[a]Detection of $p210^{bcr\text{-}abl}$ by protein kinase assay in vitro.

worthy that the 389–403 mouse sequence (DEVEKELGKRGTRGG) differs significantly from the human sequence (DEVEKELGK<u>Q</u>G<u>V</u>RG<u>A</u>), yet the antibodies to the mouse sequence efficiently detected the human *bcr-abl* protein (17). In contrast, the 260–283 mouse sequence is identical to the human *abl* segment, yet the antibody to this segment, although able to detect the viral $p120^{gag\text{-}abl}$, was unable to detect $p210^{bcr\text{-}abl}$. At this point we have prepared more than 10 different site-directed antipeptide antibodies, both polyclonal rabbit antisera and mouse monoclonal antibodies, that are useful in the detection of *bcr-abl* proteins (Table 1). Of these 10 antibodies, 8 are derived from *bcr* sequences upstream of the *bcr-abl* junction and 2 are from *abl* sequences downstream of the junction. These results support the original report that $p210^{bcr\text{-}abl}$ is in fact composed of both types of sequences.

p210 EXPRESSION IN UNCULTURED PATIENT CELLS FROM Ph^1-POSITIVE CML PATIENTS

The simplest and most sensitive method of detecting p210 is the immune complex kinase assay. This assay can be performed on crude cytoplasmic extracts of cells; it measures the phosphorylation of p210 transferred from the γ phosphate of ATP. Briefly, immune complexes containing p210 are incubated for a short time on ice in buffered solution containing divalent cation and about 10 μCi [γ-^{32}P] ATP. Both autophosphorylation of p210 and transphosphorylation of exogenous substrates (such as enolase) can be done in these reactions. The resulting products are visualized on a polyacrylamide gel containing sodium dodecyl sulfate (SDS, Figure 1). The specificity of the test can be easily determined by assaying immunoprecipitates generated with antibodies competed with excess homologous peptide.

Protein kinase-induced phosphorylation of p210 can be most easily observed in such cell lines as K562 (13,15) and EM2 cells (17) derived from Ph^1-positive patients with CML. Uncultured cells from patients also score positive in this test, but only if such samples are enriched in cells with blast morphology (17). Cells from chronic-phase patients usually contain less than 30% blasts and score negative, probably due to the presence of factors in mature cells that either degrade or dephosphorylate p210 in cell extracts during preparation or incubation (17). However, cells from chronic-phase patients have been found to express p210 with its associated kinase activity, as demonstrated by the detection of functional p210 in B cells from a chronic-phase patient (17). Therefore, it should be possible to design a simple test that detects and quantitates p210 in extracts of cells derived from patients in chronic, accelerated, and acute phases of disease. Such tests, which we are currently developing, will be valuable aids to the clinician treating patients.

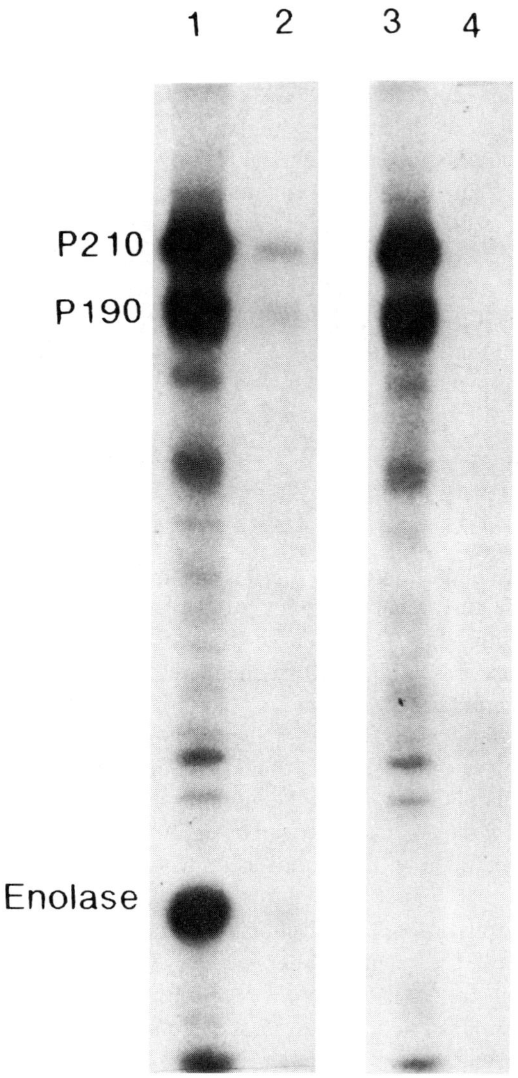

Figure 1 Autophosphorylation of $p210^{bcr\text{-}abl}$ and transphosphorylation of enolase by $p210^{bcr\text{-}abl}$. Total cytoplasmic extracts of K562 cells were lysed with detergent, and the high-speed supernatant fluid was immunoprecipitated with either anti-*bcr*(989–911) (lanes 1 and 3) or anti-*bcr*(898–911) blocked with cognate peptide (lanes 2 and 4). Washed immunoprecipitated proteins were collected on protein A-Sepharose beads and assayed for protein kinase activity in vitro. The immunoprecipitates were incubated with [γ-^{32}P] ATP and 5 μg enolase (Sigma Chemical Co., St. Louis, MO) (lanes 1 and 2) or without enolase (lanes 3 and 4) for 3 minutes before resolving by 6.5% SDS-polyacrylamide gel electrophoresis. The exposure time was 3 h.

ph-p53 FORMS A COMPLEX WITH p210*bcr-abl*

A key step toward understanding the role of protein tyrosine kinases in cell transformation is to identify the relevant protein substrates of these kinases. One method of identifying possible substrates of p210 is to search for intracellular complexes that contain p210 in association with normal cellular proteins. In two previous reports (17,18), we have detected a 53 kD protein (termed ph-p53) associated with p210*bcr-abl* in a putative complex with an estimated molecular weight of 300,000 that sediments in glycerol gradients. ph-p53 was found in two blast crisis CML cell lines (K562 and EM2) and in fresh blood cell preparations from CML patients in blast crisis (17). ph-p53 was phosphorylated on serine and tyrosine residues in immune complex protein kinase assays generated with antisera raised against an A-MuLV peptide (v-*abl* 389–403). V8 peptide mapping suggested that ph-p53 was not related to p210*bcr-abl*.

We subsequently investigated further the properties of ph-p53 and its association with p210*bcr-abl* (18). Our results have established that ph-p53 is complexed with p210*bcr-abl* and that ph-p53 is not a breakdown product of p210*bcr-abl*. The p210-ph-p53 complex is detectable by several different *bcr* and *abl* antipeptide antibodies and can be observed in nonreducing SDS-polyacrylamide gels. Under these conditions the proteins in the complexes can be recovered by treatment with room temperature SDS in the absence of 2-mercaptoethanol; these complexes can be detected in glycerol gradients, which sediment in the 100–400 kD size range. Regarding its identity, ph-p53 is recognized neither by a polyclonal antibody made against a large protein fragment derived from the viral *abl* protein (unpublished results) nor by two site-directed antipeptide antibodies [*abl*(51-64) or *bcr*(898-911)] in immunoblotting experiments. Lastly, one-dimensional patterns of fragments of ph-p53 produced by partial V8 protease treatment and separated on SDS gel fail to show structural homology with p210 (17).

Three lines of evidence support the interpretation that pH-p53 forms a complex with p210*bcr-abl*. First, a 20-fold range of antipeptide antibody concentration immunoprecipitated a constant ratio of ph-p53 to p210*bcr-abl*. A similar approach was used to demonstrate a complex between the large T antigen of simian virus 40 (SV40) and the nonviral T antigen (19). Second, SDS gel analyses of immunoprecipitates of p210*bcr-abl* under nonreducing conditions revealed at least two differently sized complexes containing p210 and ph-p53. More important, a ph-p53 sized band was absent from the nonreducing gels but could be recovered from higher molecular weight complexes by complete denaturation. Major ph-p53 spots were recovered from protein complexes with molecular weights higher than 210,000, including over 500,000, 275,000, and 240,000 kD.

The third piece of evidence that ph-p53 and p210 exist in a complex comes from their cosedimentation after glyerol gradient centrifugation. The complexes

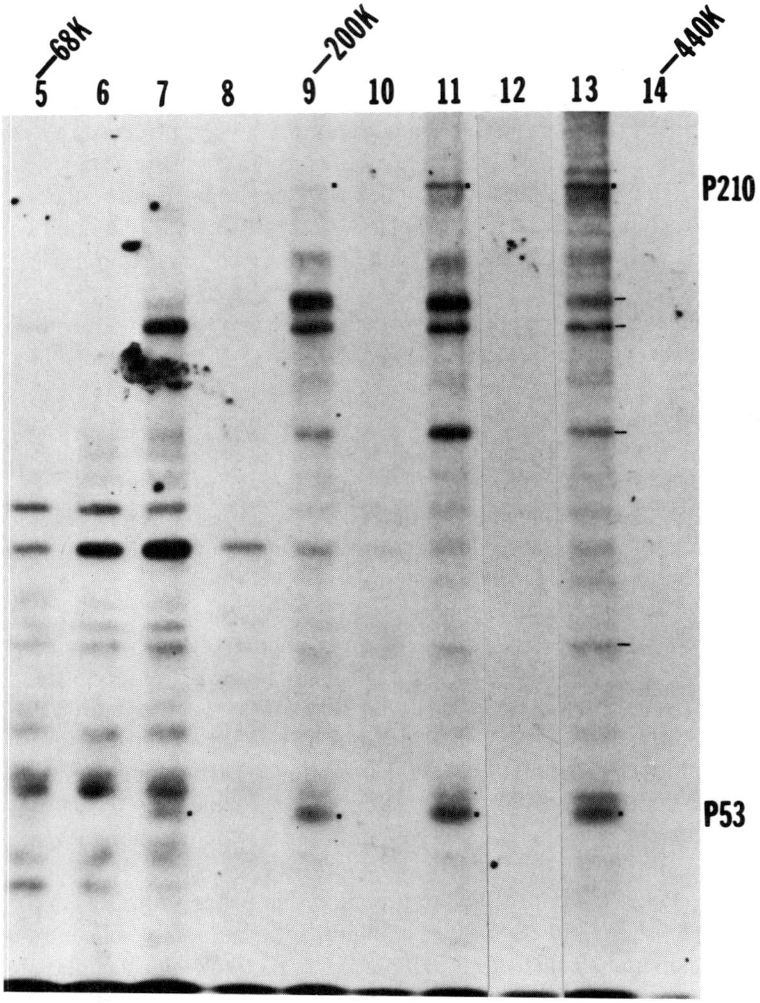

Figure 2 Glycerol gradient centrifugation of [^{35}S] methionine-labeled K562 cell lysates. A 10–50% glycerol gradient centrifugation was carried out on a 3 h in vivo [^{35}S] methionine-labeled K562 lysate followed by immunoprecipitation. The fractions (20 in total) were collected and reacted with monoclonal anti-*abl* (51–64) (P6D, odd number), and P6D was blocked with cognated peptide (even number). The immunoprecipitates were finally subjected to electrophoresis in a 6.5% SDS-polyacrylamide gel. Serum albumin (BSA, 68-kD), amylase (200 kD), and ferritin (440 kD) were used as molecular mass markers and were run on a parallel gradient. Exposure time was 20 h.

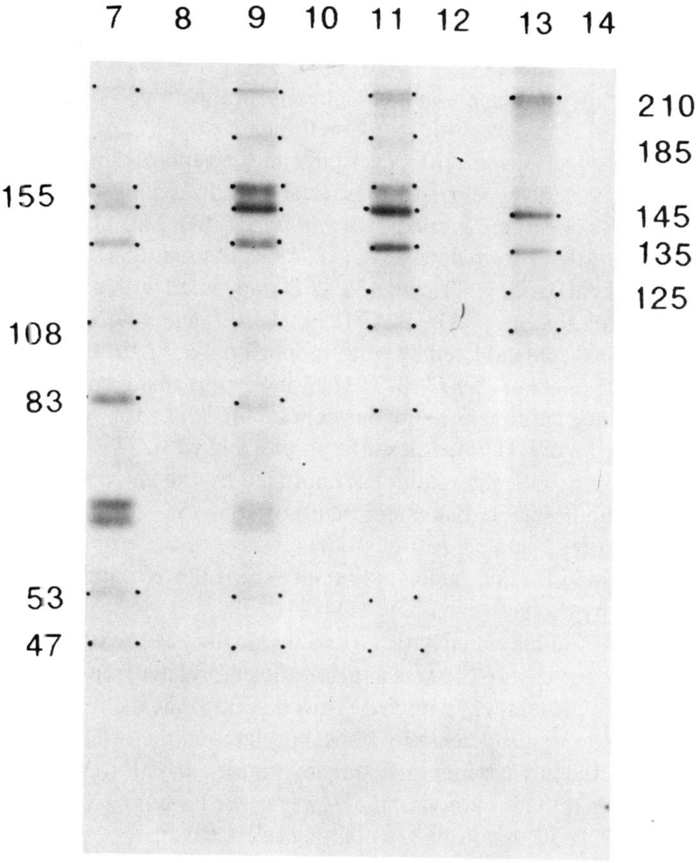

Figure 3 Metabolic labeling of *bcr* proteins in K562 cells. K562 cells (10^8) were labeled with 0.25 mCi/ml of [^{35}S] methionine (500–1000 Ci/mmol, ICN Radiochemical, Irvine, CA) in methionine-free culture medium for 3 h at 37°C. Cells were lysed in a detergent-containing buffer, and the cytoplasmic extract was run on a 10–50% glycerol gradient as usual. Each fraction was processed by immunoprecipitation with monoclonal anti-*bcr*(898–911) (P5C antibody). Lanes 7–12 represent the fraction number from the 10–50% glycerol gradient. Anti-*bcr*(898–911) was reacted with each fraction either preincubated with peptide (even number) or without (odd number) cognate peptide. Exposure time was 2 days.

sedimented slightly faster than amylase (200 kD) and slower than ferritin (440 kD). Therefore, our previous estimation of the molecular size of the complex as 300 kD seems reasonably accurate (17).

To better characterize the protein components present in the ph-p53-p210 complexes, we labeled K562 proteins with [^{35}S] methionine for 3 h. The cells were lysed and clarified by high-speed centrifugation, and the supernatant fluid was fractionated on a 10-50% glycerol gradient as usual (18). Fractions were immunoprecipitated with the anti-*abl* monoclonal antibody (P6D, Fig. 2). p210$^{bcr\text{-}abl}$ and ph-p53 proteins were detected in fractions sedimenting between the 200 and 440 kD markers (lanes 9, 11, and 13). P6D prereacted with excess *abl* peptide did not detect either ph-p53 of p210 (lanes 10, 12, and 14). Similarly, p210-ph-p53 proteins were detected by both monoclonal *bcr* (P5C) antibody (Figure 3) and polyclonal anti-*bcr* (738-753) antibodies in analogous fractions from parallel gradients, and the homologous peptide-blocked antibody did not detect either protein (Figure 3). In addition to ph-p53 and p210$^{bcr\text{-}abl}$, several other proteins were specifically immunoprecipitated by the anti-*abl* and anti-*bcr* monoclonal antibodies, including major bands of 165, 155, 145, 135, 125, 108, and 83 kD (Figures 2 and 3). Although the identity of these proteins is still under study, our initial findings indicate that all except the 165 and 145 kD proteins are encoded by the *bcr* gene (20).

Similarly, the phosphoproteins were characterized by labeling cells with [^{32}P] orthophosphate. In this case, p210 was a major phosphorylated band, but no phosphorylated ph-p53 protein was detected. Thus it seems that the ph-p53 present in the p210 complex is not detectably phosphorylated in the cell but becomes phosphorylated in the in vitro immune complex kinase assay. Further studies are needed to explain these observations. However, we have now detected a phosphorylated ph-p53 in non-Ph^1-containing cells (20).

We conclure from all these results that ph-p53 and p210$^{bcr\text{-}abl}$ are closely associated in a macromolecular complex with an estimated mass of 275-300 kD. Furthermore, several *bcr* proteins plus several other proteins of unknown identity are also present in this complex. Our recent findings indicate that ph-p53 forms complexes with several *bcr* proteins in non-Ph^1 cells. We have proposed a model that involves insertion of p210$^{bcr\text{-}abl}$, as an activated tyrosine kinase, into an otherwise normal *bcr*-ph-p53 complex containing a serine-threonine protein kinase (see Figure 5).

What is the identity of ph-p53? ph-p53 does not appear to be immunologically related to either *bcr* or *abl* gene products, as determined by Western immunoblotting experiments performed with several antibodies, including anti-*bcr*(898-911) and anti-*abl*(51-64), or by an anti-v-*abl* antibody made against a fragment of the v-*abl* protein. These results agree quite well with the one-dimensional peptide mapping studies that indicate that phosphorylated ph-p53 is not related to phosphorylated p210$^{bcr\text{-}abl}$ (17).

Experiments were also done to determine whether ph-p53 is the in vitro phosphorylated immunoglobulin heavy chain of the anti-peptide antibody. Antipeptide antibody cross-linked to Affi-gel 10 immunoprecipitated p210 and ph-p53, and both proteins could be released from the bound antibody by standard procedures under conditions in which the heavy chain remained bound to the Affi-gel. Therefore, ph-p53 is not the heavy chain of IgG that could have been phosphorylated in the immune complex kinase assay.

Several phosphotyrosine-containing proteins with a size similar to that of ph-p53 have been reported by different investigators. Using antiphosphotyrosine antibody, p210$^{gag\text{-}abl}$, a 54 kD protein, and two other proteins were immunoprecipitated from extracts of A-MuLV-transformed cells (21). In addition to p210$^{bcr\text{-}abl}$, a 53 kD phosphotyrosine-containing protein was also detected by anti-phosphotyrosine antibody in K562 cells (22). Whether either of these proteins is related to the ph-p53 protein complexed with p210$^{bcr\text{-}abl}$ is unknown.

The size of ph-p53 is similar to the 53 kD protein known as the nonviral T antigen or p53. Our experiments employed a broadly reacting monoclonal antibody (PAb 421, Reference 23) that can recognize large T antigen complexed with p53 in SV40-transformed cells of mouse, human, and rat origin (24). In our immune kinase assays, PAb 421 recognized a 53 kD nonviral T antigen and a 94 kD large T antigen in SV40-transformed mKSA mouse cells (25). However, neither ph-p53 nor p210$^{bcr\text{-}abl}$ was detected by this antibody in K562 cells (20). The control, P6D, recognized ph-p53 and p210$^{bcr\text{-}abl}$ in K562 cells but not in mKSA cells, indicating that ph-p53 in K562 cells has properties different from those of human p53 (non-viral T) antigen. Furthermore, nonviral T antigen has been shown to be phosphorylated on serine and threonine residues (26), whereas ph-p53 associated with p210 is phosphorylated on tyrosine and serine residues (17). Despite these differences, ph-p53 may yet be related to the nonviral T p53 antigen. This possibility is of interest since the chromosome region that encodes nonviral T p53 protein is located on the 1 arm of chromosome 17, a region that frequently (20% of the cases) becomes altered in blast crises of Ph^1-positive CML patients (27). Whether the gene for the *p53* oncogene becomes affected by this chromosomal change is not yet known. Could ph-p53 be a special form of the p53 nonviral T antigen that is expressed only in certain Ph^1-positive cell lines? This seems unlikely because ph-ph53 has been detected in non-Ph^1-positive cells in complexes with *bcr* proteins (see later).

It was reported previously that several complexes of viral and cellular proteins are associated with cell transformation. As mentioned earlier, the large T antigen of SV40 is complexed with a cellular protein termed p53 (19). pp60$^{v\text{-}src}$ forms a complex with two cellular phosphoproteins of 50 and 70 kD (28). Middle T antigen is the transformation protein of polyomavirus and essential to the transformation of cells grown in culture (29). Middle T antigen has been found to form complexes with pp60$^{c\text{-}src}$ (30,31) and p62$^{c\text{-}yes}$ (32). Also 81 kD protein, a possible phosphatidylinositol kinase, was reported to form a complex with middle T antigen and pp60$^{c\text{-}src}$ in cells transformed with middle T antigen (33).

Whether ph-p53 in the complex of p210$^{bcr\text{-}abl}$ represents a potential substrate of p210$^{bcr\text{-}abl}$ or is itself a protein kinase is unknown. However, the possibility exists that ph-p53 binds to p210$^{bcr\text{-}abl}$ and stabilizes and/or activates the kinase activity associated with p210$^{bcr\text{-}abl}$. Earlier work by Maxwell et al. detected ph-p53-p210$^{bcr\text{-}abl}$ complexes in K562 and EM2 CML cell lines and in uncultured blast cells from acute-phase CML patients. Thus, the association of ph-p53 with p210$^{bcr\text{-}abl}$ is a general phenomenon in Ph^1-positive CML cells. Further studies are underway to understand the physiologic importance of the interaction of ph-p53 with p210$^{bcr\text{-}abl}$ in the leukemic process.

DIFFERENTIAL EFFECTS OF PHORBOL ESTER TREATMENT ON p210$^{bcr\text{-}abl}$ EXPRESSION IN TWO DIFFERENT CELL LINES DERIVED FROM Ph^1-POSITIVE CML PATIENTS

Altered expression of several proto-oncogenes upon exposure of certain cells to various growth and differentiation conditions has been reported. Upon incubation with all-*trans*-retinoic acid or dimethylsulfoxide, HL-60 cells undergo irreversible myeloid differentiation (34,35), whereas exposure to 12-*O*-tetradecanoylphorbol-13-acetate (TPA) induces the formation of monocytic macrophages (36,37). HL-60 cells induced with TPA undergo a rapid and transient stimulation of c-*fos* gene transcription. Detection of p55$^{c\text{-}fos}$ first occurs 20 minutes after TPA induction and disappears 2 h later (38). The c-*myc* gene is amplified in HL-60 cells (39,40) and is transcribed at relatively high levels (41). TPA induction stimulates c-*myc* transcription fourfold by 90 minutes and then drops to nearly undetectable levels 5 h later. Stimulated transcription of a third proto-oncogene, the c-*fms* gene, is first detected 6 h after TPA induction and increases through 24 h after treatment (42,43).

K562 cells differentiate in culture in response to various chemical agents. Incubation of K562 cells with all-*trans*-retinoic acid induces myeloid lineage markers, whereas exposure to TPA induced megakaryotic markers, not the expected monocytic markers (44,45). However, K562 cells display markers of the erythroid, megakaryotic, and myeloid lineages. Our previous observations have shown that exposure of Ph^1-positive cell lines to TPA reduced steady-state p210$^{bcr\text{-}abl}$ levels in K562 cells but, in contrast, increased *bcr-abl* protein levels in EM2 cells (46). Similar effects were observed upon exposure of cells to low levels of mezerein, another tumor promoter structurally unrelated to TPA (47). Both these compounds are known to activate protein kinase C by acting as diglyceride surrogates (48).

Surprisingly the end result of TPA or mezerein treatment was dependent on the type of cell line examined (47). K562 cells were down-regulated by such treatment, and the production, steady-state level, and tyrosine kinase activity of p210*bcr-abl* were all markedly decreased. In sharp contrast, EM2 cells were stimulated to proliferate and showed an increase in p210 production, its steady-state level, and its associated protein kinase activity. Although these experiments employed long and continuous treatments, exposure to the protein kinase C inducer for times as short as 5 minutes was sufficient to increase p210*bcr-abl* synthesis in EM2 cells. For this reason, it is likely that a very brief exposure to protein kinase C activators is all that is required to initiate the chain of events leading to altered p210*bcr-abl* expression.

The effects of TPA on p210*bcr-abl* steady-state levels appear to be irreversible for K562 cells. Exposure of K562 to 10 or 100 nM TPA stopped cell division and turned off p210*bcr-abl* synthesis. K562 cells incubated 24 h in 10 nM TPA and then replated in medium lacking TPA for 48 h did not recover their ability to proliferate or return p210*bcr-abl* to normal levels.

Similarly, incubation of EM2 cells in TPA-containing medium for 1 day followed by replating in TPA-deficient medium for 2 days stimulated p210*bcr-abl* synthesis in a similar manner to continuous incubation with TPA. However, after TPA-stimulated EM2 cells were placed in fresh medium and then cultured for several weeks, p210*bcr-abl* synthesis was reduced to a level identical to that of untreated EM2 cells. This apparent reversibility may be explained by the possibility that EM2 cells did not respond uniformly to TPA stimulation, allowing a minor population of nonresponding cells to re-establish the culture. Alternatively, new cells generated after the removal of TPA may have subsequently reversed the effects of TPA.

In K562 cells, TPA reduced the production of new p210 in pulse-labeling experiments and eliminated detectable steady-state levels of p210, as measured by immunoblotting or the more sensitive autophosphorylation assay. These findings confirm and extend the findings reported by Alitalo (49), who showed a decrease in p210 kinase activity in K562 cells. This report also showed that the 8.5 kb *bcr-abl* mRNA remains unchanged in TPA-treated cells (49). Considering our results together with these findings, it seems likely that TPA drastically inhibits either the translation of p210*bcr-abl* mRNA or sharply increases the turnover of p210 during TPA-induced differentiation.

Mezerein (47), although structurally unrelated to TPA, is also a potent activator of protein kinase C but has less tumor promoter activity. Exposure of K562 cells to 5, 20, or 100 nM levels of mezerein for 72 h dramatically reduced p210*bcr-abl* levels in K562 cells. In contrast, EM2 cells similarly treated showed a strong increase in p210*bcr-abl*. These results confirm the results obtained with TPA on each of these cell lines.

These findings raise the possibility that protein kinase C regulates the expression of *bcr-abl* and that, depending on the cell lineage, the expression may be up-regulated or down-regulated. How this regulation occurs is unknown, but our studies suggest that the turnover of p210*bcr-abl* could be affected. Thus TPA treatment of K562 cells decreased p210 and simultaneously increased amounts of degraded forms of active *abl* kinase forms. In contrast to these results, EM2 cells responded with increased levels of p210, apparently by preventing the breakdown of p210*bcr-abl*. In this case, p210*bcr-abl* is the usual product detected in EM2 cells, but p210*bcr-abl* becomes the predominant product after TPA treatment. Thus it appears that stimulation of protein kinase C can stabilize p210 in some cells (EM2) but cause increased turnover in others (K562).

Another issue concerns whether the differential effects on cell proliferation and differentiation observed are in any way connected to the level of p210*bcr-abl* expression. Taken together, these results are consistent with the hypothesis that implicates the *bcr-abl* gene product as the key factor in maintaining the immortalized state of the Ph^1-positive CML tumor cell. However, it is also possible that TPA and mezerein up-regulate EM2 cells and down-regulate K562 cells. Therefore, it is possible that TPA and mezerein do not limit their effects solely to p210; rather, they may up- or down-regulate the synthesis of numerous proteins. Of interest, a report by McLaughlin et al. (50) showed that infection of fresh bone marrow cells from balb/c mice with a retroviral construct expressing p210*bcr-abl* stimulated the proliferation of immature lymphoid cells.

The expression of cellular proto-oncogenes in K562 during TPA induction has also been studied in other laboratories. Tumor growth factor (TGF-β) and c-*sis* RNA levels were increased in K562 cells treated with TPA, and c-*src* tyrosine kinase activity remained unchanged (49,51). In addition, c-*abl* proteins from mice and humans were specifically phosphorylated at a unique site in TPA-treated cells and by protein kinase C phosphorylation in vitro (52). These results raise the possibility that TPA treatment, through its activation of protein kinase C, may directly alter the p210*bcr-abl* protein. This regulation is quite complex, however, since diverse effects can be seen. Therefore, further studies with this system should increase the understanding of both the regulation of p210*bcr-abl* expression and its role in leukemogenesis.

bcr PROTEINS EXPRESSED IN HUMAN CELL LINES

Four *bcr* genes have been mapped to chromosome 22 (53). These include one intact gene (*bcr* 1) and three incomplete copies lacking 5′ sequences. The order of *bcr* genes on chromosome 22 is centromere, *bcr* 2, *bcr* 4, *bcr* 1, and *bcr* 3. The *bcr* 1 gene extends over 90 kb of DNA and is composed of multiple exons. The first exon is large and is located more than 20 kb from the second exon. The *bcr* 1 gene is transcribed into mRNAs of 7.0 and 4.5 kb. Smaller transcripts of 4.0, 3.0, and 1.0 kb have also been detected in some cell lines and tissues (11,54, 55). The relationship between these major and minor mRNA species is unknown. The 7.0 and 4.5 kb RNAs hybridize with probes spanning the entire *bcr* gene. However, the 4.0 kb RNA lacks some central sequences.

The structures of molecularly cloned *bcr* cDNAs have been determined by sequence analysis. The data indicate a single long open reading frame of 3813 nucleotides encoding a protein of 1271 amino acids. Amino acids 164–194 contain a sequence that resembles a consensus ATP binding site (55), consistent with *bcr* gene products having an associated protein kinase activity, as reported previously (12).

The previous results of others suggest that *bcr* involvement is critical to the development of CML and, as reported more recently, of Ph[1]-positive acute lymphoblastic leukemia (ALL). However, because little is known regarding the normal *bcr* gene products, these data are controversial. Because of this, we studied *bcr* expression in normal and leukemia cells.

Detection of *bcr* Proteins in Hematopoietic Cells

Several hematopoietic cell lines, including the Ph-positive CML cell line K562 (16), the Ph-negative leukemic cell line HL-60 (56), and the normal B lymphoid cell line SMS-SB (57), have been examined for the presence of *bcr* proteins. Because a 160 kD *bcr* protein was reported to have an associated serine-threonine kinase activity (12), proteins were tagged first by incubation of immune complexes with [γ-^{32}P] ATP in our protein kinase assay (18). To confirm and extend these studies, *bcr* proteins were labeled with [^{35}S] methionine and [^{32}P] orthophosphate as well. Immunoprecipitation of crude cytoplasmic extracts of such cells as SMS-SB gives patterns of *bcr* proteins containing significant nonspecific protein contamination (20). Therefore, enrichment of *bcr* proteins by partial purification procedures was found necessary to improve sensitivity. Based upon our previous findings (17), we began these studies by fractionating cytoplasmic extracts by ultracentrifugation on glycerol gradients. Each fraction, ranging in molecular weight between 100,000 and 300,000, was processed by immunoprecipitation with two different site-directed anti-*bcr* peptide antibodies made against *bcr* residues 898-911 and 738-753.

The results of these studies indicate that at least seven *bcr* gene products exist in non-Ph[1]-positive cells (20). These proteins have apparent molecular weights ranging from 190 to 83 kD. Yet another even larger protein of about 220–240 kD has been detected in crude extracts. The evidence for this conclusion comes from a variety of experiments, including peptide maps, immunoblots, immunoprecipitation with two different site-directed antipeptide antibodies, and serial double immunoprecipitation with two different antipeptide antibodies.

One-dimensional V8 protease mapping experiments in which only partial proteolytic cleavage was performed on in vitro phosphorylated, gradient-purified proteins indicate that proteins with estimated sizes of 190/185, 155, 135, 125 and 108 kD (designated p190, p155, and so on) share primary structural determinants. Two-dimensional separation of in vitro phosphorylated proteins following exhaustive digestion with trypsin established that p155, p125, p108, and p83 share three tyrptic peptides but contain different phosphopeptides as well (20).

Immunoblotting with anti-*bcr*(898-911) antibody detected p190, p185, p155, p125, and p108. Sequential immunoprecipitation with two different anti-*bcr* antibodies (after complete denaturation of the first immunoprecipitate) detected p185 and p155 and a trace amount of p125. Considered together, these data suggest that there are at least seven *bcr* gene products (p190/p185, p155, p135, p125, p108, and p83).

The issue of protein degradation has been considered a possible explanation for the presence of multiple *bcr* gene products. However, a careful review of our results argues against this interpretation. First, $p210^{bcr\text{-}abl}$ does not appear to degrade in any of our studies. This is clear from the experiments described previously (18) in which anti-*abl*(51-64) monoclonal antibody was used to detect *bcr-abl* proteins in glycerol gradient-fractionated K562 cell extracts (see Figure 6a in Reference 18). Second, unfractionated cytoplasmic extracts from several different cell lines contained multiple *bcr* proteins. Third, Western immunoblots prepared directly from cells also detect multiple *bcr* proteins, as do immunoblots of gradient-fractionated cell extracts. We conclude from these results that protein degradation does not play a significant role in generating the array of observed *bcr* gene products. However, our results do not eliminate a process of rapid autocatalytic protein cleavage of primary *bcr* gene products (i.e., p220 and p190 from 7.0 kb and p155 and p125 from 4.5 kb transcripts).

Metabolic labeling experiments of SMS-SB cells using [^{32}P] orthophosphate or of both K562 and HL-60 cells using [^{35}S] methionine (Figures 2 and 3) gave similar patterns of anti-*bcr*-precipitable proteins compared with proteins labeled with [γ-^{32}P] ATP in the immune complex kinase assays. In addition, pulse-chase studies done with [^{35}S] methionine failed to identify putative precursor proteins (20). All the *bcr*-related or associated proteins were detected after a 20 minute pulse labeling, and the pulse-chase experiment did not significantly affect the protein pattern. These data failed to give evidence of a precursor-product relationship between any of the *bcr* proteins and furthermore suggest that these proteins have a relatively slow turnover rate in cells.

Our findings indicate that neither protein degradation nor posttranslational processing is involved in generating multiple *bcr* protein products. Therefore, a logical alternative to explain our results is that multiple functional *bcr* transcripts exist in hematopoietic cells. These transcripts could originate from the four different *bcr* loci, by alternative splicing from the known functional *bcr* gene or by a combination of both processes. Further studies are obviously needed to determine which of these possibilities explains our results.

bcr proteins appear to exist in cytoplasmic complexes that cosediment in glycerol gradient fractions ranging in molecular weight from 100,000 to 300,000. These cosedimenting proteins were specifically immunoprecipitated by two different site-directed anti-*bcr* antibodies derived from *bcr* peptide sequences 898–911 (P5C monoclonal antibody) and 738–753 (rabbit 709 serum) located 145 amino acid residues apart, as predicted from the *bcr* gene sequence (58). These putative complexes were found in several different cell lines, including HL-60, SMS-SB, K562, HeLa, and A498 (20).

Several other proteins were routinely detected in the 100–300 kD fractions of the glyerol gradient. These proteins are currently considered *bcr*-associated proteins; they include 165, 145, 47, and 53 kD proteins, the last being identical in size and one-dimensional peptide maps to ph-p53. It is of interest that the 145 kD protein has the size of the normal c-*abl* protein (14). Experiments are underway to determine the identity of these proteins, particularly the 145 and 53 kD *bcr*-associated proteins.

Only limited reports describing candidate *bcr* proteins have been published. Three phosphoproteins have been described, including one of 190 kD in K562 and HeLa cells (59), one of 180 kD in K562 cells, and one of 160 kD in K562 and A498 cells (12). In the latter study, p160 had an associated serine-threonine protein kinase activity. The p190, p180, and p160 proteins could be related to the p190, p185, and p155 proteins identified in this study. The reason that others have failed to detect the additional proteins may be due to several factors, including the antibodies used and the glycerol gradient centrifugation fractionation procedure, among others.

The expression of *bcr* and *bcr*-associated proteins varied among the cell lines tested. p135 and p47 were preferentially expressed in SMS-SB and HL-60 cell lines. Moreover, the size of some *bcr*-related proteins was slightly different in some cell lines. For example, the p125 expressed in K562 and SMS-SB cell lines may be equivalent to p120 in the HL-60 cell line. Similar *bcr* proteins were also detected in two other cell lines: in HeLa cells, p155, p135, p125, p108, p83, and p47 were detected; and in A498 cells (12), p190, p185, p160, p125, and p47 were found (20).

Phosphorylation sites of *bcr* proteins phosphorylated in vitro using extracts of SMS-SB cells were assessed by alkali treatment. The results showed that p185, p155, p125, p108, and p83 contain alkali-sensitive phosphate bonds indicating the presence of serine and threonine and the absence of phosphotyrosine in these proteins. Direct analyses of phosphoamino acids revealed that *bcr* proteins contain phosphoserine-threonine (20). These results are consistent with those previously reported by Stam et al. (12), who showed that a 160 kD *bcr* gene product has an associated serine-threonine protein kinase activity.

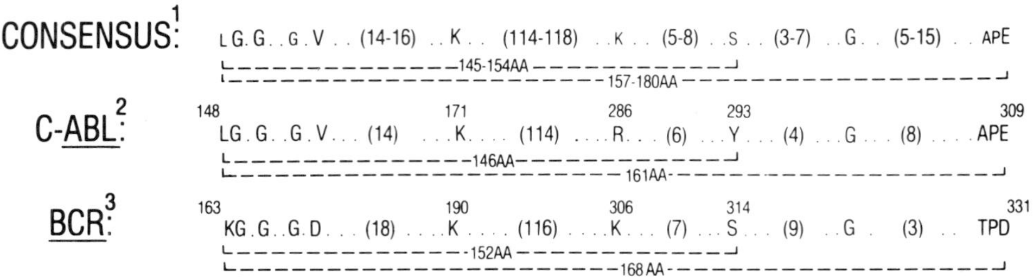

Figure 4 Comparison between consensus protein kinase domains and putative domains in the *abl* proto-oncogene and *bcr* gene. The consensus protein kinase is from Hunter (3), c-*abl* domians from Shtivelman et al. (64), and *bcr* domains from Hariharan and Adams (58).

Although none of these *bcr* proteins contained phosphotyrosine when phosphorylated in immune complexes from cells lacking Ph^1, phosphotyrosine was detected in certain of these proteins (p185, p155, and p108) phosphorylated in immune complexes from K562 cells. The presence of phosphotyrosine in these proteins indicates that they have phosphotyrosine sites, thereby suggesting that these proteins may themselves be targets of p210*bcr-abl*.

Does *bcr* Encode a Protein Kinase?

A recent report (55) identified a sequence pattern in *bcr* that is characteristic of the ATP binding site domain found in a variety of nucleotide-binding proteins and protein kinases (3,60). Considering the findings of Stam et al. (12) and our results, the presence of an ATP binding site in *bcr* raises the possibility that *bcr* proteins are protein kinases. Therefore, we compared *bcr* sequences to consensus protein kinase sequences and to those in the *abl* proto-oncogene (Figure 4). The *bcr* sequences in the first exon defined by residues 163–190 are similar to the consensus pattern of ATP binding site sequences. The Lys (K) at position 190 is suitably positioned within an apparent ATP binding domain. However, protein kinases are typically characterized by hydrophobic residues at positions 1 and 7 upstream from the first Gly (G) in the consensus sequence and by a Val (V) two positions downstream from the last Gly (Hanks of the Salk Institute, personal communication). At residues 306–331, downstream from the sequence that has ATP binding site characteristics, is a pattern of sequences that weakly resembles the consensus phosphoatransferase domain of protein kinases. Although the 114-118 residue gap in *bcr* between the putative ATP binding and phosphotransferase domains is typical of protein kinases, several sequences conserved among various protein kinases do not appear to be present in the *bcr* putative phospho-

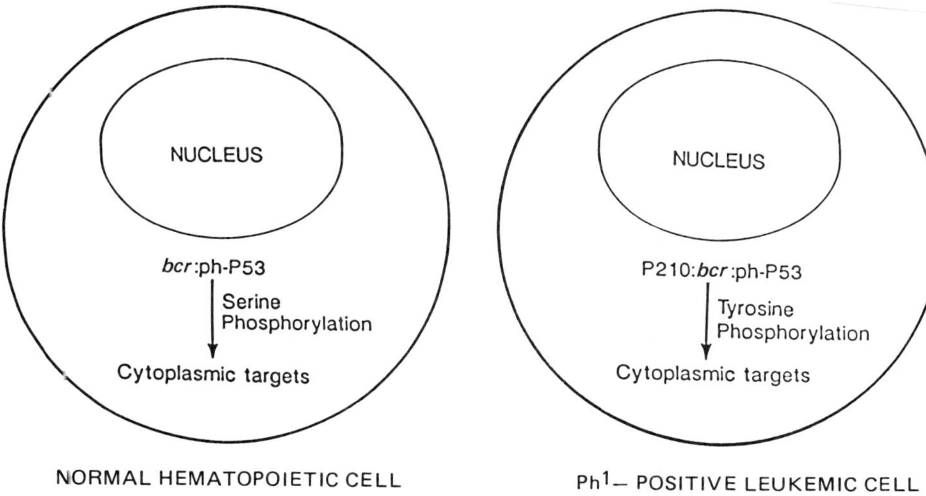

Figure 5 A model for *bcr-abl*-induced leukomogenesis.

transferase domain, as recently reviewed by Hanks et al. (61). For example, the Asp-Cys-Gly sequence (DVG, residues 323–325) domain differs from the consensus Asp-Phe-Gly romain. Similarly, Thr-Pro-Asp (TPD) at residues 329–331 differs from the consensus Ala-Pro-Glu (APE) domain in protein kinases (Hanks, personal communication). Other sequence differences also exist. Nevertheless, the sequence comparisons are intriguing and have prompted us to explore further the possibility that *bcr* gene products are protein kinases. If *bcr* does encode a protein kinase, it is certainly an evolutionary offshoot. Obviously, other interpretations are possible. For example, any one of several proteins present in the observed *bcr* complexes may be the kinase that carries out the phosphorylation.

If *bcr* proteins do in fact turn out to have serine-threonine protein activity and if the 5′ part of *bcr* contains a protein kinase domain, *bcr-abl* fusion proteins would contain two distinct functional protein kinase catalytic domains within the same polypeptide chain: one kinase domain in exon 1 of the *bcr* portion of the *bcr-abl* protein and the other in the c-*abl* domain (4). Alternatively, because of the presence of the ATP binding sitelike domain described earlier, *bcr* proteins may not function as protein kinases but as nucleotide binding proteins. The presence of a "second ATP binding domain" (the other in the *abl* portion of the *bcr-abl* protein) would have important regulatory consequences for the protein kinase activity of the *bcr-abl* proteins. Because *bcr-abl* proteins appear to play an important role in the leukemia process of CML and ALL and because both CML-specific p210 and ALL-specific p185 contain *bcr* exon 1 sequences (62), the putative *bcr* ATP binding and kinase activities may be an important factor in the leukemogenic activity of *bcr-abl* proteins.

Do *bcr*-ph 53 Complexes That Contain p210*bcr-abl* Play a Crucial Role in the Leukemic Process?

We have proposed a working model (Figure 5) that defines the role of *bcr-abl* proteins in Ph[1]-positive leukemias; the model describes the insertion of an activated *abl* tyrosine kinase into *bcr*-containing cytoplasmic complexes. Of interest, the *gag-abl* protein of A-MuLV may have a nuclear location (63), raising the possibility that c-*abl* proteins also function in the nucleus. In this model (Figure 5) we propose that *bcr*-containing cytoplasmic complexes provide the framework for a protein kinase that regulates the activities of one or more of the proteins that play key roles in several signal pathways involved in growth and differentiation. *bcr* proteins may be kinase themselves, but it is also possible that one of the proteins that associate with *bcr* proteins (i.e., ph-p53) is in fact the active kinase. In this view, the complex would house the active kinase, and the complex would physically interact with other proteins facilitating the phosphorylation of important cellular targets. We further propose that because of the fusion of *bcr* to *abl* sequences in Ph[1]-positive leukemias, p210*bcr-abl* becomes incorporated into these *bcr* complexes, thereby inserting an "unusual" and highly activated tyrosine kinase that causes the phosphorylation of targets on tyrosine instead of serine-threonine. The aberrant phosphorylation of these targets may result in uncontrolled growth of the cell as well as other changes leading to a malignant leukemic cell.

SUMMARY

Leukemic cells from patients with Philadelphia chromosome (Ph[1])-positive chronic myelogenous leukemia contain a 210 kD protein (p210*bcr-abl*) with a protein tyrosine kinase activity that is a product of fused *bcr* and *abl* genes. We prepared several polyclonal and monoclonal antipeptide antibodies for use in the isolation and characterization of *bcr* and *bcr-abl* proteins. In this review, we summarized our recent findings regarding the expression of *bcr* and *bcr-abl* proteins, their association with a 53 kD cellular protein (ph-p53), their regulation by agents that activate protein kinase C, and their possible functions. Based upon our findings, we have proposed a model that begins to address the role of p210*bcr-abl* in Ph[1]-positive leukemias.

ACKNOWLEDGMENTS

This work was supported by Public Health Services grants CA 47372, CA 16672 from the National Institutes of Health, and a grant (G1118) from The Welch

Foundation. Ralph B. Arlinghaus is an Abell-Hanger Professor. We thank Ms. Tammy Trlicek and Ms. Linda Jackson for assistance in manuscript preparation.

REFERENCES

1. Bishop, J. M. (1985). Viral oncogenes. *Cell 42*:23.
2. Goff, S. P., Gilboa, E., Witte, O. N., and Baltimore, D. (1980). Structure of the Abelson murine leukemia virus genome and the homologous cellular gene. Studies with cloned viral DNA. *Cell 22*:777.
3. Hunter, T. (1987). A thousand and one protein kinases. *Cell 50*:823.
4. Witte, O. N., Dasgupta, A., and Baltimore, D. (1980). Abelson murine leukemia virus protein is phosphorylated in vitro to form phosphotyrosine. *Nature 283*:826.
5. Prywes, R., Haag, J., Rosenberg, N., and Baltimore, D. (1985). Protein stabilization explains the *gag* requirement for transformation of lymphoid cells by Abelson murine leukemia virus. *J. Virol. 54*:123.
6. Nowell, P. C., and Hungerford, D. A. (1960). Chromosome studies on normal and leukemic human leukocytes. *JNCI 25*:85.
7. Rowley, J. D. (1973). A new consistent chromosomal abnormality in chronic myelogenous leukemia identified by quinacrine fluorescence and giemsa staining. *Nature 243*:290.
8. Groffen, J., Stephenson, J. R., Heisterkamp, N., de Klein, A., Bartram, C. R. and Grosveld, G. (1984). Philadelphia chromosomal breakpoints are clustered within a limited region, *bcr*, on chromosome 22. *Cell 36*:93.
9. Heisterkamp, N., Stephenson, J. R., Groffen, J., Hansen, P. I., de Klein, A., Bartram, R., and Grosveld, G. (1983). Localization of the c-*abl* oncogene adjacent to a translocation breakpoint in chronic myelogenous leukemia. *Nature 306*:239.
10. Gale, R. P., and Canaani, E. (1984). An 8-kilobase *abl* RNA transcript in chronic myelogenous leukemia. *Proc. Natl. Acad. Sci. USA 81*:5648.
11. Shtivelman, E., Lifshitz, B., Gale, R. P., and Canaani, E. (1985). Fused transcripts of *abl* and *bcr* genes in chronic myelogenous leukemia. *Nature 315*:550.
12. Stam, K., Heisterkamp, N., Reynolds, F. H., Jr., and Groffen, J. (1987). Evidence that the Ph-1 gene encodes a 160,000-dalton phosphoprotein with associated kinase activity. *Mol. Cell. Biol. 7*:1955.
13. Konopka, J. B., Watanabe, S. M., and Witte, O. N. (1984). An alteration of the human c-*abl* protein in K562 leukemia cells unmasks associated tyrosine kinase activity. *Cell 37*:1035.
14. Konopka, J. B., and Witte, O. N. (1985). Detection of c-*abl* tyrosine kinase activity in vitro permits direct comparison of normal and altered *abl* gene products. *Mol. Cell. Biol. 5*:3116.
15. Kloetzer, W., Kurzrock, R., Smith, L., Talpaz, M., Spiller, M., Gutterman, J., and Arlinghaus, R. (1985). The human cellular *abl* gene product in the chronic myelogenous leukemia cell line has an associated tyrosine protein kinase activity. *Virology 140*:230.

16. Lozzio, C. B., and Lozzio, B. B. (1975). Human chronic myelogenous leukemia cell line with positive Philadelphia chromosome. *Blood 45*:321.
17. Maxwell, S. A., Kurzrock, R., Parson, S., Talpaz, M., Gallick, G. E., Kloetzer, W. S., Arlinghaus, R. B., Kouttab, N. M., Keating, M. J., and Gutterman, J. U. (1987). Analysis of p210$^{bcr\text{-}abl}$ tyrosine kinase activity in various myelogenous leukemia patients. *Cancer Res. 47*:1731.
18. Li, W. J., Kloetzer, W. S., and Arlinghaus, R. B. (1988). A novel 53-kDa protein complexed with p210$^{bcr\text{-}abl}$ in human chronic myelogenous leukemia cells. *Oncogene 2*:559.
19. Lane, D. P., and Crawford, L. V. (1979). T antigen is bound to a host protein in SV40-transformed cells. *Nature 278*:261.
20. Li, W., Dreazen, O., Kloetzer, W., Gale, R. P., and Arlinghaus, R. B. (1989). Characteization of *bcr* gene products in hematopoietic cells. *Oncogene 4*:127.
21. Seki, J., Owada, M. K., Sakato, N., and Fujito, H. (1986). Direct identification of phosphotyrosine-containing proteins in some retrovirus transformed cells by use of anti-phosphotyrosine antibody. *Cancer Res. 46*:907.
22. Huhn, R. D., Posner, M. R., Ruyter, S. I., Gordon, J. J., and Frackelton, A. R., Jr. (1987). Cell lines and peripheral blood leukocytes derived from individuals with chronic myelogenous leukemia display virtually identical proteins phosphorylated on tyrosine residues. *Proc. Natl. Acad. Sci. USA 84*:4408.
23. Harlow, E., Crawford, L. V., Pim, D. C., and Williamson, N. M. (1981). Monoclonal antibodies specific for Simian virus 40 tumor antigens. *J. Virol. 39*:861.
24. Rotter, V., and Wolf, D. (1979). Biological and molecular analysis of p53 cellular encoded tumor antigen. *Adv. Cancer Res. 43*:113.
25. Kit, S., Kurimura, T., and Dubbs, D. R. (1969). Transplantable mouse tumor line induced by injection of SV40-transformed mouse kidney cells. *Int. J. Cancer 4*:384.
26. Jay, G., Khoury, G., Deleo, A. B., Dippold, W. G., and Old, L. J. (1981). p53 transformation-related protein: Detection of an associated phosphotransferase activity. *Proc. Natl. Acad. Sci. USA 78*:2932.
27. Rowley, J. D., and Testa, J. R. (1982). Chromosome abnormalities in malignant hematologic diseases. *Adv. Cancer Res. 36*:103.
28. Brugge, J. S., Erikson, E., and Erikson, R. L. (1981). The specific interaction of the Rous sarcoma virus transforming protein, pp60^{src}, with two cellular proteins. *Cell 25*:363.
29. Smith, A. E., and Ely, B. K. (1983). The biochemical basis of transformation by polyoma virus. *Adv. Virol. Oncol. 3*:3.
30. Courtneidge, S. A., and Smith, A. E. (1983). Polyoma virus transforming protein associated with the product of the c-*src* cellular gene. *Nature 303*:435.
31. Courtneidge, S. A., and Smith, A. E. (1984). The complex of polyoma virus middle-T antigen and pp60$^{c\text{-}src}$. *EMBO J. 3*:585.

32. Kornbluth, S., Sudal, M., and Hanafura, H. (1987). Association of the polyomavirus middle-T antigen with C-*yes* proteins. *Nature 325*:171.
33. Courtneidge, S. A., and Heber, A. (1987). An 81 Kd protein complexed with middle-T antigen and pp60$^{c\text{-}src}$: A possible phosphatidylinositol kinase. *Cell 50*:1031.
34. Breitman, T. R., Collins, S. J., and Keene, B. R. (1981). Terminal differentiation of human promyelocytic leukemic cells in primary culture in response to retinoic acid. *Blood 57*:1000.
35. Collins, S. J., Ruscetti, F. W., Gallagher, R. E., and Gallo, R. C. (1978). Terminal differentiation of human promyelocytic leukemia cells induced by dimethyl sulfoxide and other polar compounds. *Proc. Natl. Acad. Sci. USA 75*:2458.
36. Huberman, E., and Callahan, M. F. (1979). Induction of terminal differentiation in human promyelocytic leukemia cells by tumor-promoting agents. *Proc. Natl. Acad. Sci. USA 76*:1293.
37. Rovera, G., Santoli, O., and Damsky, C. (1979). Human promyelocytic leukemia cells in culture differentiate into macrophage-like cells when treated with a phorbol ester. *Proc. Natl. Acad. Sci. USA 76*:2779.
38. Mitchell, R. L., Zokas, L., Schreiber, R. D., and Verma, I. M. (1985). Rapid induction of the expression of proto-oncogene *fos* during human monocytic differentiation. *Cell 40*:209.
39. Collins, S., and Groudine, M. (1982). Amplification of endogenous *myc*-related DNA sequences in a human myeloid leukemia cell line. *Nature 298*: 679.
40. Dalla Favera, R., Wong-Staal, F., and Gallo, R. C. (1982). *Onc* gene amplification in promeylocytic leukemia cell line HL-60 and primary leukemic cells of the same patient. *Nature 299*:61.
41. Westin, E. H., Wong-Staal, F., Gelmann, E. P., Dalla Favera, R., Papas, T. S., Lautenberger, J. A., Eva, A., Reddy, E. P., Tronick, S. R., Aaronson, S. A., and Gallo, R. C. (1982). Expression of cellular homologous of retroviral onc genes in human hematopoietic cells. *Proc. Natl. Acad. Sci. USA 79*:2490.
42. Gonda, T. J., and Metcalf, D. (1984). Expression of *myb, myc*, and *fos* proto-oncogenes during the differentiation of a murine myeloid leukemia. *Nature 310*:249.
43. Sariban, E., Mitchell, T., and Kufe, D. (1985). Expression of the c-*fms* proto-oncogene during human monocytic differentiation. *Nature 316*:64.
44. Fududa, M. (1981). Tumor promoting phorbol diester induced specific changes in cell surface glycoprotein profile of K562 human leukemic cells. *Cancer Res. 41*:4621.
45. Tabilio, A., Pelicci, P. G., Vinci, G., Mannoni, P., Civin, C. I., Vainchenker, W., Testa, U., Lipinski, M., Rochant, H., and Breton-Gorius, J. (1983). Myeloid and megakaryocytic properties of K562 cell lines. *Cancer Res. 43*: 4569.
46. Smith, L., Kabat, K., Arlinghaus, R. B., and Kloetzer, W. S. (1987). C kinase activators alter p210$^{bcr\text{-}abl}$ expression in cell lines derived from chronic

myelogenous leukemia patients. In: *Recent Advances in Leukemia and Lymphoma* (R. P. Gale and D. Golde, eds.), UCLA Symposia on Molecular and Cellular Biology. Alan R. Liss, New York, p. 95.

47. Li, W., Smith, L. A., Kabat, K. G., Kloetzer, W. S. and Arlinghaus, R. B. (1989). Differential effects of tumor promoters on $p210^{bcr\text{-}abl}$ expression. *Hematologic Pathology 3*:113.
48. Rando, R. R. (1988). Regulation of protein kinase C activity by lipids. *FASEB J. 2*:2348.
49. Alitalo, R. (1987). The *bcr-abl* tyrosine kinase activity is extinguished by TPA in K562 leukemic cells. *FEBS Lett. 222*:293.
50. McLaughlin, J., Chianese, E., and Witte, O. N. (1987). In vitro transformation of immature hematopoietic cells by the $p210^{bcr\text{-}abl}$ oncogene product of the Philadelphia chromosome. *Proc. Natl. Acad. Sci. USA 84*:6558.
51. Alitalo, R., Anderson, L. C., Betscholtz, C., Nilsson, K., Westermark, B., Heldin, C.-H., and Alitalo, K. (1987). Induction of platelet-derived growth factor gene expression during megakaryoblastic and monocytic differentiation of human leukemia cell lines. *EMBO J. 6*:1213.
52. Pendergast, A. M., Traugh, J. A., and Witte, O. N. (1987). Normal cellular and transformation-associated *abl* protein share common sites for protein kinase C phosphorylation. *Mol. Cell. Biol. 7*:4280.
53. Croce, C. M., Huebner, K., Isobe, M., Fainstein, E., Lifshitz, B., Shtivelman, E., and Canaani, E. (1987). Mapping of four distinct *bcr*-related loci to chromosome region 22q11: Order of *bcr* loci relative to chronic myelogenous leukemia and acute lymphoblastic leukemia breakpoints. *Proc. Natl. Acad. Sci. USA 84*:7174.
54. Collins, S., Coleman, H., and Groudine, M. (1987). Expression of *bcr* and *bcr-abl* fusion transcripts in normal and leukemic cells. *Mol. Cell. Biol. 7*: 2870.
55. Lifshitz, B., Fainstein, E., Marcelle, C., Shtivelman, E., Amson, R., Gale, R. P., and Canaani, E. (1987). *bcr* genes and transcripts. *Oncogene 2*:112.
56. Collins, S. J., Gallo, R. C., and Gallagher, R. E. (1977). Continuous growth and differentiation of human myeloid leukemic cells in suspension culture. *Nature 270*:347.
57. Smith, R. G., Dev, V. G., and Shannon, W. A., Jr. (1981). Characterization of a novel human pre-B leukemia cell line. *J. Immunol. 126*:596.
58. Hariharan, I. K., and Adams, J. M. (1987). cDNA sequence for human *bcr*, the gene that translocates to the *abl* oncogene in chronic myelogenous leukemia. *EMBO J. 6*:115.
59. Ben-Neriah, Y., Daley, G. Q., Mes-Masson, A., Witte, O. N., and Baltimore, D. (1986). The chronic myelogenous leukemia-specific p210 protein is the product of the *bcr-abl* hybrid gene. *Science 233*:212.
60. Hunter, T., and Cooper, J. A. (1986). Viral oncogenes and tyrosine phosphorylation. *Enzymes XVII*:191–245.
61. Hanks, S. K., Quinn, A. M., and Hunter, T. (1988). The protein kinase family: Conserved features and deduced phylogeny of the catalytic domains. *Science 241*:42.

62. Hermans, A., Heisterkamp, N., von Lindern, M., van Baal, S., Meijer, D., van der Plas, D., Wiedemann, L. M., Groffen, J., Bootsma, D., and Grosveld, G. (1987). Unique fusion of *bcr* and c-*abl* genes in Philadelphia chromosome positive acute lymphoblastic leukemia. *Cell 51*:33.
63. Bell, J. C., Mahadevan, L. C., Colledge, W. H., Frackelton, A. R., Jr., Sargent, M. G., and Foulkes, J. G. (1987). Abelson-transformed fibroblasts contain nuclear phosphotyrosyl-proteins which preferentially bind to murine DNA. *Nature 325*:552.
64. Shtivelman, E., Lifshitz, B., Gale, R. P., Roe, B. A., and Canaani, E. (1986). Alternative splicing of RNAs transcribed from the human *abl* gene and from the *bcr-abl* fused gene. *Cell 47*:277.

PART IV
Cellular Models for Chronic Myelogenous Leukemia

13
Marrow Stromal Cells, Growth Factors, and the c-*abl* Proto-Oncogene

Jack W. Singer, D. Frank Andrews III, and John J. Nemunaitis *University of Washington and Fred Hutchinson Cancer Research Center, Seattle, Washington*

INTRODUCTION

Much of current knowledge regarding the regulation of normal and neoplastic hematopoiesis has resulted from studies of colony formation by hematopoietic progenitor cells in semisolid media (1). These studies were instrumental in the identification and cloning of hematopoietic growth factors and to our current concepts of the processes of commitment and differentiation of hematopoietic progenitor cells. Nevertheless, it is important to realize some of the limitations of the colony-forming cell assays. These culture systems, which rely on the ability of single progenitor cells to proliferate and differentiate in the presence of appropriate growth factors in a semisolid supporting medium, have uncertain relevance to physiologic hematopoiesis, which occurs within the marrow cavity at high cell density, within a complex extracellular matrix, and in the presence of many types of accessory cells that together can be termed the hematopoietic microenvironment.

The importance of a specific hematopoietic microenvironment in vivo is suggested by several observations:

1. Under most conditions, nonneoplastic hematopoiesis is restricted to such hematopoietic organs as the bone marrow and spleen despite the presence of circulating, transplantable progenitor cells. Even following bone marrow transplantation, hematopoietic cellular proliferation is restricted to the marrow cavity.

2. When bone marrow cells are transplanted ectopically, hematopoiesis develops only after a stroma has formed (2-4).
3. Marrow stroma transplanted to spleen exerts a local effect on spleen colony growth (5,6).
4. Histologic studies of in vivo hematopoiesis show hematopoietic cells always proliferate in intimate association with poorly characterized cell populations that include adventitial reticular cells as well as endothelial cells and macrophages (7).

In 1977, Dexter et al. described a murine liquid marrow culture system that allowed both colony-forming and reconstituting hematopoietic progenitors to be propagated for many months (8). Unlike systems measuring colony-forming cells, long-term marrow cultures allowed self-renewal as well as differentiation to proceed in a manner not dissimilar to in vivo hematopoiesis. This system was adapted for the propagation of human marrow by Gartner and Kaplan in 1980 (9). A unique feature of these systems was the development of an in vitro microenvironment consisting of diverse cells with features of endothelial cells, fibroblastic cells, adipocytes, and macrophages. Hematopoietic cell proliferation occurs in intimate contact with these adherent cells, which are termed "stromal cells" in the remainder of this chapter.

Stromal cells are defined as the heterogeneous-appearing collection of adherent cells that form and are necessary to support hematopoiesis in long-term marrow cultures. In human cultures, they consist of mixtures of developing and immature hematopoietic cells along with a predominant population of elongated, plump mesenchymal cells that form a syncytium (10). Some cells accumulate lipid, and others have an endothelial appearance and express factor VIII-associated antigen. Macrophages are present but comprise fewer than 10% of the adherent cell population in active cultures (11).

The essential nature of stromal cells for the maintenance of hematopoiesis in both murine and human long-term marrow cultures can be demonstrated by several types of studies. If long-term cultures are initiated in siliconized flasks, which prevents the formation of adherent cell layers, hematopoietic cell growth is abrogated. Isolated precursors of colony-forming cells (see later) proliferate only in the presence of stromal cells (12,13). Certain interleukin-3 (IL-3)-dependent cell lines proliferate in the absence of IL-3 if stromal cells are present (14). Thus, stromal cells exert effects on both survival and proliferation of early hematopoietic progenitor cells. A demonstration of the manner in which stromal cells can influence hematopoietic cell differentiation is provided by the demonstration that changes in culture conditions in long-term marrow cultures can determine whether myeloid or pre-B cells are expressed (15). However, the mechanism by which stromal cells support and control hematopoiesis remain to be elucidated. Although growth factors produced by hematopoietic and nonhematopoietic accessory cells can exert major modulating effects on hematopoiesis and are instrumental in response to hematopoietic stress, their role in the basal hematopoiesis remains speculative. It is possible that transcripts for such growth factors as the granulocyte-macrophage- and granulocyte colony-stimulating factors (GM-CSF and G-CSF) are synthesized at below detectable levels or are rapidly degraded under basal conditions. Since proteoglycans produced by stromal cells can actively bind growth factors (16), it is possible that levels below detectability can still be physiologically active. In actively hematopoietic long-term marrw cultures, only M-CSF and transforming growth factor β (TGF-β) mRNA transcripts can be detected in stromal cells (unpublished data). However, neither M-CSF nor any other growth factor nor combination of growth factors yet identified can substitute for stromal cells in allowing self-renewal of early hematopoietic progenitor cells in liquid culture.

In this chapter, aspects of the cellular and molecular biology of human marrow stromal cells are reviewed. Particular emphasis is given to studies of the response of stromal cells to hematopoietic growth factors, to control of elaboration of hematopoietic growth factors by stromal cells, and to their expression of proto-oncogenes. Recent data concerning the relationship of c-*abl* proto-oncogene transcripts to expression of growth factor mRNAs in marrow stromal cells is reviewed.

CELLULAR BIOLOGY OF STROMAL CELLS

The studies described here use two systems for the in vitro culture of stromal cells. The initial studies relied on the mixed population of stromal cells and hematopoietic cells in the adherent cell layers from active long-term marrow cultures (9). Since it proved impossible to generate clones of stromal cells from these cultures to characterize stromal cells free of admixed hematopoietic cells, the adherent cells from long-term marrow cultures were transformed with simian virus 40 (SV-40) (17). The cell lines that resulted were clonable yet had many of the characteristics of the elongated cell population found in the nontransformed adherent cells. In addition, the transformed stromal cells developed the potential for anchorage-independent growth in the presence of hematopoietic growth factors (18).

Characterization of Stromal Cells in Long-Term Marrow Cultures

Expression of Cell Surface Antigens

The surface antigens expressed by marrow stromal cells are similar to those of other mesenchymal cells. HLA type 1 antigens are expressed, but stromal cells do not react with monoclonal antibodies to HLA-DR framework determinants (Reference 11 and unpublished data). Cell sorting experiments demonstrate that stromal cell precursors express the CD34 antigen, which is also found on 10–20%

elongated cells in confluent adherent cell layers from long-term marrow cultures and on cultured endothelial cells (Reference 11 and unpublished data). The common acute lymphocytic leukemia antigen (CALLA) is expressed by most stromal cells and is characterized by faint, punctate fluorescence with anti-CALLA monoclonal antibodies (19). Passaged stromal cells do not express other determinants characteristic of mycloid or lymphoid cells (11).

Cytoskeletal Proteins

When marrow stromal cells were examined with a series of monoclonal antibodies to cytoskeletal proteins, they were found to express vimentin (antibody 43BE8) and a type of actin found only in smooth muscle and myoepithelial cells recognized by monoclonal antibody CGA-7 (20,21). Stromal cells did not react with antibodies to neurofilaments (31A11) or cytokeratin (35BH11). Importantly, neither cultured marrow fibroblasts nor cultured endothelial cells produce the actin molecule recognized by antibody CGA-7 (20), suggesting that marrow stromal cells were most closely related to smooth muscle cells and that fibroblasts, if present in the stroma, constitute a minority population. The CGA-7 monoclonal antibody is thus useful in the identification of marrow stromal cells and was used to demonstrate that SV40-transformed cell lines derived from long-term marrow culture adherent cells were stromal cells rather than fibroblasts (17).

Extracellular Matrix

Marrow stromal cells produce a complex matrix consisting of connective tissue proteins and proteoglycans, which in vivo may have a significant role in hematopoietic cell lodgment, proliferation, differentiation, and egress. A brief summary of studies of matrix molecules produced by human marrow stromal cells follows.

Matrix proteins

Analyses of proteins of the extracellular matrix produced by lcng-term marrow culture adherent cells demonstrated the presence of collagen types I, III, IV, and V, fibronectin, laminin, and thrombospondin (References 10, 22, and 23 and unpublished data). These findings are in contrast with passaged marrow fibroblasts from other sources, which synthesize only collagen types I and III. The presence of basal laminar collagens (types IV and V) in long-term marrow cultures provides further evidence for a relationship between marrow stromal cells and cultured smooth muscle cells. However, marrow stromal cells do not express myosin (unpublished data). These data suggest that marrow stromal cells have unique characteristics along with a unique function (support of hematopoiesis) and therefore should be considered an independent cell lineage.

Proteoglycans

Proteoglycans are complex macromolecules that consist of a protein core to which glycosaminoglycans and oligosaccharides are covalently attached. They can influence many cellular functions, including proliferation, differentiation, and migration. Several studies have shown their importance as regulatory molecules in hematopoiesis (24–26). For example, when proteoglycan synthesis in murine long-term marrow cultures was perturbed by treatment with β-D-xyloside, the cultures produced increased numbers of stem cells (25). The effect of β-D-xyloside is to increase free glycosaminoglycans but decrease overall proteoglycan synthesis. Proteoglycans synthesized by human marrow stromal cells from long-term marrow cultures differ significantly from those in the murine system (26). A large chondroitin sulfate proteoglycan predominates in both the medium and the cell layer. This class of proteoglycans is synthesized by many cell types, including smooth muscle cells, glial cells, and lung fibroblasts. The second major proteoglycan is hydrodynamically smaller and has glycosaminoglycans that contain about 10% idouronic acid residues. A third species found in both the medium and cell layers consists of dermatan sulfate. About 5% of the [^{35}S] sulfate labeled is heparan sulfate. Both the structural and compositional characteristics of the proteoglycans synthesized by marrow stromal cells strongly resemble those of arterial smooth muscle cells and are significantly more complex than those synthesized by marrow fibroblasts. A unique feature of long-term marrow cultures is the presence of a thick, matlike layer of proteoglycan-containing material above the stromal cell layer in which hematopoiesis cell proliferation occurs (26).

Recent data suggest that certain proteoglycan molecules, such as heparan sulfate, can specifically bind such growth factors as GM-CSF (16,27,28) and thus act as nurturing macromolecules as well as providing a physical niche for stem cell development. It is also of interest that another major component of the extracellular matrix, fibronectin, can bind TGF-β, a major hematopoietic proliferation inhibitor constitutively produced by stromal cells (29). Moreover, IL-1, another potentially important regulatory molecule produced by stimulated stromal cells and macrophages, can bind to endothelial cells (30).

Stromal Cell-Associated Hematopoiesis

Stromal cells and the extracellular matrix they produce are essential for the maintenance of hematopoiesis in long-term marrow cultures. If long-term marrow cultures are initiated in siliconized flasks, hematopoiesis declines rapidly. If an inhibitor of collagen synthesis is added, hematopoiesis is not sustained (22). The unique nature of stromal cells in supporting hematopoiesis can be shown using two-stage long-term cultures. This system employes enriched populations of hematopoietic cell progenitors (see later) cocultured with irradiated adherent cell layers from long-term marrow cultures or other test cells (12,13). The loosely adherent cells are removed weekly and tested for colony-forming progenitor cells. Stromal cells are capable of maintaining the formation of multipotent, erythroid, and granulocyte-macrophage colong-forming cells (CFU-GM) for more than 4 weeks in cultures initiated with marrow cells depleted of nearly all colony-forming cells following complement-mediated lysis using monoclonal antibodies to CD33 (13). Passaged marrow fibroblasts, umbilical vein endothelial cells, and collagen-coated flasks are ineffective at sustaining the recovery of colony-forming cells in long-term cultures from CD33-negative marrow cells (Reference 13 and unpublished data). In the following section, the growth of normal and leukemic hematopoietic cells in long-term culture is briefly reviewed to indicate interactions between hematopoietic and stromal cells.

Long-Term Marrow Cultures

Studies on normal marrow donors

When human marrow cells are placed in liquid culture in a complex medium containing fetal calf serum, horse serum, and hydrocortisone, an adherent stromal cell layer forms that supports the proliferation of multipotent hematopoietic progenitor cell for 1-2 months and committed granulopoietic progenitors for up to 4 months (9). Studies have shown that the progenitors that form the largest colonies and most multipotent colony-forming progenitors (CFU-MIX) are tightly bound to stromal cells and can only be measured following enzymatic treatment of the adherent cell layer (31). The longevity of long-term marrow cultures suggests that they allow immature progenitors, with greater self-renewal potential than colony-forming cells, to proliferate. Data on long-term cultures of hematopoietic progenitor cells isolated on the basis of cell surface phenotype support this contention (see Regulation of matrix protein mRNA).

Hematopoietic growth factors in long-term cultures. The role of hematopoietic growth factors in long-term marrow cultures is controversial. Most studies have shown that there are low levels of colony-stimulating activity in the supernatant medium of murine and human long-term marrow cultures (32). Moreover, as discussed earlier, the matrix proteoglycans of these cultures may specifically bind such growth factors as GM-CSF and thus provide relatively high local concentrations despite low levels in the medium. Studies of growth factor production by stromal cells at the RNA level are discussed in the following section.

Long-term culture of enriched progenitor cells. Antibodies recognizing differentiation antigens on myeloid cells have been used to define antigens on both colony-forming cells and a colony-forming cell precursor that proliferates in long-term culture. The antigens that have been useful in this regard are designated CD33 and CD34. CD33 is a 67 kD cell surface molecule of unknown function recognized by monoclonal antibodies L4F3 and MY9 (13). It is expressed on nearly all multipotent and committed colony-forming cells as well as more mature cells in the granulocytic lineage. When marrow cells are treated with L4F3 and rabbit complement to remove cells expressing CD33, nearly all colony-forming cells are lost. Nevertheless, if the remaining cells are cocultured with irradiated marrow stromal cells from long-term cultures, recovery of colony-forming cells occurs within 2–3 weeks and sustained hematopoiesis is observed (13). In contrast, if marrow cells expressing CD33 are positively selected by fluorescence-activated cell sorting (FACS), although colony-forming cells are greatly enriched, CFU-GM can only be detected in long-term cultures for 1–2 weeks. However, when $CD33^-$ cells are collected by FACS and cocultured with marrow stromal cells, large numbers of colony-forming cells are generated for 8 weeks or more (13). In the absence of stromal cells, regeneration of colony-forming cells does not occur. These data suggest that the CD33 antigen is not present on the progenitors capable of proliferating in long-term cultures but is acquired at the level of differentiation associated with the ability to form colonies in the presence of hematopoietic growth factors.

A second antigen that has proven useful in defining the cell surface determinants on colony-forming cell precursors is designated CD34. This is a 115 kD cell surface molecule recognized by monoclonal antibodies 12.8 and MY10. Unlike CD33, it is present on both colony-forming cells and the progenitor cells that generate colony-forming cells in long-term marrow cultures (12). Recent data have shown that CD34 is expressed on transplantable stem cells in baboons (33). When $CD34^+$ cells are separated by FACS, colony-forming cells are greatly enriched, and large numbers of colonies are produced over several months when these cells are cocultured with irradiated marrow stromal cells. $CD33^-$ cells contain no colony-forming cells and do not produce them in long-term cultures.

When two-color FACS is performed using antibodies CD33 and CD34, a non-colony-forming cell population consisting of $< 0.1\%$ of starting mononuclear marrow cells can be selected that is $CD33^-CD34^+$ with low forward light-scattering properties. When these cells are placed in long-term cultures with irradiated marrow stromal cells at limiting dilutions, colony-forming cells can be detected after several weeks from cultures initiated with as few as 10 cells (unpublished data). In a series of experiments, neither individual recombinant growth factors, such as IL-3, GM-CSF, IL-1, or IL-6, nor combinations of these factors were able to substitute for marrow stromal cells in supporting the proliferation of $CD33^-$ $CD34^+$ cells (unpublished data).

These data suggest that $CD33^-CD34^+$ is the likely phenotype for stem cells that have the following properties: (1) they are multipotent for at least the myeloid and erythroid lineages; (2) they have substantial in vitro differentiative and possibly self-renewal capabilities; (3) they have an absolute requirement for the presence of stromal cells and/or the extracellular matrix produced by stromal cells or for an as yet unidentified growth factor produced by stromal cells for proliferation.

Growth of leukemic marrow in long-term cultures. Studies by Coulombel et al. have demonstrated that long-term marrow cultures select against the growth of leukemic progenitor in samples from patients with either chronic myelogenous leukemia (CML) (34) or acute nonlymphocytic leukemia (ANL) (35). Similar data have been obtained from this laboratory using marrow from patients who were heterozygous for the X-linked enzyme glucose-6-phosphate dehydrogenase (G6PD) (Reference 36 and unpublished data). When long-term marrow cultures are established from marrow from some but not all patients with ANL or CML, after 3-4 weeks an increasing proportion of colonies express the G6PD enzyme not associated with the leukemic clone. Whether this phenomenon is due to a direct antileukemic effect of stromal cells or to a leukemic inhibitory growth factor they produce, such as transforming growth factor β (see later), has not been established.

Use of differentiation antigens to select normal progenitor cells that proliferate in long-term cultures from leukemic cells in untreated patients with ANL. When cells from G6PD heterozygous patients with newly diagnosed ANL were analyzed, two patterns of differentiative expression of clonal cells became apparent. In each of 26 cases, blast cells manifested only a single enzyme type, indicating that the disease was clonal at the time of testing (37). G6PD studies showed that in 5 elderly patients with FABM2 or FABM4 ANL, none of whom had the Philadelphia chromosome (Ph), red cells, platelets, and leukemic blast cells were derived from a common clonal progenitor cell. In contrast, in studies of 21 younger individuals, red cells and platelets appeared to be derived predominantly from normal stem cells. Thus it appeared that ANL is a heterogeneous disease; in some patients the disease either arises in or is expressed predominantly in a committed granulocyte-monocyte progenitor cell, or in other patients, as in CML, ANL originates in a multipotent stem cell.

Since CD33 is a differentiation antigen in normal marrow that distinguishes colony-forming progenitors, including multipotent colony-forming cells from their precursors, we hypothesized that if some cases of ANL either originated in or were predominantly expressed in cells at the level of committed myeloid progenitors, removal of CD33-expressing cells might purge the marrow samples of leukemic cells without affecting normal hematopoietic stem cells. Two types of experiments were performed to test this hypothesis. In the first, blood cells from seven patients with ANL were treated with monoclonal antibody L4F3 to the CD33 antigen and rabbit complement and then grown in long-term cultures with irradiated stromal cells from normal long-term cultures (38). Despite a percentage lysis that varied from 70 to 99, in four of seven G6PD heterozygous patients studied, the outgrowth of substantial numbers of normal colony-forming cells was detected within 2–3 weeks from cultures initiated with $CD33^-$ cells. Cultures from cells treated with an irrelevant control antibody grew poorly and produced only leukemic colonies. These studies have recently been confirmed in two cases studied after blood cells were separated by two-color FACS analysis using antibodies to CD33 and CD34 (submitted for publication). When blood cells from these patients were sorted on the basis of expression of CD33 and CD34 antigens and then grown in long-term cultures with irradiated long-term marrow culture adherent cell layers, only the <0.5% of cells that expressed CD34 but not CD33 proliferated and produced normal colony-forming cells. Cells that expressed both CD33 and CD34 grew only leukemic colony-forming cells. These data indicate that in some patients with ANL, early hematopoietic precursors derived from normal stem cells circulate and have the $CD33^- CD34^+$ phenotype. These cells, like their counterparts from normal bone marrow, have an absolute growth requirement for stromal cells.

$CD33^-CD34^+$ cells in patients with CML. To contrast the findings from patients with ANL whose diseases were expressed in a restricted lineage cell with a disease that originates in a pluripotent stem cell, cells with a $CD33^- CD34^+$ phenotype were isolated by FACS from peripheral blood mononuclear cells from a G6PD heterozygous patient with CML. It was possible to identify a minor cell population with a $CD33^-CD34^+$ phenotype that represented <0.01% of the starting cells. As has been described in normal marrow and in ANL blood, cells of this phenotype contained progenitor cells that have substantial proliferative capacity in two-stage long-term cultures. Approximately 3×10^3 CFU-GM-derived colonies were harvested weekly for 10 weeks from 10^4 $CD33^-$ $CD34^+$ peripheral blood cells derived from a patient 6 months after diagnosis with CML in chronic phase. The ability of these CML progenitors to produce colony-forming cells exceeded that of similarly selected marrow or blood progenitors from normal individuals by approximately 2 logs, suggesting a greatly enhanced capacity for self-renewal, a stem cell characteristic long postulated to be abnormal in CML. In contrast to similar studies on ANL, nearly all colonies obtained from the CML patient, even after 2 months in long-term culture, were derived from leukemic progenitors when analyzed by G6PD, and all colonies examined manifested the Ph chromosome (146 colonies manifested G6PD type A and 4 were G6PD type B in this patient whose CML clone was G6PD type A). Unlike direct long-term marrow cultures of CML bone marrow, two-stage long-term cultures of CML blood cells appear only rarely to selectively express colony-forming cells derived from normal stem cells. It has been shown by Eaves et al. (29), in a similar system employing CML whole-blood mononuclear cells, that CML progenitors, unlike normal progenitors, were constantly in cell cycle. They postulated that CML cells failed to respond to normal inhibitors of cell cycle that accumulate between medium replenishment in long-term marrow cultures. The present data extend these observations and suggest that isolated early progenitor cells from a single CML patient possessed greater self-renewal potential than do normal progenitors with a similar phenotype.

Table 1 Stromal Cell Production of Growth Factor and Matrix Protein mRNA[a]

Group[b]	Stimulus	mRNA Expression								
		TP	COL1	GM-CSF	IL-1β	TNF-α	G-CSF	M-CSF	IL-6	TGF-β
I*	None	++	+++	0	±	0	0	++	0	++
	IL-1	++	+	0	+	0	0	++	+	++
	TNF	++	+	0	+	0	0	++	+	++
	TNF + IL-1	++	+	0	+	+	0	++	++	++
	5AZA	-	+	0	0	0	0	-	++	-
II*	None	++	+++	0	0	0	0	++	++++	+
	IL-1	++	0	++	+	0	++	++	++	+
	TNF	++	+	++	0	+	++	++	++	+
	IL-1 + TNF	++	0	++++	+++	+++	+++	-	++++	+
	IL-6	++	0	0	0	0	0	-	0	+++
	TGF-β	++	++++	0	0	0	0	-	0	+++
	5AZA	-	+	0	0	0	0	-	+++	-
III*	-	++	+	++	++	++	+	++	++	+

[a]The exogenous growth factors applied to the cell lines were recombinant human factors and were used at the following concentrations; IL-1α, 10 U/mL; TNF-α, 1000 U/mL; IL-6, 500 U/mL; and TGF-β, 0.3 ng/mL. (IL-1α and IL-6 were kindly donated by Immunex Corporation; TNF-α was donated by Genentech Corporation.) 5-Azacytidine was used at a concentration of 10 μM. TP, thrombospondin; COL1, collagen I; 5AZA, 5-azacytidine.

[b]Group I cells were passaged stromal cells from long-term marrow cultures exposed to various stimuli. Group II cells were native SV40-transformed stromal cell lines. Group III cells were SV40-transformed stromal cell lines derived from colonies. The cell lines were tested between passages 8 and 14 from the time of derivation, which was between 2 and 4 months from the time of exogenous stimulation. Growth factor and matrix protein expression in the colony-derived cell lines were similar regardless of whether the colonies originally were autonomous or stimulated by added growth factors. All studies were performed on RNA from passaged cell lines. For studies of group I and group II cells, the dose of the stimulating factor used was one that caused maximal stimulation of colony growth in semisolid medium. The amount of mRNA present on a Northern blot was estimated semiquantitatively on a 0 to ++++ scale. Probes used were full-length cDNAs except for collagen I, which was a 1.8 kb fragment. Probes were hybridized to the blots after random priming.

MOLECULAR BIOLOGY OF STROMAL CELLS

Regulation of Expression of Growth Factor Genes in Stromal Cells

Adherent Cells from Long-Term Marrow Cultures

The adherent cell layers in long-term marrow cultures are heterogeneous and contain stromal cells, macrophages, and developing hematopoietic cells. Therefore, studies of growth factor expression by these cells can prove misleading if large amounts of a growth factor are produced by a small subpopulation of cells. Therefore, before concluding that stromal cells themselves produce a growth factor, it is necessary to confirm the finding on cloned cell lines, as described here.

When RNA was extracted from hematopoietically active long-term marrow culture adherent cells, run on Northern blots, and analyzed with cDNA probes to hematopoietic growth factor genes, only transcripts for M-CSF and transforming growth factor β were detected (summarized in Table 1). Transcripts for IL-1β, tumor necrosis factor α (TNF-α), GM-CSF, IL-6, IL-3, and G-CSF were not found even when blots were run using poly A-selected RNA. However, more sensitive techniques, such as nuclease protection assays, may demonstrate growth factor transcripts not seen on Northern blots. Therefore, the present data can be taken only as indicative of either low levels or absent growth factor expression.

When mesenchymal cells closely related to marrow stromal cell, such as cultured fibroblasts or endothelial cells, are exposed to the inflammatory lymphokines IL-1 and/or TNF, the expression of growth GM-CSF is up-regulated (39–44). In contrast, when adherent cells from long-term marrow cultures were exposed to IL-1 and/or TNF and mRNA was extracted between 30 minutes and 120 h, although transcripts for IL-6 became detectable within 2 h and expression peaked at 3 days, no transcripts for IL-1, TNF, or GM-CSF were detected (unpublished data). Adherent cells from long-term marrow cultures constitutively produce M-CSF and TGF-β transcripts. These data correlated the findings of extremely low levels of colony-stimulating activity in supernatant medium from either long-term marrow cultures or from passaged, nontransformed marrow stromal cells even after exposure to IL-1 and/or TNF. It is still possible that growth factors are transcribed by a small percentage of marrow stromal cells or that the transcripts produced by marrow stromal cells are too unstable to be detected by Northern blot analysis. There are no published data examining growth factor transcription in marrow stromal cells using the nuclear run-on technique. Data from studies of transformed marrow stromal cells suggest that a low frequency of stromal cells may constitutively produce multiple growth factors. However, the ability to detect these cells is hampered by the inability to clone nontransformed human stromal cells.

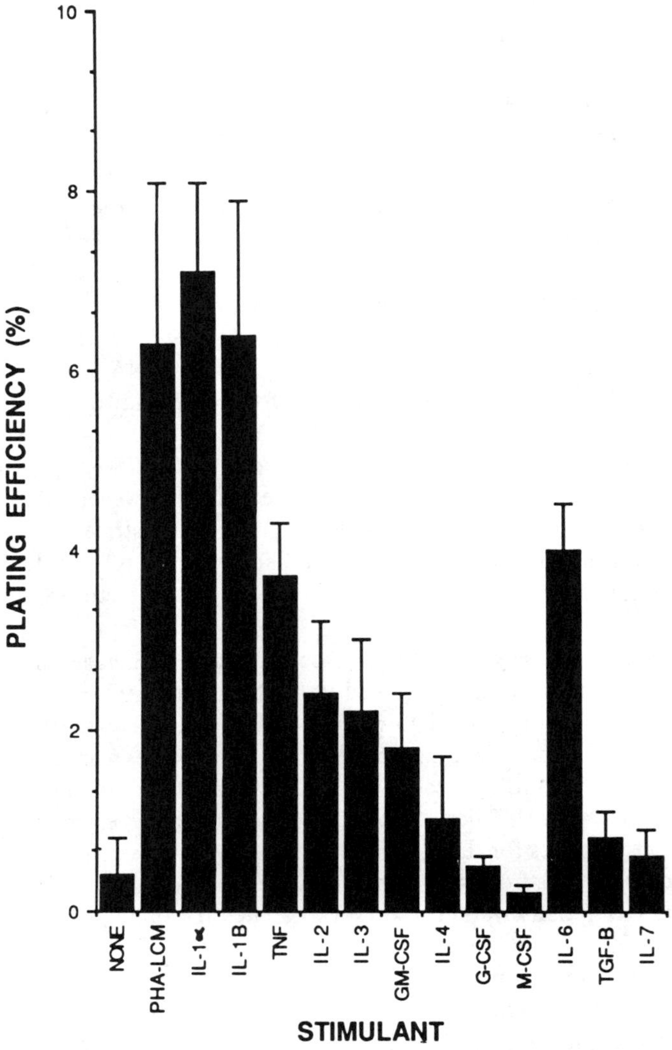

Figure 1 The effect of recombinant growth factors on colony formation by transformed marrow stromal cells. Stromal cells were seeded into semisolid medium at 10^4 cells per mL in the presence of the maximally effective concentration of various growth factors as determined by dose-response experiments. These data represent the means of at least three experiments on independently derived stromal cell lines.

Transformed Marrow Stromal Cell Lines

To further examine the properties of marrow stromal cells, SV40 was used to develop semipermanent, clonable cell lines (17). These transformed cells retained many of the characteristics of nontransformed stromal cells but acquired an apparently new potential to differentiate into "round cells," which expressed certain hematopoietic determinants, such as the T-200 antigen, and had the electron and light microscopic appearance of large, undifferentiated "blast cells" (17). An additional novel feature of the transformed cell lins was their ability to form colonies in semisolid medium. The frequency of colony formation was greatly enhanced in the presence of recombinant hematopoietic growth factors (18). In order of activity, the recombinant factors that stimulated transformed stromal cell body formation were IL-α or β, TNF-α, IL-6, IL-2, IL-3, and GM-CSF. With IL-1, a mean of 7% of plated cells formed colonies, but with GM-CSF, approximately 1% of cells did so (see Figure 1). G-CSF, M-CSF, IL-4, TGF-β, and IL-7 were without activity in this assay. The appearance of the colonies was similar regardless of which factor was used to stimulate their growth.

When individual transformed stromal cell colonies were plucked, placed in suspension culture, and assayed for expression of growth factor mRNAs, constitutive up-regulation of IL-1β, TNF-α, G-CSF, GM-CSF, and IL-6 transcripts was noted regardless of whether the colonies had grown spontaneously or in the presence of growth factors (see Table 1) (18). No transcripts for these factors were detectable in the parental cell lines, IL-3 transcripts were not found in either parental or colony-derived cell lines, but M-CSF was present at similar levels in both. Transforming growth factor β was barely detectable in the colony-derived cell lines but it was highly expressed in the native cell lines (unpublished data). The colony-derived cell lines maintained this pattern of growth factor expression without further stimulation for as long as they were maintained (over 4 months). When a colony-derived cell line was treated with actinomycin D to block transcription, the half-life for IL-6 transcripts was estimated to be in excess of 4 h, suggesting that transcript stabilization played a role in up-regulation of expression of growth factor genes.

Thus, using transformed marrow stromal cell lines, it has been possible to develop a model system to examine the regulation of growth factor gene expression in a hematopoietically relevant cell population. The data indicate that under basal conditions only M-CSF and TGF-β are constitutively expressed. However, a low frequency of transformed stromal cells spontaneously up-regulate multiple growth factor genes and form spontaneously growing anchorage-independent colonies. Cell lines developed from these colonies or from colonies stimulated by exogenous growth factors have constitutive up-regulation of expression of GM-CSF, G-CSF, IL-6, IL-1β, and TNF-α and have down-regulated TGF-β. The mechanism by which this up-regulation is achieved and its physiologic significance await further study. Studies of other mesenchymal cells suggest that both

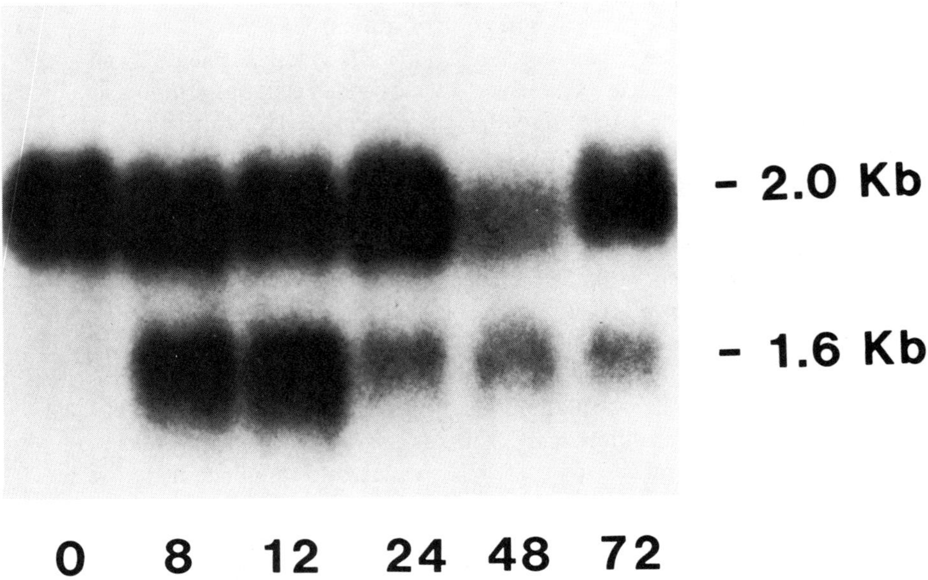

Figure 2 The effect of 20% PHA-LCM on the expression of IL-6 by transformed marrow stromal cells. Lanes represent 0, 8, 12, 24, 48, and 72 h after stimulation. Whole cellular RNA was extracted and probed on a Northern blot with a full-length cDNA for human IL-6 (1.6 kb) (courtesy of Immunex Corporation); and actin (2.0 kb).

transcriptional and posttranscriptional regulation may play a role in the up-regulation of growth factor gene expression (45).

Regulation of Matrix Protein mRNA

Marrow stromal cells produce a large number of different matrix molecules, including collagens I, III, IV, and V, fibronectin, thrombospondin, laminin, and proteoglycans (10). Using the model systems described earlier, the effect of anchorage-independent growth and exogenous growth factors on the expression of collagen types I and IV mRNA were studied. The data suggest that the expression of collagen I and TGF-β are similarly regulated and their expression bears an inverse relationship to levels of IL-6 transcripts.

When adherent cells from long-term marrow cultures were exposed to rhIL-1, IL-6 expression was up-regulated within 8 h. Somewhat later, down-regulation of collagen I and IV was observed. By 96 h, collagen transcripts were barely

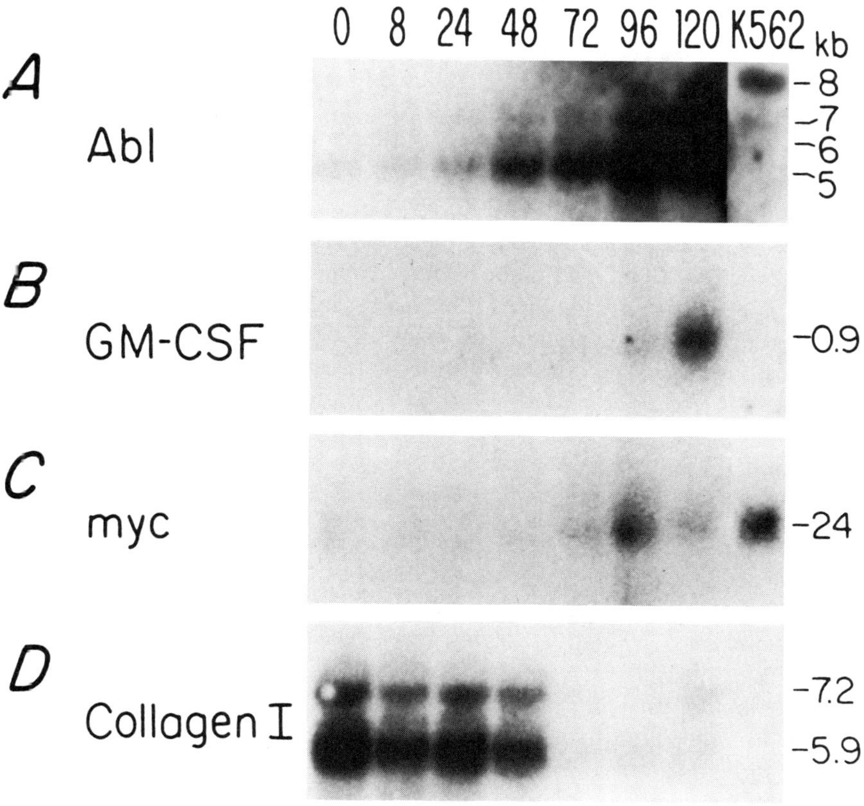

Figure 3 Northern blot of whole cellular RNA extracted at indicated times after the exposure of transformed marrow stromal cells to PHA-LCM. Each lane contains 20 μg RNA. The same blot was sequentially hybridized to a v-*abl* fragment (A); a full-length cDNA for GM-CSF (courtesy of Immunex Corporation) (B); a c-*myc* fragment (C); and a procollagen I fragment (D).

detectable (submitted for publication). Similarly, when these cells were exposed to the DNA demethylating agent 5-azacytidine, up-regulation of IL-6 was observed at 12 h and down-regulation of collagen I was noted after 72 h (submitted for publication).

Similar results were obtained using cloned SV40-transformed stromal cell lines. Induction with phytohemagglutinin- (PHA-LCM), IL-1, and/or TNF resulted in the up-regulation of IL-6 as well as G-CSF and GM-CSF with concurrent transient down-regulation of TGF-β and prolonged down-regulation of collagen (Figures 2 and 3) (18). When transformed stromal cells were grown as colonies and cell lines subsequently derived that constitutively expressed IL-6, IL-1, GM-CSF, and G-CSF, only low levels of collagen I and TGF-β transcripts were expressed (Reference 18 and unpublished data). In contrast, the parental cell lines had nondetectable expression of IL-6, G-CSF, and GM-CSF RNA when examined by Northern blot analysis but had high levels of expression of TGF-β and collagen I. M-CSF, thrombospondin, and collagen IV were equivalently expressed in parental and colony-derived cell lines.

The colony-derived cell lines are morphologically different from the native stromal cell lines. The former produce larger numbers of round cells and appear more epitheloid than the fibroblastic native cell lines. Taken together, these data are consistent with the hypothesis that transformed stromal cells have two differentiative pathways, one associated with round cells and the other with fibroblastic cells.

Regulation of c-*abl* Proto-Oncogene Expression in Marrow Stromal Cells

The process of cell differentiation from primordial embryonic cells to differentiated tissues entails the successive activation of certain basic genes, some of which control the responses to environmental factors, such as growth factors, adhesion proteins, and matrix proteins. Proto-oncogenes have physiologic roles at every level of cellular response and development. These genes, although designated proto-oncogenes, are involved in cellular processes so fundamental that their perturbation leads to cataclysmic consequences, such as malignant transformation. Proto-oncogenes have been identified that are cell surface receptors (*erb*A, *erb*B, *sis*, and *fms*), a cell membrane ion channel (*mas*), a probable signal transducer (*ras*), and DNA transcription factors (*jun* and *fos*) (46). The roles of some proto-oncogenes have been identified, but the normal role of the *abl* oncogene has remained elusive. Studies of c-*abl* expression in marrow stromal cells have led to several unique observations regarding the control of c-*abl* mRNA expression and its relationship to expression of other genes.

c-*abl* was initially isolated as the cellular homolog of an animal-transforming retrovirus, the Abelson murine leukemia retrovirus (A-MuLV) (47). In the human, the gene covers an expanse of genomic DNA spanning in excess of 200 kb at the q34.1 band of chromosome 9 (48). Interest in human c-*abl* was aroused when it was found to be involved in the 9;22 translocation of CML, where it is translocated from its normal location at 9q34 to the 3′ end of the *bcr* (breakpoint cluster region) gene located at chromosome 22 band q11 (49). Human c-*abl* has alternative first exons, designated Ia and Ib, which are found in the primary transcripts of 6 and 7 kb, respectively (50). Although two transcripts are found, only one protein product, $p145^{c\text{-}abl}$, has been described in human cells (51). Although structurally the protein possesses a tyrosine kinase domain, this activity is weak. In contrast, the p210*bcr-abl* found in CML cells has readily detectable tyrosine kinase activity (52).

The evolutionary conservation of c-*abl* is apparent from the description of a corresponding gene in *Drosophila* (53). The organization of c-*abl* in the mouse shares common features with that of the human gene. In the mouse, predominant transcripts of 5 and 6 kb are found. The murine genomic c-*abl* sequence extends over an expanse of greater than 40 kb and, like its human homolog, contains alternative first exons, each of which is spliced onto a common second exon (54). Alternative splicing of these first exons is responsible for the production of the predominant mouse c-*abl* transcripts designated type I (5 kb) and type IV (6 kb). Type I represents the predominant transcript in most tissues; type IV represents the less abundant of the two transcripts (54,55). Together, types I and IV constitute roughly 75% of c-*abl* transcripts in a given murine cell (55). The types II and III transcripts compose less than 30% of murine c-*abl* transcripts (54,55). The types II and III transcripts represent alternative splicing products of the two abundant transcripts, I and IV, and have no apparent counterparts in human cells (56).

An interesting analogy between mouse and human c-*abl* transcript expression arises when examining the relative levels of two major transcripts. Renshaw et al. have shown in the mouse that throughout various tissues the expression of higher molecular weight type IV transcript remains relatively constant but the type I may show tissue-specific expression (55). However, the rates of transcription for the two mouse c-*abl* RNAs are the same, indicating that the absolute transcript concentration is likely dependent on differential transcript stability. It is intriguing to consider in conjunction with this that the *Drosophila abl* homolog (the *dash* gene), which is most homologous with the mouse IV or human Ib transcript, possesses a 3′ untranslated region that contains multiple copies of the AUUUA motif, which designates transcripts of short duration in vertebrates (57).

This leads to the hypothesis that the high-molecular-weight c-*abl* transcript (7 kb in human or 6 kb in the mouse) in vertebrate species may be regulated by a posttranscriptional mechanism that greatly reduces its half-life but the lower molecular weight transcript is more stable. The presence of different promoters for the two transcripts and apparent variability in expression for only one transcript implies differing functions for the two translational protein products. It appears that one c-*abl* protein product (type IV), although not possessing a transmembrane region, possesses a myristylation site and is likely to be membrane bound but the type I protein product is cytoplasmic (58).

A further analogy between mouse and human c-*abl* arises when comparing low-molecular-weight transcripts. Lower molecular weight human c-*abl* transcripts besides the 6 and 7 kb transcripts have been reported (59). A human 5 kb c-*abl* transcript was found in RNA derived from blast cells of patients in the blast crisis phase of CML and also in RNA derived from marrow stromal cells

(References 60 and 61 and submitted for publication). Ponzetto and Wolgemuth described the presence of a so-called testis-specific 4 kb transcript in the mouse (62). Later, the work of two separate groups determined that this third transcript is the splice product of the mouse 5 kb transcript. That is, the mouse 4 kb testis-specific transcript arises from a truncation of a 1.2 kb portion from the 3′ untranslated region of the mouse 5 kb c-*abl* transcript (63,64).

c-abl *Expression in Marrow Stromal Cells*

In examining the level of expression of several proto-oncogenes in marrow stromal cells, high levels of expression of c-*abl* were found. Of interest, unlike the pattern in normal T lymphocytes, the 5 kb transcript was found as well as the 6 and 7 kb transcripts. The effect of growth factors that affected stromal cell proliferation on the expression of c-*abl* transcripts were then examined.

When PHA-stimulated T cell-conditioned medium was added to transformed marrow stromal cells, the level of expression of the 5 and 6 kb *abl* transcripts increased starting at about 24 h (Figure 3). A similar response was observed when IL-1α and TNF-α were used in combination. Striking up-regulation predominantly of the 5 kb c-*abl* proceeded over the ensuing 120 h (submitted for publication). This modulation of c-*abl* expression was made more intriguing by the correlation of c-*abl* up-regulation with the up-regulation of multiple growth factor genes and down-regulation of expression matrix proteins, such as collagen I, as described earlier.

*Effect of 5-Azacytidine on c-*abl *Expression*

5-Azacytidine, a cytidine analog, has been shown to affect the differentiation of murine fibroblasts to myoblasts by inducing the expression of a controlling gene (65). The exact mechanism of action of 5-azacytidine remains obscure, but one likely mechanism by which it affects certain genes is through the de facto demethylation of genes that possess G + C-rich promoters. The promoter of the c-*abl* Ia exon is G + C rich. Therefore, if 5-azacytidine affects c-*abl* expression, this may provide an opportunity to examine the effect of changes in c-*abl* expression on other genes. When either marrow stromal cells from long-term marrow cultures or transformed marrow stromal cell lines were cultured with 5-azacytidine, a rapid up-regulation of the 6 kb c-*abl* transcript was observed, with a peak effect at approximately 12 h (Figure 4). The 5 and 7 kb transcripts were unaffected. When Southern blots were prepared from stromal cell DNA restricted with methylation-sensitive restriction endonucleases, evidence for the demethylation of genomic c-*abl* was found. Thus 5-azacytidine selectively and rapidly upregulated the c-*abl* 6 kb transcript.

When the Northern blots obtained after 5-azacytidine were probed with cDNAs for growth factors, up-regulation of IL-6 was found. However, transcripts for GM-CSF, G-CSF, IL-1β, and TNF were not detectable. 5-Azacytidine-treated cultures also substantially down-regulated the expression of collagen I. These

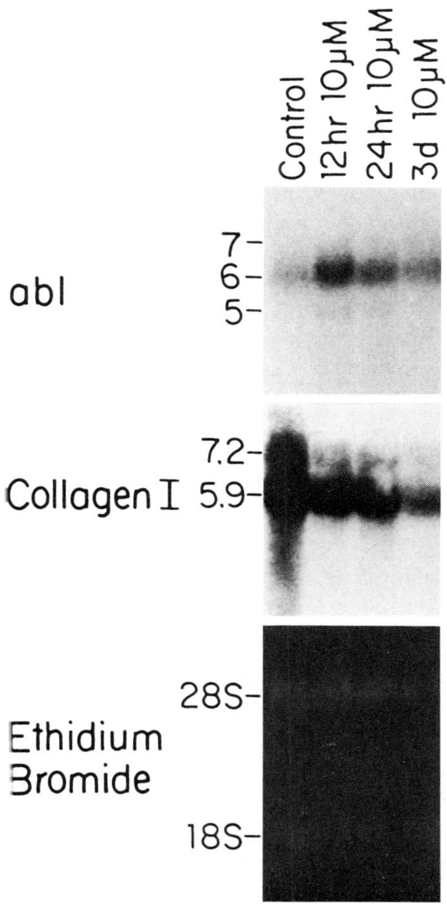

Figure 4 c-*abl* and collagen I transcript expression in transformed marrow stromal cells following treatment with 5-azacytidine. Whole cellular RNA was extracted at the indicated times. Equivalence of loading was evaluated by staining with ethidium bromide prior to transfer to nitrocellulose. The resulting blot was hybridized with a 1.5 kb *Bgl*II fragment isolated from the v-*abl* insert of the pABI sub 9 plasmid (82) (upper panel) or with a 1.8 kb collagen fragment isolated from Hf677 (83) (lower panel).

data suggest a potential direct or indirect role for the c-*abl* 6 kb transcript in increasing the expression of IL-6 and down-regulating matrix proteins.

When the effects of 5-azacytidine and IL-1 or TNF on c-*abl* expression are compared, there are two major differences. First, 5-azacytidine rapidly up-regulated c-*abl* but the effect of TNF and IL-1 occurs over several days. Second, 5-azacytidine affects only the 6 kb transcript, but the growth factors up-regulate both the 5 and 6 kb transcripts. It is of potential interest that up-regulation of either the 5 or 6 kb c-*abl* transcripts is associated with up-regulation of IL-6. However, up-regulation of other growth factors, such as GM-CSF, G-CSF, IL-1β, and TNF-α is associated only with up-regulation of the 5 kb c-*abl*, which is observed following stimulation with PHA-LCM or IL-1 and TNF. The finding of a linkage between the expression of IL-6, a B cell growth factor (66), and c-*abl* is particularly intriguing since the c-*abl*-specific sequences of the Abelson murine leukemia virus (v-abl) induce a B cell neoplasm in mice (67).

Although *abl* is expressed at low levels in many cell types, it is most highly expressed in fibroblasts (68). Nevertheless, variations in its level of transcript expression have not been shown except in murine fetal tissues and during fetal hematopoietic development (55,69). The specificity of the c-*abl* gene in transforming hematopoietic precursors has been demonstrated in two ways. First, it has been shown that expression vectors containing the *bcr-abl* fusion gene can transform pre-B cells but not fibroblasts (70–72). It has also been shown that the c-*abl* sequences of A-MuLV specify the pre-B cell-transforming qualities of the virus rather than virus-specific sequences, such as long terminal repeat (LTR) (67,73). It is likely, then, that modulation in c-*abl* transcript expression relates to the differentiative level and type of the cell affected. Additionally, the expression of the third, lower molecular weight c-*abl* transcript, which is expressed in the mouse testis, suggests tissue-specific expression. An analogous human lower molecular weight c-*abl* transcript has been found in leukemic blasts from patients in the blast crisis of CML and in transformed marrow stromal cells (60, 61). Thus, expression of the lower molecular weight transcript may be present only in primitive or transformed cell types, such as germ cell tissues, hematopoietic blasts, and transformed cell lines.

In CML, the *bcr-abl* fusion transcript is the most highly expressed of the *abl* transcripts (74,75). In normal tissues, it is possible that high expression of c-*abl* is required to produce sufficient *abl* gene product (p145) to titrate out intrinsic cellular mechanisms that inhibit that protein's tyrosine kinase activity. Such dose-dependent behavior has been proposed to explain the mechanisms of similar cytoplasmic protein kinases that are the products of the oncogenes *src* and *crk* (76,77). The possibility of such a titration mechanism is suggested by the finding that the tyrosine kinase activity of the related oncogene product $pp60^{c\text{-}src}$ is greatly enhanced after the level of the protein surpasses a certain, well-defined threshold (77). However, the ability to increase c-*abl* expression may be restricted to particular cell types at specific levels of differentiation.

As a cytoplasmic oncogene, the activated *abl* gene may be involved in anchorage independence of cells as are other cytoplasmic oncogenes (78). For example, *v-src*, another tyrosine kinase, is involved with organization of the cytoskeletal matrix (79). The present studies with c-*abl* imply a direct or indirect role for c-*abl* in the control of the extracellular matrix proteins, such as type I collagen. The implications of c-*abl* interaction with matrix proteins are myriad given the known functions of the marrow matrix. For instance, it has been shown that hematopoietic matrix proteins are capable of sequestering hematopoietic growth factors (16). It has also been shown that certain matrix elements are necessary for the differentiation of murine erythroid cells (80). Gordon et al. have shown that CML progenitors have a diminished capacity to adhere to marrow stroma and speculated that one defect in CML may be the phosphorylation of proteins involved in cell–cell adhesion by the enhanced *bcr-abl* kinase (81).

Thus, preliminary studies suggest a potential role for the c-*abl* gene product in the regulation of growth factor and matrix protein production by marrow stromal cells. It is not unreasonable to assume that similar relationships may be present in hematopoietic cells at some level of differentiation. The role of the three different c-*abl* transcripts awaits elucidation. However, the present studies suggest that they may be associated with activation of different sets of genes and affect different aspects of cell differentiation in stromal cells. It is therefore possible that c-*abl* acts as a master controlling gene for certain restricted differentiative programs.

To summarize, the findings with regard to c-*abl* mRNA expression in marrow stromal cells include (1) the presence of a 5 kb c-*abl* transcript, (2) the differential up-regulation of different c-*abl* transcripts depending upon the inducing agent used, (3) a correlation of c-*abl* up-regulation with IL-6 transcript up-regulation, and (4) a correlation of an increase in c-*abl* transcript with a decrease in collagen I transcript. Although these observations fall short of a complete mechanism to explain such interactions, they nevertheless represent new avenues to be explored in explaining the physiologic and pathophysiologic role of c-*abl* in the cell. Given the relationship of this proto-oncogene to hematopoietic cells, it is reasonable to assume that it may play a pivotal role in their proliferative or differentiative processes by interacting with specific growth factors and certain matrix or adhesion proteins.

ACKNOWLEDGMENTS

Supported by grant numbers HL31782, CA18029, CA1033, and CA 16448 from the National Institutes of Health and by research funds from the Veterans Administration.

REFERENCES

1. Metcalf, D. (1984). *The Hemopoietic Colony Stimulating Factors*. Elsevier, Amsterdam.
2. Friedenstein, A. J., Chailakhyan, R. K., Latsinik, N. V., Panasyuk, A. F., and Keiliss-Borok, I. V. (1974). Stromal cells responsible for transferring the microenvironment of hematopoietic tissues. Cloning and retransplantation in vivo. *Transplantation 17*:331–340.
3. Tavassoli, M., and Crosby, W. H. (1968). Transplantation of marrow to extramedullary sites. *Science 161*:54–56.
4. Wolf, N. S. (1983). The hematopoietic microenvironment: Current status. In *Frontiers in Experimental Hematology. Serono Symposium* (U. Torelli, P. Bagnava, M. A. Brunelli, C. Castaldini, and A. V. DiPrisco, eds.). Rome, p. 233.
5. Trentin, J. J. (1971). Determination of bone marrow stem cell differentiation by stromal hemopoietic inductive microenvironments (HIM). *Am. J. Pathol. 65*:621–627.
6. Wolf, N. S., and Trentin, J. J. (1968). Haemopoietic colony sites. V. Effect of haemopoietic organ stroma on differentiation of pluripotent stem cells. *J. Exp. Med. 127*:205–214.
7. Lichtman, M. A. (1981). The ultrastructure of the hematopoietic environment of marrow. A review. *Exp. Hematol. 9*:391–410.
8. Dexter, T. M., Allen, T. D., and Lajtha, L. G. (1977). Conditions controlling the proliferation of haemopoietic stem cells in vitro. *J. Cell. Physiol. 91*: 335–344.
9. Gartner, S. M., and Kaplan, H. S. (1980). Long term culture of human bone marrow cells. *Proc. Natl. Acad. Sci. USA 77*:4756–4761.
10. Singer, J. W., Keating, A., and Wight, T. N. (1985). The human haematopoietic microenvironment. In *Recent Advances in Haematology*, Vol. 4 (A. V. Hoffbrand, ed.). Churchill Livingstone, Edinburgh, p. 1.
11. Charbord, P., and Singer, J. W. (1986). Long-term cultures of human marrow cells. A review. *Nouv. Rev. Hematol. 28*:65–72.
12. Andrews, R. G., Singer, J. W., and Bernstein, I. D. (1986). Monoclonal antibody 12.8 recognizes a 115 kd molecule present on both unipotent and multipotent hematopoietic colony-forming cells and their progenitors. *Blood 67*:842–845.
13. Andrews, R. G., Takahashi, M., Segal, G. M., Powell, J. S., Bernstein, I. D., and Singer, J. W. (1986). The L4F3 antigen is expressed by uini- and multipotent colony forming cells but not by their precursors. *Blood 68*:1030–10035.
14. Li, C. L., and Johnson, G. R. (1985). Stimulation of multipotential, erythroid, and other murine hematopoietic progenitor cells by adherent cell lines in the absence of detectable multi-CSF (IL-3). *Nature 31*:633–635.
15. Whitlock, C. A., and Witte, O. N. (1982). Long-term culture of B lymphocytes and their precursors from murine bone marrow. *Proc. Natl. Acad. Sci. USA 79*:3608–3614.

16. Roberts, R., Gallagher, J., Spooncer, E., Allen, T. D., Bloomfield, F., and Dexter, T. M. (1988). Heparan sulfate-bound growth factors: A mechanism for stromal cell-mediated haemopoiesis. *Nature 332*:376–378.
17. Singer, J. W., Raugi, G., Charbord, P., Wight, T. N., Lopez, J., Roth, G., and Keating, A. (1987). Simian virus-40 transformed adherent cell lines from human long-term marrow cultures: Cloned cell lines produce cells with "stromal" and hematopoietic characteristics. *Blood 70*:464–474.
18. Nemunaitis, J. J., Andrews, D. F., Crittenden, C., Kaushansky, K., and Singer, J. W. (1989). The response of simian virus 40 (SV40) transformed, cultured marrow stromal cells to hematopoietic growth factors. *J. Clin. Invest.* in press.
19. Keating, A., Whalen, C. K., and Singer, J. W. (1983). Cultured marrow stromal cells express common acute lymphoblastic leukemia antigen (CALLA): Generation of long-term cultures with antibody-treated marrow. *Br. J. Haematol. 55*:623–628.
20. Gown, A. M., and Vogel, A. M. (1982). Monoclonal antibodies to intermediate filament proteins of human cells: Unique and cross-reacting antibodies. *J. Cell Biol. 95*:414–424.
21. Chabord, P., Gown, A. M., Keating, A., and Singer, J. W. (1985). CGA-7 and HHF, two monoclonal antibodies that recognize muscle actin and react with adherent cells in human long-term marrow cultures. *Blood 66*:1138–1142.
22. Zuckerman, K. S. (1984). Composition and function of the extracellular matrix in the stroma of long-term bone marrow cell cultures. In *Long-Term Bone Marrow Culture* (D. G. Wright and J. S. Greenberger, eds.). Alan R. Liss, New York, p. 157.
23. Zuckerman, K. S., and Wicha, M. S. (1983). Extracellular matrix production by the adherent cells of long-term marrow murine bone marrow cultures. *Blood 61*:540–547.
24. Gallagher, J. T., Spooncer, E., and Dexter, T. M. (1983). Role of extracellular matrix in haemopoiesis. I. Synthesis of blycosaminoglycans by mouse bone marrow cultures. *J. Cell Sci. 63*:155–171.
25. Spooncer, E., Gallagher, T. J., Kriza, F., and Dexter, T. M. (1983). Regulation of haemopoiesis in long term bone marrow cultures. IV. Glycosaminoglycans synthesis and the stimulation of haemopoiesis by β-d-xylosides. *J. Cell Biol. 96*:510–514.
26. Wight, T. N., Kinsella, M. G., Keating, A., and Singer, J. W. (1986). Proteoglycans in human long-term marrow cultures: Biochemical and ultrastructural analyses. *Blood 67*:1333–1343.
27. Gordon, M. Y., Riley, G. P., Watt, S. M., and Greaves, M. E. (1987). Compartmentalization of a haematopoietic growth factor (GM-CSF) by glycosaminoglycans in the bone marrow microenvironment. *Nature 326*:403–405.
28. Gordon, M. Y. (1988). Annotation: Extracellular matrix of the marrow microenvironment. *Br. J. Haematol. 70*:1–4.
29. Eaves, A. C., Cashman, J. D., Gaboury, L. A., Kalousek, D. K., and Eaves, C. J. (1986). Unregulated proliferation of primitive chronic myeloid leu-

kemia progenitors in the presence of normal marrow adherent cells. *Proc. Natl. Acad. Sci. USA 83*:5306–5310.
30. Thieme, T. R., Hefeneider, S. H., Wagner, C. R., and Burger, D. R. (1987). Recombinant murine and leukemia Il-1 bind to human endothelial cells with equal affinity but have an unequal capacity to induce endothelial cell adherence of lymphocytes. *J. Immunol. 139*:1173–1178.
31. Coulombel, L., Eaves, A. C., and Eaves, C. J. (1983). Enzymatic treatment of long-term marrow cultures reveals the preferential location of primitive hemopoietic progenitors in the adherent layer. *Blood 6*:291–297.
32. Lipschitz, D. A., Udupa, K. B., Taylor, R. K., Shadduck, R. K., and Waheed, A. (1987). Role of colony stimulating factor in myelopoiesis in murine long-term marrow cultures. *Blood 69*:1211–1217.
33. Berenson, R. J., Andrews, R. G., Bensinger, W. I., Kalamasz, D., Knitter, G., Buckner, C. D., and Bernstein, I. D. (1988). Antigen CD34+ marrow cells engraft lethally irradiated baboons. *J. Clin. Invest. 81*:951–955.
34. Coulombel, L., Kalousek, D. K., Eaves, C. J., Gupta, C. M., and Eaves, A. C. (1983). Long-term marrow culture reveals chromosomally normal hematopoietic progenitor cells in patients with Philadelphia chromosome positive chronic myelogenous leukemia. *N. Engl. J. Med. 308*:1493–1498.
35. Coulombel, L., Eaves, A. C., Kalousek, D., Gupta, C., and Eaves, A. (1985). Long term marrow culture of cells from patients with acute myelogenous. *J. Clin. Invest. 75*:961–969.
36. Singer, J. W., Bernstein, I. D., Davis, P. C., Walters, T. R., Raskind, W. R., and Fialkow, P. J. (1988). The effect of long-term marrow culture on the origin of colony-forming cells in acute myeloblastic leukemia: Studies of two patients heterozygous for glucose-6-phosphate dehydrogenase. *Leukemia 2*:148–152.
37. Fialkow, P. J., Singer, J. W., Raskind, W. H., Adamson, J. W., Jacobson, R. J., Bernstein, I. D., Dow, L. W., Najfeld, V., and Veith, R. (1987). Clonal development, stem cell differentiation and the nature of clinical remission in acute nonlymphocytic leukemia: Studies of patients heterozygous for glucose-6-phosphate dehydrogenase. *N. Engl. J. Med. 317*:468–473.
38. Bernstein, I. D., Singer, J. W., Andrews, R. G., Keating, A., Powell, J. S., Bjornson, B. H., Cuttner, J., Najfeld, V., Reaman, G., Raskind, W., Sutton, D. M. C., and Fialkow, P. J. (1987). Treatment of acute myeloid leukemia cells in vitro with a monoclonal antibody recognizing a myeloid differentiation antigen allows normal progenitor cells to be expressed. *J. Clin. Invest. 79*:1153–1159.
39. Bagby, G. C., Dinarello, C. A., Wallace, P., Wagner, C., Hefeneider, S., and McCall, E. (1986). Interleukin-I stimulates granulocyte-macrophage colony-stimulating activity release by vascular endothelial cells. *J. Clin. Invest. 78*: 1316–1323.
40. Broudy, V. C., Kaushansky, K., Segal, G. S., Harlan, J. N., and Adamson, J. W. (1986). Tumor necrosis factor stimulates human endothelial cells to produce granulocytic-macrophage colony stimulating factor. *Proc. Natl. Acad. Sci. USA 83*:7467–7480.

41. Fibbe, W. E., Van Damme, J., Billau, A., Duinkerken, N., Lurvink, E., Ralph, P., Altrock, B. W., Kaushansky, K., Wilemeze, W., and Falkenburg, J. H. F. (1988). Human fibroblasts produce granulocyte-CSF, macrophage-CSF, and granulocyte-macrophage-CSF following stimulation by interleukin-1 and poly(rI)·poly(rC). *Blood 72*:860–866.
42. Fibbe, W. E., Van Damme, J., Billau, A., Goselink, H. M., Voogt, P. J., Van Eeden, G., Ralph, P., Altrock, B. W., and Falkenburg, J. H. F. (1988). Interleukin-1 induces human marrow stromal cells in long-term culture to produce G-CSF and M-CSF. *Blood 71*:430–435.
43. Kaushansky, K., Lin, N., and Adamson, J. W. (1988). Interleukin 1 stimulates fibroblasts to synthesize granulocyte-macrophage and granulocyte colony-stimulating factors. *J. Clin. Invest. 81*:92–97.
44. Zsebo, K. M., Yuschenkoff, V. N., Schiffer, F., Chang, D., McCall, E., Dinarello, C. A., Brown, M. A., Altrock, B., and Bagby, G. C., Jr. (1988). Interleukin-1 stimulates human endothelial cells to produce granulocyte-macrophage colony-stimulating factor and granulocyte colony-stimulating factor. *Blood 71*:99–103.
45. Koeffler, H. P., Gasson, J., and Tobler, A. (1988). Transcriptional and post-transcriptional modulation of myeloid colony-stimulating factor expression by tumor necrosis factor and other agents. *Mol. Cell. Biol. 8*:3432–3438.
46. Bishop, J. M. (1987). The molecular genetics of cancer. *Science 235*:305–311.
47. Heisterkamp, N., Groffen, J., and Stephenson, J. (1983). The human v-*abl* homologue. *J. Mol. Appl. Genet. 2*:57–68.
48. Bernards, A., Rubin, C. M., Westbrook, C. A., Paskind, M., and Baltimore, D. (1987). The first intron in the human c-*abl* gene is at least 200 kilobases long and is a target for translocations in chronic myelogenous leukemia. *Mol. Cell. Biol.* 7:3231–3236.
49. de Klein, A., van Keessel, G., Grosveld, G., Bartram, C., Hagemeijer, D., Bootsma, D., Spurr, N., Heisterkamp, N., Groffen, J., and Stephenson, J. (1982). A cellular oncogene is translocated to the Philadelphia chromosome in chronic myelogenous leukaemia. *Nature 300*:765–767.
50. Shtivelman, E., Lifschitz, B., Gale, R. P., Roe, B., and Canaani, E. (1986). Alternative splicing of RNA's transcribed from the human abl gene and from the *bcr-abl* fuser gene. *Cell 47*:277–284.
51. Witte, O. N., Rosenberg, N., and Baltimore, D. (1979). A normal cell protein cross reactive to the major Abelson murine leukaemia virus gene product. *Nature 281*:396–398.
52. Davis, R. L., Konopka, J. B., and Witte, O. N. (1985). Activation of the c-*abl* oncogene by viral transduction or chromosomal translocation generates altered c-*abl* proteins with similar in vitro kinase activity. *Mol. Cell. Biol. 5*: 204–213.
53. Hoffman-Falk, H., Einat, P., and Shilo, B. Z. (1983). *Drosophila melanogaster* DNA clones homologous to vertebrate oncogenes: Evidence for a common ancestor to the *scr* and *abl* cellular genes. *Cell 32*:589–598.
54. Ben-Neriah, Y., Bernards, A., Paskind, M., Daley, G. Q., and Baltimore, D. (1986). Alternative 5′ exons in c-*abl* mRNA. *Cell 44*:577–586.

55. Renshaw, M. W., Capozzo, M. A., and Wang, J. W. J. (1988). Differential expression of type-specific c-*abl* mRNAs in mouse tissue and cell lines. *Mol. Cell. Biol. 8*:4547–4551.
56. Bernards, A., Paskind, M. T., and Baltimore, D. (1988). Four murine c-*abl* mRNA's arise by usage of two transcriptional promoters and alternative splicing. *Oncogene 2*:297–304.
57. Henkemeyer, M. J., Bennett, R. L., Gertler, F. B., and Hoffman, F. M. (1988). DNA sequence, structure, and tyrosine kinase activity of the *Drosophila melanogaster* Abelson proto-oncogene homolog. *Mol. Cell. Biol. 8*: 843–853.
58. Pendergast, A. M., Traugh, J. A., and Witte, O. N. (1987). Normal cellular and transformation-associated *abl* proteins share common sites for protein kinase C phosphorylation. *Mol. Cell. Biol. 7*:4280–4298.
59. Westin, E. H., Wong-Staal, F., Gelmann, E. P., Eva, A., Reddy, E. P., Tronick, S. R., Aaronson, S. A., and Gallo, R. C. (1982). Expression of cellular homologs of retroviral *onc* genes in human hematopoietic cells. *Proc. Natl. Acad. Sci. USA 79*:2490–2494.
60. Andrews, D. F., and Collins, S. J. (1987). Heterogeneity in expression of the *bcr-abl* fusion transcript in CML blast crisis. *Leukemia 1*:718–724.
61. Andrews, D. F., Nemunaitis, J. J., and Singer, J. W. (1988). Cultured human marrow stromal cells increase the expression of the c-*abl* proto-oncogene and GM-CSF but down-regulate collagen I in response to tumor necrosis factor and interleukin 1. submitted.
62. Ponzetto, C., and Wolgemuth, D. J. (1985). Haploid expression of a unique c-*abl* transcript in the mouse male germ line. *Mol. Cell. Biol. 5*:1791–1794.
63. Oppi, C., Shore, S. K., and Reddy, E. P. (1987). Nucleotide sequence of testis-derived c-*abl* cDNA's: Implications for testis-specific transcription and *abl* oncogene activation. *Proc. Natl. Acad. Sci. USA 84*:8200–8204.
64. Meijer, D., Hermans, A., von Lindern, M., van Agthoven, T., de Klein, A., Mackenback, P., Grootegoed, A., Talarico, D., Valle, G., and Grosveld, G. (1987). Molecular characterization of the testes-specific c-*abl* mRNA in mouse. *EMBO J. 6*:4041–4048.
65. Pinney, D. F., Pearson-White, S. H., Konieczny, S. F., Latham, K. E., and Emerson, C. P. (1988). Myogenic lineage determination and differentiation: Evidence for a regulatory pathway. *Cell 53*:781–793.
66. Kohase, M., Henriksen-DeStenfano, D., May, L. T., Vilcek, J., and Sehgal, P. B. (1986). Induction of beta 2-interferon by tumor necrosis factor: A homeostatic mechanism in the control of cell proliferation. *Cell 45*:659–664.
67. Mathey-Prevot, B., and Baltimore, D. (1988). Recombinants within the tyrosine kinase region of v-*abl* and v-*src* identify a v-*abl* segment that confers lymphoid specificity. *Mol. Cell. Biol. 8*:234–240.
68. Wang, J., and Baltimore, D. (1983). Cellular RNA homologous to the Abelson murine leukemia virus transforming gene: Expression and relationship to the viral sequence. *Mol. Cell. Biol. 3*:773–779.

69. Muller, R., Slamon, D. J., Tremblay, J. M., Cline, M. J., and Verma, M. (1982). Differential expression of cellular oncogenes during pre- and post-natal development of the mouse. *Nature 299*:640–644.
70. Daley, G. Q., McLaughlin, J., Witte, O. N., and Baltimore, D. (1987). The CML-specific p210 *bcr/abl* protein, unlike v-*abl*, does not transform NIH/3/3 fibroblasts. *Science 237*:532–535.
71. McLaughlin, J., Chianese, E., and Witte, O. N. (1987). In vitro transformation of immature hematopoietic cells by the p210 *bcr/abl* oncogene product of the Philadelphia chromosome. *Proc. Natl. Acad. Sci. USA 84*:6558–6562.
72. Young, J., and Witte, O. N. (1988). Selective transformation of primitive lymphoid cells by the *bcr/abl* oncogene expressed in long-term lymphoid or myeloid cultures. *Mol. Cell. Biol. 8*:4079–4087.
73. Green, P. L., Kaehler, D. A., McKearn, J., and Risser, R. (1988). Substitution on the LTR of Abelson murine leukemia virus does not alter the cell type of virally induced tumors. *Oncogene 2*:585–592.
74. Collins, S. J., and Groudine, M. (1983). Rearrangement and amplification of c-*abl* sequences in the human chronic myelogenous leukemia cell line K-562. *Proc. Natl. Acad. Sci. USA 80*:4813–4817.
75. Shtivelman, E., Lifshitz, B., Gale, R. P., and Canaani, E. (1985). Fused transcripts of *abl* and *bcr* in chronic myelogenous leukemia. *Nature 315*:550–554.
76. Mayer, B. J., Hammaguchi, M., and Hanafusa, H. (1988). A novel viral oncogene with structural similarity to phospholipase C. *Nature 332*:272–275.
77. Kmiecik, T. E., Johnson, P. J., and Shalloway, D. (1988). Regulation by the autophosphorylation site in overexpressed pp60c-*src*. *Mol. Cell. Biol. 8*:4541–4546.
78. Weinberg, R. A. (1985). The actions of oncogenes in the cytoplasm and nucleus. *Science 230*:770–776.
79. Rohrschneider, C. R. (1980). Adhesion plaques of Rous sarcoma virus transformed cells contain the *src* gene product. *Proc. Natl. Acad. Sci. USA 77*:3514–3518.
80. Patel, V. P., and Lodish, H. F. (1987). A fibronectin matrix is required for differentiation of murine erythroid cells into reticulocytes. *J. Cell Biol. 105*:3105–3118.
81. Gordon, M. Y., Dowding, C. R., Riley, G. P., Goldman, J. M., and Greaves, M. E. (1987). Altered adhesive interactions with marrow stroma of haematopoietic progenitor cells in chronic myeloid leukemia. *Nature 328*:342–344.
82. Wang, A. M., Creasey, A. A., Ladner, M. B., Lin, L. S., Strickler, J., Van Arsdell, J. N., Yamamoto, R., and Mark, D. F. (1985). Molecular cloning of a cDNA for human tumor necrosis factor. *Science 228*:149–154.
83. Chu, M. L., Myeres, J. C., Bernard, M. P., Ding, J. F., and Ramirez, F. (1982). Cloning and characterization of five overlapping cDNAs specific for human proAl(I) collagen chain. *Nucleic Acids Res. 10*:5925–5933.

14

Hematopoietic Regulation of Stem Cell Dynamics in Chronic Myelogenous Leukemia

Susan C. Guba and Stephen G. Emerson *The University of Michigan Medical Center, Ann Arbor, Michigan*

INTRODUCTION

Stable-phase chronic myelogenous leukemia (CML) is a disease characterized by an unexplained phenotypic presentation. The peripheral blood white blood cell count is elevated and includes immature myeloid forms. The bone marrow is hypercellular, and the cells derive almost entirely from a single leukemic clone, marked by the Philadelphia chromosome (Ph). The cellular and molecular mechanisms that allow both the expansion of the CML clone within the bone marrow and the increased production of myeloid cells by that clone are not yet known. In this chapter, we explore a possible molecular basis that explains these dynamic features of CML.

PARADOXICAL BEHAVIOR OF IN VIVO AND IN VITRO CML STEM CELLS AND PROGENITOR CELLS

CML cells behave paradoxically in vivo and in vitro. In vivo, CML cells have a clear proliferative advantage over normal bone marrow cells. This proliferative advantage results in a gradual overwhelming of the bone marrow hematopoietic cells compartment by the CML clone (1). Premature, exuberant release of the CML cells results in a left-shifted peripheral blood leukocytosis.

In contrast, in vitro CML bone marrow progenitor cells have no proliferative advantage over normal hematopoietic bone marrow cells. Two general categories of in vitro hematopoietic cell culture techniques exist: short-term and long-term cultures. Short-term cultures consist of a semisolid nutrient medium, such as methylcellulose, to which appropriate cell numbers and colony-stimulating factors have been added. When plated in short-term methylcellulose cultures, CML progenitor cells differentiate with the same kinetics as do normal progenitor cells. Moreover, their quantitative dose response to colony-stimulating factors [granulocyte-macrophage colony-stimulating factor (GM-CSF) and interleukin 3 (IL-3)] is identical to that of normal bone marrow progenitor cells (2).

Long-term (Dexter) cultures consist of a stromal layer capable of producing CSF as well as providing a surface for cell-cell interaction. In long-term liquid cultures, the hematopoietic bone marrow cells are suspended in an appropriate liquid nutrient medium and then layered onto the stromal layer (3). The stromal layer produces the colony-stimulating activity required for progenitor cell proliferation and differentiation. When bone marrow samples from CML patients are cultured in such a long-term Dexter culture, cells derived from the malignant Philadelphia-positive (Ph^+) clone not only have no proliferative advantage over normal (Ph^-) stem cells but actually proliferate less well then the normal stem cells. In fact, over the course of 2-3 months in Dexter culture, CML stem cell growth disadvantage results in the disappearance of the Ph^+ clone from the cultures and resurgence of the normal Ph^- cells (4-6).

What is the molecular basis or explanation for the in vivo growth advantage and the in vitro growth disadvantage of CML (Ph^+) stem cells? Does a predictable, manipulatable cell marker exist that explains the aberrant behavior of Ph^+ stem cells? Can the abnormal in vivo behavior of CML stem cells be identified by a specific in vitro assay? Can specific therapeutic modalities be tested by this in vitro assay to predict a clinical response? These questions serve as the basis for our discussion.

HYPOTHETICAL EXPLANATION OF THE IN VIVO AND IN VITRO PARADOXICAL DYNAMICS OF CML

The paradox of in vivo CML proliferative advantage and in vitro proliferative disadvantage could have several explanations, including two that take into account the particular features of Dexter cultures. First, by disrupting the normal, tightly packed three-dimensional bone marrow architecture, the effective local concentration of matrix proteins and stroma around stem cells is reduced. Thus, in vivo, a defect in stem cell receptors for adhesive stromal proteins would permit anomalous quantitative regulation of CML stem cells, leading to uncontrolled proliferation and release of early myeloid forms into the peripheral blood. In contrast, defective stem cell receptors in vitro could result in the total failure of sufficient stem cell adhesion, leading to irreversible failure of Ph^+ hematopoiesis.

A second, alternative mechanism to explain the in vivo-in vitro paradox is in vivo stem cell regulation by T lymphocytes. If a subset of bone marrow T cells suppresses normal stem cell proliferation but is unable to suppress Ph^+ stem cell proliferation, then CML cells would have a strong in vivo proliferative advantage. If this T cell subset failed to survive in vitro, then no proliferative advantage of CML stem cells would be observed. Thus, it is possible that CML progenitor cells achieve their in vivo proliferative advantage by escaping from this autologous immune regulatory system. As we discuss later, several lines of evidence suggest that such an immune surveillance mechanism may exist and may be subverted in CML. Specific experiments to substantiate or disprove such a mechanism are directly available.

HEMATOPOIETIC REGULATION BY T LYMPHOCYTES

Hematopoiesis is a tightly regulated process. Normal blood counts are maintained within a tight range even when violent disruptions of the system, such as bone marrow transplantation, are imposed (7,8). The mechanism of this self-regulation is unknown; however, DR-recognizing T cells, suppressive to progenitor cells, may mediate the process. This hypothesis is based upon clinical observation: monoclonal T cell proliferations that suppress either erythropoiesis or myelopoiesis have been widely described and characterized. Furthermore, such lineage-specific regulation has, in some cases, been shown to be DR restricted (9–13).

To explain in more detail the cellular and molecular basis of T cell-progenitor cell regulation, we have developed an in vitro model system that demonstrates aspects of specific T cell-progenitor cell recognition and regulation, which we term the autologous T cell proliferative response (APLR) (14). The autologous proliferative T lymphocyte response is an autostimulatory response in which bone marrow mononuclear cells enriched for progenitor cells stimulate the proliferation of a subset of peripheral autologous T lymphocytes.

The in vitro model system is a coculture between bone marrow progenitor cells and peripheral blood T lymphocytes. To obtain the progenitor cells, bone marrow mononuclear cells are separated on a Ficoll gradient, thrice washed, and adherence depleted to remove stromal cells. The nonadherent cells are then labeled with a panel of murine monoclonal antibodies. The panel is designed to remove nonprogenitor cells that stimulate immune responses: B cells [anti-B_1, anti-CALLA, (common acute lymphocytic leukemia antigen) and anti-DQ), monocytes (adherence, anti-Leu M1,and anti-DQ), dendritic cells (anti-Leu 6 and anti-DQ), endothelial cells and fibroblasts (adherence and anti-DQ), and T cells (anti-Leu 1 and anti-Leu 5). The antibody-coated cells are removed by adherence to rabbit antimouse Ig-coated plastic dishes ("panning"). The nonadherent cells are enriched approximately 100-fold for progenitor cells. Anti-HLA-DQ is

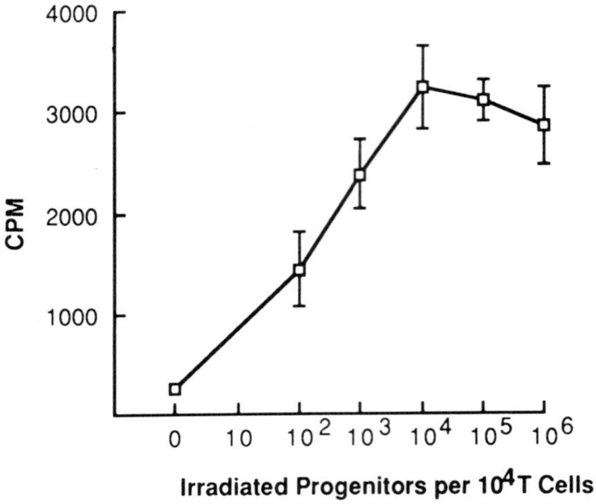

Figure 1 The stimulator cell-responder cell dose-response curve for the APLR. [^{3}H] thymidine uptake by 10,000 Leu 1$^+$ T cells stimulated by 100–1,000,000 cells measured on day 8. The data shown are means ± SD of triplicate samples and are from one of five similar experiments. (Reprinted from *The Journal of Immunology 142*:766–772, 1989, with permission courtesy of the American Association of Immunologists.)

Table 1 Proliferation of Multiply Autostimulated T Cells to Autologous and Allogeneic Targets

Stimulator cells	T cell proliferation (CPM)	Mean stimulation index
0	543 ± 173[a]	–
Autologous progenitors	9205 ± 1420	16.1 ± 3.1
Autologous macrophage	1043 ± 120	1.8 ± 0.9
Autologous B cells	832 ± 75	1.5 ± 0.7
Allogeneic PBLs	2400 ± 725	4.4 ± 2.4
Allogeneic B cells	3225 ± 922	5.0 ± 2.4
Allogeneic macrophages	1900 ± 425	3.1 ± 1.6

[a]Peripheral Leu 1$^+$ T cells were cultured with irradiated enriched autologous progenitor cells and then restimulated with frozen-thawed irradiated autologous progenitor cells on days 14 and 28. On day 42 the cells were collected, separated on Ficoll, washed, and rechallenged with irradiated autologous progenitors, B cells, or macrophages or allogeneic peripheral blood lymphocytes, B cells, or macrophages. The data are presented both as raw cpm ± SD from one representative experiment (of three) and as mean SI ± SD from all three experiments. [^{3}H] thymidine incorporation in control cultures containing 10^4 progenitors alone was always less than 150 cpm.

Source: Reprinted from *The Journal of Immunology 142*:766–772, 1989, with permission courtesy of the American Association of Immunologists.

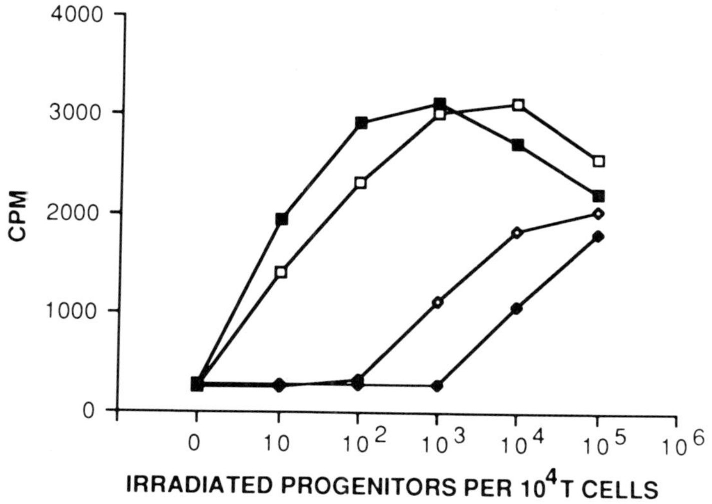

Figure 2 An My $10^{+}DR^{+}$ cell is required to stimulate the APLR. Enriched progenitor cells were prepared by adherence depletion and panning utilizing the standard cocktail of monoclonal antibodies (antiglycophorin A, Leu 1, Leu 5, Leu 6, DQ, Leu M1, Leu 12, CALLA, and My 8, □). In parallel aliquots, saturating quantities of anti-HLA-DR (◇), anti-My 10 (◆), or anti-LFA-1α + 1β (■) were included in the panning cocktail. The resultant negatively selected cells (100–1,000,000) were irradiated and cocultured with 10^4 autologous Leu 1^+ T cells, and [^{3}H] thymidine uptake was measured on day 8. Reprinted from the Journal of Immunology 142:766–772, 1989, courtesy of the Americal Association of Immunologists.

especially useful since progenitors are the only known HLA-DR^+, DQ^- cells. Peripheral blood T cells are isolated in a similar fashion. Adherence-depleted peripheral blood mononuclear cells are incubated with anti-Leu 1 and then exposed to the rabbit antimouse Ig-coated plastic dish. Adherent Leu 1^+ T cells are then recovered by scraping with a rubber policeman.

Utilizing the enriched bone marrow progenitor cells and peripheral blood T cells, one-way stimulatory cocultures are established to directly measure T cell proliferation stimulated by autologous progenitor cells. The bone marrow progenitor cells are irradiated (20 Gy) and cultured with the peripheral blood T cells in 10% autologous serum. T cell proliferation is then assessed by [^{3}H] thymidine incorporation, following a 16 h pulse, at 4, 8, and 12 days. Under these conditions, optimal stimulation occurs when T cells and progenitor cells are mixed in a 1:1 ratio (Figure 1) and is seen at 8 days of coculture. This primary autologous proliferative T lymphocyte response to progenitor cells is stronger than the APLR to B cells or macrophages. Of particular interest, these progenitor-responsive T cells are specifically expanded, resulting in a population of T

Table 2 Inhibition of Progenitor-Stimulated T Cell Proliferation by Monoclonal Antibodies Binding Progenitor Cell and T Cell Determinants

Stimulator cells	Antibodies	T cell proliferation CPM	Mean stimulation index
0	0	437 ± 125[a]	–
Progenitor cells	0	3480 ± 760	8.2 ± 2.9[a]
	CD3	9520 ± 1242	22.2 ± 4.9
	CD2	250 ± 85	0.5 ± 0.2
	CD4	1825 ± 325	4.3 ± 3.4
	CD8	3560 ± 842	8.4 ± 3.4
	LFA-1α	3240 ± 520	6.9 ± 2.7
	LFA-1β	3654 ± 830	9.0 ± 4.0
	IL-2R	3404 ± 423	8.5 ± 2.6
	DR	429 ± 109	1.2 ± 0.3
	My 7	3642 ± 859	9.3 ± 3.6
	My 9	3423 ± 645	7.8 ± 3.3
	LFA-3	452 ± 89	1.1 ± 0.2

[a]Saturating quantities of individual monoclonal antibodies were added to APLR reactions containing 10^4 Leu 1^+ peripheral T cells and 10^4 irradiated bone marrow progenitor cells or without progenitor cells. Microcultures were pulsed on day 7 and harvested on day 8. The data shown are raw cpm ± SD from an individual representative experiment (of four) and mean stimulation indices ± SD from all four experiments. Stimulation indices were calculated by comparing [^{3}H] thymidine incorporation in experimental samples with control samples containing only T cells. [^{3}H] thymidine incorporation in cultures containing only 10^4 irradiated enriched progenitor cells was always less than 150 cpm.

Source: Reprinted from *The Journal of Immunology 142*:766–772, 1989, with permission courtesy of the American Association of Immunologists.

cells that proliferates strongly and relatively specifically to autologous progenitor cells (Table 1).

Since not all the cells remaining following bone marrow panning were progenitor cells, we modified the panning antibody cocktail to remove progenitor cells as well. The cocktail of monoclonal antibodies (antiglycophorin A, Leu 1, Leu 5, Leu 6, DQ, Leu M1, Leu 12, CALLA, and My 8) used to pan the bone marrow mononuclear cells also contained saturating quantities of anti-HLA-DR, anti-My 10, or anti-LFA-1α and anti-LFA-1β. The panned bone marrow mononuclear cells and T cells were then coincubated and T cell proliferation was assessed by [^{3}H] thymidine incorporation. These experiments showed that inclusion of either anti-HLA-DR or anti-My 10 antibodies in the panning cocktail, but not anti-LFA-1α plus anti-LFA-1β antibodies, attenuated the autostimulation of T lymphocytes by over 99% (Figure 2). DR and My 10 are present on hematopoietic

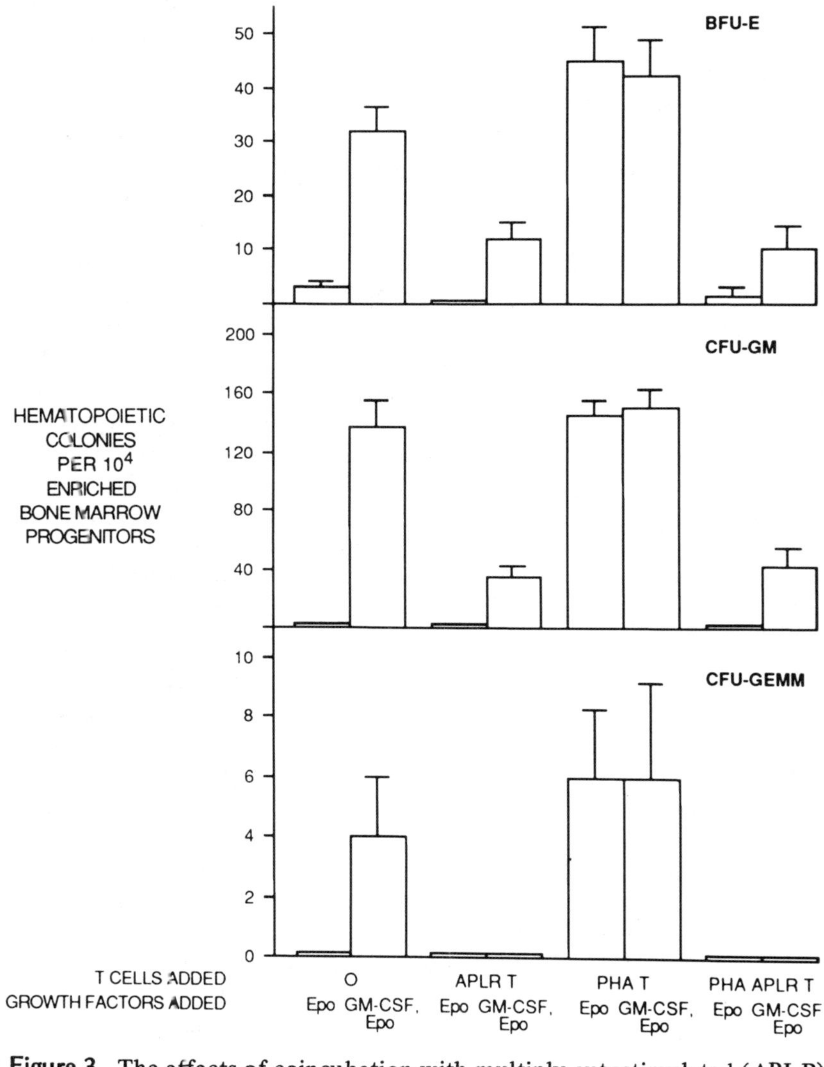

Figure 3 The effects of coincubation with multiply autostimulated (APLR) T cells on the proliferation and differentiation of hematopoietic progenitors. Enriched progenitor cells were cultured overnight either alone or with an equal number of APLR T cells, PHA-stimulated T cells, or PHA-stimulated APLR T cells and then plated in methylcellulose. Colonies were counted on days 14 and 17. Mean colony counts are from one of three experiments. (Reprinted from *The Journal of Immunology 142*: 766–772, 1989, with permission courtesy of the American Association of Immunologists.)

progenitor cells, DQ is not, and LFA-1 is widely expressed on bone marrow cells except progenitors. These data indicate, then, that the DR^+ My 10^+ DQ^- $LFA\text{-}1^-$ cells—that is, progenitor cells—from the incubation coculture are responsible for the generation of a suppressive T cell subset.

What molecular characteristics of the progenitor cells or T lymphocytes are required for the autostimulation and T cell proliferation to occur? Asked another way, are specific T cell and specific progenitor cell surface receptors required for normal autostimulation? To answer this question, blocking experiments were performed. In these experiments, murine monoclonal antibodies directed against the progenitor cell surface receptors HLA-DR, LFA-3, My 7, and My 9 were coincubated with irradiated, enriched bone marrow progenitor cells and peripheral blood T lymphocytes. Blocking the HLA-DR and LFA-3 receptors with their monoclonal antibody results in abrogation of the APLR, but blocking with My 7 or My 9 had no effect (Table 2). Similarly, known T cell surface markers potentially required for progenitor cell recognition were tested for their role in the stimulation of T cells. T cell surface proteins CD2, the LFA-3 receptor, CD4, CD8, and LFA-1 were blocked with their corresponding monoclonal antibody. Anti-CD2 was completely inhibitory to T cell proliferation. Anti-CD4 was partially inhibitory to T cell proliferation, but anti-CD8, anti-LFA-1α,β, and anti-IL-2R were ineffective blockers of the APLR. Finally, anti-CD3 was directly mitogenic to T cells (Table 2).

We then asked about the characteristics of the autostimulated T cells. Specifically, were the T cells suppressive or stimulatory to autologous progenitor cell proliferation? Four parallel experiments were performed to determine the effect of the autostimulated T lymphocytes on autologous progenitor cells. Unirradiated progenitor cells were incubated overnight either alone or with autostimulated T cells, phytohemagglutinin (PHA)-stimulated T cells, or PHA-autostimulated T cells. The cells were then plated on short-term methylcellulose culture and growth was supported with the growth factors granulocyte-macrophage colony-stimulating factor and erythropoietin. Colonies were counted on days 14 and 17. The results of this experiment showed that, nonspecifically, PHA-stimulated T cells replaced the requirement for added GM-CSF and did not suppress maximally stimulated cultures. However, the APLR stimulated T cells did not replace the GM-CSF requirement and actually significantly decreased the proliferation of autologous progenitor cells (Figure 3). Thus, APLR T cells are a specific subset of T cells that have a suppressive effect on autologous progenitor cell proliferation. Moreover, this subset of T cells is specifically stimulated and appears to require recognition of HLA-DR and LFA-3 for proliferation of the appropriate T cell subset.

This information has profound implications for normal hematopoietic regulation. A T cell subset exists that proliferates in response to DR^+ cycling progenitor cells. Once activated, these autoreactive T cells are responsible for the autoregulation of progenitor cells. The autoregulation is suppressive and thereby ensures that blood count homeostasis is maintained. Generation of the appropriate T cell subset requires interaction between bone marrow LFA-3+, DR+, progenitor cells and peripheral blood T lymphocytes. Interference with this interaction could result in the loss of homeostatic control if the suppressive T cell subset is not generated.

APPLICATION OF THE APLR MODEL TO CML

The APLR model we have developed is exciting not only because it explains hematopoietic homeostasis in normal bone marrow, but also because it may be useful in explaining hematopoietic hyperproliferation in myeloproliferative disorders, such as CML. As we have discussed, CML is a disease characterized by hyperproliferation in the bone marrow. Based upon the APLR model, the hyperproliferation of CML could be explained as a result of progenitor cell escape from T cell autoregulation.

To test this hypothesis, CML bone marrow and peripheral blood are panned for progenitor cells and T lymphocytes, respectively. The irradiated progenitor cells and T lymphocytes are coincubated, and T cell proliferation is measured by [^{3}H] thymidine incorporation. When this experiment is performed, no T cell proliferation occurs (15). The lack of the autologous proliferative lymphocyte response suggests that stimulation of CML T lymphocytes with autologous CML progenitor cells does not result in generation (proliferation) of a suppressive T cell subset. As a result, in vivo, unsuppressed or hyperproliferative growth of progenitor cells occurs.

Furthermore, the lack of the APLR suggests that CML Ph+ progenitor cells are deficient, structurally or functionally, in the cell surface receptors required for generation of the suppressive T cell subset. In other words, CML Ph+ progenitor cells lack either or both DR or LFA-3 cell surface markers. When the presence of these cell surface markers on progenitor cells is evaluated by panning and methylcellulose cultures, CML progenitor cells appear to be LFA-3 deficient (15). Thus, absence of the LFA-3 cell surface receptor would prevent the autoproliferation of regulatory, suppressive T cells and explain the exuberant hyperproliferation of the CML clone in vivo. In addition, the absence of these regulatory T cells in vitro removes the proliferative advantage of the CML Ph+ progenitor cells and results in the observed re-establishment on normal Ph− progenitor cells.

The therapeutic implications of these data are exciting. If treatment of Ph+ cells with a specific drug produces resurgence of the LFA-3+ surface marker, then normalization of the APLR is expected. Thus, a clinical in vivo response could be predicted in vitro in patients whose APLR is normalized. α-Interferon (IFN-α) has been shown to induce a clinical in vivo response in some CML patients manifested by normalization of the bone marrow and peripheral blood as well as disappearance of the Philadelphia chromosome. In addition, IFN-α normalizes the APLR in some CML patients. Thus, the APLR may be a powerful tool to predict, in vitro, a response of CML cells to specific therapies.

SUMMARY

Normal hematopoiesis is an autoregulated process. Abnormal hematopoiesis, as exemplified by CML, represents an escape from this normal autoregulation. This lack of autoregulation in CML may well be due to loss of the LFA-3 cytoadhesion molecules on progenitor cells, which are necessary for stimulation of autosuppressive T cells. This lack of stimulation results in no proliferation of a suppressive T cell subset and thereby allows hyperproliferation of the CML clone in vivo. The possible lack of autoregulatory T cells in vitro decreases the CML clone proliferative advantage, so the CML clone dies. Finally, the loss of the LFA-3 cytoadhesion molecule on Ph^+ CML progenitor cells may result from a change in the genetic message coding for the cytoadhesion molecules. This mutation is likely a result of the *bcr-abl* translocation via an as yet undetermined mechanism. Exploitation of this model system should yield new insight into the pathogenesis of the phenotype of CML and should define new roles for cytoadhesion molecules in the regulation of hematopoiesis.

REFERENCES

1. Adamson, J. W. (1984). Analysis of haemopoiesis: The use of cell markers and in vitro culture techniques in studies of clonal haemopathies in man. *Clin. Haematol. 13*:489–502.
2. Clark, S. C., and Kamen, R. (1987). The human hematopoietic colony-stimulating factors. *Science 236*:1229–1237.
3. Dexter, T. M., Spooncer, E., Toksoz, D., and Lajtha, L. G. (1980). The role of cells and their products in the regulation of in vitro stem cell proliferation and granulocyte development. *J. Supramol. Struct. 13*:513–524.
4. Coulombel, L., Kalousek, D. K., Eaves, C. J., Gupta, C. M., and Eaves, A. C. (1983). Long-term marrow culture reveals chromosomally normal hematopoietic progenitor cells in patients with Philadelphia chromosome-positive chronic myelogenous leukemia. *N. Engl. J. Med. 308*:1493–1498.
5. Coulombel, L., Eaves, C., Kalousek, D., Gupta, C., and Eaves, A. (1985). Long-term marrow culture of cells from patient with acute myelogenous leukemia: Selection in favor of normal phenotypes in some but not all cases. *J. Clin. Invest. 75*:961–969.
6. Dube, I. D., Kalousek, D. K., Coulombel, L., Gupta, C. M., Eaves, C. J., and Eaves, A. C. (1984). Cytogenetic studies of early myeloid progenitor compartments in Ph^1-positive chronic myeloid leukemia. II. Long-term culture

reveals the persistence of Ph^1-negative progenitors in treated as well as newly diagnosed patients. *Blood 63*:1172–1177.
7. Lemischka, I. R., Raulet, D. H., and Mulligan, R. C. (1986). Developmental potential and dynamic behavior of hematopoietic stem cells. *Cell 45*:917–927.
8. Emerson, S. G., and Gale, R. P. (1987). The regulation of hematopoiesis following bone marrow transplantation. *Int. J. Cell Cloning 5*:432–449.
9. Rammbaldi, A., Pelicci, P., Allavena, P., Knowles, D. M., Rossini, S., Bassan, R., Barbui, T., Dalla-Favera, R., and Mamtovami, A. (1985). T cell receptor β chain gene rearrangements in lymphoproliferative disorders of large granular lymphocytes/Natural killer cells. *J. Exp. Med. 162*:2156–2162.
10. Koizumi, S., Seki, H., Tachinami, T., Taniguchi, M., Matsuda, A., Taga, K., Nakarai, T., Kato, E., Taniguchi, N., and Nakamura, H. (1986). Malignant clonal expansion of large granular lymphocytes with a Leu-11^+, Leu-7^- surface phenotype: In vitro responsiveness of malignant cells to recombinant human interleukin 2. *Blood 68*:1065–1073.
11. Loughran, T. P., and Hammond, W. P. (1986). Adult onset cyclic neutropenia is a benign neoplasm associated with clonal proliferation of large granular lymphocytes. *J. Exp. Med. 164*:2089–2094.
12. Lipton, J. M., Nadler, L. M., Canellos, G. P., Kudisch, M., Reiss, C. S., and Nathan, D. G. (1983). Evidence for genetic restriction in the suppression of erythropoiesis by a unique subset of T lymphocytes in man. *J. Clin. Invest. 72*:694–706.
13. Torok-Storb, B. J., and Hansen, J. A. (1982). Modulation of in vitro BFU-E growth by normal Ia-positive T cells is unrestricted by HLA-DR. *Nature 298*:473–474.
14. Emerson, S. G., and Antin, J. H. (1989). Bone marrow progenitor cells induce a regulatory autologous proliferative T lymphocyte response. *J. Immunol. 142*:766–772.
15. Upadhyaya, G., Deisseroth, A. B., and Emerson, S. G. (1988). CML progenitor cells are deficient in cell surface LFA-3: Modulation by alpha-interferon in vitro and in vivo. (Abstract). *Blood 72*(Suppl. 1):836a.

15
The *bcr-abl* Protein of Philadelphia Chromosome-Positive Leukemias

Tracy Gross Lugo and Owen N. Witte *Howard Hughes Medical Institute*
University of California, Los Angeles, California

INTRODUCTION

The *bcr-abl* protein is the product of rearranged genes on the Philadelphia chromosome (Ph^1). This reciprocal translocation between chromosomes 9 and 22 is seen in the leukemic cells of >95% of patients with chronic myelogenous leukemia (CML) and of 10-20% of patients with acute lymphocytic leukemia (ALL) (1-3). The striking reproducibility of their appearance suggests that Ph^1 and its abnormal gene product play a role in the pathogenesis of these diseases.

RELATIONSHIP OF *bcr-abl* PROTEINS TO THEIR NORMAL CELLULAR COUNTERPARTS

In CML the translocation breakpoint on chromosome 22 occurs within a limited region of about 5 kilobases (kb), the breakpoint cluster region (*bcr*), which lies within a gene of unknown fuction (4,5). The *bcr* gene is a member of a small gene family located on chromosome 22, and it encodes a phosphoprotein of 160,000 molecular weight (6,7). The translocation joins the 5′ half of *bcr* to downstream sequences from the proto-oncogene, c-*abl,* on chromosome 9 (8-10). The consequence is fusion of the *bcr* and c-*abl* transcription units and production of a hybrid *bcr-abl* messenger RNA (11-15). The resulting hybrid pro-

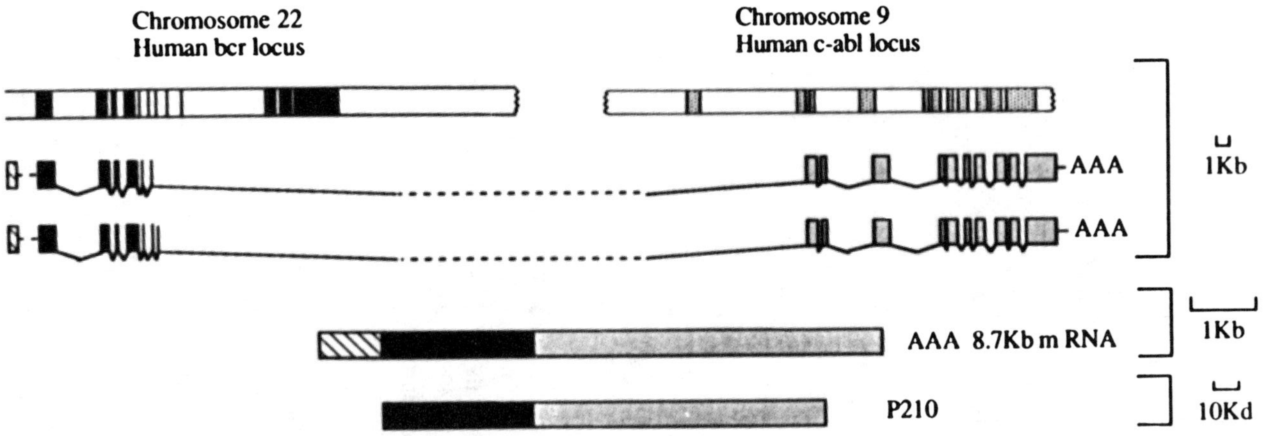

Figure 1 Production of p210 from the Philadelphia chromosome in CML. In ALL, the breakpoint on chromosome 22 occurs within the first *bcr* intron.

tein has an apparent molecular weight of 210,000 and is designated p210 (Figure 1) (16–18).

The Ph[1] seen in ALL is karyotypically indistinguishable and has a very similar molecular structure. The breakpoints on chromosome 22 cluster within a 12 kb region in the first intron of *bcr*, closer to the 5′ end of the *bcr* gene, with the consequence that a larger portion of the *bcr* gene is deleted from the hybrid transcript (5,19–23). The resulting protein, p185, is smaller and lacks *bcr*-derived serologic determinants that are present in p210 (22,24).

The unrearranged c-*abl* gene consists of at least 13 exons (13,25,26). The carboxy-terminal portion of the protein is encoded by a single large exon. This is preceded by 11 smaller exons, 8 of which specify the highly conserved region essential for the protein's tyrosine kinase activity. A set of alternative first exons (two in humans and four in the mouse) are joined by differential splicing to the second exon to produce a set of mRNAs with distinct protein-coding sequences (12,26). The first exon sequences are separated from the common splice acceptor exon by unusually large distances, up to 200 kb. On Ph[1] the chromosome 9 breakpoint may occur over a fairly large region upstream of the second exon (27).

Two major c-*abl* mRNAs (designated types a and b in humans, corresponding to types I and IV in the mouse) are expressed at low copy number in a variety of cell types (28). These include both proliferating (thymus) and post-mitotic (brain) tissues. A unique c-*abl* mRNA species is found highly expressed in haploid germ cells in mouse testis (29). This smaller message is formed by utilization of an alternative termination site in the type I transcript (30,31).

The alternative c-*abl* proteins encoded by the two major mRNAs differ from each other by 19 amino acids at the amino terminus and cannot be separated by sodium dodecyl sulfate-polyacrylamide gel electrophoresis (32). They migrate as a single band with apparent molecular weights of 150,000 for murine c-*abl* and 145,000 for the human form. In both species one of the alternative forms of c-*abl* protein has a putative myristylation site at the N-terminus and is probably associated with cellular membranes; the other form is soluble (References 33 and 34 and Clark, Pendergast, and Witte, unpublished data). Both c-*abl* proteins contain a canonical nuclear localization signal (amino acid sequence KKKKK), and in the NIH-3T3 cells that overexpress the form with the myristylation site, a substantial fraction of the protein is found in the nucleus (98).

The c-*abl* proteins can serve as both catalysts and substrates in intracellular phosphorylation reactions. Both forms possess an intrinsic tyrosine kinase activity and are capable of in vitro autophosphorylation on tyrosine at a single major site (17). However, c-*abl* proteins that are labeled in vivo with inorganic phosphate contain no phosphotyrosine (16,35). There are two serine residues in c-*abl* and *bcr-abl* proteins that can serve as sites of phosphorylation by protein kinase C (36). Phosphorylation and dephosphorylation cascades are a feature of several intracellular signaling pathways (for reviews see References 37 and 38), indicating a possible normal function of the c-*abl* proteins.

The normal *bcr* protein, on the other hand, has no tyrosine kinase activity and its sequence has no homology to other tyrosine or serine kinases. It has been reported to have serine kinase activity, but this may be a property of a separate, associated molecule (7). Two *bcr* mRNAs of 7.0 and 4.5 kb are expressed in a wide variety of human cell types and, like c-*abl* mRNAs, show no particular pattern of expression related to the proliferative state of the cells (39,40). In CML cells, messages from both the intact *bcr* gene and the rearranged *bcr-abl* locus can be detected (41).

MODELS OF *bcr-abl* BIOLOGIC FUNCTION

Abelson Disease

The c-*abl* gene was first detected as the cellular counterpart of v-*abl*, the transforming gene of Abelson murine leukemia virus (A-MuLV). A-MuLV was isolated in 1970 from a tumor arising in a Balb/c mouse that had been infected with Moloney murine leukemia virus (Mo-MuLV) (42,43). It causes a disease that is quite distinct from that associated with Mo-MuLV (44).

Mice injected with Mo-MuLV develop a thymic lymphoma after a latent period of several months. A-MuLV, on the other hand, is an acutely transforming virus that causes thymus-independent lymphoma within 3-5 weeks of injection into susceptible mice. The tumor arises in the marrow of the vertebrae and often spreads to secondary sites in the central nervous system, a pattern again distinct from that of Mo-MuLV tumors. A-MuLV also infects bone marrow cells in culture. The outgrowths have altered growth properties and are tumorigenic in syngeneic animals (45).

Molecular analysis of Abelson virus revealed that it is a derivative of Mo-MuLV in which 6.3 kb of the Moloney genome, comprising the *pol* and *env* genes and a portion of the *gag* gene, have been replaced by 3.5 kb of exogenous sequences (46,47). This novel transcription unit is designated v-*abl*. The source of the nonviral DNA was determined to be the cellular gene c-*abl*. Due to the loss of viral genes, A-MuLV is replication defective, and propagation of A-MuLV stocks requires the presence of Mo-MuLV helper virus to provide replication functions in *trans* (48).

A similar transduction event was involved in the generation of Hardy-Zuckerman-2 feline sarcoma virus (HZ2-FeSV), which causes fibrosarcomas in cats (49). In this instance the recombination occurred within the second exon of the cat c-*abl* gene. In HZ2-FeSV the carboxy-terminal portion of c-*abl* has also been deleted, so that the feline virus oncogene encodes a *gag-abl-pol* fusion protein (50).

There are structural and biochemical similarities between v-*abl* and the *bcr-abl* gene products. In v-*abl*, the amino-terminal portion of c-*abl* has been replaced by sequences from the *gag* gene of Mo-MuLV; the break occurred in the third exon of c-*abl*, so the common splice acceptor is not present in v-*abl*. The portion of *gag* included in v-*abl* includes a putative N-terminal myristylation signal, but an analogous site does not exist in *bcr-abl* (25).

The domains of c-*abl* that encode the tyrosine kinase activity are retained in v-*abl* and are essential for its transforming ability. Both v-*abl* and the *bcr-abl* proteins possess an enhanced tyrosine autophosphorylation activity and are phosphorylated on tyrosine in vivo (17,36,51). The site of v-*abl* phosphorylation in vivo corresponds to the tyrosine residue that is phosphorylated in vitro by c-*abl*; v-*abl* and the *bcr-abl* proteins are phosphorylated at several novel sites in vitro (17).

Franz et al. (52) have reported studies on the structural requirements for conversion of c-*abl* to a protein with transforming activity. Using deletion mutants and defined recombinants between c-*abl* and v-*abl* they established three requirements for oncogenic activation of c-*abl*: (1) the deletion of N-terminal amino acids between the *Pst*I site in the first exon and the *Hinc*II site in the second, (2) the provision of an N-terminal myristylation site, and (3) overproduction of the mutant protein. These alterations reportedly shift the subcellular localization of c-*abl* from partially nuclear to predominantly cytoplasmic (98). The N-terminal region that appears to have an inhibitory effect on transformation by c-*abl* contains a domain with homology to other tyrosine kinases, including *src* and *fps*, which may negatively regulate tyrosine kinase activity. However, this domain is included in both p210$^{bcr\text{-}abl}$ and p185$^{bcr\text{-}abl}$.

Thus two different mechanisms that activate the oncogenic potential of c-*abl*, chromosome translocation and viral transduction, both result in the replacement of the amino terminus of the protein with exogenous sequences and lead to an alteration in its enzymatic properties. This clearly suggests a significant role for these changes in the pathogenic process. However, there are also important differences between the pathology of Abelson disease and the two human leukemias associated with *bcr-abl*.

CML, in particular, takes a strikingly different time course (3,53,54). This disease is characterized by a long chronic phase with a usual duration of 3–5 years. During this phase there is an increase in the Ph^1-positive myeloid stem cells, but their progeny continue to differentiate, and they respond appropriately to GM-CSF (granulocyte-macrophage colony-stimulating factor) and other regulatory factors. The leukemic cells have a growth advantage and eventually predominate in the bone marrow Following a more or less gradual transition into the acute phase of the disease, the leukemic cells lose the ability to mature and proliferating blast cells invade the periphery. Lymphomagenesis by A-MuLV, on the other hand, occurs very rapidly; the leukemic cells can be detected in the bone marrow as early as 15 days after infection. In this respect, it may represent a better model of ALL.

There may also be different target cells for transformation by *bcr-abl* or v-*abl*. CML is caused by malignant transformation in a pluripotent hematopoietic progenitor cell and involves predominantly the myeloid elements of the blood. During the chronic phase, Ph^1 is evident in all the myeloid lineages. In about 75% of blast crises the dividing cells resemble myeloblasts or, less frequently, erythroblasts or megakaryocytes ;in the remaining 25% of cases the blasts resemble pre-B cells. (T cell outgrowth during the acute phase of CML occurs very infrequently.) The target cell in ALL has not been as clearly defined.

In contrast to the leukemic cells in CML, Abelson virus-infected cells derived from typical tumors most closely resemble pre-B lymphocytes (55,56). They have undergone DNA rearrangements at their immunoglobulin gene loci and frequently produce μ heavy-chain proteins. They also display other markers of B lymphoid differentiation, including expression of B220 and *lyb*-2 antigens. Cloned pre-B cells isolated in culture can be transformed by A-MuLV in vitro, and at least some of the transformants are capable of proceeding to gene rearrangement at the κ light-chain locus (57).

However, under appropriate circumstances a variety of tumors can be evoked by A-MuLV. Direct intrathymic injection of virus causes the development of thymomas (58). Intraperitoneal injection into pristane-primed animals leads to the appearance of plasmacytomas (59). Cell lines resembling macrophages and mast cells have been derived as outgrowths of Abelson lymphomas (60,61). The only common ancestor of all these cell types is the pluripotent hematopoietic progenitor. It thus remains possible that at least part of the tissue specificity of transformation in Abelson disease is the outcome of selective pressures operating on the population of infected cells.

bcr-abl Retroviruses

Retroviral vectors that can be used to introduce the expression of human *bcr-abl* oncoproteins into rodent cells provide an important alternative model system for the study of *bcr-abl* functions. The structure of two such viruses is diagrammed in Figure 2. In both constructs, the Moloney virus long terminal repeats (LTRs) direct integration of the provirus and transcription of *bcr-abl*. These vectors can be used to introduce *bcr-abl* genes into a wide variety of cell types at high efficiency. Stocks of virus that do not contain Moloney helper virus can be prepared in packaging cell lines, such as ψ 2 cells (62). The sequences of these vectors can be readily manipulated in vitro to study the effects of defined alterations in *bcr-abl* molecules.

Infection of cultured mouse bone marrow cells with *bcr-abl* retroviruses leads to the outgrowth of cell lines with altered growth properties (63,64). When uninfected bone marrow is plated under conditions that favor the growth of lymphoid cells, the cultures pass through a series of reproducible stages (65,66). A layer of adherent bone marrow stromal cells is formed first, followed in 3-4 weeks by the appearance of nonadherent cells with many characteristics of pre-B cells. A healthy culture maintains a density of approximately 10^5 cells per mL. Examination of DNA rearrangement at the immunoglobulin heavy-chain

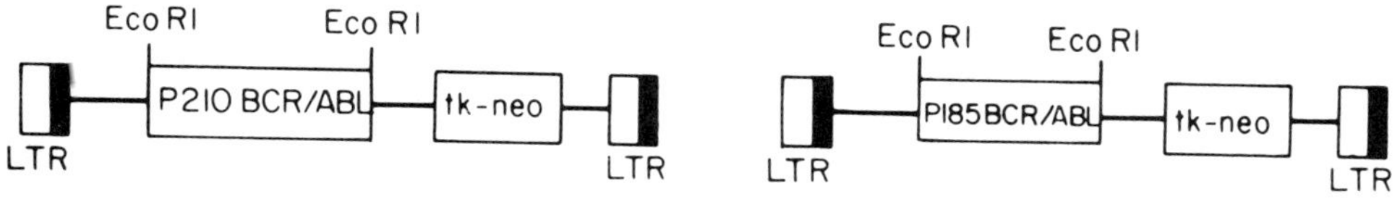

Figure 2 *bcr-abl* retroviral vectors. LTR, long terminal repeat; tk-*neo*, neomycin-resistance gene driven from the herpes simplex virus thymidine kinase gene promoter, which serves as an independent selectable marker. Details of the construction of these viruses are given in References 64 and 72.

loci has shown that the nonadherent cells are polyclonal in early cultures but that after 10–12 weeks the cultures become predominated by one or a few clones of cells.

Bone marrow cells infected with the p210*bcr-abl* virus pJW-RX frequently attain much higher saturation densities (10^6 cells per mL). They may also acquire additional characteristics of transformed cells, such as loss of dependence on stromal feeder cells and the ability to form foci in soft agar. A small fraction are tumorigenic. Cells infected with the analogous virus expressing p185*bcr-abl* generally undergo a more rapid shift to high saturation density and are significantly more efficient at forming tumors in syngeneic animals. Neither virus is as potent as A-MuLV at causing these changes in lymphoid cells.

When p210*bcr-abl*-infected cells are plated under conditions that favor the growth of myeloid cells, outgrowths rarely occur (67). Cell lines obtained in this fashion have characteristics of lymphoid rather than myeloid cells and express truncated forms of p210. This indicates that a high level of p210 expression may have deleterious effects in mouse myeloid cells; a similar phenomenon has been well-documented in fibroblasts (68).

Introduction of transgenes encoding v-*abl* or *bcr-abl* into the mouse germline leads to disease syndromes that depend on the enhancers and promoters used to direct expression. Transgenic mice bearing v-*abl* or *bcr*-v-*abl* transgenes expressed from promoters specific to hematopoietic tissues develop T- or B-cell lymphomas at high frequency (99). Mice that carry a p185 *bcr-abl* transgene under the control of the metallothionein promoter, which directs ubiquitous expression, develop both lymphoid and myeloid malignancies (100).

The injection of *bcr-abl* virus into mice is pathogenic. The diseases that develop are variable in nature and are strongly influenced by the transcriptional and translational control elements included in the vector (Gishizsky and Witte, unpublished results). Animals injected with stocks of pJW-RX virus containing replication-competent Moloney helper virus develop splenic tumors with a long latent period (>60 days). The tumorigenicity of the virus is significantly diminished by truncation of the *bcr* 5′ untranslated sequence preceding the coding region from a length of 447 base pairs to 113 base pairs or fewer.

A more promising approach is the infection of bone marrow, which is then used to reconstitute lethally irradiated mice (101,102). This permits the introduction of p210 expression into very primitive stem cells. These reconstituted animals develop a variety of hematopoietic malignancies, including pre-B lymphomas, macrophage-like tumors, or a myeloproliferative syndrome that strongly resembles human CML. Both p210 and v-*abl* are capable of producing myeloid tumors via this route. Considered together with the behavior of transforming *abl* genes in transgenic mice (above), these results indicate that expression in the appropriate target cell, rather than the structure of the protein, may determine the cell specificity of transformation.

Rodent fibroblasts, such as NIH 3T3 cells and Rat 1 cells, have been surprisingly useful for studying *abl* gene effects. NIH 3T3 cells infected with Abelson virus undergo morphologic transformation and lose anchorage dependence (69). A growth-suppressive or toxic effect is also associated with Abelson infection in fibroblasts; many transformed clones die out, and outgrowths frequently undergo deletions of a carboxy-terminal portion of *abl* distinct from the tyrosine kinase domain (68). A-MuLV has similar effects on Rat 1 cells, a line of immortalized rat fibroblasts established in a manner similar to NIH 3T3 cells (70).

Rat 1 cells and NIH 3T3 cells respond differently to infection by p210*bcr-abl* and p185*bcr-abl* (71). NIH 3T3 cells are not transformed by p210, although the addition of a small region of *gag* to the amino terminus of p210 converts it into a protein capable of transforming NIH 3T3 cells (72). Rat 1 cells infected with p210*bcr-abl* exhibit a range of partially transformed characteristics. They undergo a subtle change in shape, they form tumors in nude mice, and they form foci in soft agar in 20% fetal calf serum. Rat 1 cells infected with p185*bcr-abl* exhibit an overtly transformed morphology and form foci in soft agar with high efficiency. p185*bcr-abl*-infected NIH 3T3 cells do not undergo morphologic transformation and form only microscopic foci in soft agar.

The differential response of these two lines of fibroblasts provides an important tool for the study of *bcr-abl* intracellular functions. It may be that the subcellular localization of p210 and p185 is different in Rat 1 cells and NIH 3T3 cells; this is suggested by the fact that the *gag-bcr-abl* protein that transforms NIH 3T3 cells lack some crucial intracellular substrate for phosphorylation by that may direct the protein to the cell membrane. Another possibility is that nih 3T3 cells lack some crucial intracellular substrate for phosphorylation by *bcr-abl* that is present in Rat 1 cells. Biochemical approaches to these questions would be quite difficult in hematopoietic cell cultures, which are complex mixtures of several cell types and grow relatively slowly, but they are quite feasible in cultures of fibroblasts.

bcr-abl PROTEINS AND MALIGNANT PROGRESSION IN CML

Nothing is known about what triggers the transition from the chronic to the acute phase of CML. The appearance of Ph^1 occurs early in CML, and p210*bcr-abl* is expressed throughout both the chronic and the acute phases.

Comparisons of p210*bcr-abl* mRNA and protein levels in cells from acute versus chronic CML have revealed no distinct patterns of changes (73,74). During the acute phase, chromosomal abnormalities in addition to Ph^1 frequently appear in the leukemic cells (75). The most common are trisomy 8, the appearance of an isochromosome 17, and duplication of the Ph^1 itself. However, there are documented instances of loss of Ph^1 and p210*bcr-abl* with persistence of CML (76). These observations suggest that one or more secondary events, such as the activation of oncogenes in addition to *bcr-abl*, are required before blast crisis ensues.

An alteration in the function of the *myc* gene is a likely possibility. Chromosomal translocations that juxtapose a portion of the c-*myc* locus to regulatory regions of the immunoglobulin genes are a consistent feature of Burkitt's lymphoma and other B cell malignancies (77). Plasmacytomas can be induced in mice by injection of Abelson virus into pristane-primed animals, and the cells of these tumors contain structural rearrangements of c-*myc* and express abundant c-*myc* and v-*abl* transcripts (78). Moreover, transgenic mice that have the v-*abl* gene linked to an immunoglobulin heavy chain enhancer (Eμ) frequently develop clonal plasmacytomas with an apprently similar *myc* translocation. Progency of crosses between these Eμ-v-*abl* mice and Eμ-*myc* transgenics rapidly develop polyclonal plasmacytomas without additional *myc* rearrangement (103). The human c-*myc* gene is located on chromosome 8, which is often trisomic in leukemic cells in advanced CML (79). DNA amplification at c-*myc* in CML cells has been observed infrequently (80).

Levels of c-*myc* mRNA are often, but not invariably, elevated in CML cells (73). The significance of this has been difficult to assess, because the expression of c-*myc* is correlated with proliferation in nonmalignant cells and high levels in leukemic cells may simply reflect the presence of a larger number of proliferating cells. However, Preisler et al. (81) used an immunochemical method to study c-*myc* protein expression at the single cell level in leukemic bone marrow and found no correlation between the percentage of dividing cells and the proportion of cells expressing c-*myc*. They found c-*myc* protein expression in the majority of leukemic cells in five patients in CML blast crisis, with variation in the amounts of protein among cells from individual patients, but in cells from three patients in the chronic phase of CML c-*myc*-expressing cells were rare.

We have obtained additional evidence for an interaction between p210*bcr-abl* and c-*myc* (71) (Lugo and Witte, unpublished results). Rat 1 cells infected with the p210*bcr-abl*-expressing retrovirus are only partially transformed. Their shape is not grossly altered, and they form foci in soft agar only in high concentrations of serum. When p210-expressing Rat 1 cells are superinfected with a second virus that directs high levels of c-*myc* (or v-*myc*) transcription, they undergo a florid morphologic transformation and have a sharply reduced serum requirement for anchorage-independent growth. Curiously, this interaction between p210*bcr-abl* and *myc* does not take place in NIH 3T3 cells; this is similar to the response of NIH 3T3 cells to p185*bcr-abl*.

Table 1 Oncogenes in Leukemia Cells Detected by NIH 3T3 Transfection Assays

	Number tested	Number with dominant transforming activity	Number with presence of activated *ras* gene:			References
			K-ras	N-ras	H-ras	
Chronic myelogenous leukemia						
Cell lines	3	1		1		91, 93
Primary tumors						
Chronic phase	27	3		1	1	91, 93–96
Acute phase	24	4		1	2	93, 95, 96
Acute lymphocytic leukemias						
Cell lines	12	7	1	5		91, 97
Primary tumors	8	2		1		93
Acute myelogenous leukemia						
Cell lines	3	3		3		95
Primary tumors	27	11		10	1	90–95

The cellular oncogene *p53* is another candidate for a role in the progression of CML. This is a nuclear phosphoprotein that was first identified by virtue of its association with SV40 T antigen in SV40-transformed cells (82). It is similar in several respects to *myc*, including its localization to the cell nucleus, and mutated forms of *p53* are able to cooperate with activated *ras* genes in transforming primary cells (83). It has been mapped to human chromosome 17, another of the chromosomes frequently involved in secondary karyotypic abnormalities in CML. Overexpression of *p53* occurs in many kinds of tumors and has been found in several types of leukemia (84). Lubbert et al. (85) screened a series of CML cell samples and found elevated *p53* mRNA levels in those that did not overexpress c-*myc*. There is very recent evidence that normal *p53* may actually function as an antioncogene in the manner of the retinoblastoma-susceptibility gene product and that oncogenicity is associated only with mutant forms of *p53* (86). The presence of altered *p53* molecules in CML cells remains to be determined.

Surveys with a variety of probes have found that mRNAs for many cellular proto-oncogenes in addition to c-*myc*, *p53*, and c-*abl* are expressed or overexpressed in leukemia cells, but no consistent relationship between diagnosis and the pattern of expression has emerged (87–89). Another approach to the identification of activated oncogenes in CML has been to transfect DNA from leukemic cells into NIH 3T3 cells and then to isolate human DNA from morphologically transformed or tumorigenic transfectants. A considerable number of such studies have now been reported (Table 1) (90–97). Activated members of the *ras* gene family are most easily detected in this type of assay, and mutant *ras* genes are found in approximately 40% of the DNA samples derived from acute leukemias. N-*ras* mutations are particularly prominent among DNAs from AML patients. However, most DNAs from CML patients do not have transforming activity in NIH 3T3 cells.

There are several possible explanations for this. Activation of *myc* or similar oncogenes are probably not detected in this assay because *myc* does not transform NIH 3T3 cells. It is also possible that CML involves secondary events that result in malignant transformation only when p210*bcr-abl* expression is present. Finally, since there is clearly a difference in the response of Rat 1 cells and NIH 3T3 cells to the synergistic effects of *bcr-abl* and c-*myc* overexpression, it may be that NIH 3T3 cells are particularly refractory to *bcr-abl*-mediated transformation. Rat 1 cells partially transformed by *bcr-abl* expression are probably a more suitable indicator cell line for this type of experiment.

CONCLUSIONS AND PROSPECTS

The *bcr-abl* proteins p210 and p185 are clearly implicated in the pathogenesis of the leukemias with which they are associated. However, they probably do not act alone. p185 is associated with an acute disease, and it is clearly a more potent carcinogen than p210. It is not as potent as its viral counterpart, v-*abl*, however, and its expression does not invariably lead to malignant transformation in vitro or tumor formation in vivo. p210 is present during the relatively benign phase of CML and may even be dispensable after full-blown malignancy has developed. The identification of secondary or accessory oncogenic events in both diseases is clearly essential. The natural animal model, Abelson disease, which provided crucial information about the nature of the molecular lesion at the c-*abl* locus, is of limited use for the investigation of progression in human leukemia because of its rapid time course. In vitro models of CML and ALL created by introducing *bcr-abl* proteins into several kinds of cultured rodent cells provide a necessary flexibility, because each different cell type offers particular experimental advantages. These tissue culture models should make it possible to define the biochemical functions of the *bcr-abl* proteins and to identify their intracellular targets.

REFERENCES

1. Nowell, P. C., and Hungerford, D. A. (1960). A minute chromosome in human chronic granulocyte leukemia. *Science 132*:1497–1499.
2. Rowley, J. D. (1973). A new consistent chromosomal abnormality in chronic myelogenous leukemia identified by quinacrine fluorescence and Giemsa staining. *Nature 243*:290–291.
3. Champlin, R. E., and Golde, D. W. (1985). Chronic myelogenous leukemia (CML): Recent advances, *Blood 65*:1039–1047.
4. Groffen, J., Stephenson, J. R., Heisterkamp, N., de Klein, A., Bartram, C. R. and Grosveld, G. (1984). Philadelphia chromosomal breakpoints are clustered within a limited region, *bcr*, on chromosome 22. *Cell 36*:93–99.
5. Hermans, A., Heisterkamp, N., von Lindern, M., Van Baal, S., Meijer, D., van der Plas, D., Wiedemann, L. M., Groffen, J., Bootsma, D., and Grosveld, G. (1987). Unique fusion of *bcr* and c-*abl* genes in Philadelphia chromosome positive acute lymphoblastic leukemia. *Cell 51*:33–40.
6. Croce, C. M., Huebner, K., Isobe, M., Fainstain, E., Lifshitz, B., Shtivelman, E., and Canaani, E. (1987). Mapping of four distinct *bcr*-related loci to chromosome region 22q11: Order of *bcr* loci relative to chronic myelogenous leukemia and acute lymphoblastic leukemia breakpoints. *Proc. Natl. Acad. Sci. USA 84*:7174–7178.
7. Stam, K., Heisterkamp, N., Reynolds, F. H., Jr., and Groffen, J. (1987). Evidence that the *phl* gene encodes a 160,000-dalton phosphoprotein with associated kinase activity. *Mol. Cell. Biol. 7*:1955–1960.
8. de Klein, A., van Kessel, A. G., Grosveld, G., Bartram, C. R., Hagemeijer, A., Bootsma, D., Spurr, N. K., Heisterkamp, N., Groffen, J., and Stephenson, J. R. (1982). A cellular oncogene is translocated to the Philadelphia chromosome in chronic myelocytic leukaemia. *Nature 300*:765–767.
9. Heisterkamp, N., Groffen, J., Stephenson, J. R., Goodfellow, P. N., Spurr, N. K., Solomon, E., Carritt, B., and Bodmer, W. F. (1982). Chromosomal localization of human cellular homologues of two viral oncogenes. *Nature 299*:747–749.

10. Bartram, C. R., de Klein, A., Hagemeijer, A., van Agthoven, T., van Kessel, A. G., Bootsma, D., Grosveld, G., Ferguson-Smith, M. A., Davies, T., Stone, M., Heisterkamp, N., Stephenson, J. R., and Groffen, J. (1983). Translocation of c-*abl* oncogene correlates with the presence of a Philadelphia chromosome in chronic myelocytic leukemia. *Nature 306*:277–280.
11. Collins, S. J., Kubonishi, I., Miyoshi, I., and Groudine, M. T. (1984). Altered transcription of the c-*abl* oncogene in K562 and other chronic myelogenous leukemia cells. *Science 225*:72–74.
12. Shtivelman, E., Lifshitz, B., Gale, R. P., and Canaani, E. (1985). Fused transcript of *abl* and *bcr* genes in chronic myelogenous leukemia. *Nature 315*:550–554.
13. Shtivelman, E., Lifshitz, B., Gale, R. P., Roe, B. A., and Canaani, E. (1986). Alternative splicing of RNAs transcribed from the human *abl* gene and from the *bcr-abl* fused gene. *Cell 47*:277–284.
14. Ben-Neriah, Y., Daley, G. Q., Mes-Masson, A.-M., Witte, O. N., and Baltimore, D. (1986). The chronic myelogenous leukemia-specific p210 protein is the product of the *bcr/abl* hybrid gene. *Science 233*:212–214.
15. Mes-Masson, A.-M., McLaughlin, J., Daley, G. Q., Paskind, M., and Witte, O. N. (1986). Overlapping cDNA clones define the complete coding region for the $p210^{c\text{-}abl}$ gene product associated with chronic myelogenous leukemia cells containing the Philadelphia chromosome. *Proc. Natl. Acad. Sci. USA 83*:9768–9772.
16. Konopka, J. B., Watanabe, S. M., and Witte, O. N. (1984). An alteration of the human c-*abl* protein in K562 leukemia cells unmasks associated tyrosine kinase activity. *Cell 37*:1035–1042.
17. Konopka, J. B., and Witte, O. N. (1985). Detection of c-*abl* tyrosine kinase activity in vitro permits direct comparison of normal and altered *abl* gene products. *Mol. Cell. Biol. 5*:3116–3123.
18. Kloetzer, W., Kurzrock, R., Smith, L., Talpaz, M., Spiller, M., Gutterman, J., and Arlinghaus, R. (1985). The human cellular *abl* gene product in the chronic myelogenous leukemia cell line K562 has an associated tyrosine kinase protein activity. *Virology 140*:230–238.
19. Chan, L. C., Karhi, K. K., Rayter, S. I., Heisterkamp, N., Eridani, S., Powles, R., Lawler, S. D., Groffen, J., Foulkes, J. G., Greaves, M. F., and Wiedemann, L. M. (1987). A novel *abl* protein expressed in Philadelphia chromosome positive acute lymphoblastic leukemia. *Nature 325*:635–637.
20. Kurzrock, R., Shtalrid, M., Romero, P., Kloetzer, W. S., Talpas, M., Trujillo, J. M., Blick, M., Beran, M., and Gutterman, J. U. (1987). A novel c-*abl* protein product in Philadelphia positive acute lymphoblastic leukemia. *Nature 325*:631–635.
21. Walker, L. C., Ganesan, T. S., Dhut, S., Gibbons, B., Lister, T. A., Rothbard, J., and Young, B. D. (1987). Novel chimaeric protein expressed in Philadelphia positive acute lymphoblastic leukaemia. *Nature 329*:851–853.
22. Clark, S. S., McLaughlin, J., Timmons, M., Pendergast, A. M., Ben-Neriah, Y., Dow, L., Crist, W., Rovera, G., Smith, S. D., and Witte, O. N. (1988). Expression of a distinctive BCR-ABL oncogene in Ph⁺ acute lymphoblastic leukemia (ALL). *Science 239*:775–777.

23. Denny, C. T., Shah, N., Ogden, S., William, C., McConnell, T., Crist, W., Carroll, A., and Witte, O. N. (1989). Localization of preferential sites of rearrangement within the *bcr* gene in Philadelphia chromosome positive acute lymphoblastic leukemia. *Proc. Natl. Acad. Sci. USA 86*:4254–4258.
24. Clark, S. S., McLaughlin, J., Crist, W. M., Champlin, R., and Witte, O. N. (1987). Unique forms of the *abl* tyrosine kinase distinguish Ph[1]-positive CML from Ph[1]-positive ALL. *Science 235*:85–88.
25. Wang, J. Y. J., Ledley, F., Goff, S., Lee, R., Groner, Y., and Baltimore, D. (1984). The mouse c-*abl* locus: Molecular cloning and characterization. *Cell 36*:349–356.
26. Ben-Neriah, Y., Bernards, A., Paskind, M., Daley, G. Q., and Baltimore, D. (1986). Alternative 5′ exons in c-*abl* mRNA. *Cell* 44:577–586.
27. Bernards, A., Rubin, C. M., Westbrook, C. A., Paskind, M., and Baltimore, D. (1987). The first intron in the human c-*abl* gene is at least 200 kilobases long and is a target for translocations in chronic myelogenous leukemia. *Mol. Cell. Biol.* 7:3231–3236.
28. Wang, J. Y. J., and Baltimore, D. (1983). Cellular RNA homologues to the Abelson murine leukemia virus transforming gene: Expression and relationship to the viral sequence. *Mol. Cell. Biol. 3*:773–779.
29. Ponzetto, C., and Wolgemuth, D. J. (1985). Haploid expression of a unique c-*abl* transcript in the mouse male germ line. *Mol. Cell. Biol. 5*:1791–1794.
30. Meijer, D., Hermans, A., von Lindern, M., van Agthoven, T., de Klein, A., Mackenbach, P., Grootgoed, A., Talarico, D., Della Valle, G., and Grosveld, G. (1987). Molecular characterization of the testis-specific c-*abl* mRNA in mouse. *EMBO J. 6*:4041–4048.
31. Oppi, C., Shore, S. K., and Reddy, E. P. (1987). Nucleotide sequence of testis-derived c-*abl* cDNAs: Implications for testis-specific transcription and *abl* oncogene activation. *Proc. Natl. Acad. Sci. USA 84*:8200–8204.
32. Witte, O. N., Rosenberg, N., and Baltimore, D. (1979). A normal cell protein cross-reactive to the major Abelson murine leukemia virus gene product. *Nature 281*:396–398.
33. Konopka, J. B., and Witte, O. N. (1985). Activation of the *abl* oncogene in murine and human leukemias. *Biochim. Biophys. Acta 823*:1–17.
34. Sefton, B. M., Trowbridge, I. S., Cooper, J. A., and Scolnick, E. M. (1982). The transforming proteins of Rous sarcoma virus, Harvey sarcoma virus, and Abelson virus contain tightly bound lipid. *Cell 31*:465–474.
35. Ponticelli, A. S., Whitlock, C. A., Rosenberg, N., and Witte, O. N. (1982). In vivo tyrosine phosphorylations of the Abelson virus transforming protein are absent in its normal cell homolog. *Cell 29*:953–960.
36. Pendergast, A. M., Traugh, J. A., and Witte, O. N. (1987). Normal cellular and transformation-associated *abl* proteins share common sites for protein kinase C phosphorylation. *Mol. Cell. Biol.* 7:4280–4289.
37. Cohen, P. (1985). The role of protein phosphorylation in the hormonal control of enzyme activity. *Eur. J. Biochem. 151*:439–448.
38. Krebs, E. G. (1986). The enzymology of control by phosphorylation. *Enzymes 17*:3–20.

39. Hariharan, I. K., and Adams, J. M. (1987). cDNA sequence for human *bcr*, the gene that translocates to the *abl* oncogene in chronic myeloid leukemia. *EMBO J. 6*:115–119.
40. Heisterkamp, N., Stam, K., Groffen, J., de Klein, A., and Grosveld, G. (1985). Structural organization of the *bcr* gene and its role in the Ph' translocation. *Nature 315*:758–761.
41. Collins, S. J., Coleman, H., and Groudine, M. (1987). Expression of *bcr* and *bcr-abl* fusion transcripts in normal and leukemic cells. *Mol. Cell. Biol. 7*:2870–2876.
42. Abelson, H. T., and Rabstein, L. S. (1970). Influence of prednisolone on Moloney leukemogenic virus in BALB/c mice. *Cancer Res. 30*:2208–2212.
43. Abelson, H. T., and Rabstein, L. S. (1970). Lymphosarcoma: Virus-induced thymic-independent disease in mice. *Cancer Res. 30*:2213–2222.
44. Risser, R. (1982). The pathogenesis of Abelson virus lymphomas of the mouse. *Biochim. Biophys. Acta 651*:213–244.
45. Whitlock, C. A., Ziegler, S. F., and Witte, O. N. (1983). Progression of the transformed phenotype in clonal lines of Abelson virus-infected lymphocytes. *Mol. Cell. Biol. 3*:596–604.
46. Goff, S. P., Gilboa, E., Witte, O. N., and Baltimore, D. (1980). Structure of the Abelson murine leukemia virus genome and the homologous cellular DNA: Studies with cloned DNA. *Cell 22*:777–785.
47. Rosenberg, N., and Baltimore, D. (1980). Abelson virus. In *Viral Oncology* (George Klein, ed.). Raven Press, New York, pp. 187–203.
48. Goff, S. P., Tabin, C. J., Wang, J., Weinberg, R., and Baltimore, D. (1982). Transfection of fibroblasts by cloned Abelson murine leukemia virus DNA and recovery of transmissible virus by recombination with helper virus. *J. Virol. 41*:271–285.
49. Besmer, P., Hardy, W. D., Zuckerman, E. E., Bergold, P., Lederman, L., and Snyder, H. W., Jr. (1983). The Hardy-Zuckerman 2-FeSV, a new feline retrovirus with oncogene homology to Abelson-MuLV. *Nature 303*:825–828.
50 Bergold, P. J., Blumenthal, A. J., D'Andrea, E., Snyder, H. W., Lederman, L., Silverstone, A., Nguyen, H., and Besmer, P. (1987). Nucleic acid sequence and oncogenic properties of the HZ2 feline sarcoma virus v-*abl* insert. *J. Virol. 61*:1193–1202.
51. Davis, R. L., Konopka, J. B., and Witte, O. N. (1985). Activation of the c-*abl* oncogene by viral transformation or chromosomal translocation generates altered c-*abl* proteins with similar in vitro kinase properties. *Mol. Cell. Biol. 5*:204–213.
52. Franz, W. M., Berger, P., and Wang, J. Y. J. (1989). Deletion of an N-terminal regulatory domain of the c-*abl* tyrosine kinase activates its oncogenic potential. *EMBO J. 8*:137–147.
53. Dreazen, O., Canaani, E., and Gale, R. P. (1988). Molecular biology of chronic myelogenous leukemia. *Semin. Hematol. 25*:35–49.
54. Clark, S. S., Crist, W. M., and Witte, O. N. (1989). Molecular pathogenesis of pH-positive leukemias. *Annu. Rev. Med. 40*:113–122.

55. Whitlock, C. A., and Witte, O. N. (1985). The complexity of virus-cell interactions in Abelson virus infection of lymphoid and other hematopoietic cells. *Adv. Immunol. 37*:73–98.
56. Rosenberg, N., and Witte, O. N. (1988). The viral and cellular forms of the Abelson (*abl*) oncogene. *Adv. Virus Res. 35*:39–81.
57. Whitlock, C. A., Ziegler, S. F., Treiman, L. J., Stafford, J. I., and Witte, O. N. (1983). Differentiation of cloned populations of immature B cells after transformation with Abelson murine leukemia virus. *Cell 32*:903–911.
58. Cook, W. D. (1982). Rapid thymomas induced by Abelson murine leukemia virus. *Proc. Natl. Acad. Sci. USA 79*:2917–2921.
59. Potter, M., Sklar, M. D., and Rowe, W. P. (1973). Rapid induction of plasmacytomas in pristane primed BALB/c mice. *Science 182*:592–594.
60. Pierce, J. H., DiFiore, P. P., Aaronson, S. A., Potter, M., Humphrey, J., Scott, A., and Ihle, J. N. (1985). Neoplastic transformation of mast cells by Abelson-MuLV: Abrogation of IL-3 dependence by a nonautocrine mechanism. *Cell 41*:685–693.
61. Raschke, W. C., Baird, S., Ralph, P., and Nakoinz, I. (1978). Functional macrophage cell lines transformed by Abelson leukemia virus. *Cell 15*:261–267.
62. Mann, R., Mulligan, R. C., and Baltimore, D. (1983). Construction of a retrovirus packaging mutant and its use to produce helper-free defective retrovirus. *Cell 33*:153–159.
63. McLaughlin, J., Chianese, E., and Witte, O. N. (1987). In vitro transformation of immature hematopoietic cells by the p210 *bcr/abl* oncogene product of the Philadelphia chromosome. *Proc. Natl. Acad. Sci. USA 84*:6558–6562.
64. McLaughlin, J., Chianese, E., and Witte, O. N. (1989). Alternative forms of the *bcr/abl* oncogene have quantitatively different potencies for stimulation of immature lymphoid cells. *Mol. Cell. Biol. 9*:1866–1874.
65. Whitlock, C. A., and Witte, O. N. (1982). Long term culture of B lymphocytes and their precursors from murine bone marrow. *Proc. Natl. Acad. Sci. USA 79*:3608–3612.
66. Whitlock, C. A., Robertson, D., and Witte, O. N. (1984). Murine B cell lymphopoiesis in long term culture. *J. Immunol. Methods 67*:353–369.
67. Young, J. C., and Witte, O. N. (1988). Selective transformation of primitive lymphoid cells by the *bcr/abl* oncogene expressed in long-term lymphoid or myeloid culture. *Mol. Cell. Biol. 8*:4079–4087.
68. Ziegler, S. F., Whitlock, C. A., Goff, S. F., Gifford, A., and Witte, O. N. (1981). Lethal effect of the Abelson murine leukemia virus transforming gene product. *Cell 27*:477–486.
69. Scher, C. D., and Siegler, R. (1975). Direct transformation of 3T3 cells by Abelson murine leukemia virus. *Nature 253*:729–731.
70. Prasad, I., Zouzias, D., and Basilico, C. (1976). State of the viral RNA in rat cells transformed by polyoma virus. I. Virus rescue and the presence of non-integrated viral DNA molecules. *J. Virol. 18*:436–444.
71. Lugo, T. G., and Witte, O. N.(1989). The *bcr-abl* oncogene transforms Rat 1 cells and co-operates with v-*myc*. *Mol. Cell. Biol. 9*:1263–1270.
72. Daley, G. Q., McLaughlin, J., Witte, O. N., and Baltimore, D. (1987). The

CML-specific p210 *bcr/abl* protein, unlike v-*abl*, does not transform NIH-3T3 fibroblasts. *Science 237*:532–535.
73. Bartram, C. R. (1985). Activation of proto-oncogenes in human leukemias. *Blut 51*:63–71.
74. Gale, R. P., and Canaani, E. (1984). A 8-kilobase *abl* RNA transcript in chronic myelogenous leukemia. *Proc. Natl. Acad. Sci. USA 81*:5648–5652.
75. Sandberg, A. A. (1980). The cytogenetics of chronic myelocytic leukemia (CML): Chronic phase and blast crisis. *Cancer Genet. Cytogenet. 1*:217–228.
76. Bartram, C. R., Janssen, J. W., Becher, R., de Klein, A., and Grosveld, G. (1986). Persistence of chronic myelocytic leukemia despite deletion of rearranged *bcr*/c-*abl* sequences in blast crisis. *J. Exp. Med. 164*:1389–1396.
77. Cole, M. (1986). The *myc* oncogene: Its role in transformation and differentiation. *Annu. Rev. Genet. 20*:361–384.
78. Ohno, S., Migita, S., Wiener, F., Babonits, M., Klein, G., Mushinski, J. F., and Potter, M. (1984). Chromosomal translocations activating *myc* sequences and transduction of v-*abl* are critical events in the rapid induction of plasmacytomas by pristane and Abelson virus. *J. Exp. Med. 159*:1762–1777.
79. Nowell, P., Finan, J., Dalla Favera, R., Gallo, R. C., ar-Rushdi, A., Romanczuk, H., Selden, J. R., Emanuel, B. S., Rovera, G., and Croce, C. M. (1983). Association of amplified oncogene c-*myc* with an abnormally banded chromosome 8 in a human leukemia cell line. *Nature 306*:494–497.
80. McCarthy, D. M., Goldman, J. M., Rassool, F. V., Graham, S. V., and Birnie, G. D. (1984). Genomic alterations involving the c-*myc* proto-oncogene locus during the evolution of a case of chronic granulocytic leukaemia. *Lancet 2*: 1362–1365.
81. Preisler, H. D., Sato, H., Yang, P., Wilson, M., Kaufman, C., and Watt, R. (1988). Assessment of c-*myc* expression in individual leukemic cells. *Leukemia Res. 12*:507–516.
82. Milner, J., and Milner, S. (1981). SV40-53K antigen: A possible role for 53K in normal cells. *Virology 112*:785–788.
83. Parada, L., Land, H., Weinberg, R. A., Wolf, D., and Rotter, V. (1984). Cooperation between genes encoding p53 tumor antigen and *ras* in cellular transformation. *Nature 312*:649–651.
84. Koeffler, H. P., Miller, C., Nicolson, M. A., Ranyard, J., and Bosselman, R. A. (1986). Increased expression of p53 protein in human leukemia cells. *Proc. Natl. Acad. Sci. USA 83*:4035–4039.
85. Lubbert, M., Miller, C. W., Crawford, L., and Koeffler, H. P. (1988). p53 in chronic myelogenous leukemia. *J. Exp. Med. 167*:873–886.
86. Hinds, P., Finlay, C., and Levine, A. J. (1989). Mutation is required to activate the p53 gene for cooperation with the *ras* oncogene and transformation. *J. Virol. 63*:739–746.
87. Blick, M., Westin, E., Gutterman, J., Wong-Staal, F., Gallo, R., McCredie, K., Keating, M., and Murphy, E. (1984). Oncogene expression in human leukemia. *Blood 64*:1234–1239.
88. Evinger-Hodges, M. J., Blick, M., Bresser, J., and Dicke, K. A. (1987). Comparison of oncogene expression in human normal bone marrow and leukemia. *Ann. N.Y. Acad. Sci. 511*:284–291.
89. Ferrari, S., Torelli, U., Selleri, L., Donelli, A., Venturelli, D., Narni, F.,

Moretti, L., and Torelli, G. (1985). Study of the levels of expression of two oncogenes, c-*myc* and c-*myb*, in acute and chronic leukemias of both lymphoid and myeloid lineage. *Leukemia Res. 9*:833–842.
90. Bos, J. L., Toksoz, D., Marshall, C. J., Verlaan-de Vries, M., Veeneman, G. H., van der Eb, A. J., van Boom, J. H., Janssen, J. W. G., and Steenvoorden, A. C. M. (1985). Amino-acid substitutions at codon 13 of the N-*ras* oncogene in human acute myeloid leukemia. *Nature 315*:726–730.
91. Eva, A., Tronick, S. R., Gol, R. A., Pierce, J. H., and Aaronson, S. A. (1983). Transforming genes of human hematopoietic tumors: Frequent detection of *ras*-related oncogenes whose activation appears to be independent of tumor phenotype. *Proc. Natl. Acad. Sci. USA 80*:4926–4930.
92. Gambke, C., Signer, E., and Moroni, C. (1984). Activation of N-*ras* gene in bone marrow cells from a patient with acute myeloblastic leukemia. *Nature 307*:476–478.
93. Hirai, H., Tanaka, S., Azuma, M., Anraku, Y., Kobayashi, Y., Fujisawa, M., Okabe, T., Urabe, A., and Takaku, F. (1985). Transforming genes in human leukemia cells. *Blood 66*:1371–1378.
94. Janssen, J. W. G., Steenvoorden, A. C. M., Collard, J. G., and Nusse, R. (1985). Oncogene activation in human myeloid leukemia. *Cancer Res. 45*: 3262–3267.
95. Janssen, J. W. G., Steenvoorden, A. C. M., Lyons, J., Anger, B., Bohlke, J. U., Bos, J. L., Seliger, H., and Bartram, C. R. (1987). *ras* gene mutations in acute and chronic myelocytic leukemias, chronic myeloproliferative disorders and myelodysplastic syndromes. *Proc. Natl. Acad. Sci. USA 84*: 9228–9232.
96. Liu, E., Hjelle, B., and Bishop, J. M. (1988). Transforming genes in chronic myelogenous leukemia. *Proc. Natl. Acad. Sci. USA 85*:1952–1956.
97. Souyri, M., and Fleissner, E. (1983). Identification by transfection of transforming sequences in DNA of human T-cell leukemias. *Proc. Natl. Acad. Sci. USA 80*:6676–6679.
98. Van Etten, R. A., Jackson, P., and Baltimore, D. (1989). The mouse type IV c-*abl* gene product is a nuclear protein, and activation of transforming ability is associated with cytoplasmic localization. *Cell 58*:669–678.
99. Hariharan, I. K., Harris, A. W., Crawford, M., Abud, H., Webb, E., Cory, S., and Adams, J.M. (1989). A *bcr*-v-*abl* oncogene induces lymphomas in transgenic mice. *Mol. Cell. Biol. 9*:2798–2805.
100. Heisterkamp, N., Jenster, G., ten Hoeve, J., Zovich, D., Pattengale, P., and Groffen, J. (1990). Acute leukaemia in *bcr/abl* transgenic mice. *Nature 344*:251–253.
101. Kelliher, M. A., McLaughlin, J., Witte, O. N., and Rosenberg, N. (1990). Induction of a chronic myelogenous leukemia-like syndrome in mice with v-*abl* and bcr-*abl*. *Proc. Natl. Acad. Sci. USA*, in press.
102. Daley, G. Q., Van Etten, R. A., and Baltimore, D. (1990). Induction of chronic myelogenous leukemia in mice by the P210$^{bcr\text{-}abl}$ gene of the Philadelphia chromosome. *Science 247*:824–830.
103. Rosenbaum, H., Harris, A. W., Bath, M. L., McNeall, J., Webb, E., Adams, J. M., and Cory, S. (1990). An Eμ-v-*abl* transgene elicits plasmacytomas in concert with an activated *myc* gene. *EMBO J. 9*:897–905.

PART V
Therapy of Chronic Myelogenous Leukemia

16

Ph-Negative Chronic Myelogenous Leukemia: Molecular Genetics and Clinical Characteristics

Razelle Kurzrock, Moshe Talpaz, and Jordan U. Gutterman *The University of Texas M. D. Anderson Cancer Center, Houston, Texas*

BACKGROUND

The cytogenetic emblem of chronic myelogenous leukemia (CML) is a shortened chromosome 22, termed the Philadelphia (Ph) chromosome (1). The Ph chromosome arises from a reciprocal translocation between chromosomes 9 and 22: t(9;22) (q34;q11) (2). Molecular studies have revealed that this exchange of cytogenetic material results in the transfer of the c-*abl* proto-oncogene from chromosome 9 to a restricted chromosome 22 segment of about 5.8 kb, termed the breakpoint cluster region (bcr) (3–7). The 5.8 kb bcr segment forms the central portion of a gene of 130 kb, designated the *bcr* gene (8). (In some publications, it has been called the *phl* gene.) The disrupted 5′ portion of the *bcr* gene, proximal to the point of breakage within the 5.8 kb bcr segment, is therefore juxtaposed to the relocated c-*abl* gene in a head-to-tail configuration, and a chimeric *bcr-abl* gene is created on chromosome 22. This anomalous gene consistently encodes a novel 8.5 kb *bcr-abl* mRNA (9,10), which is translated to a 210 kD *bcr-abl* protein ($p210^{bcr\text{-}abl}$) (11-13), in virtually all Ph-positive CML patients. Both the aberrant $p210^{bcr\text{-}abl}$ and the normal c-*abl* protein ($p145^{c\text{-}abl}$)are tyrosine kinase enzymes; $p210^{bcr\text{-}abl}$ has a much higher enzymatic activity than its normal counterpart, and the fashion in which $p210^{bcr\text{-}abl}$ interacts with substrates may be different from that of $p145^{c\text{-}abl}$ (11-14). These observations are probably of crucial significance because tyrosine phosphokinase activity is closely coupled to the function of some oncogenes and growth factor receptors. Therefore, the creation of an abnormal, enzymatically enhanced, hybrid protein may play a pivotal role in neoplastic transformation of CML stem cells.

Patients with Ph-positive CML have typical clinical and morphologic features: splenomegaly, a hypercellular bone marrow with granulocytic hyperplasia, impressive neutrophils, basophilia, frequent thrombocytosis, and a low leukocyte alkaline phosphatase (LAP) score (15). The disease course generally includes a chronic phase of 3-4 years, followed by rapid evolution to a terminal blast transformation phase (16). A minority of patients (5-10%) do not have cytogenetic evidence of the Ph chromosome (17). Ph-negative CML patients were originally reported to have distinct clinical characteristics: short survival, old age, low frequency of basophilia, only modest leukocytosis, thrombocytopenia, anemia, and a poor response to chemotherapy (17). Recent careful morphologic reassessment of this group has suggested that their disease can often be reclassified as a myelodysplastic syndrome (18,19); however, a subgroup of Ph-negative CML patients appears to have a phenotype and natural history that bears a striking resemblance to that of Ph-positive CML patients (17).

Over the last few years, our group, as well as other investigators, have described Ph-negative CML patients in whom *bcr* rearrangement was observed (20-30). Here, we summarize the reported clinical and molecular findings that characterize Ph-negative CML.

Ph-NEGATIVE CML WITH *bcr* REARRANGEMENT

Molecular Characteristics

Since 1985, about 42 patients with Ph-negative CML and *bcr* rearrangement have been reported in the world literature (Table 1) (20-30). The true incidence of this entity is difficult to determine because of patient selection. However, based on the experience at M. D. Anderson Cancer Center, approximately 5% of the total number of patients referred with a confirmed diagnosis of CML have Ph-negative, bcr rearrangement-positive disease (16). Accurate diagnosis of bcr rearrangement requires the use of a probe encompassing the entire 5.8 kb bcr segment, as deletions of a portion of this segment may occur and result in false-negative results for rearrangements if the probe used corresponds to the area deleted (29). At the genomic level, in situ hybridization studies have shown that c-*abl* is inserted next to disrupted 5′ *bcr* sequences, usually on chromosome 22q11 (22,23). However, in one case with a t(9;12) (q34;q21) anomaly, *bcr* and c-*abl* had both been moved and were juxtaposed on chromosome 12 (20). Analysis of mRNA by Northern blotting has revealed the chimeric 8.5 kb *bcr-abl* transcript in all but one case. In this exception (25), an aberrant *bcr* message without evidence of a *bcr-abl* transcript was found. Although this finding raises intriquing questions about the role of the *bcr* gene itself in CML, its significance is tempered by

Table 1 Summary of Reported Characteristics of 42 Ph-Negative CML Patients with bcr Rearrangement[a]

		Median (range)						
Female (% of cases)	Splenomegaly (% of cases)	Age (year)	WBC ($\times 10^3$ per mm^3)	Platelets ($\times 10^3$ per mm^3)	Basophils (%)	Bone marrow blasts (%)	LAP[b]	Survival[c] (months)
38	50	34	112	450	2	1	12	24+
		11–81	21–506	53–996	0–14	1–9	1–150	3–168+

[a]LAP, leukocyte alkaline phosphatase; WBC = white blood cells. Data summarized from References 20–30. Patients reported in more than one reference were counted only once.
[b]Normal range for LAP score is 40–120 units.
[c]Median survival not reached at a follow-up of 24 months.

the absence of any subsequent confirmatory reports of this phenomenon. All Ph-negative, bcr-positive CML patients examined for their protein products showed the pathognomonic p210*bcr-abl* (21,24). Therefore, the molecular fingerprint of bcr-positive CML is identical in Ph-positive and Ph-negative patients.

Clinical and Laboratory Characteristics

The phenotype of the 42 patients with Ph-negative, bcr-positive disease was similar to that of patients with Ph-positive CML (Table 1). Of the patients, 38% were women. Their median age was 34 years (range 11–81 years). Of 303 Ph-positive CML patients seen at M. D. Anderson Cancer Center, 43% were women; their median age was 46 years (16). Therefore, the male-female ratio for Ph-negative bcr-positive versus Ph-positive CML patients is similar, but the former group appears to be somewhat younger. Of Ph-negative bcr-positive patients with available data on spleen size, 50% demonstrated splenomegaly. As in Ph-positive patients, most Ph-negative bcr-positive individuals presented with high white blood cell counts, consisting predominantly of mature neutrophils. Thrombocysosis and basophilia were common. The majority of patients also exhibited a low leukocyte alkaline phosphatase score. Bone marrows were uniformly hypercellular with an increased myeloid-erythroid ratio, granulocytic hyperplasia, and a shift to the left in the myeloid compartment.

Response to Therapy and Prognosis

The follow-up period for most of the published Ph-negative, bcr-positive cases is relatively short (median 24+ months; range 3–168+ months; Table 1). Their median survival has not been reached.

In patients with available data, hematologic response to hydroxyurea and busulfan was excellent (29). Interestingly, at the time of remission, patients with a diploid karyotype appeared free of disease. However, performance of molecular studies revealed bcr rearrangement and hence persistence of the malignant clone (29), a situation analogous to that in Ph-positive CML in which the Ph chromosome is found in 100% of bone marrow metaphases despite the morphologic appearance of a remission.

Because of our previous observations of hematologic and cytogenetic remissions after 6–18 months of α-interferon therapy of newly diagnosed, Ph-positive CML patients (31), seven Ph-negative, bcr-positive patients have been treated with this agent at M. D. Anderson Cancer Center. To date, five of these patients have achieved a complete hematologic remission. In one case, significant ongoing reduction in the intensity of the rearranged bcr band is being observed, suggesting that, with time, the malignant clone is disappearing. Presumably, in this group of patients, a similar methodology would be valuable in detecting clonality of cells after allogeneic bone marrow transplantations. These findings underscore the importance of a search for bcr rearrangement as part of the work-up, as well as the follow-up, of Ph-negative CML patients.

Cytogenetic Characteristics

Cytogenetic studies revealed a normal karyotype in 32 patients (76%). Chromosomal abnormalities were discerned in 10 patients (24%) and included the following: involvement of chromosome 9q34 via translocation with chromosome 8, 11, 12, or 18, respectively, 4 patients; t(2;9), 1 patient; t(5;6), 1 patient; -Y, 1 patient; inv(2) (p13q13), 1 patient; del(22) (pter → q11:), 1 patient, and del(16) (pter → q22:), 1 patient.

Ph-NEGATIVE CML WITHOUT bcr REARRANGEMENT

Bcr rearrangement has been found to be a very sensitive test for CML. Indeed, a review of the world literature reveals that over 98% of the more than 250 published cases of Ph-positive CML have bcr rearrangement (7). In our series of 100 Ph-positive CML patients, rearrangement was detected within the 5.8 kb bcr in 99 cases and just proximal to this segment in 1 case (32). Deletions can occur within bcr and cause false-negative results for rearrangement unless a more extensive search is undertaken with the use of large probes encompassing most of the 5.8 kb bcr (33); such deletions may account for a few of the rare published cases without rearrangement. All the Ph-positive CML patients at M. D. Anderson Cancer Center who were tested produced a *bcr-abl* message. Furthermore, this unique message has never been detected in any tumor sample not representative of the Ph-positive leukemia phenotype or in any normal tissue. These data indicate that p210$^{bcr\text{-}abl}$ is the first genuine, cancer-specific marker!

The question arises as to whether all Ph-negative patients with a phenotype of CML exhibit bcr rearrangement. Intuitively, we have thought that this should be true. Even so, we have now encountered 11 patients with clinical and laboratory characteristics indistinguishable from those of chronic-phase CML who have neither a discernible bcr rearrangement nor a *bcr-abl* message (28,34). As with bcr-positive patients, these individuals present with splenomegaly, high white blood cell (WBC) counts, neutrophilia, and a hypercellular bone marrow with granulocytic hyperplasia. The dysplastic features and/or monocytosis typical of the dysmyelopoietic syndromes are absent. These patients respond to hydroxyurea, and 2 individuals have shown a favorable response to α-interferon therapy. With ongoing follow-up, the mode of disease progression has emerged as distinct from that of classic CML. bcr-positive CML patients ineluctably progress from the chronic phase to a more accelerated myeloproliferative state characterized by the appearance of increasing numbers of immature cells; in contrast, to date, bcr-negative CML patients have not developed blast transformation but rather have shown progressive organomegaly, extramedullary infiltrates, thrombocytopenia, and anemia, leading to their eventual demise, without a significant increase in bone marrow blasts. Therefore it appears that a bcr-negative, morphologic facsimile of chronic-phase CML exists. However, the presence or absence of $p210^{bcr\text{-}abl}$ may lay the groundwork for differing secondary genetic driving forces capable of directing the progression of disease.

CONCLUSIONS

Over the last few years, a series of incisive studies have uncovered prodigious amounts of information concerning the basic molecular genetic mechanisms in Ph-positive leukemogenesis. Interestingly, a subgroup of CML patients lack the Ph translocation. The following concepts have emerged regarding the Ph-negative CML state:

1. Patients with CML, but without a discernible cytogenetic abnormality on chromosome 22, often shown subchromosomal aberrations indistinguishable from those in Ph-positive CML: bcr rearrangement and expression of a hybrid *bcr-abl* message and protein.
2. Clinical and molecular studies strongly suggest that bcr-positive chronic leukemia patients have a single disease state, CML, regardless of Ph chromosome status.
3. The prognosis and response to therapy of Ph-negative, bcr-positive CML patients is indistinguishable from that of Ph-positive patients; therefore, they should be eligible for allogeneic bone marrow transplantation and α-interferon trials.
4. Diploid, bcr-positive CML patients appear free of disease at the time of hematologic remission with conventional chemotherapy; however, molecular studies for bcr rearrangement reveal the persistence of the malignant clone. Therefore, analysis of bcr status provides a crucial adjunct to morphologic investigations during the diagnostic work-up and the follow-up of these patients.
5. Deletions within bcr occur and may confound test results by suggesting false negativity for bcr rearrangement, unless a large probe encompassing most of the 5.8 kb bcr segment is utilized.
6. A bcr-negative disease process that mirrors chronic-phase Ph-positive CML appears to exist. Preliminary observations suggest that progression in these patients may manifest as increasing organ infiltrates by leukemic cells and bone marrow failure, rather than blast transformation.

Finally, unraveling the molecular genetics of CML has provided significant insights into the mechanism of development of this disease. Clinically useful diagnostic tools have arisen from these studies. The existence of a Ph-negative bcr-negative CML state suggests that an alternative pathway, perhaps involving growth factors or their receptors, may lead to a disease process similar to bcr positive chronic-phase CML. Further investigation of Ph-negative CML may help elucidate the intercellular interactions of the unique tumor marker $p210^{bcr\text{-}abl}$.

ACKNOWLEDGMENTS

Supported, in part, by the John D. and Catherine T. MacArthur Foundation. Research conducted, in part, by the Clayton Foundation for Research and the Dalis Foundation. Dr. Gutterman is a Senior Clayton Foundation Investigator.

REFERENCES

1. Nowell, P. C., and Hungerford, D. A. (1960). A minute chromosome in human chronic granulocytic leukemia. *Science 132*:1197–1198.
2. Rowley, J. D. (1973). A new consistent chromosomal abnormality in chronic myelogenous leukemia identified by quinacrine fluorescence and Giemsa staining. *Nature 243*:290–293.
3. Bartram, C. R., de Klein, A., Hageimeijer, A., et al. (1983). Translocation of the c-*abl* oncogene correlates with the presence of the Philadelphia chromosome in chronic myelocytic leukaemia. *Nature 306*:277–280.
4. Heisterkamp, N., Stephenson, J. R., Groffen, J., Hansen, P. F., de Klein, A., Bartram, C. R., and Grosveld, G. (1983). Localization of the c-*abl* oncogene adjacent to a translocation breakpoint in CML. *Nature 306*:239–241.
5. Groffen, J., Stephenson, J. R., Heisterkamp, N., de Klein, A., Bartram, C. R., and Grosveld, G. (1984). Philadelphia chromosomal breakpoints are clustered within a limited region, *bcr*, on chromosome 22. *Cell 36*:93–99.
6 Heisterkamp, N., Stam, K., Groffen, J., de Klein, A., and Grosveld, G. (1985). Structural organization of the *bcr* gene and its role in the Ph translocation. *Nature 316*:758–761.
7. Kurzrock, R., Gutterman, J. U., and Talpaz, M. (1988). The molecular genetics of Philadelphia chromosome-positive leukemias. *N. Engl. J. Med. 319*: 990–998.
8. Heisterkamp, N., Knoppel, E., and Groffen, J. (1988). The first *bcr* gene intron contains breakpoints in Philadelphia chromosome positive leukemia. *Nucleic Acids Res. 16*:10069–10081.
9. Shtivelman, E., Lifshitz, B., Gale, R. P., and Canaani, E. (1985). Fused transcript of *abl* and *bcr* genes in chronic myelogenous leukemia. *Nature 315*: 550–554.
10. Stam, K., Heisterkamp, N., Grosveld, G., et al. (1985). Evidence of a new chi chimeric *bcr*/c-*abl* mRNA in patients with chronic myelocytic leukemia and the Philadelphia chromosome. *N. Engl. J. Med. 313*:1429–1433.

11. Kloetzer, W., Kurzrock, R., Smith, L., et al. (1985). The human cellular *abl* gene product in the chronic myelogenous leukemia cell line K562 has an associated tyrosine protein kinase activity. *Virology 140*:230–238.
12. Konopka, J. B., Watanave, S. M., and Witte, O. N. (1984). An alteration of the human c-*abl* protein in K562 leukemia cells unmasks associated tyrosine kinase activity. *Cell 37*:1035–1042.
13. Kurzrock, R., Kloetzer, W. S., Talpaz, M., Blick, M., Walters, R., Arlinghaus, R. B., and Gutterman, J. U. (1987). Identification of molecular variants of p210$^{bcr\text{-}abl}$ in chronic myelogenous leukemia. *Blood 70*:233–236.
14. Maxwell, S. A., Kurzrock, R., Parsons, S. J., et al. (1987). Analysis of p210$^{bcr\text{-}abl}$ tyrosine protein kinase activity in various subtypes of Philadelphia chromosome positive cells from chronic myelogenous leukemia patients. *Cancer Res. 47*:1731–1739.
15. Koeffler, H. P., and Golde, D. W. (1981). Chronic myelogenous leukemia—new concepts. *N. Engl. J. Med. 304*:1201–1209, 1269–1274.
16. Kantarjian, H. M., Smith, T. L., McCredie, K. B., et al. (1985). Chronic myelogenous leukemia: A multivariate analysis of the associations of patient characteristics and therapy with survival. *Blood 66*:1326–1335.
17. Ezdinli, E. Z., Sokal, J. E., Crosswhite, L., and Sandberh, A. A. (1970). Philadelphia chromosome-positive and -negative chronic myelocytic leukemia. *Ann. Intern. Med. 72*:175–182.
18. Travis, L. B., Pierre, R. V., and DeWald, G. W. (1986). Ph^1-negative chronic granulocyte leukemia: A nonentity. *Am. J. Clin. Pathol. 85*:186–193.
19. Pugh, W. C., Pearson, M., Vardiman, J. W., and Rowley, J. D. (1985). Philadelphia chromosome-negative chronic myelogenous leukaemia: A morphological reassessment. *Br. J. Haematol. 60*:457–467.
20. Bartram, C. R., Kleihauer, E., de Klein, A., Grosveld, G., Teyssier, J. R., Heisterkamp, N., and Groffen, J. (1985). c-*abl* and *bcr* are rearranged in a Ph^1-negative CML patient. *EMBO J. 4*:683–686.
21. Kurzrock, R., Blick, M. B., Talpaz, M., Velasquez, W. S., Trujillo, J. M., Kouttab, N. M., Kloetzer, W. S., Arlinghaus, R. B., and Gutterman, J. U. (1986). Rearrangement in the breakpoint cluster region and the clinical course in Philadelphia-negative chronic myelogenous leukemia. *Ann. Intern. Med. 105*:673–679.
22. Morris, C. M., Reeve, A. E., Fitzgerald, P. H., Hollings, P. E., Beard, M. E. J., and Heaton, D. C. (1986). Genomic diversity correlates with clinical variation in Ph'-negative chronic myeloid leukemia. *Nature 320*:281–283.
23. Dreasen, O., Rassool, F., Sparkes, R. S., Klisak, I., Goldman, J. M., and Gale, R. P. (1987). Do oncogenes determine clinical features in chronic myeloid leukemia? *Lancet 1*:1402–1405.
24. Wiedemann, L. M., Karhi, K. K., Shivji, M. K. K., Rayter, S. I., Pegram, S. M., Dowden, G., Bevan, D., Will, A., Galton, D. A. G., and Chan, L. C. (1988). The correlation of breakpoint cluster region rearrangement and p210$^{bcr/abl}$ expression with morphological analysis of Ph-negative chronic myeloid leukemia and other myeloproliferative diseases. *Blood 71*:349–355.

25. Bartram, C. R. (1985). *bcr* rearrangement without juxtaposition of c-*abl* in chronic myelocytic leukemia. *J. Exp. Med. 162*:2175–2179.
26. Bartram, C. R., and Carbonell, F. (1986). *bcr* rearrangement in Ph-negative CML. *Cancer Genet. Cytogenet. 21*:183–184.
27. Bartram, C. R. (1988). Rearrangement of the c-*abl* and *bcr* genes in Ph-negative CML and Ph-positive acute leukemias. *Leukemia 2*:63–64.
28. Kurzrock, R., Shtalrid, M., Gutterman, J. U., and Talpaz, M. (1989). The molecular diagnostics of chronic myelogenous leukemia and Philadelphia-positive acute leukemia. *Cancer Cells 7*:9–13.
29. Shtalrid, M., Talpaz, M., Blick, M., Romero, R., Kantarjian, H., Taylor, K., Trujillo, J., Schachner, J., Gutterman, J. U., and Kurzrock, R. (1988). Philadelphia-negative chronic myelogenous leukemia with breakpoint cluster region rearrangement: Molecular analysis, clinical characteristics, and response to therapy. *J. Clin. Oncol. 6*:1569–1575.
30. Reeve, A. E., Morris, C. M., and Fitzgerald, P. H. (1988). Acquired homozygosity of the rearranced *bcr* allele during the acute leukemic phase of a patient with Ph-negative chronic myeloid leukemia. *Blood 72*:24–28.
31. Talpaz, M., Kantarjian, H. M., McCredie, K. B., et al. (1986). Hematologic remission and cytogenetic improvement induced by recombinant human interferon alpha in chronic myelogenous leukemia. *N. Engl. J. Med. 314*: 1065–1069.
32. Shtalrid, M., Talpaz, M., Kurzrock, R., Kantarjian, H., Trujillo, J., Gutterman, J. U., Yoffe, G., and Blick, M. (1988). Analysis of breakpoints within the *bcr* gene and their correlation with the clinical course of Philadelphia-positive chronic myelogenous leukemia. *Blood 72*:485–490.
33. Popenoe, D., Shaefer-Rego, K., Mears, J. G., Bank, A., and Leibowitz, D. (1986). Frequent and extensive deletion during the 9,22 translocation in CML. *Blood 68*:1123–1126.
34. Kurzrock, R., Kantarjian, H. M., Shtalrid, M., Gutterman, J. U., Talpaz, M. (1990). Philadelphia chromosome-negative chronic myelogenous leukemia without breakpoint cluster region rearrangement: A chronic myeloid leukemic with a distinct clinical course. *Blood 75*:445–452.

17
Graft-vs-Leukemia in Chronic Myelogenous Leukemia

Anna Butturini *University of Parma, Parma, Italy*

Robert Peter Gale *University of California, Los Angeles, California*

INTRODUCTION

Bone marrow transplantation (BMT) is the only potentially curative treatment of chronic myelogenous leukemia (CML). HLA-identical bone marrow transplants in chronic phase result in a 5 year relapse rate of about 10%; leukemia-free survival is about 50% (1-3). Considerable experimental and clinical data suggest that the efficacy of transplants in curing leukemia results from diverse mechanisms, including high-dose chemotherapy and radiation used for pretransplant conditioning and antileukemic effects mediated by donor immunocompetent cells infused with the graft. In this chapter we discuss the role of T lymphocytes in preventing leukemia relapse in CML after bone marrow transplantation. We suggest how this mechanism may be used to treat CML in settings other than transplantation.

IMMUNE-MEDIATED ANTILEUKEMIC EFFECT OF TRANSPLANTATION

The concept that factors other than high-dose chemoradiotherapy used for the conditioning regimen contribute to the antileukemic effect of bone marrow transplantation derives from the different relapse rates observed in animals and humans receiving syngeneic (twin) versus allogeneic transplants (4–11). In some animal models, this effect, termed "adoptive immunotherapy" or "graft versus

Table 1. Variables Associated to Different Situations of Bone Marrow Transplantation

	Syngeneic	T depleted	Allo no GVHD	Allo + GVHD
GVHD	–	–/+	–	+
Genetic disparity	–	+	+	+
T cells	+	–	+	+

leukemia" (GVL), is distinguishable from graft-versus-host disease (GVHD) (12–15).

Considerable data in humans suggest that acute and chronic GVHD are associated with a decreased risk of leukemia relapse (16-32). This is particularly true of *chronic* GVHD. The hypothesis that immune mechanisms independent of GVHD also have an antileukemic effect is based on a comparison of actuarial relapse rates in situations with diverse incidences or severity of GVHD, genetic disparity between donor and recipient, or the presence or absence or T lymphocytes in the graft (Table 1). For example, it is possible to determine the antileukemic effect of GVHD by comparing relapse rates in persons with and without GVHD, from GVHD-independent effects. The latter are determined by comparing relapse rates in recipients of HLA-identical allogeneic transplants without GVHD with those in twins and in recipients of T-depleted transplants (24).

Data from the literature and from the International Bone Marrow Transplant Registry (IBMTR) indicate an antileukemic effect of GVHD in acute myeloid leukemia (AML), acute lymphoblastic leukemia (ALL), and CML (Table 2). Also, in AML, recipients of syngeneic (twin) grafts have increased relapses compared to recipients of allogeneic transplants not developing acute or chronic GVHD. These data suggest that in AML, genetic disparity between donor and recipient may permit a specific antileukemic effect independent of (clinically detectable) GVHD. We refer to this effect as GVL.

In CML in chronic phase, allogeneic T cell-depleted transplants are associated with a high risk of leukemia relapse. This is significantly higher than the risk after syngeneic transplants or allogeneic transplants (50% versus 25 and 15%, respectively). Some of this increased relapse rate after T cell depletion may be related to the loss of GVHD and GVL effects. However, the different relapse rates in reports of allogeneic transplants without GVHD, whether or not T cells are depleted, and the higher relapse rate compared to syngeneic transplants suggest that this effect is probably linked to the absence of T lymphocytes in the graft. We term this mechanism a direct T cell effect (25). Extensive analyses from the IBMTR confirm this notion since it is detectable even when data are adjusted for GVHD (23).

Table 2 Probability of Relapse of AML and ALL in First Remission and CML in Chronic Phase in Different Clinical Setting

	T depleted (%)	Syngeneic (%)	Allo no GVHD (%)	Allo + GVHD (%)
AML	30	40	27	5
ALL	25	40	40	15
CML	40	20	20	3
	T effect		GVL	GVHD effect

The biologic bases of these immune-mediated antileukemic effects of bone marrow transplantation are unknown. The antileukemic effect of GVHD likely results from reactivity of donor lymphocytes to minor histocompatibility antigens present on recipient normal and leukemia cells (26–28). It is also possible that leukemia cells are particularly sensitive to factors released by the immune activation that accompanies GVHD. It is unclear why the antileukemic effect of GVHD is associated predominantly with chronic but not acute GVHD. Possibly different immune mechanisms underlie these diseases. Biases in data analysis, namely, misdiagnosis of acute GVHD (29), are also possible.

The GVL effect is presumed to relate to the fact that minor histocompatibility antigens and possibly leukemia-related antigens are immunogenic when present in the context of allogeneic versus syngeneic genetic background. The concept of leukemia-associated antigens is controversial. Leukemia cells may express unique antigens or may lack common recognition antigens (30–33). Cells responsible for GVL are unknown; cytotoxic T lymphocytes or natural killer (NK) cells are proposed. In rare cases, donor NK cells with specific antileukemic but not antirecipient activity are identified after bone marrow transplantation (34–36); their importance is unknown.

Explaining the T cell-mediated effect is even more complex. There are two mechanisms whereby T cell-related factors may decrease leukemia relapse in CML. The first mechanism is based on the ability of T cells to synthesize factors that affect leukemia cell growth. Proliferating donor T cells may release lymphokines or may stimulate other cells, such as NK cells, fibroblasts, and macrophages, to release lymphokines. These lymphokines may be cytotoxic or inhibit the growth of CML cells. The α-, β-, and γ-interferons tumor growth factor (TGF) β, and tumor necrosis factor (TNF) α and β inhibit leukemia growth in vitro (37–41). α- and γ-interferon induce hematologic remission and decrease the proportion of Philadelphia-positive cells in vivo in CML (42–44). The effect of lymphokines may be increased in bone marrow transplantation because there are few residual CML stem cells. Indirect support of this hypothesis is that interleukin-2 (IL-2)-stimulated autologous immune cells decrease the growth of CML cells in long-term cultures (Santucci and Butturini, unpublished).

A second possible mechanism of the T cell effect relates to the influence of donor T cells on the tempo and extent of engraftment after bone marrow transplantation (45,46). If the number of sites in the bone marrow where stem cells can replicate is limited, the likelihood of relapse may correlate with competition between donor normal stem cells and host residual CML cells for these sites. Consequently, interventions that impair engraftment, such as T cell depletion (45-48), increase the risk of relapse. This notion is supported by some data in T cell-depleted transplants in which the likelihood of relapse correlates with time of engraftments (45-47). However, these data are controversial. Furthermore, it is equally possible that the opposite relationship exists; that is, the presence of residual leukemia impairs engraftment. It is also possible that delayed engraftment and relapse result from ineffective conditioning. Recent data against the concept of spatial competition comes from an IBMTR analysis showing that after T cell-depleted transplants cyclosporin A positively affects the engraftment rate but is associated with increased relapse (23).

Finally, it is possible that the increased relapses following T cell-depleted transplants relate to synthesis by T cells of substances that stimulate normal hematopoiesis (49-51). If CML stem cells were less dependent on these factors than normal stem cells, T cell depletion would favor the growth of CML cells and thereby increase the likelihood of relapse.

GVL AS A MODEL OF IMMUNE THERAPY

Considerable data suggest that several immune mechanisms may play a role in CML eradication after bone marrow transplantation. In this chapter we described the antileukemic effect of GVHD, GVL, and a T cell effect. These mechanisms can operate simultaneously and may interact. For example, lymphokines released by activated T cells can regulate the expression of HLA antigens on normal and leukemia cells (52). The extent and type of immune-mediated antileukemic effect associated with bone marrow transplants related to several factors, including genetic disparity between donor and recipient, donor and recipient immune function, and biology of the residual leukemia cells. The relative contribution of each of these effects to leukemia eradication probably differs in each case.

How can the mechanisms we described be used to treat CML? At present there is no example of successful manipulation of the GVL effect in humans. Attempts to enhance GVL by increasing GVHD result in increased mortality (53,54). Conversely, T cell depletion and more effective GVHD prophylaxis decrease GVHD but result in a higher risk of relapse (21-23,45-48). The T cell-mediated effect is perhaps the most attractive therapeutic strategy. If autologous T cells control CML (an unproven hypothesis), then immune manipulations may influence disease characteristics, such as the WBC count or duration of chronic phase. Trials of α- and γ-interferon indicate that lymphokines can affect the growth of CML cells in vivo (References 42-44 and Tura, personal communication). The impact of this treatment on the duration of the chronic phase is unknown. The different incidence of transient cytogenetic relapse following non-T cell-depleted and T cell-depleted transplants (55) suggests that the T cell-mediated antileukemic effect is not only an early event after transplant (56). Immune-related control of CML may require a high effector-target cell ratio. Consequently, the extreme cytoreduction achieved with transplant-related conditioning regimens may be necessary for this T cell effect to operate.

The optimal strategy of immune therapy in CML is likely to be the use of bone marrow transplantation combined with the more effective GVHD prophylaxis. Perhaps this could be followed by infusion of lymphokines or alternative immune interventions. Clinical studies are in progress (47,57,58); results may be forthcoming.

REFERENCES

1. Thomas, E. D., Clift, R. A., Fefer, A., et al. (1986). Marrow transplantation for the treatment of chronic myelogenous leukemia. *Ann. Intern. Med. 104*: 155.
2. Goldman, J. M., Apperley, J. F., Jones, L., et al. (1986). Bone marrow transplantation for patients with chronic myelogenous leukemia. *N. Engl. J. Med. 314*:202.
3. McGlave, P., Arthur, D., Haoke, R., et al.(1987). Therapy of chronic myelogenous leukemia with allogeneic bone marrow transplantation. *J. Clin. Oncol. 5*:1033.
4. Barnes, D. W. H., Corp, M. J., Loutit, L. F., and Nael, F. E. (1956). Treatment of murine leukemia with X-rays and homologous bone marrow. *Br. Med. J. 2*:626.
5. Bortin, M. M., Rimm, A. A., Rose, W. C., and Saltzstein, E. C. (1974). Graft versus leukemia. V. Absence of antileukemic effect using allogeneic H-2 identical immunocompetent cells. *Transplantation 18*:280.
6. Alexander, P. (1981). Treatment of acute leukemia by whole body irradiation and marrow transplantation: 25 years from mouse to man. *Br. J. Cancer 43*:413.
7. O'Kunewich, J. P., and Meredith, R. P. (1981). *Graft Versus Leukemia in Man and in Animal Models*. CRC Press, Boca Raton, Florida.
8. Fefer, A., Buckner, C. D., Clift, R. A., et al. (1977). Cure of hematological neoplasma with transplantation of marrow from identical twins. *N. Engl. J. Med. 297*:146.

9. Gale, R. P., and Champlin, R. (1984). How does bone marrow transplantation cure leukemia? *Lancet 2*:28.
10. Gale, R. P., and Bortin, M. M. (1985). Bone marrow transplantation in leukemia: International Bone Marrot Transplant Registry (IBMTR) data. *Int. J. Cell Cloning 3*:236.
11. Fefer, A., Sullivan, K. M., Weiden, P., et al. (1987). Graft versus leukemia effect in man: The relapse rate of acute leukemia is lower after allogeneic than after syngeneic marrow transplantation. In *Cellular Immunotherapy of Cancer*. (R. L. Truitt, R. P. Gale, and M. M. Bortin, eds.). Alan R. Liss, New York, p. 401.
12. Bortin, M. M., Rimm, A. A., Saltzstein, E. C., and Rodey, G. E. (1973). Graft versus leukemia. III. Apparent independent antihost and antileukemia activity of transplanted immunocompetent cells. *Transplantation 16*:182.
13. Chester, S. J., Esparza, A. R., Flinton, L. J., Simon, J. D., Kelley, R. J., and Albala, M. M. (1977). Further development of a successful protocol of graft versus host leukemia without a fatal graft versus host disease in AKR mice. *Cancer Res. 37*:3494.
14. Bortin, M. M., Truitt, R. L., Rimm, A. A., and Bach, F. H. (1979). Graft versus leukemia reactivity induced by alloimmunization without augmentation of graft versus host reactivity. *Nature 281*:490.
15. Truitt, R. L., Shih, C. C. Y., and Le Fever, A. V. (1986). Manipulation of graft versus host disease for a graft versus leukemia effect after allogeneic bone marrow transplantation in AKR mice with spontaneous leukemia lymphoma. *Transplantation 41*:301.
16. Weiden, P. L., Sullivan, K. M., Flournoy, N., Storb, R., and Thomas, E. D. (1981). Antileukemic effect of chronic graft versus host disease: Contribution to improved survival after bone marrow transplantation. *N. Engl. J. Med. 304*:1529.
17. Zwaan, F. E., Hermans, J., and Lyklema, A. (1986). Factors influencing long term leukemia free survival after allogeneic bone marrow transplantation in acute leukemia. In *Minimal Residual Disease in Acute Leukemia*. (A. Hagenbeek and B. Lowenberg, eds.). Nijoff, Dordrecht, p. 295.
18. Clift, R. A., Buckner, C. D., Thomas, E. D., et al. (1987). The treatment of acute nonlymphoblastic leukemia by bone marrow transplantation. *Bone Marrow Transplant. 2*:243.
19. Kersey, J. H., Weisdorf, D., Nesbit, M. E., et al. (1987). Comparison of autologous and allogeneic bone marrow transplantation for treatment of high risk refractory acute lymphoblastic leukemia. *N. Engl. J. Med. 317*: 461.
20. Brochstein, J. A., Kernan, N. A., Groshen, S., et al. (1987). Allogeneic bone marrow transplantation after hyperfractionated total body irradiation and cyclophosphamide in children with acute leukemia. *N. Engl. J. Med. 317*: 1618.
21. Apperley, J. F., Mauro, F. R., Goldman, J. M., et al. (1988). Bone marrow transplantation for chronic myelogenous leukemia in first chronic phase: Importance of a graft versus leukemia effect. *Br. J. Haematol. 69*:239.

22. Goldman, J. M., Gale, R. P., Horowitz, M. M., et al. (1988). Bone marrow transplantation for chronic myelogenous leukemia in chronic phase: Increased risk of relapse associated with T cell depletion. *Ann. Intern. Med. 108*:806.
23. Horowitz, M. M., Gale, R. P., Sondel, P. M., et al. (1990). Graft-verses-leukemia reactions following bone marrow transplantation. *Blood 75*:555.
24. Butturini, A., Bortin, M. M., and Gale, R. P. (1987). Graft-versus-leukemia following bone marrow transplantation. *Bone Marrow Transplant. 2*:233.
25. Butturini, A., and Gale, R. P. (1987). The role of T cells in preventing relapse in chronic myelogenous leukemia. *Bone Marrow Transplant. 2*:351.
26. Goulmy, E., Blokland, E., Gratama, J. W., et al. (1985). Impact of mismatching for minor histocompatibility antigens on the occurrence of graft versus host disease. *Exp. Hematol. 13*(Suppl. 17):127.
27. Van Leewen, A., Schrier, P. I., Giphart, M. J., et al. (1986). TCA: A polymorphic genetic marker in leukemia and melanoma cell lines. *Blood 67*: 1139.
28. van Rood, J. J., Goulmy, E., and van Leewen, A. (1987). The immunogenetic of chronic graft versus host disease and its relevance for the graft versus leukemia effect. In: *Cellular Immunotherapy of Cancer*. (R. L. Truitt, R. P. Gale, and M. M. Bortin, eds.). Alan R. Liss, New York, p. 433.
29. Atkinson, K., Horowitz, M. M., Biggs, J. C., Gale, R. P., Rimm, A. A., and Bortin, M. M. (1988). The clinical diagnosis of acute graft versus host disease: A diversity of views amongst marrow transplant centers. *Bone Marrow Transplant. 3*:5.
30. Meredith, R. F., and O'Kunewich, J. P. (1983). Possibility of graft versus leukemia determinants independent of the major histocompatibility complex in allogeneic bone marrow transplantation. *Transplantation 33*:370.
31. Clayberger, C., Wright, A., Medeiros, L. S., et al. (1987). Absence of cell surface LFA-1 as a mechanism of escape from immunosurveillance. *Lancet 2*: 533.
32. Ozawa, H., Iwaguchi, T., and Kataoka, T. (1987). Essential requirement of IA region identical host bone marrow or bone marrow derived cells for tumor neutralization by primed L3T4 T cells. *J. Immunol. 139*:3896.
33. Karre, K., Ljunggren, H. G., Piote, K., and Kiessling, R. (1986). Selective rejection of H-2 deficient lymphoma variants suggests an alternative immune defense strategy. *Nature 319*:675.
34. Delmon, L., Ythier, A., Moingeon, P., et al. (1986). Characterization of antileukemia cells' cytotoxic effector function. *Transplantation 42*:252.
35. Hercend, T., Tavkorian, T., Nowill, A., et al. (1986). Characterization of natural killer cells with antileukemic activity following bone marrow transplantation. *Blood 67*:722.
36. Keever, C. A., Hauch, M., Barnett, L., et al. (1988). The potentiation of NK cell mediated antileukemia activity following BMT. *Blood 72*(Suppl. 1): 393a.
37. Andrews, F., Singer, J. W., and Collins, S. J. (1987). Effect of recombinant alpha interferon on the expression of the *bcr-abl* fusion gene in human chronic myelogenous leukemia cell lines. *Cancer Res. 47*:6629.

38. Carlo-Stella, C., Cazzola, M., Ganser, A., et al. (1988). Synergistic antiproliferative effect of recombinant interferon γ with recombinant interferon alpha on chronic myelogenous leukemia hematopoietic progenitor cells (CFU-GEMM, CFU-MK, BFU-E, and CFU-GM). *Blood 72*:1293.
39. Tessier, N., and Hoang, T. (1988). Transforming growth factor β inhibits the proliferation of the blast cells of acute myeloblastic leukemia. *Blood 72*:159.
40. Beran, M., Andersson, B. S., Kelleher, P., Whalen, K., McCredie, K., and Gutterman, J. (1987). Diversity of the effect of recombinant tumor necrosis factor α and β on human myelogenous leukemia cell lines. *Blood 69*: 721.
41. Beran, M., McCredie, K. B., Keating, M. J., and Gutterman, J. U. (1988). Antileukemic effect of recombinant tumor necrosis factor α in vitro and its modulation by α and β interferons. *Blood 72*:728.
42. Talpaz, M., Kantarjian, H. M., and McCredie, K. (1986). Hematologic remission and cytogenetic improvement induced by recombinant interferon alpha in chronic myelogenous leukemia. *N. Engl. J. Med. 314*:1064.
43. Talpaz, M., Kantarjian, H. K., McCredie, K. B., Keating, M. J., Trujillo, J., and Gutterman, J. (1987). Clinical investigation of human alpha interferon in chronic myelogenous leukemia. *Blood 69*:1280.
44. Kurzrock, R., Talpaz, M., and Kantarjian, H. (1987). Therapy of chronic myelogenous leukemia with recombinant inteferon γ. *Blood 7*:943.
45. Waldmann, H., and Hale, G., for the Campath Users (in press). Results of Campath-1 T cell depleted bone marrow transplantation. In *New Issues in T Cell Depletion*. (F. Grignani and F. Martelli, eds.). Serono Symposia, Rome.
46. Hale, G., Cobbold, S., and Waldman, H., for the Campath-1 Users. (1988). T cell depletion with Campath-1 in allogeneic bone marrow transplantation. *Transplantation 45*:753.
47. O'Reilly, R. J., Kernan, N. A., Cunningham, I., et al. (1988). T cell depleted marrow transplants for the treatment in leukemia. In *Bone Marrow Transplantation: Current Controversies*. (R. P. Gale and R. Champlin, eds.). Alan R. Liss, New York, p. 477.
48. Butturini, A., and Gale, R. P. (1988). Clinical trials of T cell depletion: Current controversies, future directions. In *Bone Marrow Transplantation: Current Controversies*. (R. P. Gale, and R. Champlin, eds.). Alan R. Liss, New York, p. 495.
49. Tomonaga, M., Golde, D. W., and Gasson, J. C. (1986). Biosinthetic (recombinant) human granulocyte macrophage colony stimulating factor: Effect on normal bone marrow and leukemia cell lines. *Blood 67*:31.
50. Westbrook, C. A., Gasson, J. C., Gerber, S. E., Selsted, M. E., and Golde, D. W. (1984). Purification and characterization of human lymphocytes-derived erythroid potentiating activity. *J. Biol. Chem. 259*:9992.
51. Yang, Y., Ciarletta, A. B., Temple, P. A., et al. (1986). Human IL-3 (multi CFS): Identification by expression cloning of a novel hematopoietic growth factor related to murine IL-3. *Cell 47*:3.

52. Amatruda, T. T., Boheman, R., Ranyard, J., and Koeffler, P. (1987). Pattern or expression of HLA DR and HLA DQ antigens and mRNA in myeloid differentiation. *Blood 69*:1225.
53. Sullivan, K. M., Storb, R., Buckner, C. D., et al. (1983). Graft versus host disease as adoptive inmunotherapy in patients with advanced hematologic neoplasmas. *N. Engl. J. Med. 320*:828.
54. Sullivan, K. M., Deeg, H. J., Sandres, J., et al. (1986). Hyperacute graft versus host disease in patients not given immunosuppression after allogenic bone marrow transplantation. *Blood 67*:1172.
55. Arthur, C. K., Apperley, J. F., Guo, A. P., et al. (1988). Cytogenic events after bone marrow transplantation for chronic myelogenous leukemia in chromic phase. *Blood 71*:1179.
56. Roth, M. S., Antin, J. H., Bingham, E. L., and Ginsburg, D. (1989). Detection of Philadelphia chromosome positive cells by the polymerase chain reaction following bone marrow transplantation for chronic myelogenous leukemia. *Blood 74*:577.
57. Gratwohl, A., Tichelli, A., Wursch, A., et al. (1988). Irradiated donor buffy coat following T cell depleted bone marrow transplants. *Bone Marrow Transplant 3*:577.
58. Slavin, S., Or, R., Neparstek, E., Eckerstein, A., and Weiss, L. (1988). Cellular-mediated immunotherapy of leukemia in conjunction with autologous and allogeneic bone marrow transplantation in experimental animals and man. *Blood 72*(Suppl. 1):407a.

18

Chronic Myelogenous Leukemia in Accelerated and Blastic Phases: Present Status and Future Prospects

Hagop M. Kantarjian, Moshe Talpaz, and Michael J. Keating *The University of Texas M. D. Anderson Cancer Center, Houston, Texas*

INTRODUCTION

Chronic myelogenous leukemia (CML) is a clonal myeloproliferative disorder of the hematopoietic stem cells (1-3). The multistep pathophysiologic evolution of CML (4) is characterized as a biphasic or triphasic clinical course with a chronic, an accelerated, and a blastic phase (5-12). The realization that potentially useful treatments for CML may be ineffective in the resistant blastic phase (13-16) has stressed the importance of an objective description of the poorly defined accelerated phase of CML. New regimens could then be investigated in a stage that retains relative sensitivity to treatment and in which the potential benefit-to-risk ratio of novel approaches is favorable.

Progress in understanding the molecular biology of CML, and in its therapy, has renewed interest in the entity. New therapeutic modalities have included intensive combination chemotherapy (17-19), differentiating agents (20-22), biologic response modifiers (13,14,23-29), and transplantation with allogeneic (30,31) or autologous stem cells (32,33). Although several of these approaches have produced exciting results in the earlier chronic-phase CML, studies in the blastic phase have been less encouraging.

DEFINITION AND INCIDENCE

The definitions and terminology of the accelerated and blastic phases of CML are variable. Terms describing these stages include terminal-phase CML, CML in transformation, aggressive-phase CML, and blast crisis. The original definitions referred to a broad "terminal phase," which underscores disease progression and aggressiveness (10). This was described by Karanes and Silver in 1968 as a CML stage with an increased percentage of blasts and promyelocytes in the peripheral blood of 30% or more; a triad of anemia, leukocytosis, and thrombocytopenia; or unexplained persistent fever (8). Using these criteria, the median survival of patients was 1 month, with about 10% of patients surviving 6 months. Rosenthal et al. described the "blast crisis" phase based on the presence of 30% or more blasts in the peripheral blood or bone marrow, extramedullary disease, or cytogenetic clonal evolution (11). They also defined a separate "accelerated phase" characterized by marked leukocytosis with progressive granulocytic immaturity and transformation-dependent anemia and thrombocytopenia, hypermetabolic symptoms, or refractoriness to therapy but with less than 30% blasts. Other investigators have proposed such modifications as the inclusion of blasts and promyelocytes, or a cutoff of 50% immature blasts in the peripheral blood, to define the blastic phase. Less specific features often characterized accelerated-phase CML, such as the presence of malaise, increasing splenomegaly, rising leukocyte alkaline phosphatase (34), bone marrow or peripheral blasts or basophils of 10% or more, extremes of platelet counts, and the development of myelofibrosis (35-37).

Standard definition criteria for the accelerated and blastic phases allow comparability of populations on different trials. The blastic phase of CML is now defined by 30% or more blasts in the marrow or peripheral blood or the presence of extramedullary disease (38). Peripheral blasts and promyelocytes of 30% or more are associated with an ominous prognosis reminiscent of the blastic phase (7). However, patients with a high promyelocytic percentage alone or with 30% blasts and promyelocytes in the bone marrow have a median survival of 16 months (7,37). Inclusion of such patients in trials of CML blastic phase results in longer survival independent of the treatment. A definition of accelerated-phase CML should be associated with a short subsequent survival. Based on a multivariate analysis of patient survival from the time of development of presumed features of disease acceleration (Tables 1 and 2), we have proposed the following criteria for accelerated-phase CML: peripheral blasts of 15% or more; peripheral blasts and promyelocytes of 30% or more; peripheral basophils of 20% or more; cytogenetic clonal evolution; and thrombocytopenia less than 100×10^3 per μL unrelated to therapy (7). Although myelofibrosis has been reported to indicate an ominous prognosis (36), its definition (collagen versus reticulin fibrosis) and patterns (focal or diffuse and degree of fibrosis) are impre-

Table 1 Characteristics of the Accelerated Phase of CML: Univariate Analysis of Patient Survival After Development of Characteristic

Characteristic	No. of patients developing characteristics	Median survival (months)
Peripheral blasts ≥ 15%	85	8.6
Marrow blasts ≥ 15%	34	10.9
Peripheral blasts + promyelocytes ≥ 30%	32	4.7
Marrow blasts + promyelocytes ≥ 30%	38	17.4
Peripheral basophils ≥ 20%	74	16.0
Marrow basophils ≥ 20%	25	11.6
Platelets < 100×10^3 per μL	105	14.9
Platelets > 2×10^6 per μL	76	27.2
Hemoglobin < 7 g/dL	92	16.0
Nucleated red cells ≥ 15%	60	23.5
Cytogenetic clonal evolution	54	7.0
Extramedullary disease	25	10.0

cise. Significant collagen fibrosis is usually associated with other features of disease acceleration, such as cytogenetic clonal evolution, thrombocytopenia, blastosis, or basophilia. On the other hand, considerable reticulin fibrosis is present in up to 50% of patients with CML at diagnosis (39,40); although associated with shortened survival, it is not an indication of disease acceleration. The proposed criteria for the accelerated and blastic phases are clinically relevant, objective, and reproducible in different CML populations.

The incidence of accelerated and blastic phases during the course of CML is dependent on the type and success of therapy. In the past, when no effective

Table 2 Characteristics of the Accelerated Phase of CML: Summary of the Multivariate Ananlysis and the Relative Risk of Death per Unit of Time After the Development of the Accelerated Phase Characteristics

Characteristic	Relative risk
Cytogenetic clonal evolution	3.6
Peripheral blasts ≥ 15%	1.9
Peripheral basophils ≥ 20%	1.9
Peripheral blasts and promyelocytes ≥ 30%	2.2
Platelets < 100×10^3 per μL	1.7

treatments were available, most of the patients died in chronic phase from complications related to severe leukocytosis or thrombocytosis, such as leukostasis, pulmonary failure, cerebrovascular accidents, hemorrhagic events, or infiltrative organ damage. Only 15-30% of patients developed blastic-phase CML (41,42). Disease control with chemotherapy unmasked the natural course of CML that progressed into the accelerated and blastic phases. At present, less than 5% of patients die with chronic-phase complications. The others either evolve gradually through an accelerated phase (60-70%) or suddenly develop a blastic phase (30-35%). About 20-30% of patients die with accelerated-phase or myelofibrosis-associated complications, and others progress to the blastic phase, which is invariably fatal. Myelofibrosis was reported more commonly in patients receiving busulfan therapy (5,6). Patients treated with α-interferon (IFN-α) may have a tendency to develop a lymphoid blastic phase, perhaps because of a better myeloid clonal suppression by α-interferon (13). The broader application of potentially curative regimens, such as bone marrow transplantation or biologic therapies, may further change the commonly recognized clinical course of CML (13-16,30,31).

PATHOPHYSIOLOGY

CML is hypothesized to evolve in a multistep fashion. An initial phase of proliferation of Philadelphia chromosome (Ph)-negative cells has been proposed, based on the observation of several Ph-negative CML patients who later exhibited Ph-positive disease (43,44). Similar to the lymphoproliferative disorders occurring after transplantation or severe immunosuppression, these Ph-negative cells may be initially polyclonal. Alternatively, a monoclonal process independent of the acquisition of the Ph-associated molecular abnormalities may be the primary generating event.

A second stage, the Ph-positive chronic-phase CML, is probably linked to the presence of the Ph abnormality. The balanced translocation of genetic material between chromosomes 9 and 22 results in the juxtaposition of the cellular Abelson (c-*abl*) proto-oncogene sequence from chromosome 9 to the breakpoint cluster region (*bcr*) localized to a narrow 5.8 kb fragment on chromosome 22. The new hybrid *bcr-abl* oncogene induces abnormal 8.5 kb mRNA and 210 kDa (p210) protein products with increased tyrosine kinase activity (45-48). Causality between the molecular abnormalities and CML disease is suggested by experimental studies demonstrating transformation of cells through transfection by the p210 *bcr-abl* gene product (49,50). In some instances, a myristylation site anchoring the cytoplasmic *bcr-abl* message to the cellular membrane was required (50). In vitro studies investigating the effect of antisense RNA or monoclonal antibodies directed against the *bcr-abl* sequences in chronic-phase CML cells will further support this causal association.

The third stage of CML involves the transformation from chronic phase to the accelerated and blastic phases. This is associated with the development of nonrandom chromosomal abnormalities (12,43,51,52). In some instances progression may be independent of the Ph chromosome since blastic transformation was documented in patients who have lost the Ph abnormality (53) or the associated molecular event (54). It is tempting to speculate that transformation may proceed through different pathways. In patients with duplication of the Ph chromosome (one-third of patients), this may be mediated through the amplification of the *bcr-abl* messages (55,56). In fact, the patients who evolved from Ph-positive chronic-phase CML into Ph-negative blastic phase had an unusually indolent progression suggesting a potential modulating role of the *bcr-abl* abnormality (54). Patients exhibiting trisomy 8 or isochromosome 17 may have disease acceleration through alternative pathways involving amplification of the *myc* oncogene or abnormalities related to the *p53* oncogene or the granulocyte colony-stimulating factor (G-CSF) gene (57). Recent experimental data propose that the pathophysiologic evolution of CML may involve a secondary activation of growth factors or other messages (interleukin-3 and other CSFs) (58,59).

The similarity of CML with another myeloproliferative disorder, polycythemia vera (PV), may be instructive in understanding its pathophysiology. The following observations are noted in PV: (1) normal bone marrow cells produce erythroid colony-forming units (CFU-E) in agar cultures only under the influence of erythropoietin, but those from PV patients form CFU-E colonies without exposure to erythropoietin, that is, "endogenous" CFU-E; (2) erythropoietin levels are very low in PV; and (3) antibodies to erythropoietin induce suppression of the endogenous CFU-E colonies from PV (60). This suggests that the erythroid abnormal clone in PV may be extremely sensitive to, and still under partial control of erythropoietin stimulation. A similar pathophysiologic mechanism may be operating in CML, which could be extremely sensitive to other growth factors (IL-3, G-CSF, and GM-CSF) at very low levels, and secondarily suppressing normal myeloid growth. It is anticipated that levels of growth factors may be undetectable or extremely low in CML but that the addition of growth factor antibodies to in vitro cultures may suppress CML colonies.

A pool of normal stem cells exists in the bone marrow of patients with CML, which is suppressed by the activity of the CML clones and which may undergo gradual depletion or more effective suppression with disease progression. This concept has been supported by both in vitro (61-65) and in vivo observations (66,67) demonstrating these diploid cells to be nonclonal in origin. The reasons behind the proliferative advantage of CML over normal stem cells are unclear. In vitro liquid cultures are in fact a favorable milieu for normal stem cell growth over leukemic clones (63-65). Semisolid agar systems generally exhibit an in-

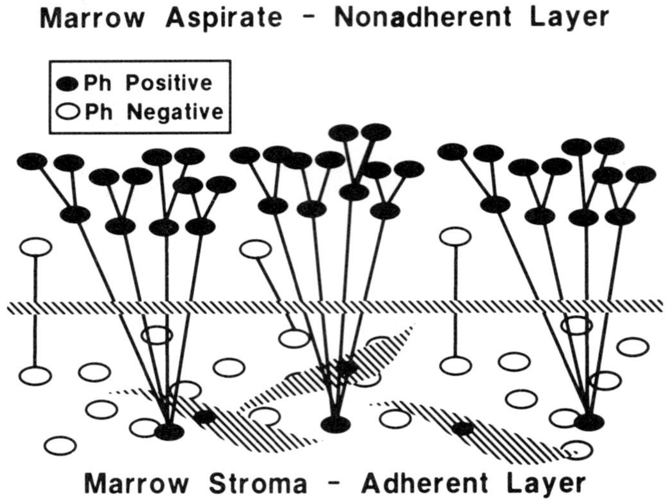

Figure 1 Hypothesis of the differential distribution of the hematopoietic Ph-positive and normal stem cells in the marrow matrix (adherent layer) and marrow fluid (nonadherent layer). The proportion of normal to Ph-positive cells is significantly higher in the hematopoietic niches of the marrow matrix or feeder layer.

creased colony formation in CML compared to normal marrow (68,69). CML cells have decreased adherence to the marrow stroma (70). Disturbance of this close cellular interaction, and earlier release of CML cells, may contribute to their growth advantage in vivo.

Based on these findings we have hypothesized a differential distribution of the hematopoietic Ph-positive and normal stem cells in the bone marrow matrix (or adherent cell layer in liquid cultures) compared to the supernatant fluid (exemplified by the nonadherent cells). Since Ph-positive cells are less adherent, the ratio of Ph-positive clones to normal cells is higher in the nonadherent compared to adherent layers. This explains several observations, including the premature release of Ph-positive clones in the peripheral blood, the finding of Ph in an overwhelming majority of patients in whom marrow aspirate is submitted for karyotypic analysis, and the more favorable selection of diploid clones in liquid culture studies of adherent (63,64) compared to nonadherent hematopoietic cells (65). Intensive chemotherapy by inducing marrow emptying provides a transient growth of diploid cells; an antiproliferative "chronic exposure" effect of interferons on the later progenitor cells (nonadherent) induces moderate but prolonged Ph suppression. This hypothesis (Figure 1) is tentative and will need modification as further data accumulate.

Other indirect mechanisms may be inducing the growth advantage of CML in vivo. The expression of Ia antigenic determinants, a signal for normal maturation of myeloid progenitor cells, is decreased on the granulocyte-macrophage colony-forming unit colonies from patients with CML. CML progenitors may thus spend a longer period in the proliferation phase before they respond to normal differentiation mechanisms (71,72). Natural killer cell activity, another important mediator of hematopoietic control, is also decreased in patients with CML (73). Although the beneficial effect of interferons in CML may be due to direct antiproliferation, indirect effects through mediation of increased Ia antigenic expression or promotion of NK cell activity are possible (74,75). An overall hypothesis incorporating these observations into a unified schema of CML pathophysiology requires further experimental data.

In chronic-phase CML, a striking proliferation of the total myeloid pool is the primary pathologic process (61). Other mechanisms of CML transformation include progressive maturational arrest, resistance to therapy, increasing inhibition of the normal stem cell pool by the leukemic activity (76), accentuated clonal expression along particular myeloid lines (7), clonal evolution (43,44,51), and secondary myelofibrosis (36).

Massive cellular proliferation produces severe leukocytosis, increased treatment requirements, organomegaly, and systemic symptoms (fever, weight loss, and poor performance). Progressive maturational arrest is associated with increased peripheral and marrow blasts. Anemia and thrombocytopenia may be due to marrow invasion by leukemic clones, leukemic inhibitory activity, or secondary myelofibrosis. Aberrant lineage commitment is manifested by excessive basophilia, eosinophilia, monocytosis, peripheral erythrocytosis, and thrombocytosis, is associated with maturational arrest, and may produce the morphologic spectrum in blastic phase, including myeloid, undifferentiated, erythroid, megakaryocytic, and mixed blastic-phase CML. Clonal evolution may occur at the cytogenetic levels with development of additional karyotypic abnormalities or clinically by extramedullary or "metastatic" clonal growth (38). Secondary myelofibrosis is thought to result from abnormalities of the *sis* oncogene, or platelet-derived growth factor (PDGF) gene, the intramedullary release of PDGF by megakaryocytes or platelets, and secondary stimulation of the marrow fibroblastic matrix (77). Significant myelofibrosis manifests by various degrees of thrombocytopenia and anemia, marrow failure, and myeloid expansion along long bones and in extramedullary sites, such as the liver and spleen. By disrupting the normal hematopoietic-matrix interaction, this process may contribute to the abnormal maturation of myeloid clones and blastic transformation.

CLINICAL MANIFESTATIONS

Unexplained fever, significant weight loss, increasing bone and joint pains, and the development of infections, bleeding, or thrombotic episodes are all suggestive of disease transformation. Occasionally, hyperhistaminic symptoms, such as skin rashes, itching, flushing, or diarrhea, may indicate basophilic transformation (78). Progressive splenomegaly despite therapy is associated with nausea, increased left upper quadrant or back pain, and palpable mass. Skin or subcutaneous nodules, lymph node enlargement, increasing jaundice, or hepatomegaly indicates extramedullary involvement. Leukemic bone involvement may be associated with severe bone pains, fractures, inflammation of surrounding tissues mimicking cellulitis or osteomyelitis, and joint effusions. Central nervous system involvement with disease transformation is observed with increasing frequency, probably because of survival prolongation with therapy (10).

LABORATORY STUDIES

Accelerated-phase CML is associated with increasing degrees of anemia and thrombocytopenia unaccounted for by bleeding or chemotherapy, cytogenetic clonal evolution, or the appearance in the peripheral blood or bone marrow of 15% or more blasts, 20% or more basophils, or 30% or more blasts and promyelocytes (7,8,37). The coexisting triad of severe leukocytosis unresponsive to therapy with significant thrombocytopenia and splenomegaly also indicates poor outcome (8). Reticulin fibrosis is not indicative of disease acceleration (39,40). However, significant marrow collagen fibrosis is reported to be an ominous sign and is associated with megakaryocytopenia, thrombocytopenia, or marrow failure, which is the terminal event in 10-20% of patients (36,79).

CML blastic phase is defined by the presence of 30% or more blasts in the peripheral blood or bone marrow. Blast cells are categorized by morphologic criteria and special stains. Myeloid blastic phase accounts for 60% of cases and shows myeloperoxidase-positive blasts. Lymphoid blasts stain negatively for myeloperoxidase and positively for terminal deoxynucleotidyltransferase (TdT) enzymatic stain; most of these cases also demonstrate the common acute lymphocytic leukemia antigen on blast cells (CALLA positive). The undifferentiated blastic phase is diagnosed when all stains on blasts are negative. In most instances, analysis by electron microscopy or immunophenotyping indicates a myeloid origin of blasts (80,81). Lymphoid and undifferentiated blastic morphologies each account for 15-20% of cases. Less than 10% of patients develop megakaryocytic or erythroid blastic phase (82,83).

Compared with chronic-phase CML, the in vitro growth of CML cells from patients with disease transformation shows absent, poor, or excessive growth with high cluster-colony ratios (84). Excessive growth of basophilic colonies has been related to poor prognosis (85). Flow cytometric studies show DNA aneuploidy in 30-40% of patients in the blastic phase (80). Cytogenetic studies reveal chromosomal abnormalities in addition to the t(9;22) $(q^{34}; q^{11})$ in 50-75% of patients in the accelerated phase and in 60-80% of those in the blastic phase. These karyotypic changes are nonrandom and frequently involve a duplication of the Philadelphia chromosome (25-30%), trisomy 8 (25-30%), an isochromosome 17 (20%), or other changes involving chromosomes 1, 3, 19, 20, and 21 (7,12). Any or a combination of the first three abnormalities is present in 40-60% of patients in blastic phase.

THERAPY

The mortality in chronic-phase CML is less than 5% with effective chemotherapy and supportive care. Most patients die from complications following disease transformation into the accelerated and blastic phases. Investigational chemotherapy trials have generally been confined to the blastic phase of CML because of the difficulty in assessing their relative efficacy in the poorly defined accelerated phase. The results of allogeneic bone marrow transplantation and biologic response modifiers in the accelerated phase were superior when compared with blastic-phase therapy and have encouraged a better definition of the accelerated phase of CML in which the benefit of newer approaches could be determined.

Despite a morphologic resemblance to de novo acute leukemia, the blastic phase of CML is probably an earlier stem cell disease that is more resistant to therapy. Prognostic factors associated with significantly worse remission rates and survivals include a nonlymphoid blast cell morphology and the presence of thrombocytopenia or cytogenetic clonal evolution (22).

The treatment strategies in the blastic phase of CML have been patterned after the successful programs in acute leukemia, including (1) intensive chemotherapy regimens aimed at emptying the bone marrow to favor normal stem cell regeneration, and (2) differentiating agents that may induce maturation of blast cells and a return to chronic-phase CML. The availability of stem cell transplantation (autologous and allogeneic), in vitro purging procedures, and biologic response modifiers have added new dimensions to therapy.

Intensive Chemotherapy

Production of marrow hypoplasia to allow normal or chronic-phase CML cell regeneration has been attempted using various intensive chemotherapy combinations, including cytosine arabinoside (ara-C), anthracyclines, amsacrine, etoposide, 5-azacytidine, cyclophosphamide, 6-mercaptopurine, and hydroxyurea. The comparative evaluation of these regimens has been extremely difficult because of the different response criteria, especially in earlier studies (42,87). Using remission criteria similar to those used in acute leukemia (88), complete remission rates of 10-30% have been reported (Table 3) (87-101). In our experience, the more recent programs evaluated since 1981 have resulted in higher remission rates (32 versus 15%; $p = 0.01$) and a significant but modest survival prolongation (24 versus 15 weeks; $p = 0.03$) (12).

Table 3 Results of Intensive Chemotherapy Trials in the Blastic Phase of CML

Study (reference)	Regimen[a]	No. patients	% CR	Median survival (weeks)
Canellos et al. (87)	VP	30	11	20
Vallejos et al. (42)	Multiple	39	15	22
Pedersen-Bjergaard (93)	Multiple	20	15	22
Hayes et al. (91)	ara-C + carmustine + VP	86	4	6
Spiers et al. (94)	TRAMPCOL	19	42	–
Coleman et al. (89)	Hydroxyurea, VP, 6-mercaptopurine	202	13	12
Kantarjian et al.	Multiple	195	23	21
	ADOAP, ROAP, COAP, AMSAOAP	48	27	–
Schiffers et al. (98)	Etoposide + 5-azacytidine	27	4	23
(99)	Etoposide + 5-azacytidine	35	3	5
Dutcher et al. (101)	Mitoxantrone + 5-azacytidine	21	10	–
		12 (accelerated)	25	–
Winton et al. (97)	DATA	30	0	5
Iacoboni et al. (95)	High-dose ara-C	22	23	16
Kantarjian et al. (96)	Mitoxantrone + high-dose ara-C	27	27	14

[a]VP, vincristine and prednisone; ara-C, cytosine arabinoside; TRAMPCOL, 6-thioguanine, daunorubicin, ara-C, methotrexate, prednisone, cyclophosphamide, vincristine, and L-asparaginase; DATA, daunorubicin, 5-azacytidine, 6-thioguanine, ara-C; OAP, vincristine, ara-C, prednisone; ADOAP, ROAP, DOAP, COAP, AMSAOAP, OAP + adriamycin, rubidazone, daunorubicin, cyclophosphamide, or amsacrine.

Many of the earlier studies have included small numbers of patients, multiple regimens, and different remission criteria (10), making their evaluation difficult. Recent large-scale trials have used combinations of an increasing number of active agents, such as the TRAMPCOL regimen consisting of 6-thioguanine, daunorubicin, ara-C, methotrexate, prednisone, and vincristine with or without L-asparaginase (87). Although a relatively high response rate was sometimes reported, survival improvement was minimal. The combination of hydroxyurea, 6-mercaptopurine, and steroids with or without vincristine was evaluated in a

Table 4 Results of Vincristine-, and Prednisone-Containing Regimens in CML Lymphoid Blastic Phase

Study (reference)	Characterization of blasts[a]	No. patients	% CR
Marks et al. (105)	Tdt-positive	13	46
Rosenthal et al. (103)	Lymphoid morphology	18	50
Janossy et al. (104)	Tdt-positive, CALLA-positive	14	71
Walters et al. (102)	Tdt positive	20	45
	CALLA-positive	12	75
	CALLA-negative	8	25

[a]Tdt, terminal nucleotidyltransferase; CALLA, common acute lymphocytic leukemia antigen.

large cooperative study that included 202 patients with CML blastic phase (89). The complete remission rate was 13%, with an overall response rate of 34%. Responders had a median survival of 7.5 months compared to 2.5 months for nonresponders; however, the median overall survival was only 3 months. When Winton et al. used a combination of daunorubicin, 5-azacytidine, 6-thioguanine, and ara-C (DATA) to treat 30 patients in blastic phase, no complete remission was observed (97). Schiffer et al. reported initial encouraging results with etoposide and 5-azacytidine: among 27 patients treated, 1 complete remission and 15 partial remissions (59%) were obtained. A subsequent trial using higher doses of both agents showed only 1 complete response among 35 patients (3%); this was attributed to the worse characteristics of the population (98).

Better results were generally noted with ara-C programs (12,95,96). Recent trials with regimens containing high-dose ara-C have yielded higher complete response rates of 20–30% (95,96,100). In our study of high-dose ara-C, the overall complete remission rate was 23% (95). The addition of mitoxantrone to high-dose ara-C did not improve the response rate or survival (96); the median survival was 3.5 months overall and 6 months among responders.

Lymphoid blastic phase defines a favorable subset of patients who have different clinical characteristics, respond favorably to therapy, and have a relatively better prognosis (12,102–106). These patients tend to develop a sudden onset of blastic phase and have a higher proportion of blasts in the marrow and higher platelet count (106). They respond favorably to vincristine- and steroid-containing programs (12,102–105) but also to other regimens (106). Complete response rates of 40–70% are observed with combinations including vincristine, anthracyclines, and steroids, especially among patients with CALLA-positive disease (Table 4).

Very few studies have extended blastic-phase intensive regimens into the accelerated phase. Dutcher et al. (101) recently treated 12 patients with accelerated-phase CML, using mitoxantrone and 5-azacytidine. The complete response rate was 25% compared to 10% for those treated in blastic phase. This supports the notion that earlier treatment may improve the results and outcome.

Differentiating Agents

Differentiation of immature blasts into mature elements is an attractive alternative concept to induction of marrow hypoplasia in CML blastic phase. Several agents induce in vitro leukemic cell differentiation, including low doses of ara-C, 6-thioguanine, homoharringtonine, 5-azacytidine, hydroxyurea, mithramycin, retinoics, and interferons (107,108). Low-dose ara-C yielded inferior results to conventional therapy in acute myelogenous leukemia, with most remissions attributed to cytoreduction rather than differentiation (109). Anecdotal reports showed low-dose ara-C activity in CML blastic phase, but the response rate in larger series was disappointing. DiRaimondo et al. reported only 1 response among 7 patients with blastic-phase CML receiving low-dose ara-C (20). Retinoics have not shown positive results in myelodysplastic syndrome or in chronic-phase CML when combined with hydroxyurea, implying they may not be beneficial in the accelerated and blastic phases. Trans-retinoic acid used alone as induction therapy in 24 patients with acute promyelocytic leukemia yielded a high response rate (110) and may be useful in the accelerated and blastic phases of CML. The combination of several differentiating agents, including low-doie ara-C, *cis*-retinoic acid, vitamin D and α-interferon produced 2 partial responses among 3 patients with CML blastic phase (111).

Mithramycin, an inhibitor of RNA synthesis, induces in vitro differentiation of blast cells and is associated with a reduction in *abl* and *myc* oncogenic expression in CML blast cells (112). Koller and Miller treated patients with CML blastic phase with low doses of mithramycin, 1 mg/m^2 intravenously two to three times weekly, together with hydroxyurea (see Table 5). The rational was that one component, mithramycin, would produce phenotypic conversion of the blast cells to differentiated chronic-phase CML cells; the other component, hydroxyurea, would suppress proliferation (21). Response, defined as a return of the peripheral counts and differential to a chronic-phase picture with less than 10% blasts, was observed in 6 of 9 patients treated, all responders exhibiting a myeloid blast cell morphology (21). A subsequent update of a larger series, using remission criteria of acute leukemia (88), resulted in 2 partial remissions among 6 patients with myeloid blastic phase (33%) but no responses in 15 patients with undifferentiated blastic phase (113). The median survival of 15 weeks for all 21 patients was not improved over previous experience. Similar low objective response rates were observed in two other studies, with only 1 complete response

Table 5 Summary of Therapy of the Blastic Phase of CML with Differentiating Agents

Study (reference)	Therapy	No. patients	No. responses (%)
DiRaimondo (20)	Low-dose ara-C	7	1 (14)
Koller and Miller (21)	Mithramycin + hydroxyurea	Myeloid, 6	6 (100)
		Other, 3	1 (33)
Koller et al. (113)	Mithramycin + hydroxyurea	Myeloid, 6	2 (33)
		Undifferentiated, 15	0 (0)
Trümper et al. (114)	Mithramycin + hydroxyurea	9	1 (11)
Antimi et al. (115)	Mithramycin + hydroxyurea	7	0 (0)
Tricot et al. (22)	Tiazofurin	5	5 (100)

obtained among 16 patients (6%) with CML blastic phase (114,115). Antimi et al. suggested, however, a possible value of the combination of mithramycin and hydroxyurea in the accelerated phase, with all 4 patients treated reverting to a second chronic phase (115). The relative contribution of mithramycin to the efficacy of the combination and the impact of the regimen on survival await further investigation.

Tiazofurin is a nucleoside analog metabolized to thiazole-4-carboxamide adenine dinucleotide (TAD). TAD acts as a false cofactor to produce potent inhibition of inosine monophosphate dehydrogenase (IMPD) activity and consequently to decrease production of guanine triphosphate (GTP) pools and inhibit cellular proliferation (116,117). TAD, the active metabolite of Tiazofurin, is concentrated 20-fold higher in leukemic cells compared with normal cells, resulting in a selective leukemic cell kill (118). Recently, Tricot et al. reported interesting results with Tiazofurin therapy in acute leukemia and CML blastic phase (22). Using a pharmacologically directed approach, they treated patients with Tiazofurin given at a dose range of 2200–7700 mg/m^2 daily for 15 days, the dose being adjusted every third day to achieve inhibition of GTP pools to less than 20% in blast cells and of IMPD activity to less than 10%. They observed partial responses in all five patients treated for CML blastic phases, response being defined as a decrease in the absolute peripheral blast count by 90% or more and in marrow blast percentages by 75% or more. Because the responses were characterized by the lack of marrow hypoplasia, differentiation was suggested as the primary antileukemic effect. However, a high ratio of blast to mature leukemic cellular kill could produce the same morphologic picture.

Table 6 Therapy of the Accelerated and Blastic Phases of CML with Interferons

Study (reference)	Interferon	No. treated	No. with hematologic remission (%) Complete	Partial
MDAH (14,27)	IFN-α	6	3 (50)	1 (17)
	IFN-α + IFN-γ	18	2 (11)	3 (17)
Alimena et al. (24)	IFN-α	9	1 (11)	2 (22)

In summary, the important observations of differentiating agents in CML blastic phase need to be confirmed using standard entry and response criteria in large population studies. Their potential value in the accelerated phase of CML has not been explored.

Biologic Agents

The positive results with interferons in the chronic phase of CML prompted their use in the later stages. Anecdotal reports had shown the capacity of α-interferon to suppress cytogenetic clonal evolution and to control disease transformation (119). A more extensive investigation of IFN-α and γ-interferon (IFN-γ) confirmed their definite but limited efficacy in producing objective complete or partial hematologic remissions (14,24,27,28). The overall remission rates ranged from 10 to 30% with IFN-α alone or in combination with IFN-γ (Table 6). Ph suppression in these stages was rare. Most patients treated were in the accelerated phase; the overall response rate in the blastic phase was 10% or less. Many patients with rapid disease proliferation experienced side effects consisting of moderate to severe muscle and bone pains related to resistance and increased white cell counts. This may be due to the release of inflammatory substances (e.g., leukotrienes) from granulocytes under the effect of interferons and has limited the duration of therapy. This peculiar syndrome seems more common in these stages than in chronic-phase CML. Although the objective response rates were low, these investigations have not addressed the issue of disease stability or the potential value of combined approaches with interferons and chemotherapy in inducing or maintaining a second chronic phase (120,121).

We have recently conducted a study using low-dose ara-C at 15 mg/m^2 daily for 3 weeks and IFN-α at 5×10^6 units daily in patients with CML. Of 10 evaluable patients with accelerated-phase CML, 7 achieved a complete hematologic remission, 2 of them showing additional minimal Ph suppression. Our experience with IFN-α and hydrea for induction and for remission maintenance in these stages is at present maturing.

Table 7 Results of Autologous Bone Marrow Transplantation in the Blastic Phase of CML

Study (reference)	No. treated	% Achieving a second second chronic phase	Median survival from transplantation (months)
Haines et al. (128)	51	94	6
Reiffers et al. (33)	45	76	4.5
Preisler et al. (130)	17	29	4
Dantas et al. (131)	11	55	7
Vellekoop et al. (129)	10	60	5

Colony-stimulating factors have produced exciting results in several tumor categories. After intensive chemotherapy or autologous bone marrow transplantation, the use of CSFs had been associated with shortening the duration of myelosuppression and a decreased incidence of infections (122,123). The in vitro observation of leukemic growth enhancement by CSFs dictated a cautious approach in trials of CSFs in myeloid tumors (124,125). The use of granulocyte-macrophage CSF in myelodysplastic syndrome resulted in a significant improvement in the granulocyte counts, with some stimulation of the erythroid and megakaryotic series (126). The leukemic marker was documented by a premature chromosome condensation technique in the mature granulocytes, indicating that GM-CSF may have differentiated leukemic cells. Variable degrees of leukemic versus normal cell enhancement were observed with a favorable leukemic over normal growth advantage in only a minority of patients (127). Our results in acute myelogenous leukemia using intensive chemotherapy followed by GM-CSF indicate regrowth of the normal stem cells. These two preliminary trials suggest a possible value of GM-CSF in reverting CML blasts into mature chronic-phase granulocytes or in inducing normal stem cell growth after intensive chemotherapy in the accelerated and blastic phases.

Autologous Stem Cell Transplantation

The hypothesis underlying autologous stem cell transplantation (marrow or peripheral blood) in the accelerated and blastic phases of CML is that the stem cells collected in chronic phase and reinfused after eradication of the accelerated or blastic phase clones with chemoirradiation re-establish a second chronic phase of equal duration to the first from the time of stem cell collection. The preparative regimens usually included total-body irradiation and high doses of cyclophosphamide (32,33,128–131). The stem cells were often harvested in

Table 8 Results of Syngeneic and Allogeneic Bone Marrow Transplantation in the Accelerated and Blastic Phases in CML

Study (reference)	No. patients	Survival % (at x year)	Leukemia relapse %
I. Syngeneic			
Thomas et al. (30)			
Accelerated phase	7	27 (6)	29
Blastic phase	8	12 (6)	50
A. Accelerated phase			
Thomas et al. (30)	42	15 (3)	40
Goldman et al. (31)	56	32 (4)	55
Int. BMT registry	202	29 (4)	54
McGlave et al. (15)	28	30 (2.5)	25
B. Blastic phase			
Thomas et al. (30)	42	14 (3)	80
Goldman et al. (31)	22	14 (4)	40
Int. BMT registry	54	16 (4)	45
C. Second chronic phase			
Thomas et al. (30)	12	58 (3)	8
Champlin et al.	17	50 (3)	12

chronic phase with a predominance of Ph-positive clones (33,128), except for few patients who had stem cell storage after chemotherapy-induced Ph suppression (129). Under these circumstances, studies of autologous stem cell transplantation have had limited success. Whereas 50–60% of patients achieved a second chronic phase, it was generally short. The median survival time from transplantation was 6 months, with less than 25% of patients surviving 1 year (Table 7). It has been proposed that the infused chronic-phase CML clones may have evolved rapidly into a blastic phase under the influence of the marrow microenvironment (132). However, serial cytogenetic studies often show recurrence of the original blastic-phase clones, indicating that most failures are from poor eradication of the blastic-phase clones by the preparative regimen, rather than enhancement of leukemic growth as postulated by the "bad soil" microenvironment theory.

Improvement of the eradicative preparative regimens (high doses of busulfan, cyclophosphamide, etoposide, and ara-C in various combinations) (133,134), the use of double autologous transplantation, the collection of autologous stem cells after partial or complete suppression of the Ph-positive clone (chemotherapy, interferons, and in vitro purging procedures) (129,135–137), and the provision for maintenance therapy (interferons and chemotherapy) after transplantation (138,139) may improve the results.

Some of these approaches have already been piloted. Reiffers et al. used a double autologous stem cell transplantation in 17 patients with CML transformation using peripheral stem cells collected at diagnosis (140). All patients engrafted promptly. Of 15 patients evaluated, 6 (40%) showed transient Ph suppression to a range of 10-84%. At the time of analysis 8 patients had relapsed after a median of 11 months, but 8 were still in a second chronic phase for a median of 11+ months, and 2 of these have a second chronic phase longer than the first. The observation of Ph suppression after infusion of predominantly Ph-positive clones is intriguing and has been observed in less than 10% of patients with CML transformation treated with a single autologous stem cell transplantation (38,128) but in a substantial fraction of those treated in chronic phase (141). Transient Ph suppression to a range of 70-80% Ph-positive metaphases was noted in 10 of 12 patients receiving ablative therapy followed by reinfusion of Ph-positive stem cells (141). This may be due to suppression of the leukemic clones by the intensive regimens, but it is possible that disruption of the marrow microenvironment produced a favorable milieu for normal over CML stem cell proliferation. This could be further exploited by the addition of maintenance therapy with interferon or hydroxyurea.

The incubation of marrow cells in long-term liquid cultures has been associated with a favorable growth advantage of the normal stem cells over the leukemic clones. This has been demonstrated for acute myeloid and lymphoid leukemias and for CML (62-65) and has encouraged the initiation of trials of autologous stem cell transplantation using autologous marrow cells "purged" by liquid cultures along or with additional in vitro incubation with γ-interferon. The number of patients is limited, but these procedures provide new ways for treating the accelerated and blastic phases of CML. The application of these programs to the earlier chronic phase of CML will also be of considerable interest.

Allogeneic Bone Marrow Transplantation

The results of syngeneic or allogeneic bone marrow transplantation in the accelerated and blastic phases of CML are less favorable than in the chronic phase. The preparative regimens, which were associated with a low incidence of leukemia relapse in acute myelogenous or lymphocytic leukemia, resulted in an unacceptably high recurrence rate of leukemia ranging from 30 to 60% in the accelerated phase and from 40 to 90% in the blastic phase of CML. Cures, however, are still possible in 10-15% of patients with blastic phase and in 15-30% of those with accelerated phase (Table 8). Thus candidate patients with available donors must be considered for syngeneic or allogeneic bone marrow transplantation despite the risks and expenses involved. Transplantation in second chronic phase has consistently yielded higher cure fractions. This could be due to the decreased tumor burden at the time of the transplantation or to the selection through induction chemotherapy of the subset of patients with intrinsically more sensitive disease or with better organ status and tolerance to therapy. Thus, although no definite recommendation can be made regarding the timing of transplantation (blastic phase or after induction of a second chronic phase), this may be a valuable therapy-associated selection procedure when risk and cost analyses are important.

As for autologous bone marrow transplantation, optimization of the preparative regimens through the use of combinations of high-dose agents with or without irradiation may decrease the incidence of leukemia relapse and improve survival (133,134).

Maintenance therapy with biologic agents or chemotherapy is a useful approach in patients at high risk of leukemia relapse after allogeneic bone marrow transplantation. This is based on several recent observations. The use of IFN-α maintenance after allogeneic bone marrow transplantation in acute lymphocytic leukemia, aimed originally at reducing the occurrence of cytomegalovirus infections, was associated with a reduction in the incidence of leukemia relapse from 74 to 36% overall ($p = 0.04$) and from 71 to 19% among first or second remission transplants ($p < 0.01$) (131). Arcese et al. (139) treated 16 patients with CML relapse after allogeneic bone marrow transplantation with IFN-α, 3×10^6 units three times weekly. Among 4 patients with hematologic relapse, 3 achieved hematologic remission, 1 of them with Ph suppression to 0% for 14+ months. Of the 12 patients treated in cytogenetic relapse, 2 achieved complete Ph suppression for 8+ and 11+ months, respectively, and 5 had a stable cytogenetic pattern. Thus, maintenance therapy using IFN-α alone or with other biologic or chemotherapeutic agents deserves investigation after allogeneic bone marrow transplantation in accelerated or blastic phases of CML in which expectations for leukemia relapse are high.

FUTURE PERSPECTIVES

Future investigations must rely on reproducible criteria for the definition of various CML stages, for patient entry to novel trials, and for response to various regimens. Objective definitions have been proposed for the accelerated and blastic phases in this review. The response criteria should probably be similar to the morphologic criteria of acute leukemia trials, which do not require disappearance of the cytogenetic clonal marker.

Although further progress with intensive chemotherapy may occur through the discovery of new agents, it is likely that these will be integrated in strategies that utilize autologous stem cell transplantation as an intensification procedure. Thus, it is anticipated that breakthroughs will occur in the field of stem cell (autologous or allogeneic) transplantation, through (1) the use of purged autologous stem cells in vivo with chemotherapy or biologic agents or in vitro via long-term liquid cultures with or without chemoimmunologic purging; (2) the improvement in preparative regimens; and (3) the application of maintenance therapy following bone marrow transplantation. Therapy of the accelerated and blastic phases with differentiating agents is currently being actively pursued. Finally, the use of growth factors in conjunction with intensive chemotherapy or biologic treatments may hold significant future promise.

ACKNOWLEDGMENTS

Dr. Kantarjian and Dr. Keating are Scholars of the Leukemia Society of America.

REFERENCES

1. Fialkow, P. J., Jacobson, R. J., and Papayannopoulou, T. (1977). Chronic myelocytic leukemia. Clonal origin in a stem cell common to the granulocyte, erythrocyte, platelet and monocyte/macrophage. *Am. J. Med. 63*: 125–130.
2. Nowell, P. C., and Hungerford, D. A. (1960). A minute chromosome in human chronic granulocytic leukemia. *Science 132*:1497–1502.
3. Rowley, J. D. (1973). A new consistent chromosomal abnormality in chronic myelogenous leukemia identified by quinacrine fluorescence and Giemsa staining. *Nature 243*:290–294.
4. Fialkow, P. J., Martin, P. J., Najfeld, V., Penfold, G. K., Jacobson, R. J., and Hansen, J. A. (1981). Evidence for a multi-step pathogenesis of chronic granulocytic leukemia. *Blood 58*:158–163.
5. Golde, D. W., and Champlin, R. E. (1985). Chronic myelogenous leukemia: Recent advances. *Blood 65*:1039–1047.
6. Goldman, J. M., and Lu Dao-Pei (1982). New approaches in chronic granulocytic leukemia-origin, prognosis, and treatment. *Semin. Hematol. 19*:241–256.
7. Kantarjian, H. N., Dixon, D., Keating, M. J., Talpaz, M., Walters, R. S., McCredie, K. B., and Freireich, E. J. (1988). Characteristics of accelerated disease in chronic myelogenous leukemia. *Cancer 61*:1441–1446.
8. Karanas, A., and Silver, R. T. (1968). Characteristics of the terminal phase of chronic granulocytic leukemia. *Blood 32*:445–459.
9. Spiers, A. S. D. (1979). Metamorphosis of chronic granulocytic leukaemia: Diagnosis, classification of management. *Br. J. Maematol. 41*:1-7.
10. Allen, S. L., and Coleman, M. (1985). Terminal-phase chronic myelogenous leukemia: Approaches to treatment. *Cancer Invest. 3*:491–503.
11. Rosenthal, S., Canellos, G. P., DeVita, V. T., Jr., and Gralnick, H. R. (1977). Characteristics of blast crisis in chronic granulocytic leukemia. *Blood 49*:705–714.

12. Kantarjian, H. M., Keating, M. J., Talpaz, M., Walters, R. S., Smith, T. L., Cork, A., McCredie, K. B., and Freireich, E. J. Chronic myelogenous leukemia in blast crisis: An analysis of 242 patients. *Am. J. Med. 83*:445–454.
13. Talpaz, M., Kantarjian, H. M., McCredie, K. B., Keating, M. J., Trujillo, J., and Gutterman, J. (1987). Clinical investigation of human alpha interferon in chronic myelogenous leukemia. *Blood 69*:1280–1288.
14. Kantarjian, H. M., Talpaz, M., and Gutterman, J. (1987). Biologic therapy of chronic myelogenous leukemia. *Oncology 1*:35–40.
15. McGlave, P., Arthur, D., Haake, R., Hurd, D., Miller, W., Vercellotti, G., Weisdorf, D., Kim, T., Ramsay, N., and Kersey, J. (1987). Therapy of chronic myelogenous leukemia with allogeneic bone marrow transplantation. *J. Clin. Oncol. 5*:1033–1040.
16. Champlin, R., Ho, W., Arenson, E., and Gale, R. P. (1982). Allogeneic bone marrow transplantation for chronic myelogenous leukemia in chronic or accelerated phase. *Blood 60*:1038–1044.
17. Cunningham, I., Gee, T., Dowling, M., Chaganti, R., Bailey, R., Hopfan, S., Bowden, L., Turnbull, A., Knapper, W., and Clarkson, B. (1979). Results of treatment of Ph^{1+} chronic myelogenous leukemia with an intensive treatment regimen (L-5 protocol). *Blood 53*:375–396.
18. Kantarjian, H. M., Vellekoop, L., McCredie, K. B., Keating, M. J., Hester, J., Smith, T., Barlogie, B., Trujillo, J., and Freireich, E. J. (1985). Intensive combination chemotherapy (ROAP) and splenectomy in the management of chronic myelogenous leukemia. *J. Clin. Oncol. 3*:192–200.
19. Hester, J. P., Waddell, C. C., Coltman, C. A., Jr., Morrison, F. S., Stephens, R. L., Balcerzak, S. P., Baker, L. H., and Chen, T. T. (1984). Response of chronic myelogenous leukemia patients to COAP-splenectomy. *Cancer 54*:1977–1982.
20. Di Raimondo, F., Milone, G., Guglielmo, P., Cacciola, E., and Giustoliso, R. (1985). Treatment of CML blast crisis with low dose ara-C. *Br. J. Haematol. 60*:773–774.
21. Koller, C. A., and Miller, D. M. (1986). Preliminary observations on the therapy of the myeloid blast phase of chronic granulocytic leukemia with plicamycin and hydroxyurea. *N. Engl. J. Med. 315*(23):1433–1438.
22. Tricot, G., Jayaram, H., Weber, G., and Hoffman, R. (1988). Tiazofurin is a potent antiproliferative agent and induced differentiation in patients with leukemia. *Am. Assoc. Cancer Res. 29*:210 (abstract 835).
23. Talpaz, M., Kantarjian, H. M., McCredie, K., Trujillo, J. M., Keating, M. J., and Gutterman, J. U. (1986). Hematologic remission and cytogenetic improvement induced by recombinant human interferon alpha A in chronic myelogenous leukemia. *N. Engl. J. Med. 314*:1065–1069.
24. Alimena, G., Morra, E., Lazzarino, M., et al. (1988). Interferon alpha-2b as therapy for Ph^1-positive chronic myelogenous leukemia: A study of 82 patients treated with intermittent or daily administration. *Blood 72*:642–647.
25. Niederle, N., Kloke, O., Osieka, K. R., Wandl, U., Opalka, B., and Schmidt, G. (1987). Interferon alpha-2b in the treatment of chronic myelogenous leukemia. *Semin. Oncol. 16*:29–35.

26. Kantarjian, H., Talpaz, M., Kurzrock, R., Keating, M., McCredie, K., Gutterman, J., and Freireich, E. (1987). Intensive combination chemotherapy and interferons in the management of chronic myelogenous leukemia. *Acta Haematol (Basel) 78*:70–74.
27. Talpaz, M., Kantarjian, H. M., Kurzrock, R., and Gutterman, J. (1988). Therapy of chronic myelogenous leukemia—chemotherapy and interferons. *Semin. Hematol. 25*:62–73.
28. Ozer, H., Mick, R., and Testa, J. (1988). Subcutaneous alpha interferon shows substantial activity in untreated chronic phase Philadelphia chromosome positive chronic myelogenous leukemia. Twenty-Second Congress of ISH Milan (Italy): 1(SYM-M-1-1).
29. Kurzrock, R., Talpaz, M., Kantarjian, H., Walters, R., Saks, S., Trujillo, J., and Gutterman, J. U. (1987). Therapy of chronic myelogenous leukemia with recombinant interferon-gamma. *Blood 70*:943–947.
30. Thomas, E. D., Clift, R. A., Fefer, A., Appelbaum, F. R., Beatty, P., Bensinger, W. I., Buckner, C. D., Cheever, M. A., Deeg, J., Doney, K., Flournoy, N., Greenberg, P., Hansen, J. A., Martin, P., MuGuffin, R., Ramberg, R., Sanders, J. E., Singer, J., Stewart, P., Storb, R., Sullivan, K., Weiden, P. L., and Witherspoon, R. (1986). Marrow transplantation for the treatment of chronic myelogenous leukemia. *Ann. Intern. Med. 104*:155–163.
31. Goldman, J. M., Apperley, J. F., Jones, L., Marcus, R., Goolden, A. W. G., Batchelor, R., Hale, G., Waldman, H., Reid, C. D., Hows, J., Gordon-Smith, E., Catovsky, D., and Galton, D. A. G. (1986). Bone marrow transplantation for patients with chronic myeloid leukemia. *N. Engl. J. Med. 314*:202–207.
32. Goldman, J. M., Catovsky, D., Hows, J., Spiers, A., and Galton, D. (1979). Cryopreserved peripheral blood cells functioning as autografts in patients with chronic granulocytic leukemia in transformation. *Br. Med. J. 1*:1310–1313.
33. Reiffers, J., Gorin, N., Michallet, M., Maraninchi, D., and Herve, P. (1986). Autografting for chronic granulocytic leukemia in transformation. *JNCI 76*:1307–1310.
34. Theologides, A. (1972). Unfavorable signs in patients with chronic myelocytic leukemia. *Ann. Intern. Med. 76*:95–99.
35. Schilling, R. F., and Crowley, J. J. (1979). Prognostic signs in chronic myelocytic leukemia. *Am. J. Hematol. 7*:1–10.
36. Clough, V., Geary, C. G., Hashmi, K., Davson, J., and Knowlson, T. (1979). Myelofibrosis in chronic granulocytic leukaemia. *Br. J. Haematol. 42*:515–526.
37. Kantarjian, H., and Talpaz, M. (1988). Definition of the accelerated phase of chronic myelogenous leukemia. *J. Clin. Oncol. 6*:180–181.
38. Terjanian, T., Kantarjian, H., Keating, M., Talpaz, M., McCredie, K., and Freireich, E. J. (1987). Clinical and prognostic features of patients with Philadelphia chromosome-positive chronic myelogenous leukemia and extramedullary disease. *Cancer 59*:297–300.
39. Dekmezian, R., Kantarjian, H. M., Keating, M. J., Talpaz, M., McCredie, K. B., and Freireich, E. J. (1987). The relevance stain-measured fibrosis at diagnosis in chronic myelogenous leukemia. *Cancer 59*:1739–1743.

40. Lazzarino, M., Morra, E., Castello, A., Inverardi, A., Coci, G. P., Magrini, U., Zei, G., and Bernasconi, C. (1986). Myelofibrosis in chronic granulocytic leukaemia: Clinicopathologic correlations and prognostic significance. *Br. J. Haematol. 64*:227–240.
41. Canellos, G. P. (1976). Chronic granulocytic leukemia. *Med. Clin. North Am. 60*:1001–1018.
42. Vallejos, C. S., Trujillo, J., Cork, A., et al. (1974). Blastic crisis in chronic granulocytic leukemias: Experience in 39 patients. *Cancer 34*:1806–1812.
43. Sandberg, A. A. (1978). Cytogenetic staging of chronic myeloid leukemia. *Boll. Ist Sieroter. Milan 57*:247–256.
44. Lisker, R., Caras, L., Mutchinick, O., Perez-Chavez, F., and Labardini, J. (1980). Late appearing Philadelphia chromosome in two patients with chronic myelogenous leukemia. *Blood 56*:812–814.
45. Heisterkamp, N., Stam, K., Groffen, J., de Klein, A., and Grosveld, G. (1985). Structural organization of the *bcr*, on chromosome 22. *Cell 36*: 93–99.
46. Shtivelman, E., Lipshitz, B., Gale, R. P., and Canaani, E. (1985). Fused transcript of *abl* and *bcr* genes in chronic myelogenous leukaemia. *Nature 315*: 550–554.
47. Stam, K., Heisterkamp, N., Grosveld, G., de Klein, A., Coleman, M., Dosik, H., and Groffen, J. (1985). Evidence of a new chimeric *bcr*/c-*abl* mRNA in patients with chronic myelocytic leukemia and the Philadelphia chromosome. *N. Engl. J. Med. 313*:1429–1433.
48. Kloetzer, W., Kurzrock, R., Smith, L., Talpaz, M., Spiller, M., Gutterman, J., and Arlinghaus, R. (1985). The human cellular *abl* gene product in the chronic myelogenous leukemia cell line K562 has an associated tyrosine protein kinase activity. *Virology 140*:230–238.
49. McLaughlin, J., Chianese, E., and Witte, O. (1987). In vitro transformation of immature hematopoietic cells by the p210 *bcr*/*abl* oncogene product of the Philadelphia chromosome. *Proc. Natl. Acad. Sci. USA 84*:6558–6562.
50. Daley, G. O., McLaughlin, J., Witte, O. N., and Baltimore, D. (1987). The CML-specific p210 *bcr*/*abl* protein, unlike v-*abl*, does not transform NIH/3T3 fibroblasts. *Science 237*:532.
51. Rowley, J. D. (1980). Ph^1-positive leukaemia, including chronic myelogenous leukaemia. *Clin. Haematol. 9*:55–81.
52. Lawler, S. D. (1977). The cytogenetics of chronic granulocytic leukemia. *Clin. Haematol. 6*:55–75.
53. Hagemeijer, A., Smith, E. M. E., Lowenberg, B., and Abels, J. (1979). Chronic myeloid leukemia with permanent disappearance of the Ph^1 chromosome and development of new clonal subpopulations. *Blood 53*: 1–14.
54. Bartram, C. R., Janssen, J. W. G., Becher, R., de Klein, A., and Grosveld, G. (1986). Persistence of chronic myelocytic leukemia despite deletion of rearranged *bcr*/c-*abl* sequences in blast crisis. *J. Exp. Med. 164*:1389–1396.
55. Collins, S. J. (1986). Breakpoints on chromosomes 9 and 22 in Philadelphia chromosome-positive chronic myelogenous leukemia (CML). Amplification

tion of rearranged c-*abl* oncogenes in CML blast crisis. *J. Clin. Invest. 78*: 1392–1396.

56. Andrews, D. F., II, and Collins, S. J. (1987). Heterogeneity in expression of the *bcr-abl* fusion transcript in CML blast crisis. *Leukemia 1*:718–724.
57. Le Beau, M., Lemons, R., Carrino, J., Pettenati, M., Souza, L., Diaz, M., and Rowley, J. (1987). Chromosomal localization of the human *G-CSF* gene to $17q_{11}$ proximal to the preakpoint of the t(15;17) in acute promyelocytic leukemia. *Leukemia 1*:795–799.
58. Chung, S. W., Wong, P. M. C., Shen-Ong, G., Ruscetti, S., Ishizaka, T., and Eaves, C. J. (1986). Production of granulocyte-macrophage colony-stimulating factor by Abelson virus-induced tumorogenic mast cell lines. *Blood 68*:1074–1081.
59. Chung, S. W., and Ruscetti, S. (1988). Formation of factor-independent hemopoietic multilineage colonies after abelson virus infections. *Blood 71*: 973–977.
60. Jandl, J. H. (1987). Polycythemia vera. In *Blood* (J. H. Jandl, ed.), Little, Brown, Boston, pp. 701–708.
61. Chervenick, P. A., Ellis, L. D., Pan, S. F., and Lawson, A. L. (1971). Human leukemic cells: In vitro growth of colonies containing the Philadelphia (Ph^1) chromosome. *Science 174*:1134–1136.
62. Coulombel, L., Kalousek, D. K., Eaves, C. J., Gupta, C. M., and Eaves, A. (1983). Long-term marrow culture reveals chromosomally normal hematopoietic progenitor cells in patients with Philadelphia chromosome-positive chronic myelogenous leukemia. *N. Engl. J. Med. 308*:1493–1493.
63. Dube, I. D., Kalousek, D. K., Coulombel, L., Gupta, C. M., Eaves, C. J., and Eaves, A. C. (1984). Cytogenetic studies of early myeloid progenitor compartments in Ph^1-positive chronic myeloid leukemia. Long-term culture reveals the persistence of Ph^1-negative progenitors in treated as well as newly diagnosed patients. *Blood 63*:1171–1177.
64. Hogge, D. E., Coulombel, L., Kalousek, D. K., Eaves, C. J., and Eaves, A. C. (1987). Nonclonal hemopoietic progenitors in a G6PD heterozygote with chronic myelogenous leukemia revealed after long-term marrow cultures. *Am. J. Hematol. 24*:389–394.
65. O'Brien, S., Kantarjian, H., Talpaz, M., Cork, A., Trujillo, J., and Beran, M. (1987). The effect of long-term marrow culture on the nonadherent Philadelphia chromosome-positive clones in chronic myelogenous leukemia in preliminary observations. *Hematol. Pathol. 1*(3):167–173.
66. Singer, J. W., Arlin, Z. A., Najfeld, V., Adamson, J. W., Kempin, S. J., Clarkson, B. D., and Fialkow, P. J. (1980). Restoration of nonclonal hematopoiesis in chronic myelogenous leukemia following a chemotherapy-induced loss of the Ph^{1+} chromosome. *Blood 56*:356–360.
67. Goto, T., Nishikori, M., and Arlin, Z. (1982). Growth characteristics of leukemia and normal hematopoietic cells in Ph^{1+} chronic myelogenous leukemia and effects of intensive treatment. *Blood 59*:793–803.
68. Moore, M. A. S., Williams, N., and Metcalf, D. (1973). In vitro colony formation by normal and leukemic human hematopoietic cells. Characterization of the colony-forming cells. *JNCI 50*:603–610.

69. Spiers, A. S. D., Bain, B. J., and Turner, J. E. (1977). The peripheral blood in chronic granulocytic leukaemia: Study of 50 untreated Philadelphia-positive cases. *Scand. J. Haematol. 18*:25–38.
70. Gordon, M. Y., Dowding, C. R., Riley, G. P., Goldman, G. M., and Greaves, M. F. (1987). Altered adhesive interactions with marrow stroma of haematopoietic progenitor cells in chronic myeloid leukemia. *Nature 328*:342–344.
71. Moore, M. A. S., Broxmeyer, H. E., Sheridan, A. P. C., Meyers, P. A., Jacobsen, N., and Winchester, R. J. (1980). Continuous human bone marrow culture: Ia antigen characterization of probable pluripotential stem cells. *Blood 55*:682.
72. Schlossman, F., Chess, L., Humphreys, R. E., and Strominger, J. L. (1976). Distribution of Ia-like molecules on the surface of normal and leukemic human cells. *Proc. Natl. Acad. Sci. USA 73*:1288.
73. Fujimiya, Y., Bakke, A., Chang, W. C., Linker-Israeli, M., Udis, B., Horowitz, D., and Pattengale, P. K. (1986). Natural killer-cell immunodeficiency in patients with chronic myelogenous leukemia. I. Analysis of the defect using the monoclonal antibodies HNK-1 (LEU-7) and B73.1. *Int. J. Cancer 37*:639–649.
74. Lyding, J., Li, W. J., Arlinghaus, R. B., and Diesseroth, A. (1987). Alpha interferon activates class I histocompatibility gene expression in chronic myelogenous leukemia cells. *Blood 70*(Suppl. 1):263a (abstract 907).
75. Riccarid, C., Giampietri, A., Migliorati, G., Cannarile, L., Adamio, L., and Herberman, R. B. (1986). Generation of mouse natural killer cell ativity: Effect of interleukin-2 and interferon on the in vivo development of natural killer cells from bone marrow progenitor cells. *Int. J. Cancer 38*:553–562.
76. Olofsson, T., and Olsson, I. (1980). Suppression of normal granulopoiesis in vitro by a leukemia-associated inhibitor (LAI) of acute and chronic leukemia. *Blood 55*:975–982.
77. Francis, G. E., Michalevicz, R., and Wickremasinghe, R. G. (1983). Chronic myeloid leukaemia and the Philadelphia translocation: Do the c-*sis* oncogene and platelet-derived growth factor provide the link? *Leuk. Res. 7*: 817–820.
78. Youman, J. D., Taddeini, L., and Cooper, T. (1973). Histamine excess symptoms in basophilic chronic granulocytic leukemia. *Arch. Intern. Med. 131*:560–562.
79. Gralnick, H. R., Harbor, J., and Vogel, C. (1971). Myelofibrosis in chronic granulocytic leukemia. *Blood 37*:152–162.
80. Polli, N., O'Brien, M., Tavares De Castro, J., Matutes, E., San Miguel, J. F., and Catovsky, D. (1985). Characterization of blast cells in chronic granulocytic leukaemia in transformation, acute myelofibrosis and undifferentiated leukaemia. I. Ultrastructural morphology and cytochemistry. *Br. J. Haematol. 59*:277–296.
81. San Miguel, J. R., Tavares De Castro, J., Matutes, E., Rodriguez, B., Poll, N., Zola, H., McMichael, A. J., Bollum, F. J., Thompson, D. S., and Goldman, J. M. (1985). Characterization of blast cells in chronic granulocytic leukaemia in transformation, acute myelofibroblasts and differentiated leu-

kaemia. II. Studies with monoclonal antibodies and terminal transferase. *Br. J. Haematol. 59*:297–309.
82. Breton-Gorius, J., Reyes, F., Vernant, J. P., Tulliez, M., and Dreyfuss, B. (1978). The blast crisis of chronic granulocytic leukaemia megakaryoblastic nature of cells as revealed by presence of platelet-peroxidase: A cytochemical ultrastructural study. *Br. J. Haematol. 39*:295–303.
83. Ekblom, M., Borgstrom, G., Willebrand, E., Gahmberg, C. G., Vuopio, P., and Andersson, L. C. (1983). Erythroid blast crisis in chronic myelogenous leukemia. *Blood 62*:591–596.
84. Saletan, S., Broxmeyer, H., Silver, R. T., Coleman, M., and Moore, M. A. (1982). Oscillations of CFU-c during the stable phase of CML. Proc. Am. Soc. Clin. Oncol. 18th Meeting, Abstract C-730.
85. Denburg, J., Wilson, W., and Bienenstock, J. (1982). Basophil production in myeloproliferative disorders—increases during acute blastic transformation of chronic myeloid leukemia. *Blood 60*:112–113.
86. Holdrinet, R., Penning, A., van Egmond, J., Wessels, J., and Haanen, C. (1983). DNA flow cytometry of blood and bone marrow in chronic myelogenous leukemia. *Acta Haematol. (Basel) 69*:98–105.
87. Canellos, G. P., DeVita, W. T., Whang-Peng, J., and Carbone, P. P. (1971). Hematologic and cytogenetic remission of blastic transformation in chronic granulocytic leukemia. *Blood 38*:671–679.
88. Keating, M. J., Smith, T. L., Gehan, E. A., McCredie, K. B., Bodey, G. P., and Freireich, E. J. (1982). A prognostic factor analysis for use in development of predictive models for response in adult acute leukemia. *Cancer 50*:457–465.
89. Coleman, M., Silver, R., Pajak, T., Cavalli, F., Rai, K. R., Lostinas, J. E., Glidewell, O., and Holland, J. F. (1980). Combination chemotherapy for terminal phase of chronic granulocytic leukemia. *Blood 55*:29–36.
90. Gomez, G. A., Sokal, J. E., and Aungst, C. W. (1976). Chemotherapy of the terminal phase of chronic myelocytic leukemia with combinations of colchicine derivatives and purine analogs. *Leuk. Res. 2*:141.
91. Hayes, D. M., Ellison, R. R., Glidewell, O., Holland, J. F., and Silver, R. T. (1974). Chemotherapy for the terminal phase of chronic myelocytic leukemia. *Cancer Chemother. Rep. 58*:233–247.
92. Mandelli, F., Amadori, S., Alimena, G., Anning, L., Nardelli, S., and Papa, G. (1977). Experience on the treatment of chronic myelocytic leukaemia (CML) in blastic crisis. *Scand. J.Haematol. 19*:495.
93. Pedersen-Bjergaard, J., Worm, A.-M., and Hainau, B. (1977). Blastic transformation of chronic myelocytic leukaemia: Clinical manifestations, prognostic factors and results of therapy. *Scand. J. Haematol. 18*:292–300.
94. Spiers, A. S., Goldman, J. M., Catovsky, D., Costello, C., Buskard, N. A., and Galton, D. A. (1977). Multiple-drug chemotherapy for acute leukemia. The TRAMPCOL regimen: Results in 86 patients. *Cancer 40*:20–29.
95. Iacoboni, S. J., Plunkett, W. K., Kantarjian, H., Estey, E., Keating, M. J., McCredie, K. B., and Freireich, E. J. (1986). High dose cytosine arabinoside: Treatment and cellular pharmacology of chronic myelogenous leukemia blast crisis. *J. Clin. Oncol. 4*:1079–1088.

96. Kantarjian, H., Walters, R., Keating, M., Talpaz, M., Andersson, B., Beran, M., McCredie, K., and Freireich, E. (1988). Treatment of the blastic phase of chronic myelogenous leukemia with mitoxantrone and high-dose cytosine arabinoside. *Cancer 62*:672–676.
97. Winton, E. F., Miller, D., and Vagler, W. R. (1981). Intensive chemotherapy and daunorubicin, 5-azacytidine, 6-thioguanine and cytarabine (DATA) for the blastic transformation of chronic granulocyte leukemia. *Cancer Treat. Rep. 6*:389.
98. Schiffer, C. A., DeBellis, R., Kasdorf, H., and Wiernik, P. (1982). Treatment of the blast crisis of chronic myelogenous leukemia with 5-azacytidine and VP-16-213. *Cancer Treat. Rep. 66*:267–271.
99. Schiffer, C. A., Anderson, K., Colman, M., and Cuttner, J. (1985). Therapy for chronic myelogenous leukemia in blast crisis with etoposide and 5-azacytidine administered by continuous infusion: A cancer and leukemia group B study. *Cancer Treat. Rep. 69*:1027–1028.
100. Herzig, R. H., Phillips, G. L., Lazarus, H. M., Wolff, S. N., Herzig, G. P. (1985). High-dose cytarabine for the treatment of blastic phase chronic myelogenous leukemia. *Cancer Treat. Rep. 69*:881–883.
101. Dutcher, J., Arlin, Z., Paietta, E., et al. (1988). Phase II study of mitoxantrone and 5 azacytidine in patients with accelerated or blastic crisis chronic myeloid leukemia. Twenty-Second Congress of ISH, Milan, Italy: 172(OP-TU-6-7).
102. Walters, R. S., Kantarjian, H. M., Keating, M. J., Talpaz, M., Childs, C. C., McCredie, K. B., and Freireich, E. J. (1987). Therapy of lymphoid and undifferentiated chronic myelogenous leukemia in blast crisis with continuous vincristine and adriamycin infusion plus high-dose Decadron (VAD). *Cancer 60*:1708–1712.
103. Rosenthal, S., Canellos, G. P., Whang-Peng, J., and Gralnick, H. R. (1977). Blast crisis of chronic granulocytic leukemia. Morphologic variants and therapeutic implications. *Am. J. Med. 63*:542–547.
104. Janossy, G., Woodruff, R. K., Pippard, M. J., Prentice, G., Hoffbrand, A. V., Paxton, A., Lister, T. A., Bunch, C., and Greaves, M. F. (1979). Relation of "lymphoid" phenotype and response to chemotherapy incorporating vincristine-prednisone in the acute phase of Ph^1 positive leukemia. *Cancer 43*:426–431.
105. Marks, S. M., Baltimore, D., and McCaffrey, R. (1978). Terminal transferase as a predictor of initial responsiveness to vincristine and prednisone in blastic chronic myelogenous leukemia. *N. Engl. J. Med. 293*:812.
106. Kantarjian, H., Keating, M., Talpaz, M., et al. (1988). Characteristics and outcome of patients with chronic myelogenous leukemia in lymphoid blast crisis. *Am. Soc. Clin. Oncol. 7*:193 (abstract 748).
107. Koeffler, H. P. (1983). Induction of differentiation of human acute myelogenous leukemia cells: Therapeutic implications. *Blood 62*:709–721.
108. Bloch, A. (1984). Induced cell differentiation in cancer therapy. *Cancer Treat. Rep. 68*:199–205.

109. Chesson, B., Jasperse, D., Simon, R., and Friedman, M. (1986). A critical appraisal of low-dose cytosine-arabinoside in patients with acute non-lymphocytic leukemia and myelodysplastic syndromes. *J. Clin. Oncol. 4*: 1857–1864.
110. Yu-Chen, Y., Shu-rong, C., and Jin-ren, C. (1988). Use of All-*trans* retinoic acid in the treatment of acute promyelocytic leukemia. *Blood 72*: 567–572.
111. Robert, K.-H., Hellstrom, E., Einhorn, S., and Gahrton, G. (1986). Acute myelogenous leukemia of unfavourable prognosis treated with retinoic acid, vitamin D^3, alpha-interferon and low doses of cytosine arabinoside. *Scand. J. Haematol. 34*(Suppl.):61–77.
112. Koller, C., Campbell, V., and Polansky, D. (1985). In vivo differentiation of blase-phase chronic granulocytic leukemia—expression of c-*myc* and c-*abl* protooncogenes. *J. Clin. Invest. 76*:365–369.
113. Koller, C., et al. (1988). ASH meeting.
114. Trümper, L., Lie, J. V. D., Goudsmit, R., Ho, A. D., and Hunstein, W. (1988). Therapy of the myeloid blast phase of chronic granulocytic leukemia with plicamycin and hydroxyurea: A retrospective analysis. 22nd Congress of ISH, Milan, Italy SYM-TU-6-6.
115. Antimi, M., Poeta, G. D., Cianciulli, P., Scimo, M. T., Stipa, E., Venditti, A., Catalano, G. F., and Papa, G. (1988). Plicamycin and hydroxyurea in the treatment of blast phase and accelerated phase of the Ph^1 chronic myelogenous leukemia. 22nd Congress of ISH, Milan, Italy OP-TU-6-6.
116. Weber, G. (1983). Biochemical strategy of cancer cells and the design of chemotherapy: G. H. A. Clowes Memorial Lecture. Cancer Res. 43:3466–3492.
117. Cooney, D. A., Jayaram, H. N., Gebeyehug, et al. (1982). The conversion of 2-β-D ribofuranosyl thiazole-4-carboxamide to an analog of NAD with potent IMP dehydrogenase inhibitory properties. *Biochem. Pharmacol. 31*:2133–2136.
118. Jayaram, H. N., Pillwein, K., Nichols, C. R., Hoffman, R., and Weber, G. (1986). Selective sensitivity to tiazofurin of human leukemic cells. *Biochem. Pharmacol. 35*(12):2029–2032.
119. Talpaz, M., Trujillo, J. M., Hittelman, W. N., Keating, M. J., and Gutterman, J. U. (1985). Suppression of clonal evolution in two chronic myelogenous leukaemia patients treatment with leukocyte interferon. *Br. J. Haematol. 60*:619.
120. Imanishi, J., and Tanaka, A. (1984). Experimental research for clinical application of interferon. *Jpn. J. Cancer Chemother. 11*:53–59.
121. Welander, C. E., Morgan, T. M., Homesley, H. D., Trotta, P. P., and Spiegel, R. J. (1985). Combined recombinant human interferon alpha2 and cytotoxic agents studied in a clonogenic assay. *Int. J. Cancer 35*:721.
122. Gabrilove, J. L., Jakubowski, A., Scher, H., Sternberg, C., Wong, G., Grous, J., Yagoda, A., Fain, K., Moore, M. A. S., Clarkson, B., Oettgen, H. F., Alton, K., Welte, K., and Souza, L. (1988). Effect of granulocyte

colony-stimulating factor on neutropenia and associated morbidity due to chemotherapy for transitional-cell carcinoma of the urothelium. *N. Engl. J. Med. 318*:1414–1422.

123. Brandt, S. J., Peters, W. P., Atwater, S. K., Kurtzberg, J., Borowitz, M. J., Jones, R. B., Shpall, E. J., Bast, R. C., Gilbert, C. J., and Oette, D. H. (1988). Effect of recombinant human granulocyte-macrophase colony-stimulating factor on hematopoietic reconstitution after high-dose chemotherapy and autologous bone marrow transplantation. *N. Engl. J. Med. 318*:869–876.

124. Vellenga, E., Delwel, H. R., Touw, I. P., and Lowenberg, B. (1987). Patterns of acute myeloid leukemia colony growth in response to recombinant granulocyte-macrophage colony-stimulating factor (rGM-CSF). *Exp. Hematol. 15*:652–656.

125. Elias, L. (1988). The basis for treatment of myelodysplastic syndrome and acute nonlymphoblastic leukemia with biologic agents. *Leukemia 2*(6): 400–402.

126. Vadhan-Raj, S., Keating, M., LeMaistre, A., Hittleman, W. N., McCredie, K., Trujillo, J. M., Broxmeyer, H. E., Henney, C., and Gutterman, J. U. (1987). Effects of recombinant human granulocyte-macrophase colony-stimulating factor in patients with myelodysplastic syndromes. *N. Engl. J. Med. 17*:1545–1552.

127. Vadhan-Raj, Hittleman, W., Ventura, C., Buescher, S., Keating, M., and Gutterman, M. (1988). Granulocyte-macrophage colony-stimulating factor in myelodysplastic syndrome (letter). *N. Engl. J. Med. 319*:51–52.

128. Haines, L. E., Goldman, J. M., Worsley, A. M., McCarthy, D. M., Wyatt, L. E., Dowding, C., Kearney, L., Th'ng, K. H., Wareham, N. J., Pollock, C., Galvin, M. C., Samson, D., Geary, C. G., Catovsky, D., and Galton, D. A. G. (1984). Chemotherapy and autografting for chronic granulocytic leukaemia in transformation: Probably prolongation of survival for some patients. *Br. J. Haematol. 58*:711–721.

129. Vellekoop, L., Zander, A. R., Kantarjian, H. M., Jagannath, S., Hester, J. P., Trujillo, J., McCredie, K. B., Zagars, G., Spitzer, G., and Dicke, K. A. (1986). Piperazinedione, total body irradiation, and autologous bone marrow transplantation in chronic myelogenous leukemia. *J. Clin. Oncol. 4*:906–911.

130. Preisler, H. D., Raza, A., Higby, D., Kirshner, J., Woll, J., Bennett, J., Winton, L., Weiner, R., Richman, C., Golomb, H., and Goldberg, J. (1984). Treatment of myeloid blastic crisis of chronic myelogenous leukemia. *Cancer Treat. Rep. 11*:1351–1355.

131. Dantas, M. E., Robinson, W. A., and Thomas, M. R. (1981). Autologous marrow infusion in blastic crisis of chronic myeloid leukemia. *Blood 58*: 1721.

132. Michallet, M., Leger, J., Chabannon, C., Cousin, F., Chauvet, M., Stephany, I., and Hollard, D. (1987). Long term bone marrow cultures in patients with chronic granulocytic leukemia before and after bone marrow

transplantation: Persistence of an altered bone marrow environment after BMT. *Blood 70*(Suppl. 1):311a (abstract 1101).
133. Tutschka, P. J., Copeland, E. A., and Klein, J. P. (1987). Bone marrow transplantation for leukemia following a new busulfan and cyclophosphamide regimen. *Blood 70*: 1382–1388.
134. Blume, K. G., Beutler, E., Bross, K. J., Chillar, R. K., Ellington, O. B., Fahey, J. L., Farbstein, M. J., Forman, S. J., Schmidt, G. M., Scott, E. P., Spruce, W. E., Turner, M. A., and Wold, J. L. (1980). Bone marrow ablation and allogeneic marrow transplantation in acute leukemia. *N. Engl. J. Med. 302*: 1041.
135. Chang, J., Moregenstern, G., Deakin, D., Testa, N. G., Coutiinho, L., Scarffe, J. H., Harrison, C., and Dexter, T. M. (1986). Reconstitution of hematopoietic system with autologous marrow taken during relapse of acute myeloblastic leukemia and grown in long term culture. *Lancet 1*: 294.
136. Degliantoni, G., Mangoni, L., and Rizzoli, V. (1985). In vitro restoration of polyclonal hematopoiesis in a chronic myelogenous leukemia after in vitro treatment with 4-hydroperoxycyclophosphamide. *Blood 65*:753–757.
137. Kaizer, H., Stuart, R. K., Colvin, M., Korbling, M., Wharam, M. D., and Santos, G. W. (1981). Autologous bone marrow transplantation in acute leukemia. A pilot study utilizing in vitro incubation of autologous marrow with 4-hydroperoxycyclophosphamide (4-HC) prior to cryopreservation (abstract). *Exp. Hematol. 9*(suppl. 9): 190.
138. Newland, A. C., Jones, L., Mir, N., and Slocombe, G. W. (1987). Alpha 2 interferon in chronic myeloid leukaemia following relapse post-allogeneic transplant. *Br. J. Haematol. 66*: 147–148.
139. Arcese, et al. (1988). European Cooperative Group for bone marrow transplantation. Chamonix, France.
140. Reiffers et al. (1988). European Cooperative Group for bone marrow transplantation. Chamonix, France.
141. Brito-Babapulle, F., Marcu, F., Rassoal, F., Ai-Pu, G., Th'ng, K.-H., Dowding, C., McCarthy, D., Catovsky, D., Galton, D. A. G., and Goldman, J. M. (1985). Transient restoration of partial Philadelphia chromosome negativity after autografting in CML in autologous bone marrow transplantation. Proceeding of the Third International Symposium, 1987. UT MD Anderson Hospital and Tumor Institute, Houston, Texas, pp. 189–194.
142. Meyers, J., Flournoy, N., Sanders, J., et al. (1987). Prophylactic use of human leukocytic interferon after allogeneic marrow transplantation. *Ann. Intern. Med. 107*:809–816.

19
Bone Marrow Transplantation for Chronic Myelogenous Leukemia

Alexander Fefer and E. Donnall Thomas *University of Washington and Fred Hutchinson Cancer Research Center, Seattle, Washington*

INTRODUCTION

The treatment of chronic myelogenous leukemia (CML) has presented a major challenge for the past 60 years. The chronic phase of the disease usually terminates in blast crisis, often preceded by a brief accelerated phase, which is usually not responsive to chemotherapy and is fatal within a few months. Conventional treatment in the chronic phase, most commonly with busulfan or hydroxyurea, has had no appreciable effect on survival because it has had little impact on the development of blast crisis (1). α-Interferon has been reported to induce a decrease or even disappearance of Philadelphia chromosome (Ph) positive cells in some patients (2), but additional patients and longer follow-up are needed to substantiate the encouraging results and to determine an effect on the course of the disease and on patient survival.

Intensive combination chemotherapy has been administered in the chronic phase in an effort to suppress the Ph-positive clone and prevent or delay the onset of the accelerated phase or blast crisis (3-5). Unfortunately, cytogenetic conversion has been uncommon, incomplete, and usually transient, without a significant or reproducible effect on the progression to blast crisis. Thus, the 3-4 year median survival time of patients from diagnosis of chronic-phase CML has not changed substantially through the years because none of the therapies have significantly altered the time to or frequency of transformation to blast crisis. However, the doses of chemotherapeutic agents used even in intensive regimens in the chronic phase have always been limited largely by marrow toxicity. The availability of normal marrow for transplantation permits the administration of much higher antileukemic doses of chemotherapy and/or radiation that may have a greater probability of eradicating the Ph-positive clone. The prime function of the transplanted donor marrow is to reconstitute the host's hematopoietic and immunologic systems destroyed by the antileukemic chemoradiotherapy and to exert an antileukemic effect (6). Indeed, during the past decade bone marrow transplantation (BMT) has been convincingly demonstrated to be potentially curative for all stages of CML but most especially when it is performed in the chronic phase. BMT however, is associated with significant morbidity and mortality, which vary with the patient and the donor. This presents the physician with practical problems and with ethical and philosophic dilemmas in deciding which patients should be offered the option of BMT and when in the course of the disease such an option should be exercised.

This chapter briefly reviews the current status of BMT for all phases of CML, including the results obtained with syngeneic and allogeneic donors who represent varying degrees of histoincompatibility. An attempt is made to identify the major problems that must be resolved to make BMT more successful and more widely applicable to patients with CML. The results of the Seattle Team at the Fred Hutchinson Cancer Research Center are highlighted.

METHODS AND PROCEDURES IN BMT

Marrow Aspiration and Infusion (7)

Marrow is obtained by multiple (about 150) marrow aspirations performed on the anterior and posterior iliac crests under general or spinal anesthesia. Approximately 500–1000 mL marrow mixed with blood is collected in tissue culture medium containing heparin, screened to remove fat and large particles, and administered intravenously. Between 10^8 and 10^9 nucleated marrow cells per kilogram body weight are usually infused within 24 h after total-body irradiation (TBI). The marrow stem cells pass through the pulmonary circulation and home to the marrow cavities. The donor is usually hospitalized overnight. Potentially life-threatening complications, largely due to anesthesia, have rarely been observed. Several days of local soreness represent the principal side effect for the donor.

Histocompatibility (8)

The human leukocyte antigens (HLA) are encoded by a series of closely linked genes that map on the short arm of chromosome 6. The chromosomal region is known as a haplotype. The histocompatibility loci most critical for transplantation are HLA-A, B and D. Although the HLA chromosomal region is genetically quite polymorphic, with over 122 different HLA antigens, matching for HLA within a family is relatively simple. A person inherits one haplotype from each parent. Since there can be only four haplotypes within a family, a patient has a 25% probability of being genotypically HLA identical to a given sibling. Syngeneic BMT is that performed between monozygotic genetically identical twins who, of course, are matched not only for HLA but for all genetic loci. Allogenic BMT is that performed between different nonsyngeneic individuals.

The vast majority of allogeneic marrow transplants have been performed between siblings who were documented to be HLA identical. Attempts have recently been made to identify other types of family members who may be acceptable as donors. Thus, transplants are being performed using as donors members from the immediate and extended family who are documented to be genotypically identical to the recipient for one shared HLA haplotype but different at one, two, or three of the HLA loci on the nonshared haplotype. The relative importance of the various genetic loci and the "strength" of the various alleles can thus be investigated. Moreover, in an effort to make marrow donors available for even more recipients, transplants are being performed using marrow from unrelated donors who are phenotypically HLA identical with the recipient or who are mismatched at only one antigen.

ABO compatibility between donor and recipient is not essential. Isoantibodies in the recipient that react against donor red cells can be removed by plasma exchange.

Treatment Regimens in Preparation for BMT

The preparative regimen for a recipient of a syngeneic marrow graft must have potent antileukemic activity. The regimen for an allogeneic marrow graft must, in addition, be sufficiently immunosuppressive to prevent rejection of the allogeneic marrow. The most common regimen used in BMT for CML and for other hematologic malignancies has included cyclophosphamide (CY), 60 mg/kg on each of 2 days, followed by total-body irradiation. TBI was used because it kills leukemic cells, penetrates privileged sites, such as testes and the central nervous system, and is quite immunowuppressive. Dose rates of 3-85 cGy/minute have been delivered by opposing ^{60}Co sources or, more often, by linear accelerator. A variety of TBI regimens have been used. Originally, 920–1000 cGy administered at a single exposure was used in Seattle. More recently, regimens of fractionated TBI, most commonly 200–225 cGy/day administered for 6–7 consecutive days, or "hyperfractionated" TBI delivered at 125-330 cGy at intervals of 3-24 h, for a total dose of up to 1575 cGy, have been used in the hope that toxicity is reduced and the antileukemic effect increased. Other chemotherapeutic agents have been added to various CY-TBI regimens, including cytosine arabinoside, etoposide, and BCNU. Moreover, a regimen of CY and high-dose busulfan, without TBI, has recently been reported to yield very encouraging preliminary results in patients with acute nonlymphocytic leukemia or with CML (9,10).

Prevention and Treatment of Graft-Versus-Host Disease

Posttransplant immunosuppressive therapy is essential for prophylaxis of graft-versus-host disease (GVHD), even in recipients of HLA-identical sibling marrow. Without such prophylaxis, hyperacute GVHD occurs and kills. Although a variety of immunosuppressants have been used, including CY, prednisone, and antithymocyte globulin (ATG), the most common regimen has been intermittent methotrexate (MTX) for 100 days, cyclosporin (CSP), or, more recently, MTX plus CSP (11). Patients who, despite prophylactic therapy, developed severe acute GVHD have usually been treated with ATG, glucocorticoids, or CSP (11). Extensive chronic GVHD has usually been treated with either glucocorticoids or glucocorticoids combined with a variety of immunosuppressive agents, most commonly azathioprine, CY, or procarbazine (12).

Cytogenetics

For cytogenetic studies, marrow samples were processed after 1.5 and 24 h in culture without the presence of mitogen. Cultures of blood were incubated for 72 h in the presence of phytohemagglutinin (PHA). Chromosome banding was done using acrinyl or quinacrine mustard hydrochloride for Q bands and Giemsa stain for G bands. Cytogenetic studies were usually performed before transplantation, on days 13, 21, 28, 56, and 84 after BMT, and at least annually thereafter.

Data Analysis

A variety of statistical techniques have been used for data analysis. Probability estimates were obtained by the Kaplan-Meier method (13), and differences between survival patterns were evaluated by log-rank statistics (14). Multivariate proportional hazards regression analyses were done by the method of Cox (15). Covariates were added to the model in a stepwise fashion. The covariate most significant in a univariate analysis was added first, followed by the covariates in the order in which they added the most information to the adjusted model. All covariates that added information to the model at the 0.05 significance level, as measured by the maximum likelihood ratio tests, were included.

RESULTS OF BMT FOR CML

Syngeneic BMT (Between Genetically Identical Twins)

The rare patient who has a normal syngeneic marrow donor provides an opportunity to assess the antileukemic effect of a given chemoradiotherapy regimen as well as its toxicity to normal tissue, without the complications posed by the immunologic barrier represented by donor-host histoincompatibility. The prin-

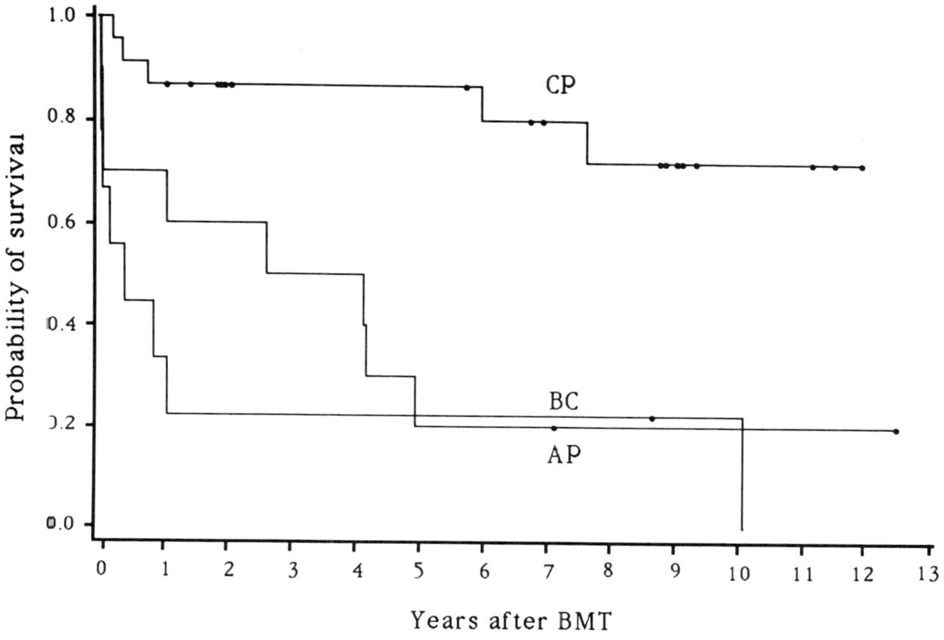

Figure 1 Kaplan-Meier product limit estimates for survival after monozygotic identical twin (syngeneic) BMT as a function of phase at BMT. CP, chronic (n = 23); AP, accelerated (n = 10); BC, blast crisis (n = 9). Dots represent surviving patients.

cipal problem in this setting is therefore not that of transplantation immunology but the presence of the leukemia. Syngeneic BMT was performed in Seattle on nine patients in blast crisis using a variety of chemoradiotherapy regimens (16,17). Only one patient became a long-term tumor-free survivor; the rest died of BMT-related complications or leukemia.

The possibility was entertained, and began to be tested in 1976, that syngeneic BMT performed earlier in the course of CML, that is, before progression to blast crisis, would yield better results than BMT performed in blast crisis because the patient would likely be in better clinical condition and be able to better tolerate BMT and the leukemia would be more sensitive to chemoradiotherapy. The goal in the chronic phase was to eradicate the Ph-positive clone and thereby test the hypothesis that such eradication would prevent or delay the development of blast crisis, prolong survival, and possibly cure the patient (18). Accordingly, syngeneic BMT was performed in patients who were still in the chronic or accelerated phase (17–19), using the chemoradiotherapy regimens that were demonstrably curative when used in syngeneic BMT for patients with acute leukemia and lymphoma refractory to conventional chemotherapy (20).

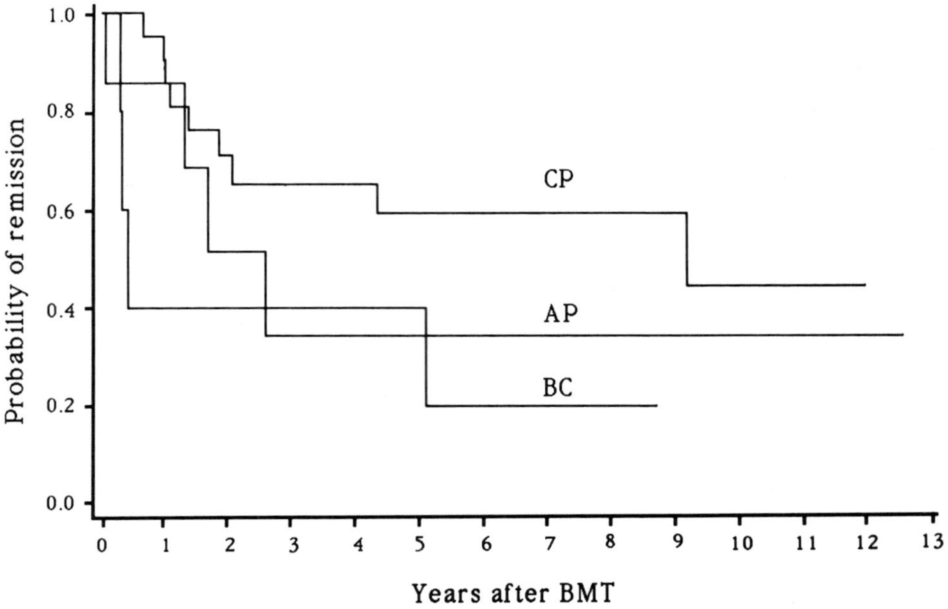

Figure 2 Kaplan-Meier product limit estimates for remission after syngeneic BMT as a function of phase at BMT.

BMT in the chronic phase presented an ethical dilemma because it was not yet known whether BMT would even be beneficial, much less curative, and whether the morbidity and the incidence of-BMT-related mortality would be significant. Moreover, for any given patient, the prognosis with conventional management without BMT is not known. However, since BMT-related mortality was rare in patients who underwent syngeneic BMT for acute leukemia while in complete remission (CR) (21), it was expected to be rare in patients transplanted in the chronic phase of CML. Moreover, it was hoped that syngeneic BMT performed in the accelerated phase would be as effective as BMT performed in the chronic phase, in which case BMT could be postponed until the first sign of the accelerated phase, thereby resolving the dilemma. Unfortunately, the results of syngeneic BMT in the accelerated phase turned out to be far worse than BMT in the chronic phase and were not much better than BMT in blast crisis (17,19).

An updated retrospective analysis of patient survival as a function of the phase of CML at BMT is shown in Figure 1. The results of BMT in the chronic phase were significantly better than those of BMT in the accelerated or blast phases. Among patients transplanted in blast crisis, 4 died of leukemia and 4 of BMT-related complications. Only two patients benefited from BMT: 1 patient had a complete hematologic and cytogenetic remission for 65 months after BMT, at which time CML recurred as a chronic phase and evolved into fatal blast crisis 116 months after BMT; 1 patient had a recurrence of blast crisis 10 months after BMT, was treated with combination chemotherapy, CY and TBI, and a second twin marrow transplant, and remains in complete hematologic and cytogenetic remission approximately 9 years after the second transplant. Similarly, among patients transplanted in the accelerated phase, 3 of 10 died of BMT-related causes and 2 of 10 remain alive. By contrast, among patients transplanted in the chronic phase, 2 of 23 died of BMT-related causes and 17 of 23 remain alive up to 13 years after BMT.

The probability of remaining in remission as a function of phase at BMT is presented in Figure 2. Of 10 patients transplanted in the accelerated phase, 5 exhibited rapid cytogenetic and hematologic relapse (3 others died early while still at risk for relapse), whereas of 23 patients transplanted in chronic phase, 9 eventually relapsed, some of them rather late.

Thus, BMT performed in blast crisis or in the accelerated phase was associated with significantly worse results than BMT performed in the chronic phase, with respect to both a higher leukemic death rate and a higher incidence of BMT-related deaths. Although no specific reason for the difference has been established, it is thought that the increased leukemic death may reflect an intrinsic resistance of the leukemia to the chemoradiotherapy and that the increase in BMT-related deaths may reflect the poor clinical status of patients in the advanced stages of CML, a longer interval from diagnosis to BMT, or a greater exposure to chemotherapy before referral for BMT—all factors known to predispose patients to BMT-related complications.

All recipients of syngeneic marrow for chronic-phase CML entered a complete hematologic and cytogenetic remission. Since some of them represented the first such effect reported and all of them represented the largest group ever induced into a complete cytogenetic remission by any therapy, they provided a rare opportunity to follow the natural history of the subsequent relapses. Of the nine patients who relapsed, one relapsed in blast crisis and died, six relapsed cytogenetically and at the same time or a few months later exhibited hematologic evidence of chronic-phase CML, and two continued to exhibit only cytogenetic evidence of relapse: one relapse was documented at 16 months after BMT and has been followed for only 5 months thereafter, and one was documented cytogenetically at 11 months after BMT and remains without clinical evidence of relapse at 32 months. Although most of the relapses occurred within 2 years, one occurred at 4½ years and another at 9 years after BMT. There may therefore be no plateau on the relapse curve of this small group of patients followed longer than any other. Moreover, no data are yet available on attempts to use the polymerase chain reaction (PCR) to detect the chimeric *bcr-abl* RNA transcipt unique to Ph-positive CML cells in cells from the long-term cytogenetically normal survivors. Therefore, additional patients and longer follow-up are still required to identify the disease-free interval of BMT that may define a "cure."

Finally, relapse does not necessarily require therapeutic intervention, since some of the patients who relapsed with clinical chronic-phase CML lived longer than expected (without a second transplant). Of six such patients who relapsed, one who relapsed at 1 year lived for 5 years more, one who relapsed at 2 years lived for 6 additional years, and another who relapsed at 2 years remains alive 8½ years after the relapse.

The conditioning regimen for syngeneic BMT in the chronic phase of CML strongly influenced the results. Fourteen patients were conditioned with intravenous dimethylbusulfan (DMB), CY for 2 days, and 920 cGy at a single exposure. Although the results were, overall, gratifying, fatal interstitial pneumonia (ISP) deprived 2 patients of whatever time they would have had without BMT. Since ISP had not been observed in over 20 patients who had undergone syngeneic BMT for acute leukemia in CR using the CY/TBI regimen *without* DMB, the possibility was considered that DMB contributed to the morbidity and mortality, a possibility that was subsequently validated by a retrospective analysis of patients undergoing syngeneic and allogeneic BMT for hematologic malignancies, which showed that conditioning regimens that included DMB were associated with greater morbidity and mortality than those that did not include DMB (22). Therefore, DMB was deleted from the conditioning regimen used for the 9 subsequent recipients of syngeneic marrow for chronic-phase CML. In addition, the TBI regimen was altered from a single-exposure TBI to fractionated TBI (200 cGy/day × 6). Fractionated TBI was used because in a randomized trial of allogeneic BMT for acute nonlymphocytic leukemia in first CR, a regimen of CY and 200 cGy/day × 6 was found to be less toxic yet no less effective than CY and 1000 cGy at a single exposure (23).

The results for the 14 patients conditioned with DMB, CY, and 920 cGy were compared with those of the subsequent group of nine patients conditioned with Cy and 200 cGy × 6. The two groups were quite comparable in their pretransplant clinical characteristics. Given the small number and the relatively short follow-up time of the non-DMB group, no statistically significant difference in disease-free survival between the two groups was detected. However, Figure 3, which presents the probability of remaining in remission as a function of the conditioning regimen, reveals a statistically significant increase in remission duration in the group conditioned with DMB. Since the antileukemic effect of CY plus fractionated TBI does not differ significantly from that of CY plus single-exposure TBI, the longer remission duration in the first group is most likely attributable to the antileukemic effect of DMB. The encouraging results recently reported with high doses of busulfan in combination with CY for allogeneic BMT for CML is consistent with this view (10).

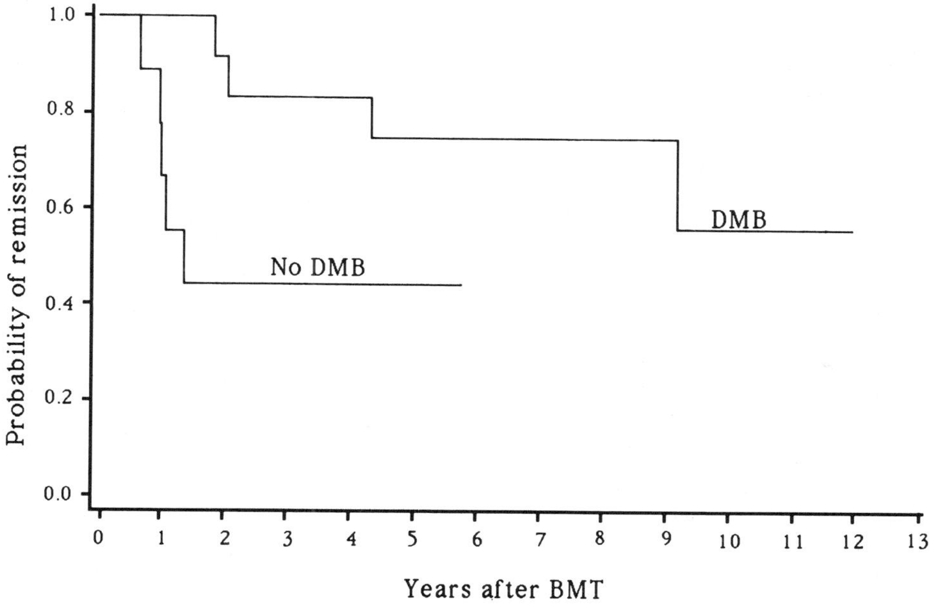

Figure 3 Kaplan-Meier product limit estimates for remission after syngeneic BMT for chronic-phase CML as a function of the conditioning regimen. DMB refers to patients treated with dimethylbusulfan, 5 mg/kg IV; cyclophosphamide, 60 mg/kg per day X 2; and TBI as 920 cGy at a single exposure (n = 14). No-DMB refers to patients treated with cyclophosphamide, 60 mg/kg per day X 2, and TBI as 200 cGy/day X 6 (n = 9).

The overall results show that syngeneic BMT can "cure" some patients in the accelerated phase or even in blast crisis, patients for whom no alternative therapy exists, and a substantial proportion of patients transplanted in the chronic phase. Since syngeneic BMT for hematologic malignancies has been performed in Seattle for patients as old as 68, the results suggest that a patient of almost any age in blast crisis or accelerated phase who has a normal genetically identical twin should undergo a marrow transplant, but that the transplant should preferably be carried out in the chronic phase at the earliest opportunity before any change to the accelerated phase has occurred.

Allogeneic BMT

BMT from HLA-Identical Sibling Donors

Given the dismal prognosis of blast crisis treated conventionally and the morbidity and mortality associated with allogeneic BMT for other hematologic malignancies, allogeneic BMT for CML was initially limited to patients in blast crisis. A 14% long-term, disease-free survival with an actuarial probability of relapse of 80% was reported from Seattle (19,24,25). Of these patients, five remain in hematologic and cytogenetic complete remission more than 5 years after BMT (26). Similar results were reported by the International Bone Marrow Transplant Registry (IBMTR) (27,28). The survival curves from Seattle and the IBMTR show an apparent plateau on the actuarial analysis plot, suggesting that a small proportion of these patients may have been cured.

As with syngeneic BMT, the possibility was considered that better results would be obtained with allogeneic BMT performed at an earlier stage of CML, that is, before evolution to blast crisis occurred. Accordingly, allogeneic BMT was performed in patients who were in the accelerated phase of CML and those who were still in the chronic phase. The criteria for categorizing a patient in the accelerated phase consisted of any one of the following: major perturbation of the white blood count; hematocrit or platelet count uncontrolled by hydroxyurea or busulfan; progressive splenomegaly despite chemotherapy; extramedullary leukemia; more than 10% but less than 30% blasts in the marrow or peripheral blood; persistent fever, bone pain, or both; or presence or appearance of cytogenetic abnormalities in addition to a single Ph chromosome, the most common abnormality being the duplication of the Ph chromosome. Since there is no effective therapy for the accelerated phase of CML and since such patients usually die within months, patients in the accelerated phase were considered appropriate for allogeneic BMT.

The most detailed analysis of the Seattle results of allogeneic BMT for CML in accelerated phase was reported by Martin et al., who treated 66 such patients with genotypically HLA-identical marrow (29). Their median age at BMT was 32, and the median time from diagnosis of CML to BMT was 2 years. The conditioning regimen for most patients was CY and TBI administered as 200 cGy/day × 6 or 225 cGy/day × 7. As prophylaxis for GVHD, 15 patients received marrow depleted of T cells without posttransplant immunosuppressive therapy. The other 51 patients received unmodified marrow followed by a regimen of MTX or CSP.

The projected 5 year survival rate was estimated by the product limit method as 18%, and the projected 5 year relapse-free survival was estimated as 11%. Within 100 days of BMT 48% of the patients died, largely from interstitial pneumonia and infection. Later deaths were largely due to leukemic relapse.

Multivariate analyses and proportional hazard regression were used to identify disease-related and BMT-related factors associated with posttransplant mortality and relapse. Splenomegaly (>4 cm below the left costal margin) at diagnosis and a >18 month interval between diagnosis of CML and BMT were associated with an increased risk of death after BMT. The increased mortality associated with splenomegaly was largely due to *nonleukemic* causes, especially infection. The status of the spleen at the time of BMT had no effect on survival. The longer interval from diagnosis to BMT was associated with increased mortality both before and after the first 100 days after BMT.

A total of 16 patients relapsed 1–52 months after BMT (median 16 months). All who relapsed cytogenetically also relapsed clinically. An interval of >18 months from diagnosis to BMT and T cell depletion of the infused marrow were each associated with an increased risk of relapse. At 3.5 years, the actuarial risk of relapse was 72 and 33%, respectively, for patients transplanted >18 months or <18 months from diagnosis. T cell-depleted marrow was associated with an 18-fold increase in the relapse rate when compared with unmodified marrow. Of the 16 relapses, 10 occurred among the 15 patients who received T cell-depleted marrow.

Cytogenetic abnormalities were categorized according to Przepiorka and Thomas (30). Non-Ph chromosomal abnormalities were observed in 44 of 66 patients. Solely based on the presence of additional chromosomal abnormalities other than a single Ph, 21 patients were categorized in the accelerated phase. Their BMT-related mortality and their relapse rate were similar to those observed in patients who were placed in the accelerated-phase category by the other standard criteria. These results, as well as those reported elsewhere, suggest that BMT in accelerated-phase patients is only marginally more effective than BMT performed in blast crisis (24,25,27–29,31–33). However, since *some* factors have been identified that may predispose to better results, it is suggested that patients meeting any of the criteria for the accelerated phase should undergo BMT at the earliest opportunity and that the marrow should not be T cell depleted.

Better results were predicted for allogeneic BMT performed in the *chronic* phase of CML. Allogeneic BMT, however, posed a greater ethical dilemma than did syngeneic BMT because allogeneic BMT would be expected to cause significant morbidity and mortality and would therefore shorten the lives of some patients.

Nevertheless, a decision to perform allogeneic BMT for patients in the chronic phase of CML was made and was supported by two major observations: (1) syngeneic BMT in the chronic phase induced long-term complete hematologic and cytogenetic remissions in a substantial proportion of patients (18,20); and (2) allogeneic BMT for patients with acute nonlymphocytic leukemia (ANL) in first CR was associated with significantly fewer BMT-related deaths and a far lower incidence of post-BMT leukemic relapse than was BMT for patients with ANL in relapse (34,35), a finding with encouraging implications if the situation is analogous to chronic- versus advanced-phase CML.

Detailed initial results using HLA-matched sibling BMT in 155 CML patients in the three phases of CML were reported from Seattle in 1986 (19). All patients received CY and TBI. Some also received DMB. For patients in the chronic phase, the TBI regimen was usually 920–1000 cGy as a single exposure or 200 cGy/day × 6. For patients in the other phases, the most common regimen was 1575 cGy given as seven daily fractions of 225 cGy. GVHD prophylaxis consisted of either intermittent MTX for 100 days or daily CSP for 180 days.

Using multivariate proportional hazards regression analysis, disease phase at BMT, patient age, acute GVHD, time from diagnosis to BMT, and spleen status at BMT were examined for their influence on survival and relapse. The main finding was that BMT during the chronic phase was associated with far better survival than BMT performed in the later phases. Thus, the probability of long-term survival was 49, 15, and 14% for BMT performed in the chronic, accelerated, and blast phase, respectively (19). Relapse was also least likely to occur in patients transplanted in chronic phase. For patients transplanted in the chronic phase the probability of cytogenetic relapse at 3 years was 0.31 and the probability of clinical relapse was 0.22. (The difference reflects that in six patients, cytogenetic relapse was the only evidence of disease.) In contrast, actuarial analyses suggested that 40% of patients in the accelerated phase and over 80% of patients in blast crisis would have had a clinical relapse and died of leukemia by 3 years after BMT had there been no competing causes of death. Phase of disease at the time of BMT was the only factor significantly influencing relapse.

For patients who underwent BMT in the chronic phase, the actuarial survival was higher for patients under age 30 than for those over age 30, higher for those with mild or no GVHD than for to those with moderate to severe GVHD, and higher for those who underwent BMT within 1 year after diagnosis than for those who underwent BMT 3 years of more after diagnosis. Spleen status at BMT did not influence survival. Increasing age at BMT was significantly associated with the development of moderate to severe acute GVHD. Allogeneic BMT during the chronic phase of CML was associated with about 20% mortality in the

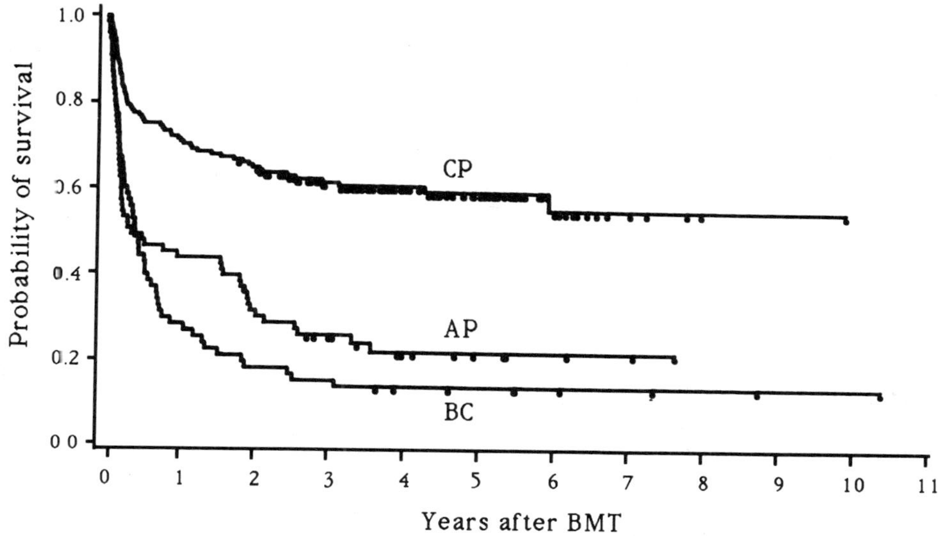

Figure 4 Kaplan-Meier product limit estimates for survival after HLA-identical sibling BMT as a function of phase at BMT. CP, chronic (n = 164); AP, accelerated (n = 75), BC, blast crisis (n = 69). Dots represent surviving patients.

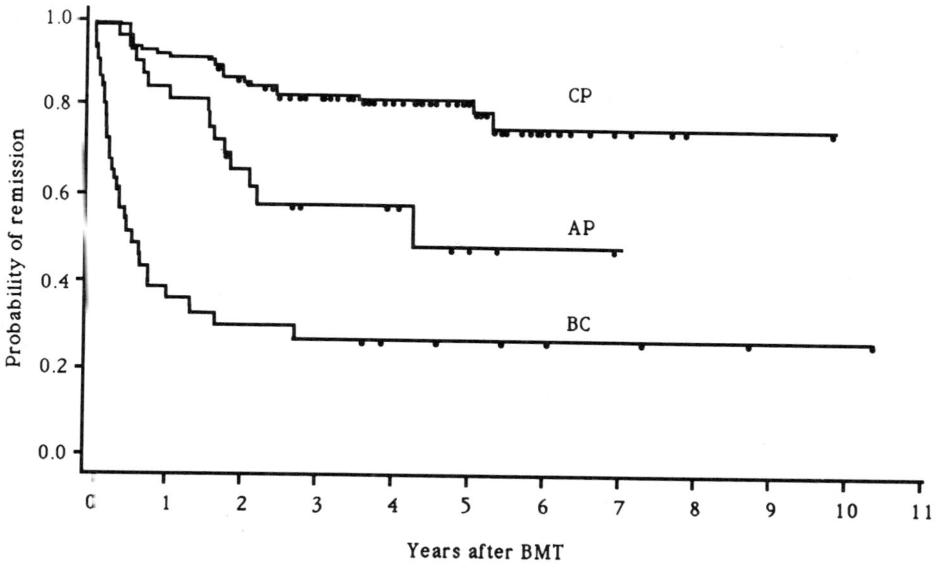

Figure 5 Kaplan-Meier product limit estimates for remission after HLA-identical sibling BMT as a function of phase at BMT. Dots representing surviving patients.

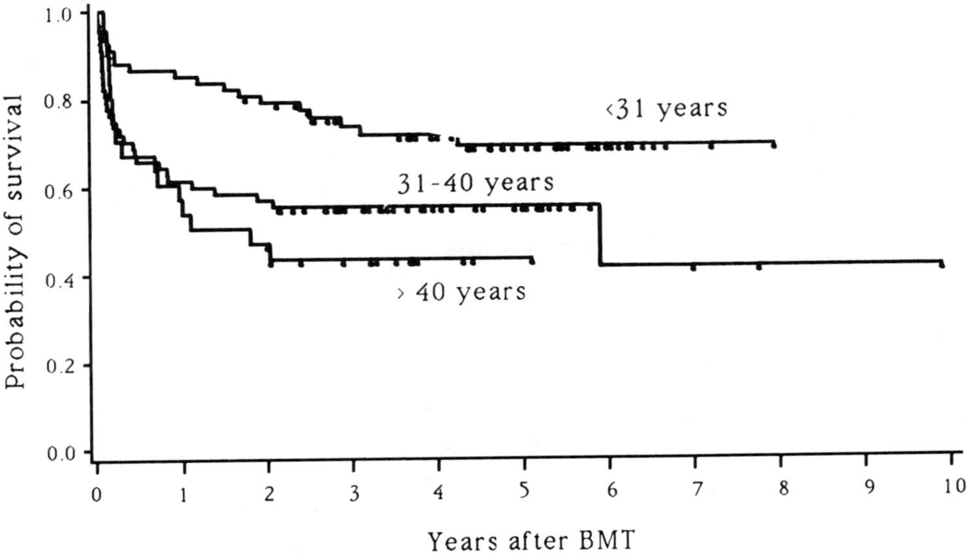

Figure 6 Kaplan-Meier product limit estimates for survival after HLA-identical sibling BMT for CML in the chronic phase as a function of age at BMT. Age < 31 years, n = 70; 31–40 years, n = 68, >40 years, n = 30. Dots represent surviving patients.

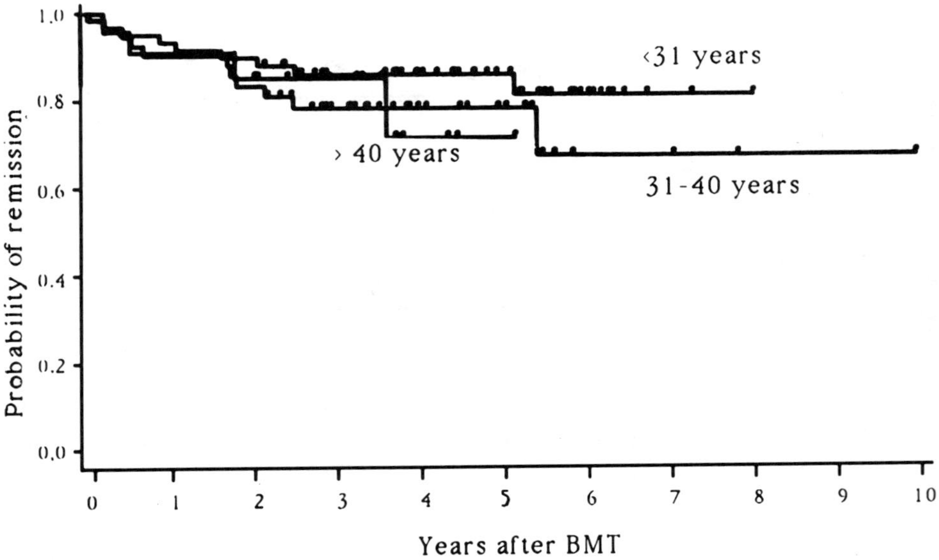

Figure 7 Kaplan-Meier product limit estimates for remission after HLA-identical sibling BMT for CML in the chronic phase as a function of age at BMT. Dots represent surviving patients.

first 100 days and up to 30% mortality during the first year, a mortality far greater than expected without BMT.

An updated analysis of the Seattle results on 308 patients in various stages of CML treated with unmodified HLA-matched sibling marrow is presented in Figures 4 through 11. They confirm the previous reports from Seattle and other centers (24,27,31,36,37) by demonstrating that the results of BMT in the chronic phase are significantly better than the results of BMT performed at a later stage.

The probability of survival as a function of phase at BMT is shown in Figure 4. Approximately 15, 22, and 60% remain long-term survivors after BMT in blast crisis, accelerated phase, or chronic phase of CML, respectively.

Figure 5 presents the probability of remaining in remission as a function of phase at BMT. That probability is approximately 75, 50, and 25% for patients transplanted while in blast, accelerated, or chronic phase, respectively.

The causes of death after BMT varied with the phase of the disease at BMT. The main causes of death after BMT in the chronic phase were BMT related, that is, GVHD, CMV pneumonia, and veno-occlusive disease (VOD) of the liver. In contrast, the main cause of death after BMT for blast crisis and, to a lesser extent, for accelerated phase was leukemic relapse. As with syngeneic BMT, the basis for both the higher leukemic relapse rate and the higher incidence of BMT related deaths in patients transplanted in the accelerated phase than in those transplanted in the chronic phase has not yet been established. A poorer clinical status, longer interval from diagnosis to BMT, and/or exposure to more chemotherapy may contribute to the poorer results in patients in the accelerated phase.

For patients who underwent BMT for CML in the chronic phase, multivariate proportional hazards regression analysis substantiated the prognostic significance of age at BMT, splenomegaly at diagnosis, and time from diagnosis to BMT. Figure 6 presents survival as a function of age at BMT. The probability of survival was significantly greater for younger than for older patients. Thus, the actuarial probability of survival at 5 years after BMT was approximately 75% for chronic-phase patients transplanted at age 31 or less but only 45% for those transplanted at age 40 or older. The lower survival of older patients is also supported by IBMTR data (33,38). Figure 7 shows that patient age did not significantly influence the probability of remission after BMT. Thus, the lower survival of the older patients presented in Figure 6 did not reflect a higher relapse rate but a higher incidence of BMT-associated mortality, largely due to a higher incidence of moderate to severe acute GVHD, as previously reported (19). Older age is not, however, an absolute contraindication to BMT. The most recently reported Seattle series included 18 patients aged 41-55 years, 11 of whom remain alive in remission (38).

An earlier analysis (19) suggested that splenomegaly at diagnosis may be associated with a worse prognosis after BMT. The updated results, presented in

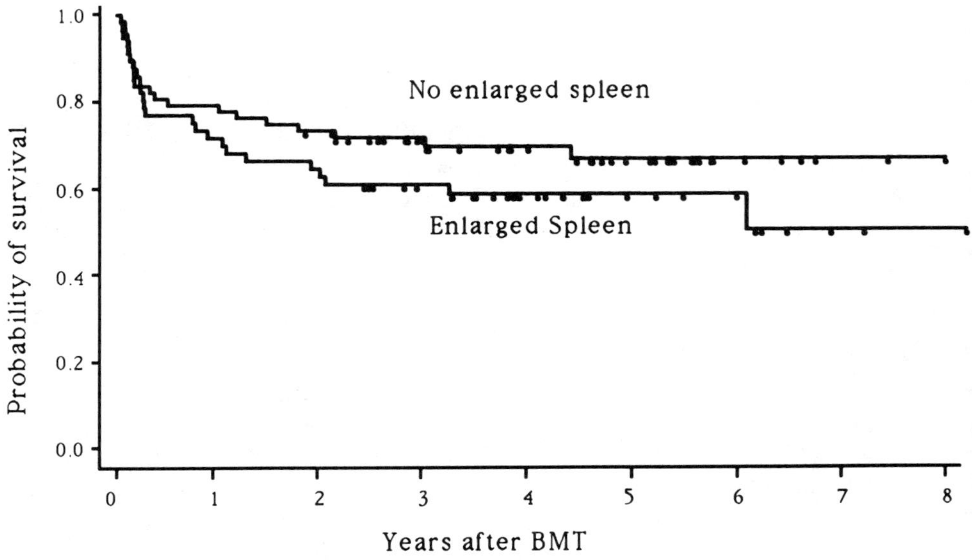

Figure 8 Kaplan-Meier product limit estimates for survival after HLA-identical sibling BMT for CML in chronic phase as a function of splenomegaly ($n = 55$) or no splenomegaly ($n = 71$) at diagnosis. Dots represent surviving patients.

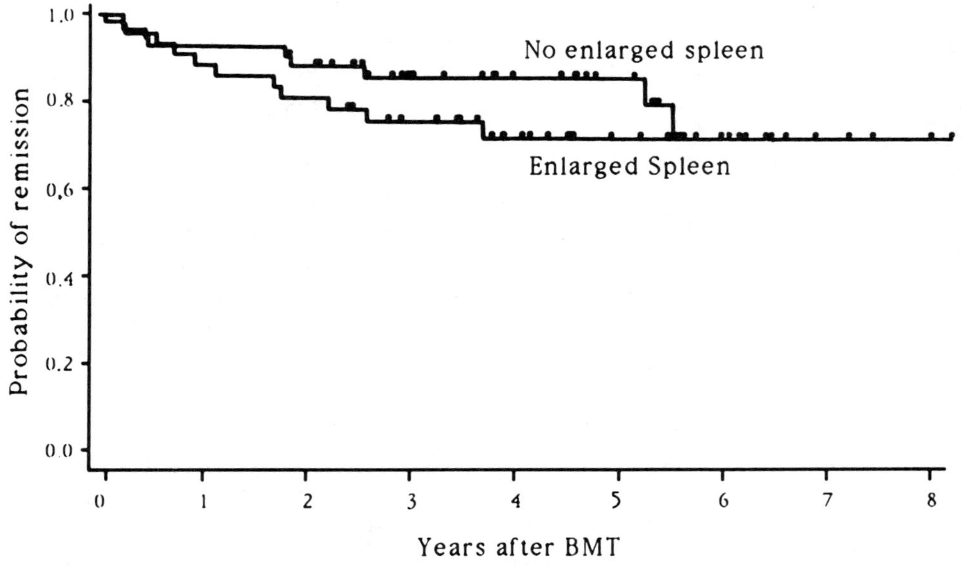

Figure 9 Kaplan-Meier product limit estimate for remission after HLA-identical sibling BMT for CML in chronic phase as a function of splenomegaly at diagnosis. Dots represent surviving patients.

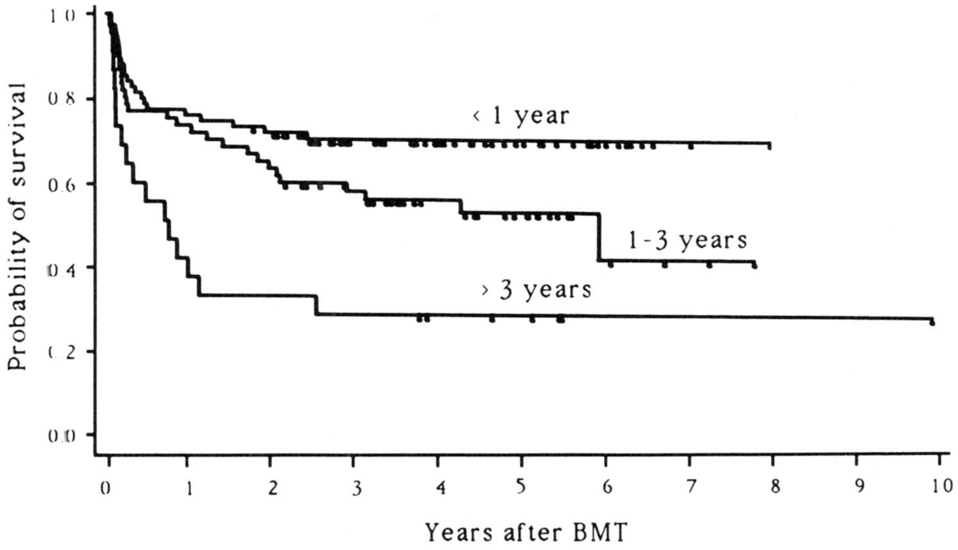

Figure 10 Kaplan-Meier product limit estimates for survival after HLA-identical sibling BMT for CML in the chronic phase as a function of the interval from diagnosis to BMT. Interval <1 year, $n = 79$; 1–3 years, $n = 61$; >3 years, $n = 35$. Dots represent surviving patients.

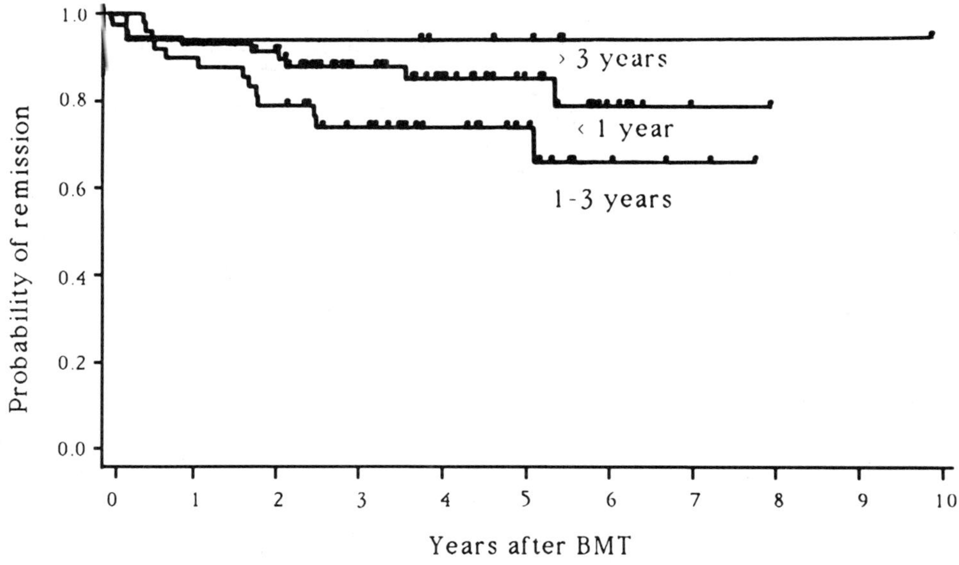

Figure 11 Kaplan-Meier product limit estimate for remission after HLA-identical sibling BMT for CML in the chronic phase as a function of the interval from diagnosis to BMT. Dots represent surviving patients.

Figure 8, support that conclusion. It reflects an increase in BMT-related mortality. Splenomegaly is not associated with a significant decrease in the probability of remission (Figure 9). Splenectomy or splenic radiation prior to BMT has not been reported to significantly increase patient survival or decrease leukemic recurrence after BMT (19,28,40–42).

The time from diagnosis to BMT has been identified as a significant risk factor for survival after BMT. This variable is especially important because it can often be controlled by the physician and the patient. The initial Seattle data suggested strongly (19) that BMT performed for chronic-phase CML within 1 year of diagnosis was associated with a significantly greater probability of survival than BMT performed later. The updated Seattle results, presented in Figure 10, continue to substantiate the original association. Figure 11 shows that the better survival with earlier BMT does not reflect a significantly greater probability of remission but a significant decrease in BMT-related deaths.

Although the results in a small series of patients in Germany (43) support the existence of a relationship between earlier BMT and improved survival, the IBMTR data do not (28,33,38). The discrepancy in the results reported from Seattle and those from the IBMTR cannot be easily explained. The patients at the one center in Seattle are not necessarily comparable to the patients represented by the many centers in the IBMTR in terms of clinical history and characteristics, the conventional therapy used before BMT, the preparative regimens used for BMT, and the nature of the follow-up evaluation after BMT. Moreover, the Seattle series included only recipients of unprocessed marrow, whereas the IBMTR series included recipients of T cell-depleted marrow. Finally, a comparison of actuarial survival data from Seattle and from the IBMTR reveals that BMT performed 17 months or more after diagnosis was associated with a 54–57% probability of survival in both series, whereas BMT performed less than 17 months after diagnosis was associated with a survival probability of 73% in the Seattle series but only 54% in the IBMTR series. Thus, the main difference was that patients transplanted earlier had a better survival in the Seattle series than did patients transplanted earlier in the IBMTR series (39).

The overall results of HLA-identical sibling BMT from other centers have been mostly, but not totally, consistent with those reported from Seattle (27, 31,28,33). IBMTR data from 36 transplant centers (27) showed that the actuarial probability of survival at 3 years for 39 patients transplanted in chronic phase, 56 patients transplanted in accelerated phase, and 22 transplanted in blast crisis was 63, 36, and 12%, respectively. With a relatively short follow-up period, the corresponding actuarial probability of relapse at 3 years was 7, 41, and 41%, respectively. Patients under age 25 had a significantly greater probability of survival than those over 25.

Goldman et al. reported on 52 patients in the chronic phase of CML and 18 patients in the advanced stages treated with HLA-identical sibling marrow in several hospitals in the United Kingdom (28). All received CY and TBI, 20 cGy/day for 5-6 days. Of the chronic-phase patients, 3 also received high-dose busulfan and 49 received daunorubincin, 60 mg/m^2. Patients with advanced CML received the same regimens. All patients in their series either underwent splenectomy or received splenic radiation before BMT; 35 patients in the chronic group and 12 in the advanced group received unmodified marrow, whereas the other patients received T cell-depleted marrow. All patients received CSP for GVHD parophylaxis, regardless of the nature of the marrow infused. The actuarial survival probability for patients transplanted in the chronic phase was 72%, in contrast to 18% for those transplanted in the advanced phases. With a median follow-up time of 25 months among the survivors, patients transplanted in the chronic phase clearly had a higher probability or survival and disease-free survival than did patients transplanted in more advance phases.

McGlave et al. reported on 29 patients transplanted in the chronic phase and 28 in the accelerated phase (32). All were prepared with CY and TBI (165 cGy twice daily × 4 days). GVHD prophylaxis consisted of MTX and ATG. The projected survival for 2.5 years was 64% for the chronic-phase patients and 30% for the accelerated-phase patients. Age less than 30 years was the only prognostic feature studied that independently predicted for better survival. With a median follow-up time of 25 months for the entire group, no relapses had been detected among the patients transplanted in the chronic phase at the time of the report.

The largest series of patients transplanted in the chronic phase of CML with HLA-identical marrow was collected from multiple centers and reported on behalf of the IBMTR (38). The median follow-up was 25 months. They were prepared with high-dose chemotherapy and TBI administered either as a single dose or in several fractions. Of the series of 405 patients evaluated, 318 patients received unmodified marrow (the other 87 patients received T cell-depleted marrow and are discussed in GVHD prophylaxis using T cell depletion). For GVHD prophylaxis the patients received MTX (30%), CSP (63%), or both (5%).

The 4 year probability of survival for the 318 recipients of unmodified marrow was 55%. Patient age was identified as a significant risk factor for survival. The 4 year probability of survival was 75% for patients under age 20 and 52% for those over 20. Older patients had higher mortaility rates due to acute GVHD and ISP than younger patients. This was not due to a higher incidence of ISP or of moderate to severe acute GVHD in patients over 20 but to a higher case fatality rate among the older patients.

Acute GVHD was also a significant risk factor for survival. For example, patients under age 20 who exhibited no or only mild acute GVHD had a projected survival probability of about 90% compared with 65% for those with moderate or severe GVHD. Corresponding probabilities for survival of patients over age 20 were 75 and 30%.

The 3 year probability for relapse for the 318 recipients of unmodified marrow was 9%. MTX did not influence the probability of relapse when compared with CSP. The interval from diagnosis to BMT did not influence the probability of relapse.

Data from all BMT centers suggest that the optimal time for BMT is in the chronic phase, before the onset of the accelerated phase or blast crisis. Data from Seattle further suggest that the optimal time is as early as possible in the chronic phase. However, the probability of long-term tumor-free survival must be weighed against the risk of BMT-related morbidity and mortality and against the indolent nature of chronic-phase CML on conventional management.

A patient's probability of survival without BMT can help in comparing the relative risks of BMT and its timing with the risks of conventional treatment. Several factors at diagnosis have been identified that are associated with prognosis and survival on conventional therapy (43,45). It is important to identify chronic-phase patients who have a poor prognosis on conventional therapy to consider the BMT option for them at an earlier date, despite its risks.

A retrospective analysis of 813 patients (44) as well as 625 (45) other patients under age 45 has identified several variables present at diagnosis of CML that predicted for survival on conventional therapy. Based on a multivariate analysis including sex, spleen size, platelet count, hematocrit, and percentage of circulating blasts, one-third of the patients were classified as having a good prognosis, with a survival rate of 90% at 2 years, an average death rate after 2 years of 20% per year, and a median survival of 5 years. Two-thirds of the patients were classified in a poor-risk group with a 5 year survival rate of 40% and with rare survivors beyond 7 years. Mathematical models that take into account factors related to conventional therapy and to allogeneic BMT have been constructed in an effort to predict survival (46). However, the value of this approach has not yet been documented in any prospective trial. The results of such statistical analyses may nevertheless help in discussing the problems and options with patients and physicians.

Most recently, a small subset of 29 patients selected for being within 1 year of diagnosis of chronic-phase CML were transplanted in Seattle, with a standard regimen of CY and 200 cGy/day × 6, followed by a combination of MTX and CSP as prophylaxis for GVHD. Although 4 of the patients experienced a cytogenetic relapse (1 is in chronic phase and 3 underwent second transplants), 28 of the 29 patients remained alive with a median follow-up of 3 years after BMT (39). The results strongly suggest that patients with CML in chronic phase who have an appropriate donor should undergo BMT as soon as possible after diagnosis. Moreover, these results coupled with the 90% projected survival of selected patients transplanted at age <20 without significant GVHD (38) highlight that in selected patients the posttransplant mortality can in fact be low and tolerable, thereby diminishing the ethical dilemma for a particular subset of patients and facilitating the decision to exercise the transplant option soon after diagnosis.

The overall results reviewed here strongly suggest that patients who are already in blast crisis or in accelerated phase should be transplanted because no better alternative exists and that the option of an allogeneic matched sibling BMT should also be offered to patients while they are still in the chronic phase of CML. The Seattle data further suggest that BMT be performed as soon as possible after the initial diagnosis, before any evidence of progression to the accelerated phase—even the appearance of a non-Ph[1] chromosomal abnormality alone—has occurred. Finally, a small series of patients who underwent allogeneic BMT after they had been induced into a second chronic phase by chemotherapy for blast crisis exhibited a 50% probability of long-term tumor-free survival (19). The results warrant an attempt to induce such a second chronic phase, especially in terminal deoxynucleotidyltransferase (TdT)-positive blast crisis (47), before proceeding with a marrow transplant.

BMT from Partially Matched or Mismatched Family Donors

Since only approximately 35% of marrow transplant candidates have a syngeneic or genotypically HLA-identical sibling donor, attempts have been made to determine the degrees of histoincompatibility between donor and recipient that might be tolerable and acceptable to increase the availability of marrow donors for patients. The Seattle team reported one study of the acceptable limits of HLA incompatibility for BMT between family members. Patients with hematologic malignancies received marrow from haploidentical family members (53 parents and 42 siblings) who shared one HLA haplotype with the patient. The unshared haplotypes differed to a variable degree for the HLA-A, B, and D antigens. A total of 12 were phenotypically but not genotypically identical for HLA-A, HLA-B, and HLA-D; 63 differed at one locus (A, B, or D); 24 at two loci; and 6 at three loci. The results of BMT in the 105 "study" patients were compared with the results of 728 similar "control" patients who concurrently received marrow from genotypically HLA-identical siblings (48). All patients in both groups were pretreated with CY and TBI and received unmodified marrow with MTX as GVHD prophylaxis.

Moderate to severe GVHD occurred earlier and with greater frequency in the study patients than in the controls. The frequency of significant GVHD increased progressively with the degree of histoincompatibility. Thus, moderate to severe GVHD, which occurred in 45% of control patients, occurred in 35, 75, 75, and 85% of recipients who were phenotypically HLA identical or incompatible at one, two, or three HLA loci, respectively.

Animal studies have suggested that incompatibility for class II antigens of the major histocompatibility complex (MHC), as opposed to class I antigens, may be associated with an increased risk of acute GVHD (49). The clinical results, however, did not bear this out; the risk for GVHD did not correlate specifically with disparity for HLA class I (A or B) or HLA class II (D region) loci. There is therefore no rationale, at least for haploidentical patient-donor pairs, for preferential selection of class II (mixed leukocyte culture-compatible) donors as opposed to class I-compatible donors (serologically compatible) in clinical BMT. A higher proportion of study patients exhibited delayed engraftment, prolonged granulocytopenia, or increased incidence of graft rejection. Although it occurred in only 0.1% of recipients of genotypically identical sibling marrow, it occurred in 5% of the study patients.

The importance of HLA incompatibility for graft rejection has been further substantiated by a recent comparison between 269 recipients of partially matched family marrow (study patients) and 930 recipients of HLA-identical sibling marrow (control patients) (50). All patients received CY and TBI and unmodified marrow. Whereas the rate of graft failure was 2% among the controls, it was 12% in the study group. Graft failure varied with degree of histoincompatibility. Thus, 7, 9, and 21% of recipients were phenotypically HLA matched, incompatible for one HLA locus, or incompatible for two loci, respectively. Graft failure was also associated with a positive cross-match for antidonor lymphocytoxic antibody (50). Moreover, residual host lymphocytes were detected in mose (11 of 14) patients with graft failure, which suggested that graft failure represented host-mediated immune rejection (50). Thus, donor HLA incompatibility and prior alloimmunization were considered significant risk factors for graft failure. It is possible that more potent immunosuppressive regimens could decrease graft rejection, but the possibility also exists that they exacerbate GVHD.

Despite the higher incidence of GVHD and graft failure, there was no statistically significant difference between the survival of recipients of marrow from donors incompatible for only one locus and that of recipients of genotypically HLA-identical sibling marrow, at least for patients transplanted for acute leukemia in remission (the only group large enough for analysis). In contrast, recipients of marrow from donors incompatible at two or three loci exhibited a far higher incidence of severe GVHD and a significant decrease in the probability of long-term survival (48,51). Based on those results, BMT from family donors phenotypically matched or mismatched at only one locus should be considered acceptable therapy for any CML patient who is a candidate for an HLA-identical sibling marrow transplant. The results with greatest degrees of histocompatibility are too poor to be recommended.

BMT from Unrelated Donors

In the United States, with only 1.7 siblings per family, only about 35% of BMT candidates turn out to have a genotypically HLA-matched sibling marrow donor available. An additional 10% of patients turn out to have an acceptable family member with one HLA haplotype genotypically identical to one haplotype of the patient and the other haplotype incompatible for only one of the three major histocompatibility loci. The marrow donor pool could potentially be greatly expanded if appropriate HLA-compatible volunteer donors who are unrelated to the recipient could be identified and used. This approach is being intensively investigated (52-54).

The combined experience of four marrow transplant centers in using unrelated donor marrow to treat CML was recently reported (54). Although the patient group was rather heterogeneous and the follow-up time relatively short, preliminary results were quite encouraging. A total of 37 patients were treated, 22 in the chronic phase and 15 in accelerated phase or blast crisis. Of these patients, 20 received grafts from HLA-A, B, or DR phenotypically matched and MHC-compatible donors, 15 received grafts from donors mismatched at one of the three HLA loci, and 2 patients received marrow mismatched at two loci. Of these patients, 12 received T cell-depleted marrow as GVHD prophylaxis. The projected survival at 1000 days was 55% for patients transplanted in the chronic phase and 22% for patients transplanted in accelerated or blast phase. The median follow-up for surviving patients was 2 years. The oldest surviving patient was 40 years at BMT. Of patients transplanted in chronic phase, 2 are alive with reappearance of the Ph chromosome: 1 in hematologic relapse at 1125 days after BMT, the other in cytogenetic relapse at 620 days. The follow-up time, however, is too short to permit significant conclusions about relapse probabilities. Nevertheless, these preliminary results demonstrate that BMT from unrelated donors is a promising form of therapy for patients with CML. As with family member transplants, unrelated transplants mismatched at only one locus yielded results similar to those of unrelated transplants that were fully matched for A, B, and D or DR.

These findings, if validated by studies on more patients and longer follow-up, could significantly broaden the potential pool of marrow donors. The pool of 100,000 HLA-typed volunteers now available worldwide could provide an HLA-A-, B-, and D or DR-matched donor for fewer than 25% of patients. However, if a one antigen-unrelated mismatch turns out, indeed, to be acceptable, it will be possible to extend the BMT option to many more patients using donors from among the 100,000 volunteers who are already typed for HLA (55).

PROBLEMS ASSOCIATED WITH ALLOGENEIC BMT FOR CML

Opportunistic Infections

Patients who have undergone chemoradiotherapy and allogeneic BMT tend to be severely granulocytopenic for at least 2-3 weeks and immunodeficient for 3 months to a year, or even longer, if chronic GVHD develops. As a result, opportunistic infections represent a significant problem.

Bacterial and fungal infections occur frequently and are responsible for the death of 5% of marrow recipients (56). Delayed engraftment or development of GVHD increases the risk of infections.

Viral infections are very common, especially during the first 4 months after BMT (57). The most frequent viral problem is infection with or activation of herpes simplex virus and varicella zoster. These can now be prevented or treated with acyclovir. The most important viral infection, however, is caused by cytomegalovirus (CMV). The most serious complication of CMV infection is CMV-induced pneumonitis, which occurs in approximately 15% of marrow recipients, is fatal in 80–90% of them, and represents the leading infectious cause of death after allogeneic BMT (56,58). Although there is as yet no effective therapy for CMV infection, major progress has been reported in prophylaxis. In patients who are seronegative for CMV prior to BMT, exogenous CMV infection can largely be prevented by using a CMV-seronegative marrow donor and subsequently transfusing blood products strictly from seronegative donors (59). Patients thus managed were reported to have a 3% incidence of primary CMV infection, in contrast to a 32% incidence for those marrow recipients who received unscreened blood products. In the future, susceptibility to opportunistic infections may be decreased by agents that may more rapidly correct the neutropenia and the immunodeficiency state that exists after BMT (11). Thus, the incidence or lethality of such infections may be reduced by the administration of hematopoietic growth factors, such as granulocyte-macrophage colony-stimulating factor (GM-CSF) and interleukins (IL-1α and/or IL-3) to shorten the neutropenic period, and such growth factors as IL-2 and IL-4 to accelerate immunologic reconstitution.

Life-Threatening Toxicities of the Chemoradiotherapy Regimens

Veno-occlusive Disease of the Liver

VOD of the liver represents a serious toxicity of all conditioning regimens for BMT. It is manifested clinically by hepatomegaly, ascites and abdominal pain, weight gain, and jaundice. Patients with an elevated SGOT at BMT are more likely to develop VOD. Other potentially hepatotoxic agents administered before or after BMT may also predispose to VOD. About 30% of patients develop clinically significant VOD, and one-third of them die at least partly due to VOD (60). It is not yet known whether conditioning regimens that do not include TBI are associated with a lower incidence of severity of VOD.

Idiopathic Interstitial Pneumonitis

ISP occurs in 8–10% of patients conditioned with single-exposure TBI and is often fatal. The increased use of fractionated TBI has been associated with a decreased rate of incidence, to only 3% (61).

Acute GVHD

Acute GVHD remains the major and most formidable complication of BMT. It reflects an immunologic attack by donor T cells against histocompatibility antigens on host tissue. It is manifested clinically most commonly by dermatitis, hepatitis, and enteritis and marked susceptibility to infections (62). The last is due to immunosuppression by GVHD and to the development of portals of entry for infectious agents through lesions in skin and the gastrointestinal tract. Despite optimal genotypic HLA identity between a patient and an allogeneic sibling marrow donor, and despite the use of MTX and/or CSP for GVHD prophylaxis, cells from the marrow induce acute GVHD in 30–60% of recipients, presumably by reacting against minor histocompatibility antigens not detected by present techniques. The GVHD is severe in about 40% of the patients who develop GVHD and is associated with a decrease in survival. For example, among recipients of HLA-matched sibling marrow for chronic-phase CML, significantly more patients who had mild or no acute GVHD survived than did patients who had severe or moderate GVHD (19,28,33,38).

Treatment of acute GVHD, once it is established, remains relatively ineffective. Prednisone, antithymocyte globulin, CSP, and a variety of monoclonal antibodies directed against T cells have been only occasionally effective (63,64). Many antibodies are directed against T cells. It is likely that some combination of antibodies, or only those antibodies that attack the particular T cells that mediate GVHD, may turn out to be effective. In the meantime, approaches to the prevention of GVHD are emphasized (65,66). A combination of MTX and CSP appears to be more effective than CSP alone in reducing the incidence of severe GVHD and in increasing survival. Thus, in patients with CML in the chronic phase, a randomized trial showed that 52% of patients treated with CSP alone developed significant acute GVHD, in contrast to only 27% of those treated with a combination of MTX and CSP (43).

Chronic GVHD (12)

Chronic GVHD occurs in 25–45% of patients, usually 5 months or later after BMT. The clinical manifestations resemble systemic collagen vascular diseases, such as scleroderma, lupus erythematosus, and Sjögren's syndrome (12,67). There is often involvement of the skin (with skin lesions, keratoconjunctivitis, and buccal mucositis), gut (with esophageal strictures), and liver. Additional major problems are progressive contractures, wasting syndrome, pulmonary insufficiency, and bacterial infections. Chronic GVHD is usually treated with 2 years of prednisone alone (68) or prednisone in combination with CPS and responds with a significant reduction in morbidity and mortality (69). Approximately 75% of patients with chronic GVHD respond to therapy, but about 25% die, usually because of infection. About 70% of patients with chronic GVHD will have had no antecedent history of acute GVHD. However, prophylaxis of acute GVHD with MTX and CSP does not decrease the incidence or severity of chronic GVHD.

GVHD Prophylaxis Using T Cell Depletion

The most effective method for decreasing the incidence and severity of acute GVHD is the removal of T cells from allogeneic marrow prior to infusion using a variety of techniques (38,70–77). The techniques have included soybean agglutination, E rosetting, elutriation, or exposure to monoclonal antibodies directed against T cells and used with complement or bound to immunotoxins. These methods have significantly reduced the incidence and severity of acute GVHD. The beneficial results, however, are counterbalanced by a significant increase in graft rejection and leukemic relapse (11,73). Thus, among recipients of HLA-identical marrow, the incidence of graft rejection is 2% with unmodified but 15% with T-depleted marrow. Moreover, in recipients of HLA-nonidentical marrow, the rejection rate is 5% with unmodified marrow but 35% with T cell-depleted marrow.

The increase in the leukemic relapse rate in recipients of T-depleted marrow has been documented most dramatically in patients transplanted in chronic-phase CML. For example, in a study of 87 recipients of T cell-depleted marrow from 82 transplant centers in 27 countries (38), the incidence of relapse was 50% in recipients of T-depleted marrow who had no or mild acute GVHD, in contrast to 10% in 318 recipients of non-T cell-depleted marrow who had moderate to severe acute GVHD. A more recent report (72) of 208 chronic-phase CML patients who received unmodified or T-depleted HLA-matched sibling marrow at eight transplant centers in Europe and the United States substantiated the observation that T cell-depleted marrow was associated with a decreased incidence of GVHD but at the cost of a higher incidence of graft rejection and a higher rate of leukemic relapse. The end result may be a lower probability of disease-free survival. For example, in a British study (71), the disease-free survival at 2 years for patients with chronic-phase CML who had received unmodified marrow was 62% compared with only 42% for those treated with T cell-depleted marrow.

Leukemic Relapse

Leukemic relapse represents a major cause of death among recipients of unmodified HLA-matched sibling marrow for CML. Except for one case report in which the recurrence of Ph^{1+} leukemia after BMT for chronic-phase CML occurred in donor cells (78), all other recurrences studied have been documented to be of host origin as determined by erythrocyte and sex marker studies or analysis of DNA restriction fragment length polymorphisms.

The definition of leukemic relapse after BMT for chronic-phase CML is fraught with problems. Although hematologic evidence of relapse is virtually always accompanied by cytogenetic relapse, that is, reappearance of Ph^+ metaphases, and is therefore easy to document, a cytogenetic relapse is not always accompanied by clinical evidence of relapse. Cytogenetic relapse occasionally precedes hematologic evidence of relapse by months or even years and may even be transient and disappear (79). This is demonstrated by the results of the Seattle chronic-phase CML series (26) of 160 recipients of unmodified marrow from HLA-matched siblings. A total of 8 patients exhibited reappearance of Ph^+ metaphases in the marrow, which spontaneously disappeared, and the patients remain without any evidence of disease. Of the 8 transient relapses, 5 were detected within 3 months, and all 8 occurred within the first year after BMT. Similar results have been reported by others (72,80,81), who observed transient cytogenetic relapses as well as cytogenetic relapses that preceded by months or years hematologic evidence of relapse. Since cytogenetic relapse may be transient or sustained or may progress to hematologic evidence of disease, cytogenetic relapse alone does not necessarily represent an indication for therapeutic intervention.

Until recently, the only basis for the diagnosis of relapse of CML consisted of the reappearance of the Ph^{1+} metaphases and, at times, the reappearance of clinical manifestations of relapse. Additional methods for documenting relapses after BMT are becoming available.

Since *bcr* rearrangement can serve as a clonal marker for CML, restriction enzyme analysis of blood DNA with a *bcr* probe is likely to be the most sensitive test for post-BMT relapse even in patients who are apparently in cytogenetic remission. The technique can also determine whether a relapse represents the appearance of the original clone or an emergence of a new clone. This technique was used to demonstrate that relapses after BMT in a small number of patients represented persistence of the original leukemic clone (82).

Roth et al. (83) reported on 16 patients who had received allogeneic BMT for CML and were then evaluated by the polymerase chain reaction (PCR) for the *bcr-abl* specific RNA transcript at various times after BMT. In reconstitution experiments, 1 CML cell per 10^6 normal mononuclear cells could be detected by direct agarose gel visualization of a *bcr-abl*-specific band following PCR. The *bcr-abl* message was found in 10 of 16 patients after BMT. PCR-positive *bcr-abl* was present only transiently in 3 patients and correlated with relapse in 3. A single patient died in clinical remission, and 2 patients remained in remission despite the persistence of *bcr-abl*-positive cells at 180 days. Long-term follow-up of *bcr-abl* patients in clinical remission may provide insight into the fate of residual Ph^+ cells after BMT. This approach may aid in the identification of patients at high risk for relapse after BMT.

Most of the attempts to reduce leukemic relapses have involved alterations in the conditioning regimens for BMT. A variety of regimens involving CY and TBI and additional chemotherapy, such as busulfan, dimethylbusulfan, or daunorubicin, have been used, without documented evidence of additional benefit (11,38, 84). Very encouraging results, however, have been reported with a combination of high-dose busulfan and CY without TBI (9,10). Most recently, busulfan, 16 mg/kg, and CY, 120 mg/kg, were used as a conditional regimen for HLA-matched sibling BMT in 13 with CML in accelerated phase and 8 in blast crisis (10). The regimen was very well tolerated. All but 1 patient achieved a complete remission. With a median follow-up time of 29 months, only 1 patient relapsed; 7 of 13 patients transplanted in the accelerated phase and 5 of 8 in blast crisis are alive without evidence of relapse 8–48 months after BMT. The estimated probability of relapse-free 3 year survival is 55%. Although this is a small series of patients followed for a relatively short time, the virtual absence of BMT-related mortality in patients considered at high risk for it is extremely encouraging. The low relapse rate is also quite encouraging and must be validated with more patients and longer follow-up.

Graft-Versus-Leukemia (GVL) Effect

One approach to decreasing the posttransplant leukemic relapses that is receiving increasing attention is to induce or potentiate and effect of infused donor marrow against the leukemia. In rodent models, a GVL effect can be induced by a graft-versus-host (GVH) reaction (85). There is some evidence that in clinical BMT allogeneic marrow may also exert a GVL effect and contribute to some of the cures observed (86–89).

The most cogent evidence for this possibility is circumstantial and statistical. In patients with acute lymphocytic or nonlymphocytic leukemia treated in relapse with BMT, the relapse rate was lower in recipients of allogeneic marrow who exhibited a moderate to severe acute GVHD than in recipients of allogeneic marrow who exhibited no or mild GVHD or than recipients of syngeneic marrow who would not experience significant GVHD (86,87). Patients who developed chronic GVHD exhibited a lower leukemic relapse rate than those who did not develop chronic GVHD; those who exhibited both acute and chronic GVHD experienced the lowest leukemic relapse and the greatest possibility of long-term tumor-free survival (90,91). Indeed, the most recent analysis of the Seattle data involving a total of 1202 patients given unmodified HLA-identical sibling marrow for ANL, ALL, and CML revealed that the incidence of leukemic relapse in patients transplanted for acute leukemia in relapse was 74% in those without GVHD but only 34% in those with chronic GVHD (90). Moreover, in the same study (90), among patients transplanted for CML in the accelerated phase or in blast crisis, the probability of relapse was 65% without GVHD and

36% with acute and/or chronic GVHD. The most persuasive evidence for the existence of a GVL effect in clinical BMT is provided by the observation that recipients of allogeneic unmodified marrow for chronic-phase CML had a significantly lower probability of leukemic relapse than did recipients of T cell-depleted marrow (38,70,71,72).

The latter association suggests that T cells from the donor marrow contribute to the antileukemic effect of chemoradiotherapy, thereby reducing the leukemic relapse rate. Studies in murine models suggest that a GVL effect can in fact be separated or distinguished from GVHD. Similarly, in humans the GVL effect may be separable from GVHD. The donor T cells that react against histocompatibility antigens expressed on normal host tissue and thus induce GVHD may or may not be the same T cells as those that react against the normal histocompatibility antigens and/or the putative tumor-specific antigens expressed on host leukemia cells and thus induce a GVL effect (85). A preliminary attempt was reported to induce GVHD or render it more severe by manipulating post-BMT immunosuppression in the hope that the incidence of leukemic relapse would thereby be decreased (92). The incidence of significant acute GVHD increased, but there was no effect on the incidence of chronic GVHD and no effect on the leukemic relapse rate was detected, partly because of a marked increase in the fatal complications associated with GVHD. In murine models, data have been reported that the GVL effect may or may not be enhanced without augmenting acute GVHD (85).

Chronic GVHD may be clinically more related to a potential GVL effect than acute GVHD. Thus, in one placebo-controlled clinical trial (68), the posttransplant probability of relapse was 55% among patients whose chronic GVHD remained subclinical throughout their treatment, whereas it was only 27% among patients who developed clinically apparent chronic GVHD. Thus the development of clinical chronic GVHD may be required for a GVL effect. This view is supported by a recent report from the IBMTR, in which the greatest antileukemic effect was observed in those patients who developed chronic GVHD (93). Moreover, in the IBMTR analysis of 405 chronic-phase CML patients treated with either T cell-depleted marrow or unmodified marrow, chronic GVHD was associated with a decreased risk of leukemic relapse regardless of the type of marrow received (38). These observations are likely to stimulate attempts to manipulate chronic GVHD in an effort to induce or enhance a GVL effect and decrease the relapse rates.

The mechanism for the GVL effect in humans and the lymphocyte subset that mediates it has not yet been identified. In animal models (85,94) and, increasingly, in humans, knowledge is rapidly increasing about MHC-restricted and MHC non-restricted cellular effector mechanisms and the lymphokines that influence the cellular reactivity to normal histocompatibility antigens and/or tumor antigens. Such knowledge is already stimulating an exploration of the potential use of lymphokines and/or lymphocytes for antileukemic therapy in the context of or as an adjunct to BMT.

ACKNOWLEDGMENT

Supported by PHS grant CA 18029 and CA 47748 awarded by the National Cancer Institute, DHHS.

REFERENCES

1. Fialkow, P. J., and Singer, J. W. (1989). Chronic leukemias. In *Cancer: Principles and Practice of Oncology*, 3rd ed. (V. T. DeVita, S. Hellman, and S. A. Rosenberg, eds.). J. B. Lippincott, Philadelphia, pp. 1836–1852.
2. Talpaz, M., Kantarjian, J. M., McCredie, K., Trujillo, J. M., Keating, M. J., and Gutterman, J. U. (1986). Hematologic remission and cytogenetic improvement induced by recombinant human interferon alpha$_A$ in chronic myelogenous leukemia. *N. Engl. J. Med. 314*:1065–1069.
3. Coleman, M., Silver, R. T., Pajak, T. F., Cavilli, F., Ari, K. R., Kostinas, J. E., Glidewell, O., and Holland, J. F. (1980). Combination chemotherapy for terminal-phase chronic granulocytic leukemia: Cancer and leukemia group B studies. *Blood 55*:29–36.
4. Cunningham, I., Gee, T., Dowling, M., Changanti, R., Bailey, R., Hopfan, S., Bowden, L., Turnbull, A., Knapper, W., and Clarkson, B. (1979). Results in the treatment of Ph^{1+} chronic myelogenous leukemia with an intensive treatment regimen (L-5 protocol). *Blood 53*:375–395.
5. Kantarjian, H. M., Vellekoop, L., McCredie, K. B., Keating, M. J., Hester, J., Smith, T., Barlogie, B., Trujillo, J., and Freireich, E. J. (1985). Intensive combination chemotherapy (ROAP 10) and splenectomy in the management of chronic myelogenous leukemia. *J. Clin. Oncol. 3*:192–200.
6. Cheever, M. A., Greenberg, P. D., and Fefer, A. (1980). Therapy of leukemia by nonimmune syngeneic spleen cells. *J. Immunol. 124*:2137–2142.
7. Thomas, E. D., and Storb, R. (1970). Technique for human marrow grafting. *Blood 36*:507–515.
8. Hansen, J. A., Beatty, P. G., Clift, R. A., Mickelson, E. M., Nisperos, B., and Thomas, E. D. (1984). The HLA system in clinical bone marrow transplantation. In *Advances in Immunobiology: Blood Cell Antigens and Bone Marrow Transplantation* (J. McCullough and S. G. Sandler, eds.). Alan R. Liss, New York, pp. 299–317.
9. Tutschka, P., Copelan, E. A., and Klein, J. P. (1987). Bone marrow transplantation for leukemia following a new busulfan and cyclophosphamide regimen. *Blood 70*:1382–1388.
10. Copelan, E. A., Grever, M. R., Kapoor, N., and Tutschka, P. J. (1988). Marrow transplantation following busulfan and cyclophosphamide for chronic myelogenous leukaemia in accelerated or blastic phase. *Br. J. Haematol. 71*:487–491.

11. Storb, R. (1989). Bone marrow transplantation. In *Cancer: Principles and Practice of Oncology*, 3rd ed. (V. T. DeVita, S. Hellman, and S. A. Rosenberg, eds.), J. B. Lippincott, Philadelphia, pp. 2474–2489.
12. Sullivan, K. M., Witherspoon, R., Storb, R., Appelbaum, F., Beatty, P., Bensinger, W., Bigelow, C., Buckner, C. D., Cheever, M. A., Clift, R., Doney, K., Fefer, A., Greenberg, P. D., Hansen, J., Martin, P., Matthews, K., McDonald, G., Meyers, J., Peterson, F. B., Sanders, J., Shulman, H., Singer, J., Stewart, P., and Thomas, E. D. (1988). Chronic graft-versus-host disease: Pathogenesis, diagnosis, treatment and prognostic factors. In *Bone Marrow Transplantation: Recent Advances and Future Directions*, Experimental Hematology Today, 1987, (S. J. Baum, G. W. Santos, and F. Takaku, eds.). Springer-Verlag, New York, pp. 150–157.
13. Kaplan, E. L., and Meier, P. (1958). Nonparametric estimation from incomplete observations. *J. Am. Statist. Assoc. 53*:457–481.
14. Gilks, W. R., Gore, S. M., and Bradley, B. A. (1986). Analyzing transplant survival data. *Transplantation 42*:46–49.
15. Cox, D. R. (1972). Regression models and life tables. *J. R. Statist. Soc. [B] 34*:187–200.
16. Fefer, A., Einstein, A. B., Thomas, E. D., Buckner, C. D., Clift, R. A., Glucksberg, H., Neiman, P. E., and Storb, R. (1974). Bone marrow transplantation for hematologic neoplasia in 16 patients with identical twins. *N. Engl. J. Med. 290*:1389–1393.
17. Fefer, A., Cheever, M. A., Greenberg, P. D., Applebaum, F. R., Boyd, C. N. Buckner, C. D., Kaplan, H. G., Ramberg, R., Sanders, J. E., Storb, R., and Thomas, E. D. (1982). Treatment of chronic granulocytic leukemia with chemoradiotherapy and transplantation of marrow from identical twins. *N. Engl. J. Med. 306*:63–68.
18. Fefer, A., Cheever, M. A., Thomas, E. D., Boyd, C., Ramberg, R., Glucksberg, H., Buckner, C. D., and Storb, R. (1978). Disappearance of Ph^1-positive cells in four patients with chronic granulocytic leukemia after chemotherapy, irradiation and marrow transplantation from an identical twin. *N. Engl. J. Med. 300*:333–337.
19. Thomas, E. D., Clift, R. A., Fefer, A., Appelbaum, F. R., Bensinger, W. I., Buckner, C. D., Cheever, M. A., Deeg, H. J., Doney, K., Flournoy, N., Greenberg, P., Hansen, J. A., Martin, P., McGuffin, R., Ramberg, R., Sanders, J. E., Singer, J., Stewart, P., Storb, R., Sullivan, K., Weiden, P. L., and Witherspoon, R. (1986). Marrow transplantation for the treatment of chronic myelogenous leukemia. *Ann. Intern. Med. 104*:155–163.
20. Fefer, A., Cheever, M. A., Thomas, E. D., Appelbaum, R. F., Buckner, C. D., Clift, R. A., Glucksberg, H., Greenberg, P. D., Johnson, F. L., Kaplan, H. G., Sanders, J. E., Storb, R., and Weiden, P. L. (1981). Bone marrow transplantation for refractory acute leukemia in 34 patients with identical twins. *Blood 57*:421–430.
21. Fefer, A. (1986). Current status of syngeneic transplants and its relevance to autografting. In *Clinics in Hematology: Autologous Bone Marrow Transplantation*, Vol. 15 (A. H. Goldstone, ed.), W. B. Saunders, London, pp. 49–65.

22. Kanfer, E. J., Buckner, C. D., Fefer, A., Storb, R., Appelbaum, F. R., Hill, R. S., Amos, D., Doney, K. C., Clift, R. A., Shulman, H. M., McDonald, G. B., and Thomas, E. D. (1987). Allogeneic and syngeneic marrow transplantation following high dose dimethylbusulfan, cyclophosphamide and total body irradiation. *Bone Marrow Transplant. 1*:339–346.
23. Thomas, E. D., Clift, R. A., Hersman, J., Sanders, J. E., Stewart, P., Buckner, C. D., Fefer, A., McGuffin, R., Smith, J. W., and Storb, R. (1982). Marrow transplantation for acute nonlymphoblastic leukemia in first remission using fractionated or single-dose irradiation. *Int. J. Radiat. Oncol. Biol. Phys. 8*:817–821.
24. Fefer, A., Clift, R. A., and Thomas, E. D. (1986). Allogeneic marrow transplantation for chronic granulocytic leukemia. *JNCI 76*:1295–1299.
25. Storb, R. (1988). Bone marrow transplantation for the treatment of chronic myelogenous leukemia. *Am. J. Med. Sci. 31*:87–94.
26. Thomas, E. D. (1989). Marrow transplantation for chronic myelogenous leukemia. In *Bone Marrow Transplantation: Current Controversies*. Alan R. Liss, New York, pp. 207–214.
27. Speck, B., Borin, M. M., Champlin, R. E., Goldman, J. M., Herzig, R. H., McGlave, P. B., Messner, H. A., Weiner, R. S., and Rimm, A. A. (1984). Allogeneic bone marrow transplantation for chronic myelogenous leukaemia. *Lancet 1*:665–668.
28. Goldman, J. M., Apperley, J. F., Jones, L., Marcus, R., Goolden, A. W. G., Batchelor, R., Hale, G., Waldmann, H., Reidd, C. D., Hows, J., Gordon-Smith, E., Catovsky, D., and Galton, D. A. G. (1986). Bone marrow transplantation for patients with chronic myeloid leukemia. *N. Engl. J. Med. 314*:202–207.
29. Martin, P. J., Clift, R. A., Fisher, L. D., Buckner, C. D., Hansen, J. A., Appelbaum, F. R., Doney, K. C., Sullivan, K. M., Witherspoon, R. P., Storb, R., and Thomas, E. D. (1988). HLA-identical marrow transplantation during accelerated-phase chronic myelogenous leukemia: Analysis of survival and remission duration. *Blood 72*:1978–1984.
30. Przepiorka, D., and Thomas, E. D. (1988). Prognostic significance of cytogenetic abnormalities in patients with chronic myelogenous leukemia. *Bone Marrow Transplant. 3*:113–119.
31. Champlin, R. W., Ho, W., Arenson, E., and Gale, R. P. (1982). Allogeneic bone marrow transplantation for chronic myelogenous leukemia in chronic or accelerated phase. *Blood 60*:1038–1041.
32. McGlave, P. B., Arthur, D. C., Weisdorf, D., Kim, R., Goldman, A., Hurd, D. D., Ransay, N. K. C., and Kersey, J. H. (1984). Allogeneic bone marrow transplantation as treatment for accelerating chronic myelogenous leukemia. *Blood 63*:219–222.
33. McGlave, P., Arthur, D., Haake, R., Hurd, D., Miller, W., Vercellotti, G., Weisdorf, D., Kim, T., Ransay, N., and Kersey, J. (1987). Therapy of chronic myelogenous leukemia with allogeneic bone marrow transplantation. *J. Clin. Oncol. 5*:1033–1040.

34. Thomas, E. D., Buckner, C. D., Clift, R. A., Fefer, A., Johnson, F. L., Neiman, P. E., Sale, G. E., Sanders, J. E., Singer, J. W., Shulman, H., Storb, R., and Weiden, P. L. (1979). Marrow transplantation for acute nonlymphoblastic leukemia in first remission. *N. Engl. J. Med. 301*:597–599.
35. Clift, R. A., Buckner, C. D., Thomas, E. D., Kopecky, J., Appelbaum, F. R., Tallman, M., Storb, R., Sanders, J., Sullivan, K., Banaji, M., Beatty, P., Bensinger, W., Cheever, M. A., Doney, R., Fefer, A., Greenberg, P. D., Hansen, J., Hackman, R., Hill, R., Martin, P., Meyers, J., McGuffin, R., Neiman, P., Sale, G., Shulman, H., Singer, J., Stewart, P., Weiden, P., and Witherspoon, R. (1987). Treatment of acute non-lymphoblastic leukemia by allogeneic marrow transplantation. *Bone Marrow Transplant. 2*:243–258.
36. Clift, R. A., Buckner, C. D., Thomas, E. D., Doney, K., Fefer, A., Neiman, P. E., Singer, J., Sanders, J., Stewart, P., Sullivan, K. M., Deeg, J., and Storb, R. (1982). The treatment of chronic granulocytic leukemia in chronic phase by allogeneic marrow transplantation. *Lancet 2*:621–624.
37. Schmeiser, T. H., Arnold, R., Wiesneth, M., Hertenstein, B., Bunjed, D., Anger, W., and Heimpel, H. (1988). Knochenmarktransplantation als Therapie der chronischmyeloischen Leukamie. *Dtsch. Med. Wochenschr. 113*: 6–10.
38. Goldman, J. M., Gale, R. P., Horowitz, M. M., Biggs, J. C., Champlin, R. E., Gluckman, E., Hoffmann, R. G., Jacobsen, S. J., Marmont, A. M., McGlave, P. B., Messner, H. A., Rimm, A. A., Rozman, C., Speck, B., Tura, S., Weiner, R. S., and Bortin, M. M. (1988). Bone marrow transplantation for chronic myelogenous leukemia in chronic phase: Increased risk for relapse associated with T cell depletion. *Ann. Intern. Med. 108*:806–184.
39. Thomas, E. D., and Clift, R. A. (1989). Indications for marrow transplantation in chronic myelogenous leukemia. *Blood 73*:861–864.
40. Ringden, O., Zwann, F., Hermans, J., and Gratwohl, A., for the Leukemia Working Party of the European Group for Bone Marrow Transplantation (1987). European experience of bone marrow trans-plantation for leukemia. *Transplant. Proc. 19*:2600–2604.
41. Gratwohl, A., Goldman, J., Gluckman, E., and Zwaan, F. (1985). Effect of splenectomy before bone marrow transplantation on survival of chronic granulocytic leukaemia. *Lancet 2*:1290–1291.
42. Baughan, A. S. J., Worsley, A. M., McCarthy, D. M., Hows, J. M., Catovsky, D., Gordon-Smith, E. C., Galton, D. A. G., and Goldman, J. M. (1984). Haematological reconstitution and severity of graft-versus-host disease after bone marrow transplantation for chronic granulocytic leukaemia: The influence of previous splenectomy. *Br. J. Haematol. 56*:445–454.
43. Storb, R., Deeg, H. J., Whitehead, J., Appelbaum, F., Beatty, P., Bensinger, W., Buckner, C. D., Clift, R., Doney, K., Farewell, V., Hansen, J., Hill, R., Lum, L., Martin, P., McGuffin, R., Sanders, J., Stewart, P., Sullivan, K., Witherspoon, R., Yee, G., and Thomas, E. D. (1986). Methotrexate and cyclosporine compared with cyclosporine alone for prophylaxis of acute graft versus host disease after marrow transplantation for leukemia. *N. Engl. J. Med. 314*:729–735.

44. Sokal, J. E., Cox, E. B., Baccarani, M., Tura, S., Gomez, G. A., Robertson, J. E., Tso, C. Y., Braun, T. J., Clarkson, B. D., Cervantes, F., Rozman, C., and the Italian Cooperative CML Study Group (1984). Prognostic discrimination in "good risk" chronic granulocytic leukemia. *Blood 63*:789–799.
45. Sokal, J. E., Baccarani, M., Tura, S., Fiacchini, M., Cervantes, F., Rozman, C., Gomez, G. A., Galton, D. A. G., Cannellos, G. P., Braun, T. J., Clarkson, B. D., Carbonell, F., Heimpel, H., Extra, J. M., Fiere, D., Nissen, N. I., Robertson, J. E., and Cox, E. B. (1985). Prognostic discrimination among younger patients with chronic granulocytic leukemia: Relevance to bone marrow transplantation. *Blood 66*:1352–1357.
46. Segel, G. B., Simon, W., and Lichtman, M. A (1986). Variables influencing the timing of marrow transplantation in patients with chronic myelogenous leukemia. *Blood 88*:1055–1064.
47. Marks, S. M., Baltimore, D., and McCaffrey, R (1978). Terminal transferase as a predictor of initial responsiveness to vincristine and prednisone in blastic chronic myelogenous leukemia. *N. Engl. J. Med. 298*:812–814.
48. Beatty, P. G., Clift, R. A., Mickelson, E. M., Nisperos, B., Flournoy, N., Martin, P. J., Sanders, J. E., Stewart, P., Buckner, C. D., Storb, R., Thomas, E. D., and Hansen, J. A. (1985). Marrow transplantation from related donors other than HLA-identical siblings. *N. Engl. J. Med. 313*:765–771.
49. Storb, R., Weiden, P. L., Schroeder, M. L., Graham, T. C., Lerner, K. G., and Thomas, E. D. (1976). Marrow grafts between canine littermates, homozygous or heterozygous for lymphocyte-defined histocompatibility antigens. *Transplantation 21*:299–306.
50. Anasetti, C., Amos, D., Beatty, P. G., Appelbaum, F. R., Bensinger, W., Buckner, C. D., Clift, R., Doney, K., Martin, P. J., Mickelson, E., Nisperos, B., O'Quigley, J., Ramberg, R., Sanders, J. E., Stewart, P., Storb, P., Sullivan, K. M., Witherspoon, R. P., Thomas, E. D., and Hansen, J. A (1989). Effect of HLA compatibility of engraftment of bone marrow transplants in patients with leukemia or lymphoma. *N. Engl. J. Med. 20*:197–204.
51. Hansen, J. A., Beatty, P. G., and Anasetti, C. (1987). Transplantation of hematopoietic stem cells (HSC). *Br. Med. Bull. 43*:203–216.
52. Hansen, J. A., Clift, R. A., Thomas, E. D., Buckner, C. D., Storb, R., and Giblett, E. R. (1980). Transplantation of marrow from an unrelated donor to a patient with acute leukemia. *N. Engl. J. Med. 303*:565–567.
53. McGlave, P., Scott, E., Ramsay, N., Arthur, D., Blazar, B., McCullough, J., and Kersey, J. (1987). Unrelated donor bone marrow transplantation therapy for chronic myelogenous leukemia. *Blood 70*:877–881.
54. Beatty, P., Ash, R., Hows, J. M., and McGlave, P. B. (1989). The use of unrelated bone marrow donors in the treatment of patients with chronic myelogenous leukemia: Experience of four marrow transplant centers. *Bone Marrow Transplant. 4*:253–256.
55. Beatty, P. G., Dahlberg, S., Mickelson, E. M., Nisperos, B., Opelz, G., Martin, P. J., and Hansen, J. A (1988). Probability of finding HLA-matched unrelated marrow donors. *Transplantation 45*:714–718.

56. Meyers, J. D., and Thomas, E. D. (1988). Infection complicating bone marrow transplantation. In *Clinical Approach to Infection in the Compromised Host*, 2nd ed. (R. H. Rubin and L. S. Young, eds.). Plenum Press, New York, pp. 525–556.
57. Bowden, R. A., and Meyers, J. D. (1985). Infectious complications following marrow transplantation. *Plasma Ther. Transfus. Technol. 6*:285–302.
58. Weiner, R. S., Bortin, M. M., Gale, R. P., Gluckman, E., Kay, H. E. M., Kolb, H.-J., Hartz, A. J., and Rimm, A. A. (1986). Interstitial pneumonitis after bone marrow transplantation: Assessment of risk factors. *Ann. Intern. Med. 104*:168–175.
59. Bowden, R. A., Sayers, M., and Fluornoy, N. (1986). Cytomegalovirus immunoglobulin and sero-negative blood products to prevent primary cytomegalovirus infection after marrow transplantation. *N. Engl. J. Med. 314*: 1006–1010.
60. McDonald, G. B., Shulman, H. M., Sullivan, K. M., and Spencer, G. D. (1986). Interstinal and hepatic complications of human bone marrow transplantation. *Gastroenterology 90*:460–477.
61. Meyers, D., Flournoy, N., and Thomas, E. D. (1982). Nonbacterial pneumonia after allogeneic marrow transplantation: A review of ten years' experience. *Rev. Infect. Dis. 4*:1119–1132.
62. Glucksberg, H., Storb, R., Fefer, A., Buckner, C. D., Neiman, P. E., Clift, R. A., Lerner, K. G., and Thomas, E. D. (1974). Clinical manifestations of graft-versus-host disease in human recipients of marrow from HLA-matched sibling donors. *Transplantation 18*:295–304.
63. Storb, R., and Thomas, E. D. (1985). Graft-versus-host disease in dog and man: The Seattle experiment. *Immunol. Rev. 88*:215–238.
64. Storb, R., Gluckman, E., Thomas, E. D., Buckner, C. D., Clift, R. A., Fefer, A., Glucksberg, H., Graham, T. C., Johnson, F. L., Lerner, K. G., Neiman, P. E., and Ochs, H. (1974). Treatment of established human graft-versus-host diseases by antithymocyte globulin. *Blood 44*:57–75.
65. Storb, R., Deeg, H. J., Fisher, L. D., Appelbaum, F., Buckner, C. D., Bensinger, W., Clift, R., Doney, K., Irle, C., McGuffin, R., Martin, P., Sanders, J., Schnoch, G., Singer, J., Stewart, P., Sullivan, K., Witherspoon, R., and Thomas, E. D. (1988). Cyclosporine versus methotrexate for graft-versus-host disease prevention in patients given marrow grafts for leukemia: Long-term follow-up of three controlled trials. *Blood 71*:293–298.
66. Storb, R., Deeg, H. J., Thomas, E. D., Appelbaum, F. R., Buckner, C. D., Cheever, M. A., Clift, R. A., Doney, K. C., Flournoy, N., Kennedy, M. S., Loughran, T. P., McGuffin, R. W., Sale, G. E., Sanders, J. E., Singer, J. W., Stewart, P. S., Sullivan, K. M., and Witherspoon, R. P. (1985). Marrow transplantation for chronic myelocytic leukemia: A controlled trial of cyclophosphamide versus methotrexate for prophylaxis of graft-versus-host disease. *Blood 66*:698–702.
67. Sullivan, K. M., Shulman, H. M., Strob, R., Weiden, P. L., Witherspoon, R. P., McDonald, G. B., Schubert, M. N., Atkinson, K., and Thomas, E. D.

(1981). Chronic graft-versus-host disease in 52 patients: Adverse natural course and successful treatment with combination immunosuppression. *Blood 57*:267–276.

68. Sullivan, K. M., Witherspoon, R. P., Storb, R., Weiden, P., Flournoy, N., Dahlberg, S., Deeg, H. J., Sanders, J. E., Doney, K. C., Appelbaum, F. R., McGuffin, R., McDonald, G. B., Meyers, J., Schubert, M. M., Gauvreau, J., Shulman, H. M., Sale, G. E., Anasetti, C., Loughran, T. P., Strom, S., Nims, J., and Thomas, E. D. (1988). Prednisone and azathioprine compared with prednisone and placebo for treatment of chronic graft-v-host disease: Prognostic influence of prolonged thrombocytopenia after allogeneic marrow transplantation. *Blood 72*:546–554.
69. Sullivan, K. M., Witherspoon, R. P., Storb, R., Deeg, H. J., Dahlberg, S., Sanders, J. E., Appelbaum, F. R., Doney, K. C., Weiden, P., Anasetti, C., Loughran, T. P., Hill, R., Shields, A., Yee, G., Shulman, H., Nims, J., Strom, S., and Thomas, E. D. (1988). Alternating-day cyclosporine and prednisone for treatment of high-risk chronic graft-v-host disease. *Blood 72*: 555–561.
70. Martin, P. J., Hansen, J. A., Buckner, C. D., Sanders, J. E., Deeg, J. J., Stewart, P., Appelbaum, F. R., Clift, R. A., Fefer, A., Witherspoon, R. P., Kennedy, M. S., Sullivan, K. M., Flournoy, N., Storb, R., and Thomas, E. D. (1985). Effects of in vitro depletion of T cells in HLA-identical allogeneic marrow grafts. *Blood 66*:664–672.
71. Apperley, J. F., Jones, L., Hale, G., Waldmann, H., Hows, J., Rombos, Y., Tsatalas, C., Marcus, R. E., Goolden, A. W. G., Gordon-Smith, E. C., Catovsky, D., Galton, D. A. G., and Goldman, J. M. (1986). Bone marrow transplantation for chronic myeloid leukemia: T cell depletion reduces the risk of graft-versus-host disease but may increase the risk of leukaemic relapse. *Bone Marrow Transplant. 1*:53–66.
72. Apperley, J. F., Mauro, F. R., Goldman, J. M., Gregory, W., Arthur, C. K., Hows, J., Arcese, W., Papa, G., Mandelli, F., Wardle, D., Gravett, P., Franklin, I. M., Bandini, G., Ricci, P., Tura, S., Iacone, A., Torlontano, G., Heit, G., Champlin, R., and Gale, R. P. (1988). Bone marrow transplantation for chronic myeloid leukaemia in first chronic phase: Importance of a graft-versus-host-leukaemia effect. *Br. J. Haematol. 69*:239–245.
73. Butturini, A., and Gale, R. P. (1988). T-cell depletion in bone marrow transplantation for leukemia: Current results and future directions. *Bone Marrow Transplant. 3*:185–192.
74. Apperley, J. F., Jones, L., Hale, G., Waldmann, H., Hows, J., Rombos, Y., Tsatalas, C., Marcus, R. E., Goolden, A. W. G., Gordon-Smith, E. C., Catovsky, D., Dalton, D. A. G., and Goldman, J. M. (1986). Bone marrow transplantation for patients with chronic myeloid leukemia: T cell depletion with Campath-1 reduces the incidence of graft-versus-host disease but may increase the risk of leukaemic relapse. *Bone Marrow Transplant. 1*:53–66.
75. Martin, P. J., Hansen, J. A., Buckner, C. D., Sanders, J. E., Deeg, J. J., Stewart, P., Appelbaum, F. R., Clift, R. A., Fefer, A., Witherspoon, R. P., Kennedy, M. S., Sullivan, K. M., Flournoy, N., Storb, R., and Thomas, E. D.

(1985). Effects of in vitro depletion of T cells in HLA-identical allogeneic marrow grafts. *Blood 66*:664–672.
76. Prentice, H. G., Blacklock, H. A., Janossy, G., Gilmore, M. J. M. L., Price-Jones, L., Tirman, N., Trejdosiewicz, L. K., Skeggs, D. B. L., Panjawani, D., Ball, S., Graphakos, S., Patterson, J., Ivory, K., and Hoffbrand, A. V. (1984). Depletion of T lymphocytes in donor marrow prevents significant graft-versus-host disease in matched allogeneic leukaemic marrow transplant recipients. *Lancet 1*:472–475.
77. Reisner, Y., Kapoor, R. J., Kirkpatrick, N., Pollack, M. S., Dupont, B., Good, R. A., and O'Reilly, R. J. (1981). Transplantation for acute leukaemia with HLA-A and B nonidentical parental marrow cells fractionated with soybean agglutinin and sheep red blood cells. *Lancet 2*:327–331.
78. Marmont, A., Frassoni, F., Bacigaluop, A., Podesta, M., Piaggio, G., Van-Lint, M. T., Caimo, A., and deFilippi, S. (1984). Recurrence of Ph^1-positive leukemia in donor cells after marrow transplantation for chronic granulocytic leukemia. *N. Engl. J. Med. 310*:903–905.
79. Apperley, J. F., Rassool, F., Parreira, A., Geary, C. G., Harrison, C., Stansfield, D., and Goldman, J. M. (1986). Philadelphia-positive metaphases in the marrow after bone marrow transplantation for chronic granulocytic leukemia. *Am. J. Hematol. 22*:199–204.
80. Zaccaria, A., Rosti, G., Testoni, N., Alimena, G., Arcese, W., Bandini, G., Boogaerts, M., Carbonell, F., Ferrant, A., Frassoni, F., Gahrton, G., Haas, O. A., Iacone, A., Mecucci, C., Michauz, J.-L., Palka, G., Papa, G., Pollak, C., Rosetti, A., Ricci, P., Schmeizer, T., Sessarego, M., Valenti, S., Van den Berghe, H., and Tura, S. (1987). Chromosome studies in patients with Philadelphia chromosome-positive chronic myeloid leukemia submitted to bone marrow transplantation—results of an European Cooperative Study. *Cancer Genet. Cytogenet. 26*:5–13.
81. Arthur, C. K., Apperley, J. F., Guo, A. P., Rassool, F., Gao, L. M., and Goldman, J. M. (1988). Cytogenetic events after bone marrow transplantation for chronic myeloid leukemia in chronic phase. *Blood 71*(5):1179–1186.
82. Ganesan, T. S., Min, G. L., Goldman, J. M., and Young, B. D. (1987). Molecular analysis of relapse in chronic myeloid leukemia after allogeneic bone marrow transplantation. *Blood 70*:873–876.
83. Roth, M. S., Antin, J. H., Bingham, E. L., and Ginsberg, D. (1989). Detection of Philadelphia chromosome positive cells by the polymerase chain reaction following bone marrow transplant for chronic myelogenous leukemia. *Blood 74*:882–885.
84. Blume, K. G., Forman, S. J., O'Donnell, M. R., Doroshow, J. H., Krance, R. A., Nademanee, A. P., Snyder, D. S., Schmidt, G. M., Fahey, J. L., Metter, G. E., Hill, L. R., Findley, D. O., and Sniecinski, I. J. (1987). Total body irradiation and high-dose etoposide: A new preparatory regimen for bone marrow transplantation in patients with advanced hematologic malignancies. *Blood 69*:1015–1020.

85. Truitt, R. L., LeFever, A. V., and Shih, C. C. Y. (1987). Graft-versus-leukemia reactions: Experimental models and clinical trials. In *Progress in Bone Marrow Transplantation: Proceedings of the Fourth International UCLA Symposium on Bone Marrow Transplantation* (R. P. Gale and R. Champlin, eds.). Alan R. Liss, New York, pp. 219–232.
86. Weiden, P. L., Flournoy, N., Thomas, E. D., Prentice, R., Fefer, A., Buckner, C. D., and Storb, R. (1979). Antileukemic effect of graft-versus-host disease in human recipients of allogeneic-marrow grafts. *N. Engl. J. Med. 300*:1068–1073.
87. Fefer, A., Sullivan, K. M., Weiden, P. C., Buckner, C. D., Shoch, G., Storb, R., and Thomas, E. D. (1987). Graft-versus-leukemia effect in man: The relapse of acute leukemia is lower after allogeneic than after syngeneic marrow transplantation. In *Cellular Immunotherapy of Cancer*, Vol. 244 (R. L. Truitt, R. P. Gale, and M. M. Bortin, eds.). Alan R. Liss, New York, pp. 401–408.
88. Butturini, A., Bortin, M. M., and Gale, R. P. (1987). Graft-versus-leukemia following bone marrow transplantation. *Bone Marrow Transplant. 2*:223–242.
89. Gale, R. P., and Champlin, R. E. (1984). How does bone marrow transplantation cure leukemia? *Lancet 1*:28–30.
90. Sullivan, K. M., Weiden, P., Storb, R., Witherspoon, R. P., Fefer, A., Fisher, L., Buckner, C. D., Anasetti, C., Appelbaum, F. R., Badger, C., Beatty, P., Bensinger, W., Berenson, R., Bigelow, C., Cheever, M. A., Clift, R., Deeg, H. J., Doney, K., Greenberg, P. D., Hansen, J. A., Hill, R., Loughran, T., Martin, P., Neiman, P., Peterson, F., Sanders, J., Singer, J., Stewart, P., and Thomas, E. D. (1989). Influence of acute and chronic graft-versus-host disease on relapse and survival after bone marrow transplantation from HLA-identical siblings as treatment of acute and chronic leukemia. *Blood 73*: 1720–1728.
91. Weiden, P. L., Sullivan, K. M., Flournoy, N., Storb, R., Thomas, E. D., the Seattle Marrow Transplant Team (1981). Antileukemic effect of graft-versus-host disease: Contribution to improved survival after allogeneic marrow transplantation. *N. Engl. J. Med. 304*:1529–1533.
92. Sullivan, K. M., Storb, R., Buckner, C. D., Fefer, A., Fisher, L., Weiden, P. L., Witherspoon, R. P., Appelbaum, F. R., Banaji, M., Hansen, J., Martin, P., Sanders, J. E., Singer, J., and Thomas, E. D. (1989). Graft-versus-host disease as adoptive immunotherapy in patients with advanced hematologic neoplasms. *N. Engl. J. Med. 320*:828–834.
93. Fefer, A., Cheever, M. A., and Greenberg, P. D. (1982). Overview of prospects and problems of lymphocyte transfer for cancer therapy. In *Progress in Cancer Research and Therapy: The Potential Role of T Cells in Cancer Therapy*, Vol. 22 (A. Fefer and A. L. Goldstein, eds.). Raven Press, New York, pp. 1–6.
94. Ringden, O., and Horowitz, M. M. Graft-versus-leukemia reactions in humans. *Transplant. Proc.* (in press).

20

Use of Autologous Stem Cells in Support of the Intensive Treatment of Chronic Myelogenous Leukemia

John M. Goldman *Royal Postgraduate Medical School, London, England*

INTRODUCTION

Chronic myeloid leukemia (CML) is conventionally thought of as a clonal disorder of the most primitive pluripotential hematopoietic stem cell characterized in most cases by acquisition of a readily identifiable cytogenetic marker, the Philadelphia chromosome. The comparatively recent discovery that the Ph chromosome is associated with the production of a chimeric *bcr-abl* gene, which in turn is expressed as a novel fusion protein with tyrosine kinase activity (see Chapter 10), has led to the suggestion that this protein may play a crucial role in the pathogenesis of the chronic phase of CML. It is also conventional to assume that the acquisition of the Ph chromosome by the targeted stem cell confers on its progeny a "proliferative advantage" whereby the leukemic clone expands inexorably while the proliferation of normal or nonclonal hematopoietic progenitor cells is suppressed indefinitely. Moreover, the expansion of the leukemia stem cell compartment is associated with an increased risk of further genetic (and cytogenetic) changes, which in due course lead to hematologic transformation.

However, a number of clinical observations imply that this interpretation of the pathogenesis of CML may be an oversimplification. There are, for example, cases in whom populations of Ph-positive and Ph-negative hematopoietic cells coexist for long periods in apparently stable mosaicism, implying that the Ph-positive population does not always express a proliferative advantage over what is presumed to be residual normal hematopoiesis. In other cases there is circumstantial evidence to suggest that both populations, the Ph positive and the Ph negative, may be of clonal origin and consequently part of the original neoplastic clone (1). One may wonder then why one or the other clone does not gain effective dominance. In certain cases the sequence of hematologic and cytogenetic events after allogeneic bone marrow transplantation also conflicts with the notion that the Ph-positive population has an automatic and unmodifiable proliferative advantage. For example, the now well documented observation that cytogenetic "relapses" after transplant may on occasion be transient (2-4) and the finding that recipients of donor marrow that has been depleted in vitro of lymphoid cells have a significantly increased probability of relapse (5,6) both suggest that the proliferation of leukemic stem cells may in selected cases be modified by extrinsic factors.

The use of high-dose chemotherapy or chemoradiotherapy followed by autografting with marrow- or blood-derived stem cells has also yielded results that suggest that the interaction of Ph-positive and Ph-negative hematopoiesis in CML is complex. Partial and transient Ph-negative hematopoiesis is seen in a high proportion of patients whose marrow is studied early after autografting (7). After autografting for patients still in chronic phase, the subsequent progression of clinical disease seems to be slowed in some cases (8). Particularly intriguing has been the observation in some cases that durable Ph-negative hematopoiesis is re-established after autografting in patients who appeared at diagnosis to have classic Ph-positive CML (8,9). Some of these points are considered in greater detail in this chapter.

STEM CELL COLLECTION AND MANIPULATION

There is ample evidence to suggest that the concentration of committed myeloid progenitor cells is greatly increased in the bone marrow and peripheral blood of patients with chronic myeloid leukemia at diagnosis [reviewed by Eaves and Eaves (10)]. The numbers of CFU-GEMM are also increased, although the proportional increase in the marrow is less than that of CFU-GM or BFU-E. These observations suggest that pluripotential stem cell numbers may also be increased.

There are various reasons for collecting and cryopreserving hematopoietic stem cells at diagnosis from newly diagnosed patients. Apart from the strictly scientific value of retaining stored material that can at a later date be studied by newly developed molecular and other techniques, an unscheduled autograft may on occasion be life-saving in cases of busulfan-induced marrow failure (11) or after graft failure following allogeneic marrow transplantation (8). It is extremely doubtful whether autografting for patients in overt transformation is clinically useful (7,12), but autografting after high-dose chemotherapy in chronic phase warrants further study (see later).

Timing and Source of Stem Cell Collection

There are no clear guidelines as to when hematopoietic stem cells should be collected from patients with CML or whether blood or marrow cells are preferred. In practice, collection of relatively large numbers of marrow cells from the untreated patient may be technically difficult because the marrow is often extremely hypercellular and difficult to aspirate: leukapheresis by contrast can yield 1-2 $\times 10^{11}$ or more cells during a 2 or 3 h collection procedure (13).

Once treatment has been initiated the number of committed myeloid progenitor cells in the circulation usually falls precipitously and leukapheresis for collection of stem cells presumably is then inappropriate (14). We have taken the empirical view that leukapheresis for collection of stem cells from patients with CML is probably useful only when the blood leukocyte count exceeds 100×10^9 per L; similarly we have avoided collecting bone marrow cells from patients receiving treatment with busulfan or hydroxyurea but have instead recommended that treatment with cytotoxic drugs be withheld for at least 4 weeks before marrow harvesting. It is quite possible, however, that this empirical approach favors the collection of Ph-positive progenitor cells and that the maximal proportion of Ph-negative cells could be collected from the peripheral blood of a treated patient (see later).

For patients who have been rendered completely or predominantly Ph negative as a result of treatment with α-interferon, it is logical to harvest marrow (or perhaps peripheral blood cells) with a view to performing an autograft at a later date. In practice the harvest procedure may be difficult because the marrow in such patients is often hypocellular and the cell yield consequently low. The group in Rome set an arbitrary minimum concentration of 50 committed progenitor cells per 2×10^5 nucleated marrow cells and reported that these values for CFU-GM and BFU-E were only reached at medians of 158 and 122 days, respectively, after stopping α-interferon (15).

Hematopoietic Stem Cell Numbers Required for Autografting

Whereas it is conventional to aim at a marrow cell dose of 3.0×10^8 per kg nucleated cells when undertaking marrow transplantation from an allogeneic donor, the numbers of nucleated cells or myeloid stem cells required to guarantee engraftment when using autologous blood or marrow in the nonleukemic patient are less well defined and depend in part on the amount and nature of previous treatment with cytotoxic drugs and/or irradiation. The same uncertainty applies to the use of blood- or marrow-derived stem cells from patients with CML. A major consideration is likely to be the extent to which the leukemic stem cell population has expanded, a value that can only be derived indirectly from consideration of the size of the total granulocyte mass. We have arbitrarily aimed to transfuse 10×10^8 per kg blood-derived nucleated cells on any one occasion, but in most cases this probably constitutes a considerable overdose.

Possible Approaches for Purging Marrow In Vitro

On the assumption that nucleated cells from the marrow or peripheral blood of newly diagnosed patients with CML contain a mixture of Ph-positive and Ph-negative stem cells, one may ask whether techniques can be devised that would enable selective concentration of the latter population. For the present this seems difficult to achieve. Attempts have been made to treat harvested marrow in vitro with cytotoxic drugs, such as 4-hydroperoxycyclophosphamide (16), but in general little selective killing of Ph-positive cells has been achieved. Although the surface membrane characteristics of circulating progenitor cells in CML differ from those of their normal counterparts (17), this probably reflects differences in levels of differentiation rather than fundamental differences intrinsic to the leukemia. There is no evidence that surface membrane determinants characteristic of pluripotential stem cells, such as CD34, are expressed differently on normal and CML cells.

With the knowledge that a proportion of patients with Ph-positive CML can be restored to Ph-negative hematopoiesis by treatment over prolonged periods by α-interferon, a number of attempts have been made to demonstrate selective inhibition of myeloid progenitor cells cultured in vitro in the presence of interferon (18,19). With some exceptions the majority of these studies have failed to demonstrate any selective inhibition. More recently, attempts have been made to promote the survival or proliferation of Ph-negative hematopoiesis by treating marrow cells in vitro with y-interferon. The results of the associated clinical studies are not yet fully evaluable (20).

A fundamental difference between normal and CM cells is the presence in the cytoplasm of CML cells of the p210$^{bcr\text{-}abl}$. Although the majority of normal cells probably express the normal *bcr* and *abl* genes, both of whose functions are still unknown, attempts have been made to develop antibodies that specifically recognize determinants on the *bcr-abl* protein but fail to react with either of the normal gene products (21). Whether such antibodies can be refined further and can be introduced into leukemia cells without causing irreparable damage to normal cells remains to be seen. Perhaps a little closer is the possibility that antisense oligonucleotides or ribozymes can be developed that specifically inactivate the *bcr-abl* mRNA.

Possible Short-Term Proliferative Advantage for Ph-Negative Hematopoietic Stem Cells In Vitro

Although there are no clear-cut differences in the sensitivity of normal and CML progenitor cells to known hematopoietic growth factors, it is nonetheless possible that the altered microenvironment of the Dexter-type long-term culture system favors the survival of Ph-negative progenitor cells (22). This provides a rationale for collecting marrow and subjecting it to culture in vitro for variable periods of time to transfuse to the patient a stem cell population from which Ph-positive cells have been selectively depleted. The approach has been tested by the Vancouver group (23) and the group in Manchester (24).

Possible Short-Term Proliferative Advantage for Ph-Negative Hematopoietic Stem Cells In Vivo

All methods of purging harvested marrow or peripheral blood cells would be superfluous if Ph-negative hematopoietic progenitor cells had a short-term proliferative advantage on reintroduction into the patient who had been treated with high-dose chemotherapy and if this proliferative advantage could then be maintained by further administration of cytotoxic drugs or cytokines, such as α-interferon or interleukin-2. The observation of partial but transient restoration of Ph-negative hematopoiesis in the majority of autografted patients suggests that the in vitro purging steps may not be strictly necessary.

AUTOGRAFTING IN ADVANCED PHASES OF CML

Clinical Results of Autografting with Marrow Cells

The capacity of autologous marrow cells that have been held at low temperature for variable periods of times to re-establish marrow function in various animal species, including humans, has been known for many years. In 1974, the Seattle group reported the results of treating two patients with CML in transformation by high-dose chemotherapy and total-body irradiation (TBI) followed by transfusion of autologous marrow cells that had been collected and cryopreserved sometime earlier (25). In 1978, the same authors reported the results of using a similar approach in five additional patients (26). In general, these patients showed evidence of myeloid engraftment but the quality of lymphoid cell engraftment was variable; it seemed to be best when relatively large numbers of blood-derived nucleated cells were transfused in conjunction with the marrow cells. All patients in this series died either of toxicity of the conditioning regiment or of early relapse of the transformed leukemia. The importance of these early studies lay, however, in their demonstration that autografting with marrow-derived stem cells was possible in principle in CML and that better results might be achieved if more effective cytoreductive schedules could be devised.

In 1984, the Denver group reported the results of treating 11 patients with CML in transformation with high-dose chemotherapy followed by autografting with stored marrow cells (27). Of these patients, 6 were restored to chronic-phase disease, and the median survival for all 11 patients was 33 weeks. All patients in this series eventually died of relapse of CML in transformation. Similar results were reported by the group in Roswell Park, who treated 6 patients with CML in transformation (28). A second chronic phase lasting 2-10 months was established in 3 patients. Essentially very similar results were also achieved by the Paris group (29).

Clinical Results of Autografting with Blood-Derived Stem Cells

As a result of the early experience in Seattle, we began in the early 1970s to collect and cryopreserve marrow cells at the Hammersmith Hospital in London. We rapidly discovered, however, that aspiration of marrow cells (with the aspiration needles then available) was technically difficult and the aspirated material was heavily contaminated with peripheral blood. We therefore continued to collect and cryopreserve nucleated cells from the peripheral blood without any certain knowledge that they would in fact be effective in reconstituting hematopoiesis. In 1977, we had the opportunity to treat a patient who had received high-dose chemotherapy for CML in transformation with autologous blood-derived stem cells, and the early hematopoietic regeneration was strong evidence, although not proof, that the autograft had been successful (30). Subsequently we demonstrated that regeneration of hematopoiesis could occur equally rapidly in patients treated with chemotherapy and "supralethal" TBI (31).

In 1984, we summarized the results of treating 51 patients in transformation of CML by high-dose chemotherapy or chemoradiotherapy followed by autografting with blood-derived stem cells (7). The median duration of survival for all 51 patients was 26 weeks (range 2-152 weeks). Of these patients, 48 were restored to "second chronic phase," but engraftment was feeble or absent in 3 cases. We formed the impression that engraftment of autologous cells was more rapid in patients who had previously been splenectomized (32). A total of 21 patients were autografted on a second occasion, either because their transformed disease had recurred or as consolidation for second chronic phase. For this selected group of patients the duration of survival after the original autograft was longer than for those autografted only once (median survival 51 versus 13 weeks, $p = 0.007$).

It rapidly became obvious that although the autograft itself was successful in restoring hematopoiesis after "myeloablative" therapy, the principal clinical problem was the rapid relapse of transformed leukemia. During the period from 1977 to 1988 we made many changes in the cytoreductive schedule preceding the autograft (Table 1), but none has solved the problem of eradicating or durably suppressing the transformed clone of leukemia cells.

Occasional patients have become long-term survivors after autografting in transformation. One such patient was a 50-year-old woman who presented to her hematologist in Yorkshire (England) in 1983 with Ph chromosome-positive CML

Table 1 Evolution of Cytoreductive Protocols Intended to Eradicate Transformed Leukemia Before Autografting as Used at the Hammersmith Hospital from 1977 to 1989

Year	Antileukemic regimen
1977	Daunrobubin, cytarabine, 6-thioguanine (DAT)
1978–1979	DAT plus TBI (2 Gy X 6)
1980–1981	DAT followed by high-dose melphalan
1983–1983	DAT plus etoposide over 8 days
1984–1985	High-dose cytarabine followed by high-dose melphalan
1986–1989	High-dose cytarabine-mitoxantrone followed by high-dose melphalan

in chronic phase. Peripheral blood nucleated cells were collected and cryopreserved at that time. She presented again with lethargy and increasing splenomegaly 1 year later. Her leukocyte count was 5.9×10^9 per L and platelets 9×10^9 per L. The marrow was hypercellular with 38% blast cells, which were morphologically lymphoid and positive for common acute lymphoblastic leukemia antigen (CALLA) and terminal deoxynucleotidyltransferase. She received high-dose chemotherapy with cytosine arabinoside and melphalan followed by autografting. Hematopoiesis characteristic of chronic-phase disease was re-established. She received a second course of cytotoxic drugs 6 weeks later, comprising cytosine arabinoside, melphalan, vincristine, and prednisolone at high dosage followed by a second autograft. Thereafter she remained in chronic phase, which was really controlled by hydroxyurea. She died of apparently unrelated causes 54 months after the onset of transformation. There was no hematologic evidence of transformation at the time of her death.

Other groups have reported the use of blood-derived stem cells to treat patients in transformation. In 1981, Korbling and colleagues described 1 patient in whom hematopoiesis had been restored to Ph negativity by treatment with high-dose cyclophosphamide (33). Blood stem cells were harvested and cryopreserved. These cells were used subsequently to restore hematopoiesis after intensive chemotherapy administered to transformation. The patient died relatively early after autografting, but hematopoiesis was entirely Ph negative shortly before death. The Boston group treated 7 patients in transformation and restored 5 to second chronic phase (34). The median survival for all 7 patients was 11 months. The group France Autogreffe treated 28 patients in accelerated phase or blastic transformation by autografting with blood-derived stem cells. The majority of these patients were restored to second chronic phase; the median survival from autografting was 4.5 months (range < 1 to 54+).

AUTOGRAFTING IN CHRONIC PHASE

The rationale for treating a patient in chronic phase by high-dose chemotherapy or chemoradiotherapy followed by autografting with hematopoietic stem cells (which may be predominantly Ph positive) is not immediately apparent. There are, however, a number of reasons, some or all of which may be highly speculative, that such treatment could benefit the patient. Perhaps most important is the possibility that such treatment substantially reduces the total number of leukemic stem cells and thus reduces the probability of transformation in any given time period. It is very difficult to see how this suggestion could be proved other than in a prospectively randomized study involving large numbers of patients. A second possibility is that autografting favors the restoration of Ph-negative hematopoiesis, which by analogy with results obtained after allogeneic transplantation for CML, may lead to prolonged survival. A third possibility is the suggestion that autografting may so modulate the leukemic cell population that it loses its proliferative advantage as a result of changes in the leukemic cell, in an accessory cell (e.g., a subset of the T cell population), or in the marrow microenvironment. Some of the clinical and cytogenetic results referred to in this section are in accord with this last interpretation.

Clinical Results of Autografting with Marrow Cells

The Vancouver group have recently reported the results of treating three patients with CML in chronic phase by autografting with marrow cells that had been held in liquid culture for 10 days (23). Of these patients, one was treated while in first chronic phase 5 years from diagnosis; two other patients were in second and third chronic phase, respectively. Marrow was aspirated from these patients in the conventional manner, and aliquots of 2×10^8 nucleated cells were dispensed into 175 cm^2 tissue culture flasks with added α medium, horse serum, and calf serum. The flasks were then incubated for 4 days at 37°C and for a further 6 days at 33°C without medium change. During this time the patient was treated with etoposide (1.8 g/m^2, 24 h infusion), cyclophosphamide (2.0 g/m^2 on 3 consecutive days), and TBI (10 or 12 Gy in twice daily fractions of 2 Gy each). After incubation of marrow cells for 10 days the nonadherent cells were collected together with adherent cells that had been detached from plastic with trypsin. These cells were washed, filtered, resuspended in TC 199, and transfused to the patient. All three patients showed rapid reconstitution of hematologic function, but two died relatively early (at 28 and 125 days post-autografting) of liver and pulmonary toxicity and leukemia relapse, respectively. The third patient was alive and well 12 months after autografting at the time of the initial report.

It is particularly interesting to note that hematopoiesis was predominantly or entirely Ph negative during the recovery phase in all three patients. Direct examination of marrow metaphases and cytogenetic study of hematopoietic colonies also showed only Ph-negative cells in the patient who survived 1 year. Similar results were obtained in one patient treated by cyclophosphamide and TBI followed by autografting with marrow held in liquid culture for 10 days in Manchester (24). This patient was slow to recover platelet numbers after autografting, but hematopoiesis was predominantly Ph negative during the period of follow-up. These fascinating clinical results are difficult to interpret. Although the experimental data referred to earlier provide support for the concept that medium-term culture of marrow cells in vitro favors restoration of Ph-negative hematopoiesis (22), the same clinical results might have been achieved if the marrow cells had been transfused to the patients without prior incubation.

The group in Rome have very recently reported the preliminary results of autografting for 12 patients treated previously with α-interferon for varying periods (15). Marrow cell harvesting had to be delayed for some months after stopping interferon to ensure adequate numbers of progenitor cells. Patients were treated with high-dose busulfan followed by melphalan and autografting. All patients engrafted, and all were in complete hematologic remission at a median of 5.5 months after autografting. Of the 12 patients, 2 had marrow hematopoiesis that was complete Ph negative on day 60 and 7 patients had partially Ph-negative hematopoiesis. In a patient with Ph-negative CML with M-*bcr* rearrangement who was treated with α-interferon, a reduction in the proportion of leukemic cells could be demonstrated by Southern blot analysis using a DNA probe hybridizing to the *bcr* gene (35).

Clinical Results of Autografting with Blood-Derived Cells

We have recently analyzed the results of treating 14 patients with CML by autografting with blood-derived stem cells (8). Of these patients, 3 were autografted after allogeneic marrow that had been depleted of T cells in vitro had failed to engraft. These patients had received daunorubicin, high-dose cyclophosphamide, and TBI as cytoreductive therapy before allografting but received no further chemotherapy before their autografts. Another 11 patients received high-dose busulfan (16 mg/kg) and melphalan (60 mg/m^2) before the autograft. A single patient failed to engraft and died 114 days after the autograft procedure. Trilineage hematopoiesis was established in the other 13 patients, but 2 of these subsequently became pancytopenic and required treatment with further stem cell transfusions at 3 and 40 months, respectively. A single patient entered lymphoid transformation and died 14 months after autografting. At the time of the analysis, 12 of the 14 patients survived at a median period of 41 months (range 24–53 months) after autografting. Because the patients in this small pilot series were obviously selected, one can make no useful statement about the effects of the autograft on their survival.

The cytogenetic findings in these patients were of some interest. In the early period after autografting (up to 8 months), 9 of the 13 evaluable patients had at least some Ph-negative marrow metaphase but this Ph negativity was transient in most cases. Of the patients in this series, 2 appear to have achieved a durable Ph-negative status whereby the majority of marrow metaphases were Ph negative on repeated study more than 3 years after autografting (8,9). In both cases occasional Ph-positive metaphases were identified later after autografting, but the Ph-positive population appeared (at least for the present) to have lost its proliferative advantage. Both patients have somewhat hypocellular marrows and are still moderately leukopenic, and one has persisting thrombocytopenia (10–20 $\times$ 10^9 per L).

The mechanism underlying this unusual sequence of events in these two patients is unknown, but it is reminiscent of those rare cases who achieved prolonged periods of Ph-negative hematopoiesis after recovery from busulfan-induced marrow hypoplasia. In these two patients it seems likely that hematopoiesis in the short term was re-established from autografted cells but that the later hematopoiesis associated with marrow hypocellularity reflects delayed recovery of residual Ph-negative stem cells in the marrow. The inability of the Ph-positive clone to resume its proliferative advantage could have a number of causes. First, it is possible that the leukemic stem cell population was eradicated by chemotherapy, in which case one would have to assume that the occasional Ph-positive metaphases identified after autografting are derived from a leukemic clone with a limited replicative capacity. Second, the marrow microenvironment may have been modified (as suggested earlier) in a manner that no longer supports the ready proliferation of Ph-positive cells. Perhaps the most attractive explanation is the suggestion that autografting has in certain circumstances the capacity to restore the homeostatic mechanism(s), immune or otherwise, that function physiologically to restrain malignant proliferations.

CONCLUSIONS

Although allogeneic marrow transplantation clearly cures a proportion of patients with CML, the mortality associated with the procedure remains daunting. For the present, allogeneic BMT is restricted to younger patients with HLA-identical siblings. Although high-dose chemotherapy and autografting appear to offer little benefit for patients with CML in transformation, various avenues of clinical research suggest that autografting for patients in chronic phase may restore Ph negativity and could be associated with prolongation of life in some cases. If harvested marrow can be purged of leukemic stem cells, autografting may prove an effective method for prolonging life or curing patients with CML.

REFERENCES

1. Fialkow, P. J., Martin, P. J., Najfeld, V., Penfold, G. K., Jacobson, R. J., and Hansen, J. A. (1981). Evidence for a multistep pathogenesis of chronic myelogenous leukemia. *Blood 58*:158–163.
2. Apperley, J. F., Rassool, F., Parreira, A., et al. (1986). Philadelphia positive metaphases in the marrow after bone marrow transplantation for chronic granulocytic leukemia. *Am. J. Hematol. 22*:199–204.
3. Thomas, E. D., Clift, R. A., Fefer, A., et al. (1986). Marrow transplantation for the treatment of chronic myelogenous leukemia. *Ann. Intern. Med. 104*; 155–163.
4. Arthur, C. K., Apperley, J. F., Guo, A. P., et al. (1988). Cytogenetic events after bone marrow transplantation for chronic myelogenous leukemia in chronic phase. *Blood 71*:1179–1186.
5. Apperley, J. F., Mauro, F., Goldman, J. M., et al. (1988). Bone marrow transplantation for chronic myeloid leukaemia in chronic phase: Importance of a graft-versus-leukaemia effect. *Br. J. Haematol. 69*:239–245.
6. Goldman, J. M., Gale, R. P., Horowitz, M. M., et al. (1988). Bone marrow transplantation for chronic myelogenous leukemia in chronic phase: Increased risk of relapse associated with T cell depletion. *Ann. Intern. Med. 108*:806–814.
7. Haines, M. E., Goldman, J. M., Worsley, A. M., et al. (1984). Chemotherapy and autografting for patients with chronic granulocytic leukaemia in transformation: Probable prolongation of life for some patients. *Br. J. Haematol. 58*:711–722.
8. Brito-Babapulle, F., Bowcock, S. J., Marcus, R. E., Apperley, J. F., Th'ng, K. H., Dowding, C., Rassool, F., Guo, A.-P., Catovsky, D., Galton, D. A. G., McCarthy, D., Goldman, J. M. (1989). Autografting for patients with chronic myeloid leukaemia in chronic phase: Peripheral blood stem cells may have a finite capacity for maintaining haemopoiesis. *Br. J. Haematol. 73*:76–81.
9. Brito-Babapulle, F., Apperley, J. F., Rassool, F., et al. (1987). Complete remission after autografting for chronic myeloid leukemia. *Leuk. Res. 11*: 1115–1117.
10. Eaves, C. J., and Eaves, A. C. (1987). Cell culture studies in CML. *Baillière's Clin. Haematol. 1*:931–961.
11. Bowcock, S. J., Galton, D. A. G., and Goldman, J. M. (1989). Marrow aplasia developing 3 years after treatment with busulphan for chronic myeloid leukemia. *Eur. J. Haematol. 42*:496–500.
12. Reiffers, J., Gorin, N. C., Michallet, M., Maraninchi, D., and Herve, P. (1986). Autografting for chronic granulocytic leukemia in transformation. *JNCI 76*:1307–1310.
13. Goldman, J. M., Th'ng, K. H., Park, D. S., Spiers, A. S. D., Lowenthal, R. M., and Ruutu, T. (1978). Collection, cryopreservation and subsequent viability of haemopoietic stem cells intended for treatment of chronic granulocytic leukemia in transformation. *Br. J. Haematol. 40*:185–195.

14. Norman, J. E., Shepherd, K. M., Dale, B. M., and Sage, R. E. (1981). Collection and cryopreservation of peripheral blood progenitor cells in chronic granulocytic leukaemia—a comparison of treated and untreated patients. *Pathology 13*:609–614.
15. De Fabritils, P., Sandrelli, A., Meloni, G., Alimena, G., Montefusco, E., Lo Coco, F., De Felice, L., and Mandelli, F. (1990). Prolonged suppression of myeloid progenitor cell numbers after stopping interferon treatment for CML necessitates delay in harvesting marrow cells for autografting. *Bone Marrow Transplant.* In press.
16. Degliantoni, G., Mangoni, L., and Rizzoli, V. (1985). In vitro restoration of polyclonal hematopoiesis in chronic myelogenous leukemia after in vitro treatment with 4-hydroperoxycyclophosphamide. *Blood 65*:753–757.
17. Robak, T., Nolasco, I., Hibbin, J. A., and Goldman, J. M. (1985). Antigenic characteristics of circulating CFU-GM in chronic granulocytic leukaemia resemble those of CFU-GM in normal marrow and differ from those in normal blood. *Leuk. Res. 9*:1023–1029.
18. Broxmeyer, H. E., Hu, L., Platzer, E., Feit, C., Julian, L., and Rubin, B. Y. (1983). Comparative analysis of the influences of gamma, alpha and beta interferons on human multipotential (CFU-GEMM), erythroid (BFU-E) and granulocyte-macrophage (CFU-GM) progenitor cells. *J. Immunol. 131*: 1300–1305.
19. Wandl, U. B., Kloke, O., Opalka, B., and Niederle, N. (1988). Suppressive effect of interferon alpha-2b on hemopoietic progenitor cells in patients with chronic myelogenous leukemia. In *Chronic Myelocytic Leukemia and Interferon* (D. Huhn, K. P. Hellriegel, and N. Niederle, eds.). Springer-Verlag, Berlin, pp. 84–90.
20. McGlave, P. B., Arthur, D., Miller, W. J., Lasky, L., Kersey, J. (1990). Autologous transplantation for CML using marrow treated ex vivo with recombinant human interferon gamma. *Bone Marrow Transplant.* In press.
21. van Denderen, J., Hermans, H., Meeuwsen, T., Troelstra, C., Zegers, N., Boersma, W., Grosveld, G., and van Ewijk, W. (1989). Antibody recognition of the tumor-specific *bcr-abl* joining region in chronic myeloid leukemia. *J. Exp. Med. 169*:87–89.
22. Coulombel, L., Kalousek, D. K., Eaves, C. H., Gupta, C. M., and Eaves, A. C. (1983). Long term marrow culture reveals chromosomally normal hematopoietic progenitor cells in patients with Philadelphia chromosome-positive chronic myelogenous leukemia. *N. Engl. J. Med. 306*:1493–1498.
23. Barnett, M. J., Eaves, C. J., Phillips, G. L., Kalousek, D. K., Klingemann, H.-G., Lansdorp, P. M., Reece, D. E., Shepherd, J. D., Shaw, G. J., and Eaves, A. C. (1989). Successful autografting in chronic myeloid leukemia after maintenance of marrow in culture. *Bone Marrow Transplant. 4*:345–351.
24. Chang, J. (1989). Data presented at the British Society of Haematology Meeting, Canterbury, UK, April.

25. Buckner, C. D., Clift, R. A., Fefer, A., et al. (1978). Treatment of blastic transformation of chronic granulocytic leukemia by high-dose cyclophosphamide, total-body irradiation and infusion of cryopreserved autologous marrow. *Exp. Hematol. 6*:96–109.
26. Buckner, C. D., Stewart, P., Clift, R. A., et al. (1978). Treatment of blastic transformation of chronic granulocytic leukemia by chemotherapy, total-body irradiation and infusion of cryopreserved autologous marrow. *Exp. Hematol. 6*:96–109.
27. Thomas, R., Robinson, W. A., Dantas, M., et al. (1984). Autologous marrow transplantation for patients with chronic myelogenous leukemia in blast crisis. *Am. J. Hematol. 16*:105–112.
28. Preisler, H. D., Raza, A., Higby, D., et al. (1984). Treatment of myeloid crisis of chronic myelogenous leukemia. *Cancer Treat. Rep. 68*:1351–1355.
29. Lemmonier, M. P., Gorin, N. C., and Laporte, J. P. (1986). Autologous marrow transplantation for patients with chronic myelogenous leukemia in accelerated or blastic phase: Report of 14 cases. *Exp. Hematol. 14*:654–658.
30. Goldman, J. M., Catovsky, D., and Galton, D. A. G. (1978). Reversal of blast-cell crisis in CGL by transfusion of stored autologous buffy-coat cells (letter). *Lancet 1*:437–438.
31. Goldman, J. M., Catovsky, D., Hows, J., Spiers, A. S. D., and Galton, D. A. G. (1979). Cryopreserved peripheral blood cells functioning as autografts in patients with chronic granulocytic leukaemia in transformation. *Br. Med. J. 1*:1310–1313.
32. Goldman, J. M., Johnson, S. A., Islam, A., Catovsky, D., and Galton, D. A. G. (1980). Haematological reconstitution after autografting for chronic granulocytic leukaemia in transformation: The influence of previous splenectomy. *Br. J. Haematol. 45*:223–231.
33. Korbling, M., Burke, P., Braine, H., et al. (1981). Successful engraftment of blood-derived normal hemopoietic stem cells in chronic myelogenous leukemia. *Exp. Hematol. 9*:684–690.
34. Karp, D. D., Parker, L. M., Binder, N., et al. (1985). Treatment of blastic transformation of chronic granulocytic leukemia using high-dose BCNU chemotherapy and cryopreserved autologous peripheral blood stem cells. *Am. J. Hematol. 18*:243–249.
35. Lo Coco, F., Saglio, G., De Fabritiis, P., Diverio, D., Guerrasio, A., Rosso, C., Melona, G., Mancini, M., and Mandelli, F. (1989). Molecular evidence of transient complete remission after autografting in Ph-/*bcr* rearranged chronic myelogenous leukaemia (letter). *Br. J. Haematol. 72*:285–286.

PART VI
Summary and Future Directions

21
Summary and Future Directions

Albert B. Deisseroth, O. M. Zack Howard*, Andrzej Wedrychowski, David Seong, Nikolaos J. Paslidis, Margaret F. Romine, Simon H. Sims, Tianying Yuan, Man-ling Hu, Min-Zhuang Fu, Timothy M. Lopez, and Elizabeth A. Johnson
The University of Texas M. D. Anderson Cancer Center, Houston, Texas

C. V. Herst *Oncore Analytics, Houston, Texas*

Kun Wu *The University of Nebraska Medical Center, Omaha, Nebraska*

INTRODUCTION

As outlined in Chapter 1 by Clarkson, chronic myelogenous leukemia (CML) is a disease of discordant myeloid maturation during the chronic phase, which lasts for a median of 4 years, following which the disease changes to a more fulminant form through acquisition of additional mutations. A recurrent theme that has persisted throughout the literature of CML is that there is an expansion of Philadelphia chromosome-positive late progenitor cells in CML (1). In addition, a compartment composed of Philadelphia chromosome-negative late and early myeloid progenitor cells, which is of variable size, is detectable at diagnosis in patients with Philadelphia chromosome-positive CML. Interestingly, Clarkson has reported that 25% of patients with Philadelphia chromosome-positive CML with myeloid phenotype also have Philadelphia chromosome-positive cells detectable in a fraction of the B cell lymphocytes (2).

As is well known, another reproducible finding in CML is that the adhesiveness of Philadelphia chromosome-positive cells to stromal cells is decreased. Philadelphia chromosome-positive late myeloid progenitors exhibit a decreased sensitivity to negative regulation that leads to their expansion (3,4). For some reason, the apparent proliferative capabilities of Philadelphia chromosome-positive cells do not match those of normal Philadelphia chromosome-negative diploid cells (3-5). In the setting of hematopoietic reconstitution after autologous bone marrow transplantation, diploid cells often dominate the popula-

---

**Current affiliation*: National Cancer Institute, Frederick, Maryland.

tion of cells in the marrow (6,7). Thymidine incorporation at the late progenitor level in Philadelphia chromosome-positive cells is 20% of that seen with Philadelphia chromosome-negative cells in semisolid culture systems (3,4,8). As outlined in earlier chapters, the Philadelphia chromosome translocation leads to a rearrangement of the *abl* oncogene that results in an increased level and an alteration in the type of autophosphorylation seen in vitro with the *abl* oncogene (9). This increase in tyrosine-specific protein kinase activity is due to the formation of the fusion gene between the c-*abl* and the 5′ exonic and flanking region of an open reading frame on chromosome 22 called the *bcr* gene (10,11). How the translocation leads to decreased proliferative capability, decreased responsiveness to negative regulatory signals among the Philadelphia chromosome-positive late myeloid progenitor cells, decreased adhesiveness of late and early progenitor cells to stromal cells, and an accumulation of a 50- to 100-fold excess of Philadelphia chromosome-positive myeloid cells early in the chronic phase of CML is unknown.

Experiments using retroviral constructs containing a functional full-length *bcr-abl* cDNA in a transcription unit have shown that the presence of this sequence in mouse B lymphocyte cell lines leads to increased saturation density (12). The presence of *bcr-abl* retroviral constructs within interleukin-3 (IL-3)-dependent cell lines renders them IL-3 independent (12–15). Finally, a retrovirus containing the IL-3, when introduced into normal mouse cells, produces a myeloproliferative disease that has many similarities to CML (16).

It appears, however,that the presence of *bcr-abl* abnormal tyrosine-specific protein kinase is not by itself sufficient in animal or cell model systems to generate a fully transformed phenotype that forms tumors and kills (12,17). The abnormal *bcr-abl* kinase may interact with other oncogenes to form a transformed phenotype (18). These data suggest that in the beginning of CML, the Philadelphia chromosome translocation results in an altered kinase that leads to a phenotype of decreased responsiveness to negative regulation and decreased adhesiveness in the chronic phase of the disease. The next phase of the disease arises through the acquisition of additional mutations that lead to an increase in the proliferative capability of myeloid or lymphoid progenitor cells, perhaps through interaction of the *bcr-abl* oncogene with mutations in other oncogenes, and this change constitutes blast crisis.

Genes that have been reported to be expressed abnormally in blast crisis cells include the *myc* gene and the *p53* gene (19,20). There are scattered reports of mutations in the *p53* gene in blast crisis, but the percentage of patients varies in any given series in which *p53* is rearranged (21). Curiously, one oncogene for which no detectable mutational change occurs is in the n-*ras* family (22,23), and this suggests that whatever function the *bcr-abl* gene subserves, it renders the acquisition of *ras* oncogenes irrelevant to the CML cell.

Despite the wealth of detail that exists concerning the biology of the *bcr-abl* and its impact on the phenotype of the hematopoietic cell, no information is available about the target proteins on which the *bcr-abl* acts to change the

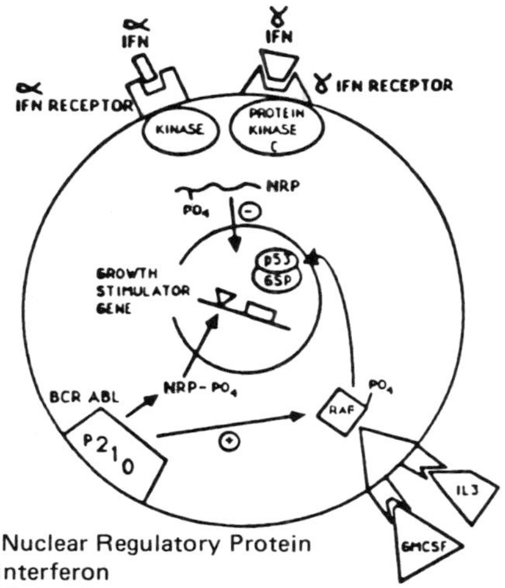

NRP = Nuclear Regulatory Protein
IFN = Interferon
RAF = Serine-Threonine Protein Kinase
GSP = Growth Stimulatory Protein

Figure 1A Signal transduction pathway on normal and leukemic myeloid cells. The p210 short circuits the dependence of the cell on extracellular growth regulatory signals.

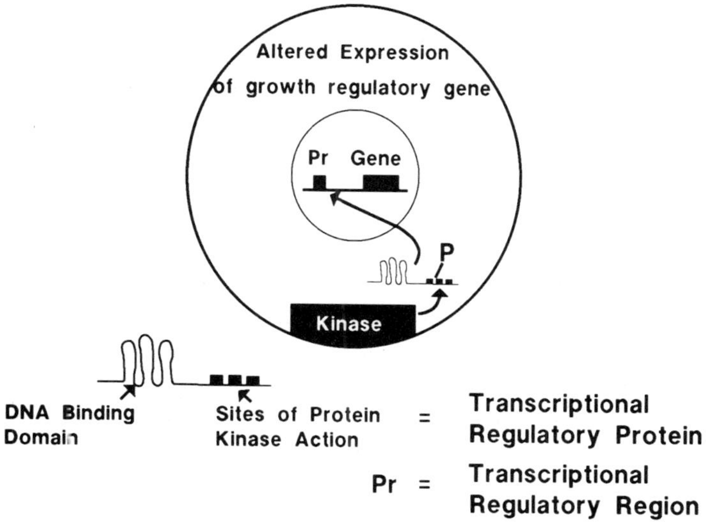

Altered Kinase adds Phosphates (B) to Proteins

Figure 1B Hypothetical mechanism of effect of p210 on the phenotype of the CML cell.

phenotype of the cells described earlier. As shown in Figure 1A, the normal myeloid cell depends on the binding of extracellular growth regulatory molecules to plasma membrane receptors for its growth. The binding of growth factors such as GMCSF and IL-3 stimulate growth of the myeloid progenitor cell by activating phosphorylation of the cytoplasmic Raf protein. This activation of Raf by phosphorylation may lead to inactivation of nuclear antioncogene proteins such as the p53 or RB (retinoblastoma) genes. As shown in Figure 1A, the abnormal *bcr-abl* protein kinase may short circuit this regulatory pathway by directly kinasing the cytoplasmic Raf protein, thus liberating the myeloid progenitor cell from the dependence on extracellular growth factors such as IL-3. The transfection experiments reviewed by Lugo and Witte (Chapter 13) suggest that this is true.

Another way in which the CML myeloid progenitor cell may loose its sensitivity to normal regulatory signals is through loss of the expression of lymphocyte function antigen-3 (LFA-3). As summarized by Guba and Emerson in Chapter 14, expression of LFA-3 is necessary on the surface of myeloid progenitor cells for the negative regulation by lymphocytes.

A third mechanism through which the abnormal p210 kinase may alter the growth and differentiation pattern of hematopoietic cells is by altering the function of nuclear transcriptional regulatory proteins as shown in Figure 1B. The effect of p210 kinase on other cytoplasmic kinases, such as Raf, and on phosphatases which affect regulation of gene expression or the sensitivity of the myeloid cell to growth factors such as GMCSF, may also be playing a role. Our laboratory has discovered a cellular phosphatase in CML cells which is present at 50 times the concentration found in normal cells, which alters the function of nuclear regulatory proteins. This phosphatase appears to be opposed by alpha-interferon in CML cells.

DISCUSSION

As summarized in Singer's chapter, data developed in his laboratory suggest that the *bcr-abl* oncogene is a "master switch" that changes the way in which hematopoietic precursor cells are regulated by stromal regulatory cells. An extension of the data presented in the chapter by Emerson's group on surface cytoadhesion protein expression in the CML myeloid cell may also be explained by the effect of the p210 protein on nuclear regulatory protein action and gene expression.

Interferon responsiveness in CML correlates with the effect of interferon on a cytoplasmic phosphatase found in interferon at higher than normal concentrations. This change in interferon-sensitive but not resistant CML cells is a basis for a potential test for interferon sensitivty. In this test, the nuclear proteins of CML patients will be isolated and studied for their binding to nuclear regulatory elements and the sensitivity of this binding to α-interferon. The evolution of CML from the chronic to the blastic phase appears to be through the acquisition of additional mutations. Candidate genes appear to include the c-myc and p53 genes. Biological therapy (interferon) as well as bone marrow transplantation (allogeneic and autologous) appear to provide the CML patient with new hope. The developing frontier of unrelated donor transplants and autologous bone marrow transplantation can only expand for the repertoire of therapeutic options open to CML patients.

The biology of CML has undergone quite a change over the past 150 years since CML was first characterized at the morphologic level. Indeed most of the progress, as evidenced in this volume, seems to have been in the last 5 years. Clearly the interaction of molecular biology and clinical investigation has led to an explosion of information concerning this disease. The major challenge is to identify the mechanism through which the presence of p210 results in the altered phenotype of the CML cell and how the acquisition of additional mutations alters the resistance to therapeutic approaches, such as interferon. Based on the progress to date in the disease, we are confident that the resolution of these questions will be forthcoming in the next few years. The dividend will be preservation of human life and a decrease in human suffering in patients with CML.

ACKNOWLEDGMENTS

The authors recognize support from the Kleberg Foundation, the Gillson-Longenbaugh Foundation, and from the American Cancer Society, and preparation of the manuscript by Rosemarie Lauzon.

REFERENCES

1. Strife, A., and Clarkson, B. (1988). Biology of chronic myelogenous leukemia. *Semin. Hematol. 25*:1–19.
2. Nitta, M., Kato, Y., Strife, A., Wachter, M., Fried, J., Perez, A., Jhanwar, S., Duigou-Osterndorf, R., Chiganti, R., and Clarkson, B. (1988). Incidence of involvement of the B and J lymphocyte lineages in CML. *Blood 66*:1053–1061.
3. Ogawa, M., Fried, J., Sakai, Y., Strife, A., and Clarkson, B. (1970). Studies of cellular proliferation in human leukemia. The proliferative activity, generation time, and emergence time of neutrophilic granulocytes in CML. *Cancer 25*:1031–1049.
4. Clarkson, B., and Rubinow, S. I. (1970). Growth kinetics in human leukemia. In *Growth Kinetics and Biochemical Regulations of Normal and Malignant Cells* (B. Drewineso and R. Humphrey, eds.). Williams & Wilkins, Baltimore, pp. 591–628.

5. Moore, M. A. S., Williams, N., and Metcalf, D. (1973). In vitro colony formation of normal and leukemic human hematopoietic cells: Characterization of the colony forming cells. *JNCI 50*:603–623.
6. Cunningham, I., Gee, T., Dowling, M., Chiganti, R., Bailey, R., Hoffan, S., Bowden, L., Turnbull, A., Knapper, W., and Clarkson, B. (1979). Results of treatment of Ph' chronic myelogenous leukemia with an intensive treatment regimen (L-5). *Blood 53*:375–395.
7. Bate-Babapulle, F., Marcus, R. E., Rassool, F., Ai-Pul, G., Th'ng, K. H., Dowding, C., McCarthy, D., Catovsky, D., Galton, D. A. G., and Goldman, J. M. (1987). Transient restoration of partial Philadelphia chromosome negativity after autografting in CML. In *Proceedings of the Third International Symposium on Autologous Bone Marrow Transplantation* (K. G. Spitzer and S. Jagannath, eds.), University of Texas, M. D. Anderson. pp. 189–195.
8. Baccarini, M., and Killman, S. A. (1972). Evidence for early presence of abnormal myeloblasts. *Scand. J. Hematol. 9*:283–292.
9. Konopka, J. B., Watanabe, S. M., and Witter, O. N. (1984). An alteration of the human c-*abl* protein in K562 leukemia cells unmarks associated tyrosine kinase activity. *Cell 37*:1035–1042.
10. Bartram, C. R., de Klein, A., Hagameister, A., van Agthoven, T., Guerts von Kessal, A., Bootsma, D., Grosveld, G., Ferguson-Smith, N. A., Davies, J. R., and Groffen, J. (1983). Translocation of c-*abl* oncogene correlates with the presence of a Philadelphia chromosome in CML. *Nature 306*: 277–280.
11. Groffen, J., Stephenson, J. R., Heisterkamp, N., de Klein, A., Bartram, C. R., and Grosveld, G. (1984). Philadelphia chromosomal breakpoints clustered within a limited region, *bcr*, on chromosome 22. *Cell 36*:93–99.
12. McLaughlin, J., Chanise, E., and Witte, O. N. (1987). In vitro transformation of immature hematopoietic cells by the p210 *bcr-abl* oncogene product of the Philadelphia chromosome. *Proc. Natl. Acad. Sci. USA 84*:6558–6562.
13. Cook, W. D., Metcalf, D., Nicola, A. A., Burgess, A. W., and Walker, F. (1985). Malignant transformation of a growth factor-independent myeloid cell line by Abelson virus without evidence of an autocrine mechanism. *Cell 41*:685–693.
14. Pierce, J. H., di Fiore, P. P., Daronson, S. A., Potter, M., Humphrey, J., Scott, A., and Ihle, J. N. (1985). Neoplastic transformation of most cells by Abelson MLV: Abrogation of IL-3 dependence by non-autocrine mechanism. *Cell 41*:677–683.
15. Haribaran, I. K., Adams, J., and Corey, S. (1988). *bcr-abl* oncogene renders myeloid cell line factor independent: Potential autocrine mechanism in CML. *Oncogene Res. 3*:387–399.
16. Wong, P. C., Chung, S. W., and Nienhuis, A. W. (1987). Retroviral transfer and expression of the interleukin-3 gene in hematopoietic cells. *Genes Dev. 1*:358–365.

17. Daley, G. Q., McLaughlin, J., Witte, O. N., and Baltimore, D. (1987). The CML specific p210 *bcr/abl* protein, unlike v-*abl*, does not transform NIH/3T3 fibroblasts. *Science 237*:532–535.
18. Lugo, T. G., and Witte, O. N. (1989). The *bcr-abl* oncogene transforms rat 1 cells and cooperates with v-*myc*. *Mol. Cell. Biol. 9*:1263–1270.
19. Andrews, D. F., Singer, J. W., and Collins, S. J. (1987). Effect of recombinant alpha-interferon on the expression of the *bcr-abl* fusion gene in human chronic myelogenous leukemia cell lines. *Cancer Res. 47*:6629–6634.
20. Lubbert, M., Miller, C. W., and Koeffler, H. P. (1988). p53 in chronic myelogenous leukemia. *J. Exp. Med. 167*:873–890.
21. Mashal, R., Shtalrid, M., Talpaz, M., Kantarjian, H., Smith, L., Beran, M., Cork, A., Trujillo, A., Gutterman, J., and Deisseroth, A. (1988). Rearrangement and expression of p53 in the chronic phase and blast crisis of CML. *Blood*, in press.
22. LeMaistre, A., Lee, M. S., Talpaz, M., Kantarjian, H., Freireich, E., Deisseroth, A., Trujillo, A., and Stass, S. (1989). *ras* oncogene mutations are rare late stage events in CML. *Blood 73*:889–891.
23. Collins, S. J., Howard, M., Andrews, D. F., Agura, E., and Rodich, J. (1989). Rare occurrence of N-*ras* point mutations in Philadelphia chromosome positive CML. *Blood 73*:1028–1032.
24. Howard, O. M. Z., Talpaz, M., Kantarjian, H., Wedrychowski, A., Turpin, J., Hester, J., Lopez-Berestein, G., Freireich, E., Gutterman, J., and Deisseroth, A. (1989). Interferon-induced binding of 84-kD nuclear protein to transcriptional regulatory site is marker for alpha-interferon sensitivity in chronic myelogenous leukemia.
25. Wedrychowski, A., Howard, O. M. Z., Paslidis, N., Talpaz, M., Kantarjian, H., Hester, J., Turpin, J., Lopez-Berestein, G., Gutterman, J., Freireich, E., and Deisseroth, A. (1989). Alpha-interferon alters binding of 84- and 50-kDa nuclear proteins from CML patients to interferon-inducible transcriptional enhancers. Submitted to *Proc. Natl. Acad. Sci. USA*.

Index